T0390830

PLANT AND ALGAL HYDROGELS FOR DRUG DELIVERY AND REGENERATIVE MEDICINE

Woodhead Publishing Series in Biomaterials

PLANT AND ALGAL HYDROGELS FOR DRUG DELIVERY AND REGENERATIVE MEDICINE

Edited by

TAPAN KUMAR GIRI

Department of Pharmaceutical Technology, Jadavpur University, Kolkata, West Bengal, India

BIJAYA GHOSH

Department of Pharmaceutical Technology, School of Health Sciences, NSHM Knowledge Campus, Kolkata Group of Institutions, Kolkata, West Bengal, India

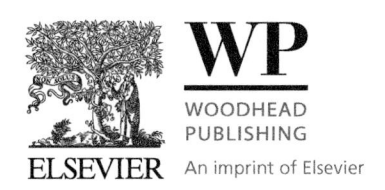

WP

WOODHEAD PUBLISHING

ELSEVIER An imprint of Elsevier

Woodhead Publishing is an imprint of Elsevier
The Officers' Mess Business Centre, Royston Road, Duxford, CB22 4QH, United Kingdom
50 Hampshire Street, 5th Floor, Cambridge, MA 02139, United States
The Boulevard, Langford Lane, Kidlington, OX5 1GB, United Kingdom

Library of Congress Cataloging-in-Publication Data

A catalog record for this book is available from the Library of Congress

British Library Cataloguing-in-Publication Data

A catalogue record for this book is available from the British Library

ISBN: 978-0-12-821649-1

ISBN: 978-0-12-821650-7

For information on all Woodhead publications
visit our website at https://www.elsevier.com/books-and-journals

Publisher: Matthew Deans
Acquisitions Editor: Sabrina Webber
Editorial Project Manager: Mariana C. Henriques
Rafael G. Trombaco
Production Project Manager: Vignesh Tamil
Cover Designer: Victoria Pearson Esser

Typeset by SPi Global, India

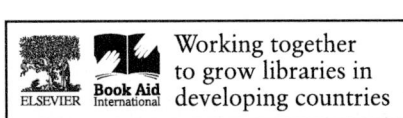

Working together to grow libraries in developing countries

www.elsevier.com • www.bookaid.org

Contents

4. Cyclodextrins-based hydrogel

Eva Pinho

5. Potential of guar gum hydrogels in drug delivery

Subhraseema Das and Usharani Subuddhi

6. Hemicelluloses-based hydrogels

Xiao-Feng Sun, Tao Zhang, and Hai-Hong Wang

7. Locust bean gum-derived hydrogels

Vipul D. Prajapati, Pankaj M. Maheriya, and Salona D. Roy

8. Inulin-based hydrogel

Moumita Das Kirtania, Nancy Kahali, and Arindam Maity

9. Hydrogels based on carrageenan

Reshma Joy, P.N. Vigneshkumar, Franklin John, and Jinu George

10. Hydrogels based on gum ghatti

Falguni Patra, Madhumita Dey, and Tapan Kumar Giri

11. Alginate-based hydrogels

Kasula Nagaraja, Kummara Madhusudana Rao, and Kummari S.V. Krishna Rao

12. Alginate-based nanocomposite hydrogels

G. Karthigadevi, Carlin Geor Malar, Nibedita Dey, K. Sathish Kumar,
Maria Sarah Roseline, and V. Subalakshmi

13. Cellulose-based stimuli-responsive hydrogels

Manuel Palencia, Arturo Espinosa-Duque, Andrés Otálora, and Angélica García-Quintero

14. Hydrogels based on cellulose nanocomposites

Neslihan Kayra, Yaprak Petek Koraltan, and Ali Özhan Aytekin

15. Composite hydrogels of pectin and alginate

Laura Sánchez-González, Kamil Elkhoury, Cyril Kahn, and Elmira Arab-Tehrany

16. Clinical applications of biopolymer-based hydrogels

Bijaya Ghosh and Moumita Das Kirtania

Contributors

Elmira Arab-Tehrany Université de Lorraine, Laboratoire Ingénierie des Biomolécules, Vandoeuvre-lès-Nancy, France

Ali Özhan Aytekin Genetics and Bioengineering Department, Engineering Faculty, Yeditepe University, Istanbul, Turkey

A.K. Bajpai Bose Memorial Research Lab, Department of Chemistry, Government Science College, Jabalpur, Madhya Pradesh, India

Madhurima Das Central Drugs Laboratory, Kolkata, West Bengal, India

Subhraseema Das Dept. of Chemistry, Ravenshaw University, Cuttack, Odisha, India

Madhumita Dey Hemraj Blood Bank, Katwa Sub-divisional Hospital, Purba Bardhaman, West Bengal, India

Nibedita Dey Department of Biotechnology, Saveetha School of Engineering, Saveetha Institute of Medical and Technical Sciences (SIMATS), Chennai, Tamilnadu, India

Pallobi Dutta NSHM Knowledge Campus, Kolkata Group of Institutions, Kolkata, West Bengal, India

Kamil Elkhoury Université de Lorraine, Laboratoire Ingénierie des Biomolécules, Vandoeuvre-lès-Nancy, France

Arturo Espinosa-Duque Research Group in Science with Technological Applications (GI-CAT), Department of Chemistry, Faculty of Natural and Exact Sciences, Universidad del Valle, Cali, Colombia

Angélica García-Quintero Mindtech Research Group (Mindtech-RG), Mindtech s.a.s., Cali, Colombia

Jinu George Biotechnology Laboratory, Department of Chemistry, Sacred Heart College, Kochi, India

Bijaya Ghosh Department of Pharmaceutical Technology, School of Health Sciences, NSHM Knowledge Campus, Kolkata Group of Institutions, Kolkata, West Bengal, India

Saumyakanti Giri NSHM Knowledge Campus, Kolkata Group of Institutions, Kolkata, West Bengal, India

Tapan Kumar Giri Department of Pharmaceutical Technology, Jadavpur University, Kolkata, West Bengal, India

Franklin John Biotechnology Laboratory, Department of Chemistry, Sacred Heart College, Kochi, India

Reshma Joy Biotechnology Laboratory, Department of Chemistry, Sacred Heart College, Kochi, India

Nancy Kahali   Sister Nivedita University, Kolkata, West Bengal, India

Cyril Kahn   Université de Lorraine, Laboratoire Ingénierie des Biomolécules, Vandoeuvre-lès-Nancy, France

G. Karthigadevi   Department of Biotechnology, Sri Venkateswara College of Engineering, Sriperumbudur, Tamilnadu, India

Neslihan Kayra   Genetics and Bioengineering Department, Engineering Faculty, Yeditepe University, Istanbul, Turkey

Moumita Das Kirtania   School of Pharmaceutical Technology, Adamas University, Kolkata, West Bengal, India

Yaprak Petek Koraltan   Biotechnology Graduate Program, Graduate School of Natural and Applied Sciences, Yeditepe University, Istanbul, Turkey

Dhanabal Kumarasamy   NSHM Knowledge Campus, Kolkata Group of Institutions, Kolkata, West Bengal, India

Pankaj M. Maheriya   Department of Formulation & Development, Ajanta Research Centre, Mumbai, India

Arindam Maity   Department of Pharmaceutical Technology, JIS University, Kolkata, West Bengal, India

Carlin Geor Malar   Department of Biotechnology, Rajalakshmi Engineering College, Chennai, Tamilnadu, India

Shubham Mukherjee   Central Drugs Laboratory, Kolkata, West Bengal, India

Kasula Nagaraja   Polymer Biomaterial Design and Synthesis Laboratory, Department of Chemistry, Yogi Vemana University, Kadapa, Andhra Pradesh, India

Andrés Otálora   Mindtech Research Group (Mindtech-RG), Mindtech s.a.s., Cali, Colombia

Manuel Palencia   Research Group in Science with Technological Applications (GI-CAT), Department of Chemistry, Faculty of Natural and Exact Sciences, Universidad del Valle, Cali, Colombia

Falguni Patra   School of Pharmacy, Techno India University, Kolkata, West Bengal, India

Eva Pinho   National Institute for Agrarian and Veterinarian Research (INIAV), Vila do Conde, Portugal

Vipul D. Prajapati   Department of Pharmaceutics, SSR College of Pharmacy, Saily, Silvassa, Union Territory of Dadra Nagar Haveli and Daman Diu, India

Kummara Madhusudana Rao   School of Chemical Engineering, Yeungnam University, Gyeongsan, Gyeongbuk, South Korea

Kummari S.V. Krishna Rao   Polymer Biomaterial Design and Synthesis Laboratory, Department of Chemistry, Yogi Vemana University, Kadapa, Andhra Pradesh, India

Maria Sarah Roseline   Department of Biotechnology, Saveetha School of Engineering, Saveetha Institute of Medical and Technical Sciences (SIMATS), Chennai, Tamilnadu, India

Salona D. Roy   Department of Pharmaceutics, SSR College of Pharmacy, Saily, Silvassa, Union Territory of Dadra Nagar Haveli and Daman Diu, India

Laura Sánchez-González Université de Lorraine, Laboratoire Ingénierie des Biomolécules, Vandoeuvre-lès-Nancy, France

K. Sathish Kumar Department of Chemical Engineering, Sri Sivasubramaniya Nadar College of Engineering, Chennai, Tamilnadu, India

Jyoti Shrivastava Bose Memorial Research Lab, Department of Chemistry, Government Science College, Jabalpur, Madhya Pradesh, India

V. Subalakshmi Department of Biotechnology, Saveetha School of Engineering, Saveetha Institute of Medical and Technical Sciences (SIMATS), Chennai, Tamilnadu, India

Usharani Subuddhi Dept. of Chemistry, NIT Rourkela, Rourkela, Odisha, India

Xiao-Feng Sun Xi'an Key Lab of Functional Organic Porous Materials, School of Chemistry and Chemical Engineering, Northwestern Polytechnical University, Xi'an, People's Republic of China

P.N. Vigneshkumar Biotechnology Laboratory, Department of Chemistry, Sacred Heart College, Kochi, India

Hai-Hong Wang Xi'an Key Lab of Functional Organic Porous Materials, School of Chemistry and Chemical Engineering, Northwestern Polytechnical University, Xi'an, People's Republic of China

Tao Zhang Xi'an Key Lab of Functional Organic Porous Materials, School of Chemistry and Chemical Engineering, Northwestern Polytechnical University, Xi'an, People's Republic of China

1

Natural polysaccharides: Types, basic structure and suitability for forming hydrogels

Saumyakanti Giri[a], Pallobi Dutta[a], Dhanabal Kumarasamy[a], and Tapan Kumar Giri[b]

[a]NSHM Knowledge Campus, Kolkata Group of Institutions, Kolkata, West Bengal, India, [b]Department of Pharmaceutical Technology, Jadavpur University, Kolkata, West Bengal, India

1.1 Background

Polymers are inorganic molecules consisting of repetitive structural units bounded by covalent bonds [1]. The term "polymer" is borrowed from a Greek word *"polys,"* which means "several or many," and *"meros"* meaning "parts or pieces" and was coined by Jöns Jacob Berzelius, a Swedish chemist in the year 1833 [2]. Polymeric materials can be produced by plants, animals, and microorganisms, termed as natural polymers, or artificially created in laboratories, which are synthetic polymers [3].

Synthetics polymers are mainly produced through controlled chemical synthesis in a controlled way, which aids the development of controlled release formulations, because it is possible to control the in vivo degradation process of the polymer to a greater extent [4]. It is possible to produce very pure polymers that reduce the risk of contamination from its monomeric precursors. Kopecek and Ulbrich indicated that synthetic polymers cannot simply be manufactured with techniques or methods that produce well-designed and unique molecular structures featured by several natural polymers. The ester bonds present in these polymers are degraded by nonenzymatic hydrolysis, resulting in water and carbon dioxide as benign products of degradation, and easily disposed of from the body. In general, synthetic polymers lack inherent biological activity and may cause adverse

Plant and Algal Hydrogels for Drug Delivery and Regenerative Medicine
https://doi.org/10.1016/B978-0-12-821649-1.00007-6

reactions, and in vivo, they tend to alter the local microenvironment, resulting in undesirable effects. Furthermore, the synthetic polymer's surface hydrophobicity denature the protein. From the biological point of view, these polymers lack highly desired biocompatibility that may lead to immune response and toxicity. So far, regulatory agencies have approved only few synthetic polymers for use in specific applications in humans.

Natural polymers are gaining interest in recent times because they are frequently found in the environment or obtained from plants or animals. Natural polymers are composed of four groups, namely polysaccharides, lipids, polypeptides, and polynucleotides, and are considered as biopolymers [5]. Such polymers are known to be well-identified in metabolic degradation in biological environments [6]. Because these materials are known to blend well with the extracellular matrix (ECM), due to their similar property, this avoids chronic immunologic reaction and toxicity stimulation, which are generally observed in the case of synthetic polymers. Natural polymers are hydrophilic in nature, and biological tissue affinity is very high. In case of controlled release formulations, these polymers can also be modified quickly and easily by attaching functional groups that further increase the controlled release properties. However, among numerous polymers from natural origin, polysaccharides are widely adopted for the pharmaceutical use.

1.2 Polysaccharides

Carbohydrates are polyhydroxy aldehydes or ketones; occasionally, other functional groups such as carboxylic acid, amine, and sulfate are also found [7]. Carbohydrates are structurally classified as monosaccharides, disaccharides, oligosaccharides, and polysaccharides. Monosaccharides are the simplest and smallest type of carbohydrates. These are either ketones or aldehydes with poly hydroxyl groups. A disaccharide comprises two monosaccharides connected together with an O-glycosidic bond. The oligosaccharides are composed of a small number of monosaccharides (usually 3–10). Polysaccharides are rather complicated carbohydrates and widely occurring biopolymers composed of numerous repetitive units of mono- or disaccharides connected through glycosidic linkages [8].

Polysaccharides are widely occurring in nature and considered as one of the major biological macromolecules [9]. They are acquired from plants (pectin, starch, and cellulose), algae (alginate), bacteria (xanthan and gellan), fungi (Pullulan), and animals (chitosan and chondroitin) [10]. Polysaccharides inherently possess a range of reactive units, in different chemical compositions, available in a broad range of molecular weights that contribute to the structural and property diversity [11–14]. Polysaccharides are widely adopted for the pharmaceutical purpose because of their exceptional physical and biological characteristics such as biodegradability, biocompatibility, can be chemically modified, cost-effective, and low immunogenicity [15–17].

Polysaccharides obtained naturally have gained greater attention in recent times for their potential application in the delivery of drug and regenerative medicine owing to their exceptional properties. Polysaccharides with a wide range of functional groups show varying physicochemical characteristics and beneficial biological activities, which make them appropriate for many pharmaceutical applications, including drug delivery [18]. These are used specifically as solid implant, beads, film, microparticle, nanoparticles, injectables, and inhalable systems [19, 20]. These materials have served various roles such as matrix-forming agents, binders, or regulators for drug release; viscosity enhancers or thickeners; disintegrants, stabilizers; emulsifiers; solubilizers; film-formers; bioadhesives; and gelling agents. Natural polysaccharides show wide biological activities such as antioxidative, antiinflammatory, immune control, antitumor, anti-HIV, and anticarcinogenic activities. In recent times, they particularly seem to be the most promising source in preparing nanometric carriers for attaching and delivering anticancer agents to the tumor site without causing drug loss and toxicity to the healthy tissues [21–23].

In case of drug delivery, hydrogels are advantageous in preventing the degradation of loaded drugs and to overcome the difficulties such as poor aqueous solubility, extreme adverse effects, and shorter half-life [24]. Polysaccharides are exceptionally advantageous among the several other macromolecules in the preparation of hydrogels because they are often produced through recombinant DNA techniques and are widely found in living organisms, which are easily accessible [25]. Hydrogels prepared with polysaccharides can be used as scaffolds for soft tissues and vehicles for the drug in controlled release formulation due to their versatile physicochemical and biological properties [26]. Hydrogels are prepared by the induction of physical bonds (hydrogen bonds, ionic gelation, etc.) and/or chemical bonds through chemical cross-linking (covalent bonds) of polysaccharides and their derivatives to form three dimensional (3D) porous networks that are extremely hydrophilic and capable of imbibing large quantities of biological fluids.

1.3 Biodegradability and digestibility of polysaccharides

1.3.1 Biodegradability of polysaccharides in the environment

Earth's 75% biomass is made up of carbohydrates [27]. The most commonly found carbohydrates are cellulose, starch, chitin, and glycogen; among all these, the most widely found carbohydrate is cellulose because it is an important structural block in plant cell wall. Xylan and other plant polysaccharides are also important structural components of plant cells. Chitin, which is the second most common structural polysaccharide, is obtained from several arthropods.

Heterotrophs are organisms that cannot produce their own food and largely depend on other sources for it. Heterotrophs have several polysaccharide-degrading enzymes such as glycoside hydrolases to degrade carbohydrates. Environmental microbes use different other enzymes along with glycoside hydrolases to degrade polysaccharides. Microbes largely depend on these polysaccharides for their energy source [28–30]. Although all microbes are not responsible for polysaccharide degradation, it is suspected that they do not have proper saccharolytic biochemical machinery [31, 32].

Soil is a good hub of major microbes such as bacteria, algae, protozoa, and fungi. The distribution of microbes in soil is influenced by several factors such as the type and extent of nutrients present in the soil, pH of the soil, temperature, amount of moisture, and favorable weather condition. The existence of root systems also influences the nature and amount of microbes in soil. Bacteria are largely present in soil. Soil bacterial population is made up of diverse bacteria such as autotrophs (photosynthetic bacteria), heterotrophs (nonphotosynthetic bacteria), mesophiles (grows in moderate temperature), thermophiles (grows at higher temperature), aerobes, anaerobes, cellulose digesters, nitrogen fixers, sulfur oxidizers, and protein digesters. Most of these bacteria have cellulose digestion ability; similarly, other natural polysaccharides are also easily degraded in the soil.

1.3.2 Digestibility of polysaccharides in human

1.3.2.1 Degradation by human digestive system

Digestion of food in humans occurs in the following order: mouth (salivary action), stomach (gastric secretion), small intestine (bile and pancreatic secretion), large intestine, and colon (microbiota). The process of human digestion can be described as a unidirectional process of oral processing, gastric processing, intestinal processing, and colonic fermentation (Fig. 1.1). Under normal process, these four processes occur in a sequence, and there is no backflow of ingested materials.

Human salivary glands are of three types: parotid gland, submaxillary gland, and sublingual gland. The main objective of human salivary gland is to secrete saliva. Saliva plays a significant role in carbohydrate digestion in humans. Saliva is mainly made up of water and mucin polysaccharides. Mucin has a big role in bolus formation. In addition, it acts as a lubricant and viscosity controller. Mucin also helps to swallow the food

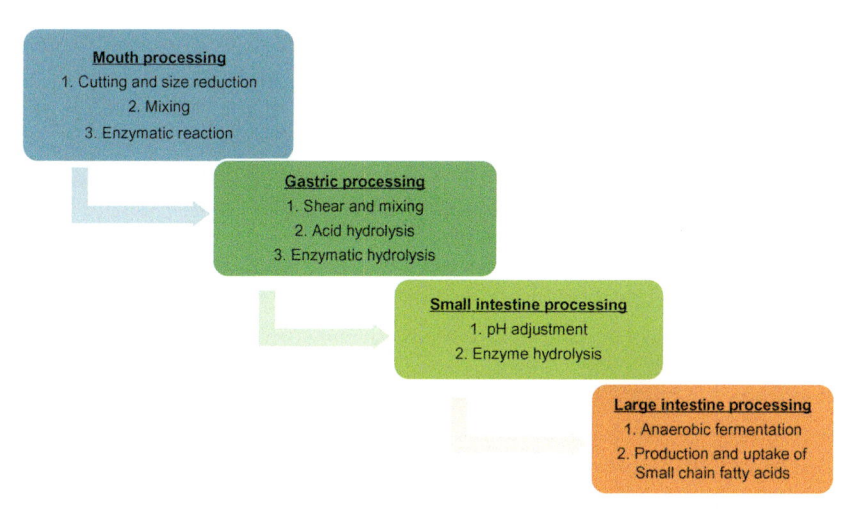

FIG. 1.1   Brief outline of digestion in humans.

and its passage through the gastrointestinal tract (GIT) [33]. The two most important salivary enzymes are salivary amylase and lysozyme. The degradation of starch is initiated by salivary amylase during mastication and is also involved in the degradation/partial digestion of other polysaccharides and oligosaccharides. The extent of salivary amylase action depends on the food residence time in the mouth. In general, the action of salivary amylase is limited because the residence of the food in the mouth is short. On the other hand, lysozyme has no such reported effect on carbohydrates, and it has antibacterial activity.

The stomach is a part of GIT, which is mainly responsible for protein degradation. Acidic environment of the stomach favors this proteolytic degradation. Two important enzymes for the digestion present in the stomach are pepsin and gastric lipase. Pepsin is obtained from pepsinogen (inactive zymogen), and it has protein degrading property. Gastric lipase is responsible for initial digestion of dietary fats. In the stomach, to a minor extent, carbohydrates are hydrolyzed by gastric acid, independent of enzymes and by the action of gastric amylase. However, in the stomach, no such major degradation of carbohydrate takes place.

The total degradation of polysaccharides happens through hydrolysis by several enzymes. In the small intestine, the major degradation of polysaccharides occurs. They are basically several monosaccharides connected through different types of glycosidic linkages. Hydrolyzing enzymes disrupt these linkages and yield monosaccharides. Collectively, these enzymes are called as glycosidases. Hehre et al. extensively studied the enzymatic degradation of glyosidic bond [34, 35]. Although the degradation initiated briefly in the mouth, mediated by salivary α-amylase, complete degradation of polysaccharides occurs at small intestine, through pancreatic α-amylase and other glycosidases, which convert polysaccharides into oligosaccharides and disaccharides. Final conversion of monosaccharides from oligosaccharides and disaccharides occur at the jejunum. Enzymes such as maltase, glucoamylase, and lactase are responsible for this conversion [36].

1.3.2.2 Degradation by bacteria present in the human gut

The human body symbiotically hosts a huge variety of microorganisms, and most of them are present in the human gut [37–39]. The human GIT microbiota comprises approximately 10^{14} microorganisms and is mostly encompassed of bacteria. In human gut, the most common bacterial phyla present are firmicutes, bacteroidates, proteobacteria, and actinobacteria [40]. Some commonly found bacterial genera in human gut are presented in Fig. 1.2 [41–43].

The human body does not have such biochemical machinery to degrade complex polysaccharides such as cellulose, xylan, and pectin, although these polysaccharides are part of food. Humans largely depend on the gut microbiota for this purpose; in turn, gut microbes also depend on humans for their nutrition and energy requirements. This mutual dependence of each other is a good example of symbiosis. One of the biggest examples of this symbiosis process is seen in *Bacteroides thetaiotaomicron*, which is a major bacterium present in the human gut and plays a critical role in the degradation of complex carbohydrates [44, 45].

The human gut bacteria secrete different types of enzymes (glycoside hydrolases, polysaccharide lyases, and carbohydrate esterases), and these enzymes functions in tandem to degrade the complex carbohydrates to simple sugars. Enzymes accountable for hydrolyzing the glycosidic bonds in polysaccharides are collectively known as glycoside hydrolases or simply glycosidase and are present in our digestive system. Apart from these gut digestive enzymes, there are several other enzymes such as polysaccharide lyases and carbohydrate esterases that are produced by human gut bacteria; they are also collectively accountable for the complete degradation of ingested polysaccharides. The group of enzymes responsible for cleaving specific portion of the glycosidic bond present in acidic polysaccharides is known as polysaccharide lyases [46]. These enzymes are also called as eliminases, and they act to cleave activated glycosidic linkages present in acidic polysaccharides. These enzymes mediate elimination mechanism-based degradation rather than hydrolysis, which results in unsaturated (olefinic) oligosaccharide products [47]. Elimination reaction produces unsaturated monosaccharides from acidic polysaccharides, and these unsaturated monosaccharides absorb 232 nm UV radiations [48]. Carbohydrate esterases are the group of enzymes that can modify,

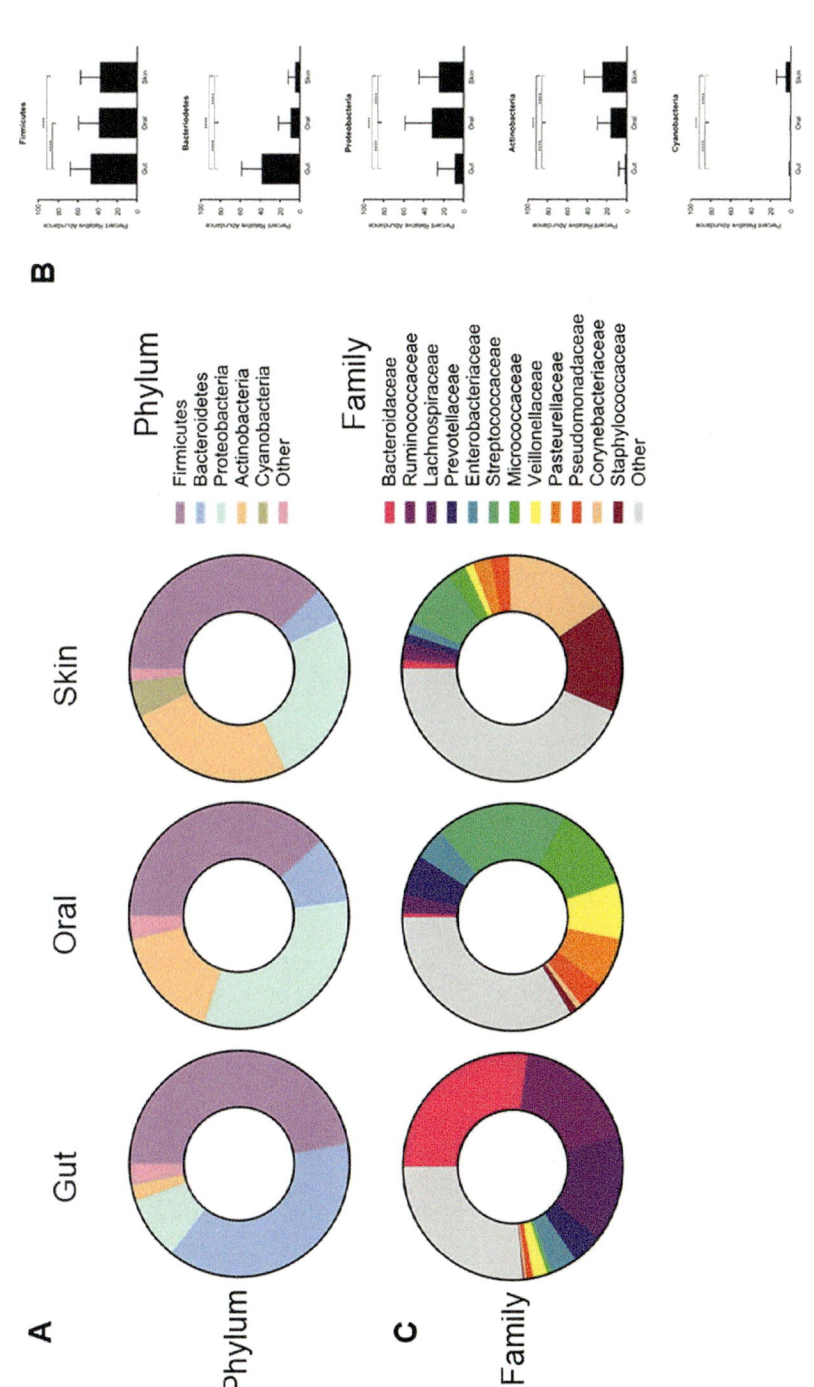

FIG. 1.2 Taxonomic composition of microbes present in different body sites. (A) Dominated microbial phylum on different body sites. (B) Percent community composition in different body sites. (C) Inhabited bacterial families in different body sites. *Reproduced from Brandwein M, Katz I, Katz I, Kohen R. Beyond the gut: skin microbiome compositional changes are associated with BMI. Hum Microb J 2019;7:100063, Copyright (2019), with permission from Elsevier.*

assemble, or break down carbohydrate esters. These enzymes basically attach ester linkage and release acyl or alkyl groups from the sugar backbone. According to carbohydrate-active enzymes database CAZy (www. cazy.org), there are total of 166 families of glycoside hydrolases, in which carbohydrate esterases are composed of 17 families, and there are 40 families of polysaccharide lyases present in all living organisms. In addition to this, there are several carbohydrate-binding modules present in the catalytic domain of carbohydrate-active enzymes.

Everyday almost 20–60 g of complex carbohydrates reach human colon escaping the digestive system [49, 50]. They are mostly of structural polysaccharide components of plant cell wall, and some are oligosaccharides; these are not degraded by human digestive machinery. One of the most common obligate anaerobic bacteria present in the human gut flora is *B. thetaiotaomicron*, which is an extensively studied gram-negative bacterium possessing a good saccharolytic machinery [51]. Utilization of polysaccharides by these bacteria can be characterized by some special features, and these features are based on enzymatic, transport, and regulatory levels. *B. thetaiotaomicron* has a large number of proteins that are responsible for complex polysaccharide binding, processing, and cleaving. Once the digestion process has been completed, then oligosaccharides are transferred to the periplasm with the help of sugar-specific outer membrane starch utilization system (Sus) proteins, SusC and SusD [52].

In starch degradation process, the first step is attachment of polysaccharide to bacterial cell surface [53]. The whole process of binding with polysaccharides, transport, and degradation is controlled by an operon system, encoded by *susRABCDEFG* gene cluster [54]. The outer membrane *susCDEFG* system is responsible for binding with starch molecule [55–58]. Several other genes such as SusE and SusF are also responsible for binding with starch. Standalone SusC cannot bind to the starch molecule and often requires the aid of SusD proteins. SusG basically codes α-amylase, which is an integral part of this starch degradation machinery. SusD acts as a critical player for targeting starch molecule and transport of oligosaccharides to SusC.

Detailed mechanism of starch degradation is as follows: At first, starch molecule is attached on the bacterial surface with the help of SusD proteins. This attachment helps in the hydrolysis of the polysaccharide molecule with the help of SusG protein. After degradation by SusG protein (α-amylase), the degraded products are transported to the periplasm by SusC protein. In periplasm, they are further degraded by SusA (neopullulanase) and SusB (α-glucosidase) proteins [59]. The whole Sus system is regulated by SusR gene in response to the inducer saccharide maltose and, consequently, orchestrate the transcription of *susABCDEFG* [60].

1.4 Classification

Polysaccharides can be classified based on their source:

(1) Plant: Polysaccharides obtained from various plant parts, for example, Guar gum (extracted from guar beans), cellulose, xyloglucan, pectins, starch, inulin, etc.
(2) Algal: These polysaccharides are obtained from various algae, for example, alginate, agar, ulvan (extracted from sea lettuces), etc.
(3) Microbial: These polysaccharides are obtained through fermentation process using bacteria and fungi. Bacterial fermentation source: for example, Xanthan gum (*Xanthomonas campestris*), Welan gum (genus *Alcaligenes*), Gellan gum (*Sphingomonas elodea*); Fungus: *Aureobasidium pullulans* is used in the production of polysaccharide pullulan using starch as substrate.
(4) Animal: These polysaccharides are obtained from animal sources; for example, chitin, chitosan, etc.

Chemical structure-based classification of polysaccharides:

(1) Homopolysaccharides or homoglycans: They are polymers of a single monosaccharide unit; for example, starch is entirely composed of α-glucose.
(2) Heteropolysaccharides or heteroglycans: These polysaccharides on hydrolysis produce a combination of monosaccharide; for example, guar gum, the hydrolytic end products are the monosaccharides galactose and mannose.

1.4.1 Plant polysaccharides

The characteristics of the polysaccharides obtained from plant sources depend on plant species, growth conditions, season, and their age at harvest [61–64]. The structural component of a typical vascular plant tissue is composed of 40%–45% cellulose, 15%–25% lignin, and 20%–30% hemicelluloses. The common storage polysaccharide found in plants is starch, and it is also the most common energy source for many organisms.

1.4.1.1 Starch

The most abundant and largest reserve of carbohydrate in plants is starch and is found in leaves, flowers, seeds, fruits, various types of roots and stems [65, 66]. Starch is used by plants as a source of carbon and energy. Commercial starches are sourced from grains, such as rice and wheat, and corn and tubers, such as arrowroot, tapioca, and potato. The starch content of most cereals and tubers on dry basis is usually about 60%–90%; thus it is economical to produce from these sources [67]. The content of starch is particularly high in rice, which is up to 88%, and in sorghum, it is variable [68]. Starch is also found in Rhodophyceae and Glaucophytes [69]. Starch comprises two types of glucose polymers, namely amylose and amylopectin. The basic unit of starch is α-D-glucopyranosyl moiety that is linked by $(1 \rightarrow 4)$ and $(1 \rightarrow 6)$ bonds. The amylose component of starch is a linear macromolecule that consists of α-D-glucopyranose units having linear α-$(1 \rightarrow 4)$ linkages, and it is lightly branched, with molecular weight in the range of 10^5–10^6. Amylopectin is highly branched biopolymer of α-D-glucopyranose units with linear α-$(1 \rightarrow 4)$ linkage and branching α-$(1 \rightarrow 6)$-linkages with the interval of 20 units.

Talaat et al. studied in detail the synthesis of superabsorbent hydrogel by grafting acrylonitrile onto starch [70]. It was prepared by combining hydrated starch with acrylonitrile (grafting); the target grafted product of starch was isolated and dried accompanied by 1h saponification at 95°C under alkaline condition, precipitation of the product with methanol, followed by washing with ethanol to make it water free, and finally dried at 60°C/h for 3h. Qunyi and Ganwei prepared superabsorbant hydrogel by using a pyrophosphate redox manganese initiation system (Fig. 1.3) [71]. The superabsorbents hydrogel were prepared by grafting 2-acrylamido-2-methylpropanesulfonic acid (AMPS) and acrylonitrile onto starch. The maximum output can be achieved under optimum saponification conditions. The water absorption capacity of the superabsorbent was 1345 g/g.

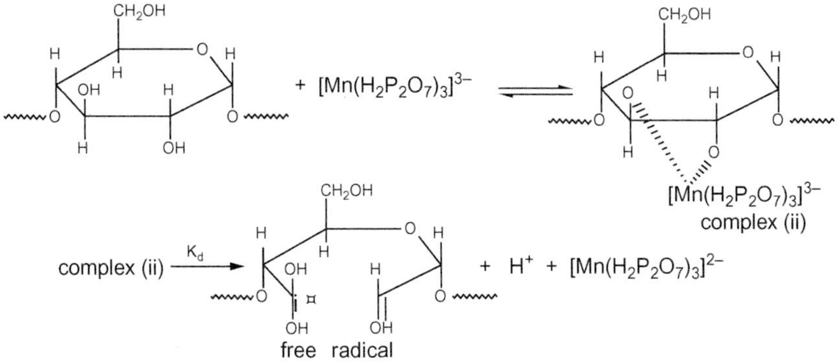

FIG. 1.3 The reaction taking place during the grafting process. *Reproduced from Qunyia T, Ganweib Z. Rapid synthesis of a superabsorbent from a saponified starch and acrylonitrile/AMPS graft copolymers. Carbohydr Polym 2005;62:74–79, Copyright (2005), with permission from Elsevier.*

1.4.1.2 Cellulose

Cellulose is a natural polysaccharide available in nature [72]. It is ubiquitous in the cell walls of higher plants as a primary structural constituent and in some types of algae [73, 74]. About 40% of wood, 90% of cotton fiber, and 80% of flax are composed of cellulose. Some bacteria such as *Acetobacter xylinum* synthesize cellulose biochemically.

Cellulose is a linear polysaccharide characterized by unbranched D-glucose residue with β (1-4)-linkage [75, 76]. Cellulose is composed of monomeric unit β-D-anhydroglucopyranose, these units are covalently linked through β-1, 4-glycosidic bonds formed between the equatorial hydroxyl group of the C4 carbon and C1 carbon [77]. In each unit (β-D-anhydroglucopyranose) of cellulose chain, three chemically reactive hydroxyl groups are present: a primary hydroxyl ($-CH_2OH$) group at C6 and two secondary hydroxyls (> C–OH) at C3 and C4 positions, which are located in the ring planes. The oxygen atoms present in the D-glucopyranose ring, the three hydroxyl groups, and the glycosidic linkage units combine with each other within the same cellulose molecule chain or with another chain resulting in multiple hydrogen bonding, leading to the creation of a crystalline structure [78, 79].

Cellulose hydrogels can be prepared by physical cross-linking of cellulose in solution [80]. Because cellulose has a variety of hydroxyl groups, it readily forms the networks linked through hydrogen bonding. Huang et al. prepared self-healing nanofiber hydrogel containing dialdehyde cellulose nanocrystals and carboxymethyl chitosan [81]. The prepared hydrogel could be repetitively extended to four times its length and had a tensile strength of 244 kPa and when compressed by 90%, it could completely come back to its original size.

Chang et al. developed double network hydrogel through diffusion of isopropylacrylamide into epichlorohydrin cross-linked cellulose hydrogels [82]. Similarly, double network hydrogels were synthesized by changing isopropylacrylamide to acrylamide ratio [83]. High stretchable cellulose hydrogels were synthesized by sequential cross-linking and dual network technique [84]. First, cellulose was dissolved in NaOH/urea system and cross-linked using epichlorohydrin as a cross-linker (Fig. 1.4). Then the prepared gels were dissolved in dilute acid that removed the residual chemicals. Moreover, $-ONa$ group was converted to $-OH$ group that enhanced the properties of hydrogel owing to the creation of hydrogen bond. Finally, the dual network hydrogel was developed by UV light-initiated polymerization process using acrylamide monomer.

1.4.1.3 Hemicellulose

Hemicelluloses are heteropolysaccharides that constitute cell walls of higher plants, which are mostly physically bound to cellulose and lignins

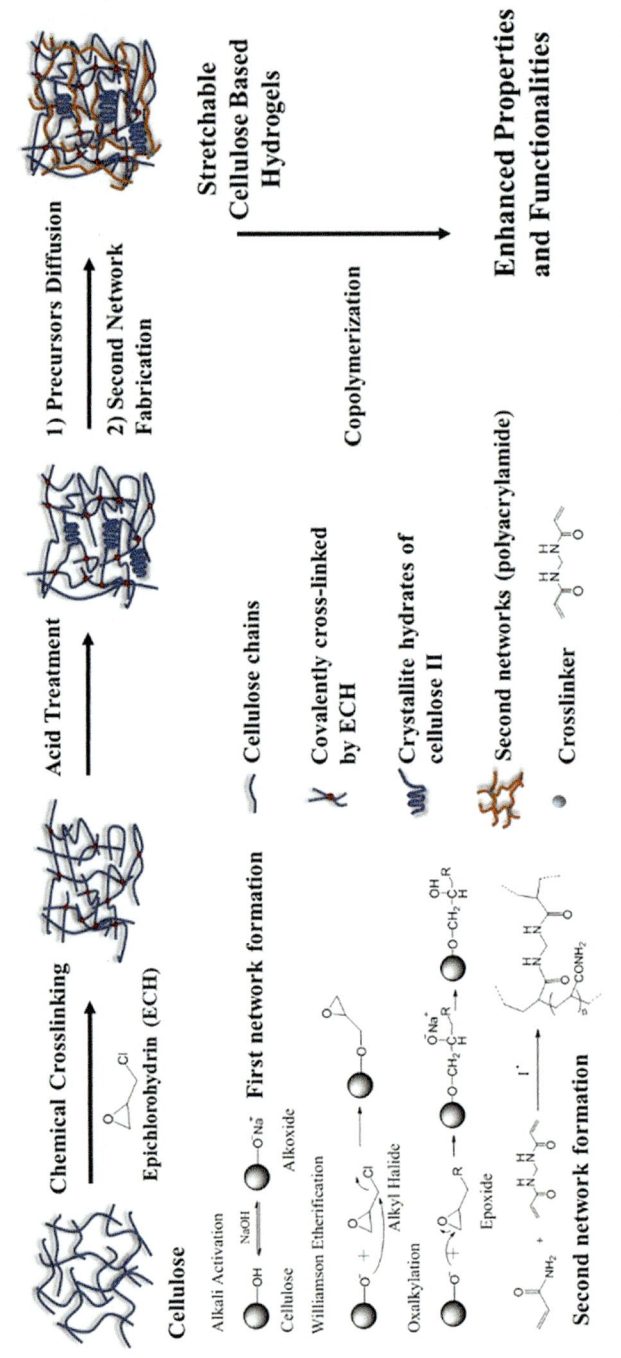

FIG. 1.4 Reaction between cellulose and epichlorohydrin, and the preparation of double network (DN) cellulose hydrogels. *Reproduced from Niu L, Zhang D, Liu Y, Zhou X, Wang J, Wang C, Chu F. Combination of acid treatment and dual network fabrication to stretchable cellulose based hydrogels with tunable properties. Int J Biol Macromol 2020;147:1–9, Copyright (2020), with permission from Elsevier.*

covalently and/or noncovalently. Approximately a one-third of wall biomass contains hemicellulose, which includes xylans, xyloglucans, and heteromannans [85]. Xylans are a group of heteropolysaccharides representing the main structural hemicellulose polysaccharides found in monocot type of cell walls (primary and secondary) and dicots (secondary cell walls) [86]. Xyloglucan is an important group of hemicellulose polymers mainly found in the primary cell wall of dicots. Xyloglucan is isolated from seeds of various species such as *Tamarindus indica, Copaifera langsdorffii,* and *Hymenaea courbaril* [87].

Galactomannan and galactoglucomannan exist in the dicot plants (primary cell wall) as minor constituents, and they may constitute as one of the most important polysaccharides of its secondary cell walls. Galactoglucomannan is present in many plants, including legumes and palms, as storage polysaccharides for many seeds and are mostly located in endosperms. Glucomannan is commercially derived from pulverized and dried root of *Amorphophallus konjac*, which is a perennial herb. Mannans are the primary hemicellulose in the gymnosperm's secondary cell wall. It is less common in spermatophytes, but some organisms may have up to 5% (w/w). The chemical structure of hemicelluloses can be classified into four groups based on their composition of the major backbone chain, that is $(1 \rightarrow 4)$-linked β-D-mannose attached to D-mannans, $(1 \rightarrow 4)$-linked β-D-xylose attached with D-xylans; $(1 \rightarrow 3)$-linked β-D-galactose attached with D-galactans; and $(1 \rightarrow 4)$-linked β-D-glucopyranoses attached with D-xyloglucans [88].

The free hydroxyls present in hemicellulose chain can easily react with various other monomeric components and cross-linkers and can be straightforwardly modified to form a 3D structure by physical or chemical cross-linking. The hydroxyl group acts as a chemically reactive site in hemicellulose in the grafting reaction. Vinyl groups that are introduced to the hemicellulose backbone enable further modification and preparation of new hemicellulose-based tunable hydrogels through graft polymerization. Cationic groups/anion groups can, therefore, be inserted into the hemicellulose backbone to ensure that hemicellulose-based hydrogels are formed.

1.4.1.4 Pectin

Pectins are commonly associated with hemicelluloses, cellulose, and lignin, along with other cell wall elements. They are present in the middle lamella and primary cell wall of many plants. Although they are present in various tissues, fruits contain the maximum concentration, and appreciable quantities are found in vegetables and young tissues [89, 90]. The concentration is more in citrus fruits such as oranges, grapes, lemons, and apples.

Pectins are heteropolysaccharides comprising predominantly galacturonic acid units [91]. The three main groups of pectins are as follows:

rhamnogalacturonan-I, rhamnogalacturonan-II, and homogalacturonan. Homogalacturonan contains $(1 \rightarrow 4)$-α-linked D-galacturonic acid units with rhamnoseresidues up to 200 units length. The backbone of rhamnogalacturonans of type I consists of alternating $(1 \rightarrow 2)$ bonded α-L-rhamnosyl and $(1 \rightarrow 4)$ bonded α-D-galacturonic acid residues. Rhamnogalacturonan II consists of α-D-galactosyluronic residues $(1 \rightarrow 4$-linked) in its backbone. It has a nonsaccharide and a side chain of octasaccharides linked to some of the backbone residues at C-2 position at approximately 30 glycosyl residues length. It also has two disaccharides that are structurally different and are attached to the C-3 of the backbone.

Pectin-based hydrogel was prepared by ionotropic gelation method [92]. On the basis of deesterification degree of carboxylic acid metabolites of galacturonic acid, pectins are divided into two groups. Pectin with demethylated degrees above 50% is known as high methoxy pectin, whereas with low demethylated degrees, it is called low methoxy pectin. The low methoxy pectin hydrogels can be formed through cross-linking between divalent cations, such as Ca^{2+}, Ba^{2+}, and Zn^{2+}, and two different pectin chains [93].

1.4.1.5 Exudate gum

Exudate gums are pathological substances generated by the rupture of cell walls after any plant injury caused by stress or fungal attack or due to adverse conditions such as drought [94]. The major exudate gums that are widely used are tragacanth, arabic, ghatti, and karaya gum [95, 96]. Tragacanth is a dried gum obtained from *Astragalus gummifer* and various other species of the genus Astragalus found in West Asia, primarily in Iran. Arabic is a natural gum obtained from acacia tree that mainly grows in Africa [97]. *Acacia senegal*, *Acacia seyal*, and *Acacia polyacantha* are major sources but some other species such as *Acacis karoo* and *Acacia laeta* can also produce small quantities of the gum. Gum ghatti is a translucent amorphous exudate from the tree of Combretaceae family named *Anogeissus latifolia* that grows in Sri Lanka and India. Gum karaya, also known as Indian tragacanth, is an exudate produced from the *Sterculia urens* tree of family Sterculiaceae cultivated in India, Pakistan, and Sudan.

Tragacanth is a highly branched polysaccharide containing water soluble and insoluble components; about 30%–40% is water soluble. The soluble portion comprised $1 \rightarrow 6$ bonded D-galactosyl backbones linked with L-arabinose side chains through $1 \rightarrow 2$, $1 \rightarrow 3$, and $1 \rightarrow 5$ links. The water insoluble part is tragacanthic acid that is composed of carbohydrates L-arabinose, L-fucose, D-galacturonic acid, D-xylose, and L-rhamnose. The α-D-galacturonopyranosyl backbone chain $(1 \rightarrow 4)$ is attached to a random xylosyl branch at the 3 location of the residues of galacturonic acid.

Gum arabic is a highly complex, heterogeneous mixture of glycoproteins and highly branched polysaccharides largely composed of the sugars arabinose and galactose. The β-D-galactopyranosyl units are linked through $(1 \to 3)$ and $(1 \to 6)$ bonds along with β-D-glucopyranosyl uronic acid units associated with $(1 \to 6)$ linkage. The side chains include β-D-glucuronic acid, α-L-arabinofuranosyl units, β-D-glucuronic acid, and α-L-rhamnopyranose involving $(1 \to 3)$, $(1 \to 4)$, and $(1 \to 6)$ glycosidic linkages.

Gum ghatti contains various monosaccharide components such as arabinose, galactose, glucuronic acid, xylose, and mannose, along with trace amounts of 6-deoxyhexoses. The main backbone polymer chain consists of a $(1 \to 6)$-linked β-D-galactopyranosyl units linked variedly with $(1 \to 4)$-D-glucopyranosyluronic acid units, L-arabinofuranosyl units, and $(1 \to 2)$-D-mannopyranosyl units.

Gum karaya comprises α-$(1 \to 2)$-linked L-rhamnosyl-related residues and α-$(1 \to 4)$-linked D-galacturonic acid. The side chain is composed of β-D-glucuronic acid having $(1 \to 3)$ linkage or β-D-galactose having $(1 \to 2)$ linkage on the main galacturonic acid unit in which approximately a half of rhamnose is replaced by β-D-galactose having $(1 \to 2)$ linkage.

The basic principle of the hydrogel forming formulation is cross-linking of the polymer chains in three dimensions [98]. This is realized either by chemically modifying the structure of the polymer with the addition of cross-linking agents or through exposing the polymer to a high-energy radiation. For the formulation of hydrogels from natural gums, both chemical and physical means of modifying the polysaccharide polymer are used. Chemical modification includes methods that lead to the creation of new covalent or ionic bonds and sometimes creating both types of bonds between the polymer chains in hydrogel. However, in a physically cross-linked hydrogel, there exists physical interlocking interactions between the polymer chains.

1.4.2 Algal polysaccharides

Marine algae are the major source of algal polysaccharides [99–103]. Algal polysaccharides have several industrial applications such as emulsifying, stabilizing, and thickening the formulation [104]. Seaweeds are rich in polysaccharides content, but they have low caloric value. These polysaccharides mostly function as dietary fibers [105]. Algal polysaccharides constitute 4%–76% of the dry weight of seaweed. Highest amount of polysaccharides is obtained from *Ulva*, *Palmaria*, and *Ascophyllum* species.

1.4.2.1 Alginate

Alginate is commercially sourced from several species of brown algae such as *Laminaria japonica*, *Laminaria hyperborean*, and *Macrocystis pyrifera*. [106]. Alginates may present in salt or acid form; salt form plays a major role in cell wall formation of brown seaweed species, and the acid form is known as alginic acid [107, 108]. Extraction of alginates is affected by using aqueous alkali solutions such as sodium hydroxide; the resultant product is sodium salt of alginic acid. Alginate was first discovered in 1880s, and the production of alginate industrially was started in 1929 at California. Structurally, alginate is made up of alternate α-L-guluronic acid (G) and β-D-mannuronic acid (M) residues that are 1,4-linked. The algae species are diverse and produce alginates with slightly different chemical sequences and composition [109, 110].

The drug delivery, biomedical, and wound healing application alginate is mostly used in the form of hydrogel preparation. The aqueous solution of alginate forms hydrogel in the existence of divalent cations (cross-linking agents). The α-L-guluronic acid residues of alginate backbone is highly susceptible for divalent cations; thus these divalent cations can form a bridge (ionic cross-linking) between two adjacent guluronate blocks belonging to different polymer chains and ultimately make an egg-box-like structure, which leads to gel formation (Fig. 1.5) [111]. The most widely used cross-linking agent for alginate is calcium chloride ($CaCl_2$).

The hydrogel uniformity is greatly influenced by the gelation rate. Slower rate of gelation leads to more homogeneous gel formation with higher mechanical strength [112, 113]. Temperature also has a great role in homogeneous gel formation because lower temperature leads to slower rate of gelation. The reactivity of cross-linkers at lower temperature is reduced, thus retarding the gelation rate [114]. In addition to this, structural variations of alginate also play a game-changing role. More G residues in alginate backbone causes highly stiff structures [115]. A typically cross-linked alginate gel can undergo plastic deformation. Plastic deformation can happen when the cross-link dissociates and the water molecule is lost from hydrogel structure. However, in case of hydrogels that are covalently cross-linked, water mitigation also occurs, but bond reformation is there that makes elastic deformation. The carboxylic acid residues present in alginate backbone makes alginate a pH-responsive polymer. The pH responsiveness is dependent on the relative position of carboxylic group in G residues and M residues. The average pKa value for alginate is 3.5, guluronic acid is 3.65,

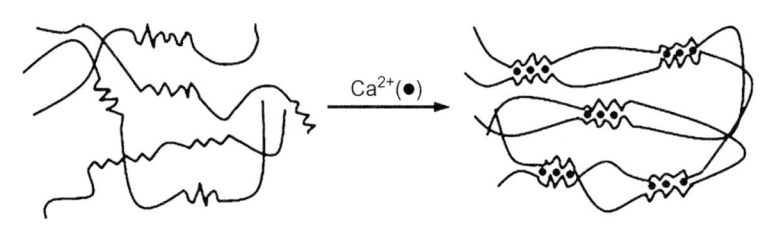

FIG. 1.5 Preparation of alginate hydrogels through ionic cross-linking (egg-box model). *Reproduced from Lee KY, Mooney DJ. Alginate: properties and biomedical applications. Prog Polym Sci 2012;37:106–126, Copyright (2012), with permission from Elsevier.*

and mannuronic acid is 3.38 [116]. Exchange of sodium ion from the guluronic acid residues of different chains with divalent cations leads to ionic cross-linking, resulting in gelation of alginate.

The native polysaccharide sodium alginate exhibited numerous shortcomings, such as low thermal stability, strong hydrophilic character, and poor mechanical properties, which significantly restrict its applications [117, 118]. Sodium alginate grafted with vinyl monomers is attempted to overcome the limitations of this natural polymer [119–123]. Alginate-grafted poly methyl methacrylate (PMMA) was developed using the grafting (polymerization) initiator ammonium persulfate (APS) under the inert atmosphere of nitrogen [124]. The mechanism of graft copolymerization is presented in Fig. 1.6. The grafting of alginate and methyl methacrylate was confirmed by the FTIR, NMR, XRD, and SEM analyses.

The developed hydrogel film has high strength. The graft copolymer, by the introduction of poly(methyl methacrylate), improves the tensile strength. The introduction of methyl carboxylate ($-COOCH_3$) function enhances the interaction force between two macromolecule chains because of the creation of newer hydrogen bonds (intermolecular) between hydroxyl ($-OH$) of alginate and the introduced methyl carboxylate functional group (Fig. 1.7). Similar enhancement of tensile strength was also observed in alginate grafted with poly(N-isopropylacrylamide) [125].

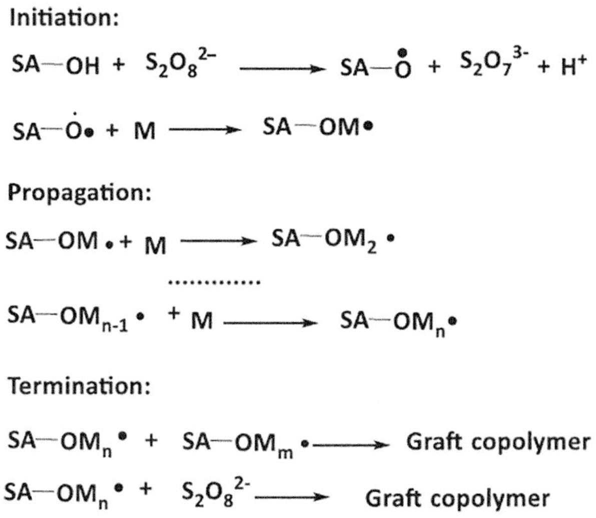

Initiation:

$$SA-OH + S_2O_8^{2-} \longrightarrow SA-\overset{\bullet}{O} + S_2O_7^{3-} + H^+$$

$$SA-\overset{\bullet}{O}\bullet + M \longrightarrow SA-OM\bullet$$

Propagation:

$$SA-OM\bullet + M \longrightarrow SA-OM_2\bullet$$

$$\cdots\cdots\cdots\cdots$$

$$SA-OM_{n-1}\bullet + M \longrightarrow SA-OM_n\bullet$$

Termination:

$$SA-OM_n\bullet + SA-OM_m\bullet \longrightarrow \text{Graft copolymer}$$

$$SA-OM_n\bullet + S_2O_8^{2-} \longrightarrow \text{Graft copolymer}$$

FIG. 1.6 The mechanism of grafting of PMMA onto alginate. *Reproduced from Yang M, Wang L, Xia Y. Ammonium persulphate induced synthesis of polymethyl methacrylate grafted sodium alginate composite films with high strength for food packaging. Int J Biol Macromol 2019;124:1238–1245, Copyright (2019), with permission from Elsevier.*

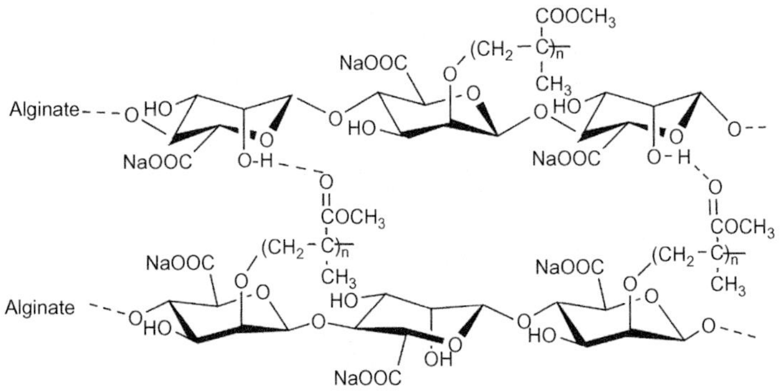

FIG. 1.7 Hydrogen bonds (intermolecular) between PMMA and SA. *Reproduced from Yang M, Wang L, Xia Y. Ammonium persulphate induced synthesis of polymethyl methacrylate grafted sodium alginate composite films with high strength for food packaging. Int J Biol Macromol 2019;124:1238–1245, Copyright (2019), with permission from Elsevier.*

1.4.2.2 *Ulvan*

Ulvan polysaccharide is sourced from edible green algae (sea let-tuces) species of the genus *Ulva*. Three other minor polysaccharides such as glucuronan, cellulose, and xyloglucan are also present in various species of *Ulva* [126, 127]. Ulvan polysaccharides are basically sulfated and highly charged polysaccharides. The average molecular weight of ulvan is between 189 and 8200 kDa [128]. The chemical structure of ulvan can be divided into four domains, a central L-rhamnose 3-sulfate backbone attached with four other structural domains such as domain A (ulvabiouronic acid A residue), domain B (ulvabiouronic acid B residue), domain C (ulvabios unit A), and domain D (ulvabios unit B) [129–131]. Chemically, domain A is D-glucuronic acid, domain B is L-iduronic acid, domain C is D-xylose 4-sulfate, and domain D is D-xylose.

Ulvan is a heteropolysaccharide, and its chemistry differs according to the taxonomic origin, growth conditions, season of harvesting, etc. [132]. The research on the chemical nature of ulvan indicates that it is mainly constituted by repeated disaccharide units [133]. The ulvan polysaccharide is endowed with both hydrophilic and hydrophobic domains in its structure that is not easily found in other natural polysaccharides and has thermoreversible gelling property in the presence of calcium ions at pH near 8. The gel creation mechanism in ulvan polysaccharide is still not explained satisfactorily [134].

1.4.2.3 *Carrageenans*

Three forms of carrageenans are present in nature such as kappa (*k*), iota (*i*), and lambda (*l*). The kappa carrageenan is sourced from *Kappaphycus alvarezii*, and iota carrageenan is produced from *Eucheuma denticulatum*.

Carrageenans are largely made up of D-galactopyranose units, which are linked with α-1,3 and β-1,4 linkages alternatively. Carrageenans are available in near about 15 different structural varieties [135]. However, only three (kappa, iota, and lambda) varieties of them are used commercially. The k-carrageenans are made up of anhydrogalactose structure linked with D-galactose-4-sulfate [136, 137]. The i-carrageenan is composed of anhydrogalactose 2-sulfate unit linked with D-galactose-4-sulfate [138]. The l-carrageenan structure consists of D-galactose 2-sulfate unit attached with D-galactose-2,6-disulfate unit [139]. Carrageenans are water-soluble, sulfur-containing polysaccharides.

Carrageenan contains hydroxyl and sulfate groups in its structure. The k-carrageenan can undergo thermosensitive sol to gel formation, and this property makes it a widely adopted ingredient in the hydrogel-forming applications. Carrageenans are principally pH-sensitive anionic polymers, characterized by the existence of sulfate functional group in their backbone. The pH-sensitive polysaccharide polymers contain either acidic or basic groups in their structure, and they can release or accept protons depending on the environmental pH [140]. If the media has higher pH value than the pKa value of ionizable group in the polysaccharide backbone, then the ionizable groups will release the proton (deprotonation). The pKa value of sulfonic acid in carrageenan is near about 2.8, and when it is placed in a media in which the pH is higher than 2.8, the ionic groups deprotonate to form sulfate anion ($-OSO_3^-$) from unionized sulfonic acid ($-OSO_3H$) group, which results in hydrogel structure. The deprotonation results in negatively charged polysaccharide backbone because protons are removed. The increase in the magnitude of negative charge increases the electrostatic repulsion among the polysaccharide backbones. Therefore this leads to an increase in polymer chain length and polymeric network and volume. This leads to more water penetration inside the knitted polymeric structure, and the system sufficiently swells and leads to the formation of hydrogel.

Carrageenan has extensive utilization in food and biomedical applications [141]. The composite hydrogel based on k-carrageenan/collagen-hydroxyapatite was prepared for bone tissue regeneration [142]. Similarly, injectable hydrogels based on carrageenan were used in tissue engineering [143]. Yegappan et al. developed carrageenan-based injectable hydrogel containing whitlockite nanoparticles (WH NPs) as bone mineral and dimethyloxallylglycine (DMOG) as an angiogenic drug [144]. The development of hydrogel is shown in Fig. 1.8. The developed hydrogel was injectable, demonstrated better protein adsorption ability, and is cytocompatible. The study exhibited sustained drug release for 7 days, which was preceded by an initial burst drug release. The developed nanocomposite hydrogel exhibited capillary tube-like structure and improved cell migration.

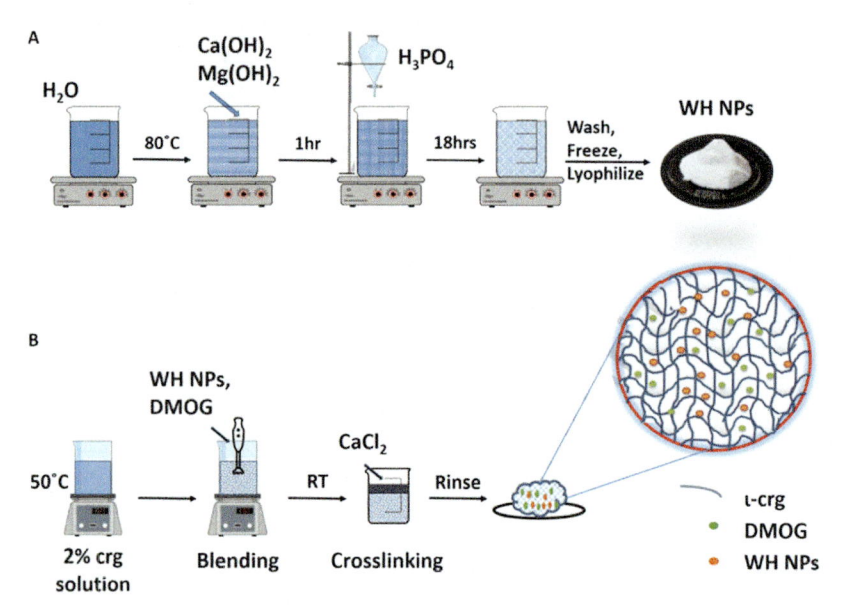

FIG. 1.8   Synthesis of (A) WH NPs and (B) hydrogel nanocomposite. *Reproduced from Yegappan R, Selvaprithiviraj V, Amirthalingam S, Mohandas A, Hwang NS, Jayakumar R. Injectable angiogenic and osteogenic carrageenan nanocomposite hydrogel for bone tissue engineering. Int J Biol Macromol 2019;122:320–328, Copyright (2019), with permission from Elsevier.*

1.4.2.4 Fucoidan

Fucoidan is a sulfated polysaccharide that was first discovered in 1913 by Kylin [145]. Fucoidans are known to possess antiinflammatory and anticoagulant property. They are hydrophilic in nature, mainly found in marine brown algae cell wall, and extracted from the species belonging to the families Laminariaceae, Chordariaceae, Fucaceae, and Alariaceae [146]. Fucoidans can also be found in some marine invertebrates such as sea urchins/eggs and sea cucumber [147].

The structure of fucoidans largely depends on several factors such as the collected sample's species, harvesting condition, and extraction method [148, 149]. Most of the fucoidans have a skeleton of repeating l-fucose units that are $1 \rightarrow 3$ and $1 \rightarrow 4$ linked. In some other minor cases, fucose molecule can also be linked through $1 \rightarrow 2$ linkages [150]. The structures of fucoidan have sulfate groups that are present in C-2, C-3, and C-4 positions. Fucoidans may have several other sugar molecules such as glucose, arabinose, xylose, and galactose. The term "fucoidan" does not reflect any specific single structure, rather a group of polysaccharides that contain fucose in their structure.

Fucoidan is also a sulfated polymer similar to carrageenan, so it can form hydrogels in a similar fashion to that of carrageenan gel formation. There is very limited information in literature about the formation of hydrogels using fucoidan alone. All the preparations were made by combining fucoidan with other polymers such as chitosan and other positively charged compounds. Sezer et al. prepared a hydrogel through the combination of negatively charged fucoidan with positively charged polysaccharide chitosan [151]. The addition of fucoidan increases the water absorption capacity in the hydrogel structure. The reason for more water absorption is attributed to the hydrophilic nature of fucoidan. It also found that the desired electrostatic interaction between chitosan cationic functional group with the anionic functional groups of fucoidan offers increased hardness to the gels in comparison with chitosan hydrogels. Among all formulations, formulation containing fucoidan (0.75%) and chitosan (2%) showed optimum cohesiveness and maximum adhesion values.

1.4.3 Animal polysaccharides

Animal polysaccharides are widely used for hydrogel preparations [152]. Most widely used animal polysaccharide is chitin. However, these polysaccharides are not used in their native form to prepare hydrogels, and they have to be chemically modified and grafted to achieve desired properties that are conductive to the desirable hydrogel formation. One of the common examples of this is native chitin that is less frequently used for hydrogel preparation, and it should be deacetylated and converted to chitosan, which has several applications in hydrogel preparation [153].

Hydrogel is essentially a cross-linked hydrophilic polymeric network able to absorb great quantities of water and can swell 100 times of its original volume. The hydrophilic polymeric backbone is altered and tuned through various chemical or physical methods in such a way to obtain the desirable physical and mechanical properties to gain control on drug release profile. In the present age, hydrogels prepared from natural polysaccharides are gaining more interest for delivery of drug owing to biocompatibility and biodegradability [154–157].

1.4.3.1 *Chitin*

Chitin is a well-known and one of the most common animal polysaccharides abundantly present in nature. It is obtained from the exoskeletons of insects and crustaceans. The common source of chitin is crab shells. The shells of the crabs are mainly formed by high amount of calcium and rigid chitin network [158]. Chitin can be obtained from the shells by demineralization process in which all other minerals are removed, and finally, chitin is obtained [159, 160].

Demineralization process is done by using dilute hydrochloric acid. On treatment with acid, calcium is converted to salts, which are easily removed by filtration process. In another process to extract chitin, deproteinization (process of removing proteins) is used by the application of bases such as sodium hydroxide [161, 162]. Chitin can also be extracted by using some specific enzymes. This process leads to the production in a much faster, safer, and controlled way.

Chitin is mainly composed of two components such as N-acetyl glucosamine and N-glucosamine, which are connected through $1 \rightarrow 4$ glycosidic bond. The most distinct difference between chitin and chitosan is the presence of highly acetylated residues in chitin molecule [163]. Chitin is rigid in structure and crystalline in nature. The molecular weight of chitin ranges from 200 to 1000 kDa and is also insoluble in water, whereas its deacetylated form chitosan has appreciable water solubility. Chitosan molecule has cationic charge owing to the presence of primary amino ($-NH_2$) functional group, which forms hydrogen bond with water molecule and shows increased water solubility [164].

1.4.3.2 Chitosan

The chitosan preparation from chitin was reported long back in 1859 by Rouget [165], and it was from 1990s that chitosan found its wide applications in pharmaceutical manufacturing and research. Chitosan is a cationic polymer extracted from the exoskeletons of insects, crustaceans, and rigid shells of crab [166]. It is a widely used natural polymer, second only to cellulose. Chemically, it is composed of two alternating units of $1 \rightarrow 4$ linked 2-acetamido-2-deoxy-β-D-glucan and $1 \rightarrow 4$ linked 2-amino-2-deoxy-β-D-glucan. Because chitosan was produced by deacetylating chitin molecules, the extent of deacetylation is the critical factor that decides the hydrophilicity of the final product [167, 168]. Solubility, viscosity, and mucoadhesiveness of the chitosan molecule depend on molecular weight and deacetylation degree of the polymer. The commercial chitosan has typical molecular mass in the range of 100–800 kDa. It can be degraded by enzymes present in our body such as lysozyme and forms biodegradable end product. Each glucosamine unit of chitosan contains a primary amino ($-NH_2$) and two hydroxyl ($-OH$) groups. The cationic amino group (protonated; $-NH_3^+$) present in chitosan is responsible for the electrostatic attraction with oppositely charged anions. Thus ionic cross-linking using anions are often used to produce ionically cross-linked chitosan hydrogels. Chitosan hydrogels are produced by chemical or physical methods. Chemically formed hydrogels have irreversible covalent bonds. On the other hand, physical method is responsible for reversible bonds formation. Physical gelation happens because of interaction between different oppositely charged electrolytes. In acidic environment, chitosan molecule shows polycationic nature, and that is why at low acidic pH, it forms complex with different anions.

Native chitosan molecule is not extensively used for drug delivery system because it is hydrophilic in nature and in native form is not useful as hydrogels. To make suitable chitosan hydrogels, chitosan molecules should be modified (grafted or cross-linked). The physical properties, mechanical

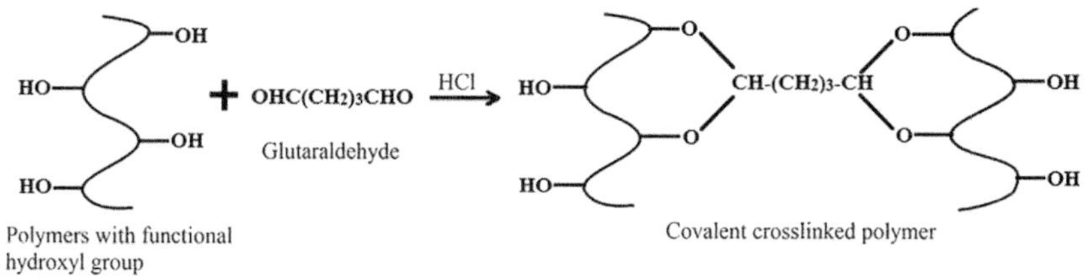

FIG. 1.9 Covalent cross-linking between glutaraldehyde and chitosan. *Reproduced from Giri TK, Thakur A, Alexander A, Ajazuddin, Badwaik H, Tripathi DK. Modified chitosan hydrogels as drug delivery and tissue engineering systems: present status and applications. Acta Pharm Sin B 2012;2:439–449, Copyright (2012), with permission from Elsevier.*

strength, swelling ratio, and temperature sensitiveness of a hydrogel can be changed or modified by altering the polymeric backbone of the hydrogel forming polymer. The ingredients used to enhance these properties are cross-linking agents (glutaraldehyde, oxalic acid, and formaldehyde). Glutaraldehyde can be cross-linked within the backbone of chitosan molecule in the following pathway (Fig. 1.9) [169]. Glutaraldehyde has –CHO functional group in its structure. Polymer containing –OH group in their structure can react with the –CHO functional group of the glutaraldehyde, and water is removed in this reaction.

Lin et al. developed [N-(2-carboxybenzyl)] chitosan (CBCS), a water-soluble chitosan derivative [170]. The hydrogel (CBCSG) was intended for colon-specific delivery of 5-fluorouracil. The hydrogel was synthesized by cross-linking CBCS with glutaraldehyde (Fig. 1.10). In this study, it was found that the release of drug was pH-sensitive.

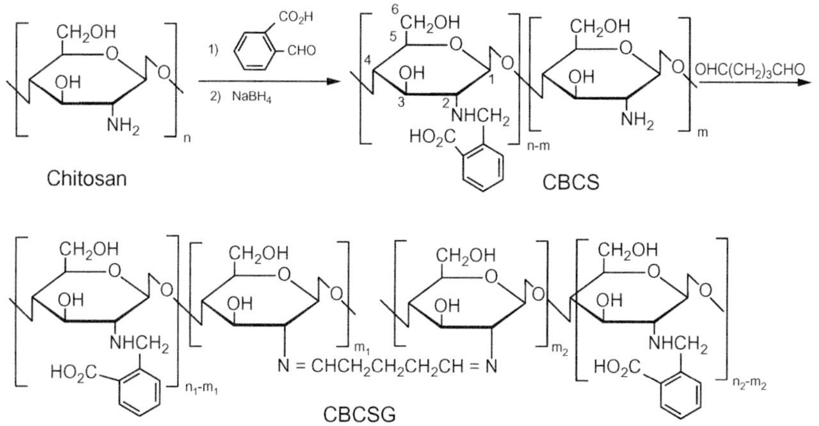

FIG. 1.10 Synthetic scheme for CBCS and CBCSG. *Reproduced from Lin Y, Chen Q, Luo H. Preparation and characterization of N-(2-carboxybenzyl)chitosan as a potential pH-sensitive hydrogel for drug delivery. Carbohydr Res 2007;342:87–95, Copyright (2007), with permission from Elsevier.*

1.4.3.3 Heparin

According to literature, heparin was discovered in 1916 [171, 172]. Heparin is sulfur-containing natural polysaccharide that is present in mast cells. The average molecular weight is between 5 and 40 kDa [173]. Heparin is an anionic polysaccharide that has repeating units of glucosamine and uronic acid. It has anticoagulant properties and can bind with different proteins and other growth factors [174–176]. Tae et al. developed a hydrogel using heparin and polyethylene glycol, which were attached with heparin-binding peptides [177]. This formulation showed sustained action.

1.4.3.4 Chondroitin sulfate

Chondroitin sulfate (CS) is the chief constituent in ECM of animals and is abundantly found in hyaline cartilage and other various tissues such as skin, blood vessels, and nerve tissues and at the site of calcification of bone [178, 179]. CS belongs to glycosaminoglycans group, and in human beings, they are linked covalently with protein core and form proteoglycan [180, 181]. Glycosaminoglycans are linear heteropolysaccharide chains with repeating units of disaccharides [182]. CS contains disaccharide units of 1,3-linked β-N-acetyl galactosamine and 1,4-linked β-glucuronic acid presenting the functionalities of hydroxyl, sulfate, and carboxylic acid with molecular weight of about 463 Da.

Barkat et al. prepared smart hydrogels loaded with oxaliplatin by using CS for targeting colorectal cancer [183]. CS is a mucopolysaccharide that contains N-acetyl-D-galactosamide linked with D-glucuronic acid. It is highly water soluble and was cross-linked with acrylic acid, which exhibited pH-sensitive properties to the polymer. The carboxylic groups of the acrylic acid chains are easily ionizable and are extremely disposed to the higher pH. These carboxylate groups are essentially having stronger affinity toward water molecules, thus extremely contributing to the swelling of polymeric chain. CS contains hydroxyl (–OH), sulfonic (–SO_3–), and carboxyl (–COOH) groups that ionize and generate repulsive forces, contributing to greater water absorbability of the hydrogel. CS with monomers in cross-linked form has been proved as a perfect candidate to target the colon.

The hydrogel was synthesized by chemically cross-linking CS, silica nanospheres (SiO_2), and casein (CAS) [184]. The synthesis of hydrogel is represented in Fig. 1.11. CAS was chemically modified using maleic anhydride to form CAS^{MA}. CS was chemically modified to form CS^{GMA}. Initially, SiO_2 nanoparticles were synthesized, and then double bond was inserted to form V-SiO_2. Finally, the hydrogel was synthesized using $Na_2S_2O_8$ and N,N,N',N'-tetramethyl ethylenediamine (TEMED). The developed hydrogels were cytocompatible and released L-dopa for 87 h.

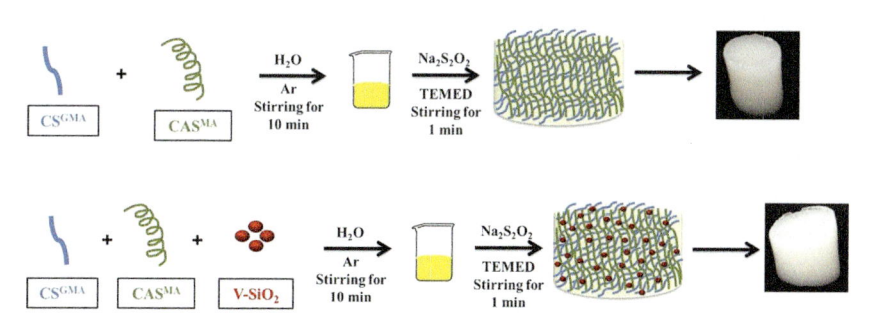

FIG. 1.11 Synthesis of CS^{GMA}/CAS^{MA} and $CS^{GMA}/CAS^{MA}/V\text{-}SiO_2$ hydrogels. *Reproduced from Simão AR, Fragal VH, Lima AMO, Pellá MCG, Garcia FP, Nakamura CV, Tambourgi EB, Rubira AF. pH-responsive hybrid hydrogels: chondroitin sulfate/casein trapped silica nanospheres for controlled drug release. Int J Biol Macromol 2020;148:302–315, Copyright (2020), with permission from Elsevier.*

1.4.3.5 Hyaluronic acid

Hyaluronic acid is a mucopolysaccharide formed in the living organisms at their ECM of connective tissues and biological fluids that bind to specific cell receptors [185–187]. It is the component of synovial fluid that acts as a lubricant. It is also found in the vitreous humor, which probably maintains the exact shape of the eye [188, 189]. Hyaluronic acid is a linear polysaccharide, which is a nonsulfated glycosaminoglycan, and is degraded by the enzyme hyaluronidases. Hydrogels using hyaluronic acid are synthesized through cross-linking. Hyaluronic acid reacts with cross-linkers through introduction of new covalent bonds between the hyaluronic acid chains [190].

Injectable hydrogel based on hyaluronic acid was synthesized for the simultaneous delivery of cancer chemotherapeutic drugs paclitaxel (PTX), 5-fluorouracil (5-FU), and cisplatin (DDP) [191]. The developed hyaluronic acid-based hydrogel showed low toxicity and released drug in a controlled manner. Approximately, 96% of free paclitaxel was released at 48h, but 80% drug was released at 168h from microspheres (Fig. 1.12A). Release of three drugs from the hydrogel beads was further studied (Fig. 1.12B). At 168h, 96% and 95% of 5-fluorouracil and cisplatin, respectively, were released, but only 40% of paclitaxel was released. Therefore dual entrapment strategy considerably slowed the drug release rate. The cytotoxicity studies of the various formulations were tested in CT26 cell line. In the presence of microsphere, 84% of the cells were viable indicating low cytotoxicity (Fig. 1.12C). Both the free and entrapped drug inhibited the growth of the cells but drug-loaded hydrogel showed enhanced cytotoxic effect in comparison with the drug alone (Fig. 1.12D). Moreover, diminished tumor growth was

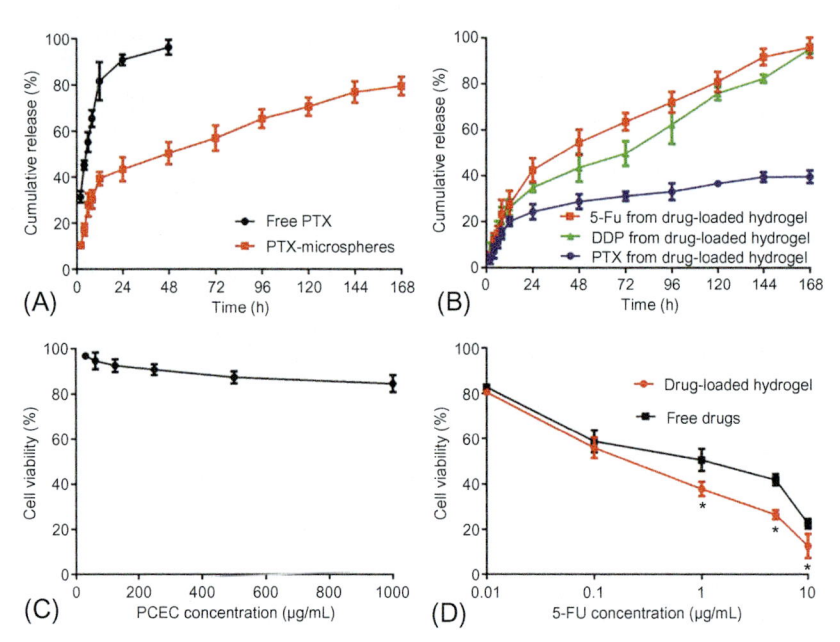

FIG. 1.12 (A) Release profile of free PTX and PTX microspheres. (B) Release profile of 5-FU, PTX, and DDP from hydrogel. (C) In vitro cytotoxicity of blank microspheres. (D) In vitro cytotoxicity of free drugs and the drug-loaded hydrogel. *Reproduced from Luo J, Wu Z, Lu Y, Xiong K, Wen Q, Zhao L, Wang B, Gui Y, Fu S. Intraperitoneal administration of biocompatible hyaluronic acid hydrogel containing multi-chemotherapeutic agents for treatment of colorectal peritoneal carcinomatosis. Int J Biol Macromol 2020;152:718–726, Copyright (2020), with permission from Elsevier.*

observed in the tumor-bearing mice model treated by injecting the drug-loaded hydrogel.

1.5 Conclusion

Hydrogels prepared with natural polysaccharides have distinguishing properties, such as biodegradability, biocompatibility, high water withholding capacity, and nontoxicity, which can be widely used in biomedical applications. In fact, polysaccharide-based hydrogels have many benefits because of their tunable composition and interconnected structure that control the release of drug embedded in the polymeric matrix. In a nutshell, hydrogel prepared with natural polysaccharides are promising carriers for delivering active ingredients to target cells. Therefore overall basic knowledge about chemistry of various naturally obtained polysaccharides, which includes sources, classification, and structural features, is attempted in this chapter, which is essential for preparing hydrogels.

References

[1] Pawar HA, Kamat SR, Choudhary PD. An overview of natural polysaccharides as biological macromolecules: their chemical modifications and pharmaceutical applications. Biol Med 2015;7(1):1–9.

[2] William BJ. Ask the historian: the origin of the polymer concept. J Chem Educ 2008;88:624–5.

[3] Shrivastava A. Introduction to plastics engineering. In: Shrivastava A, editor. Introduction to plastics engineering. William Andrew; 2018. p. 1–16.

[4] Bhatia S. Natural polymers versus synthetic polymer. In: Bhatia S, editor. Natural polymer drug delivery systems. Cham: Springer; 2016. p. 95–118.

[5] Mathur S. Understanding and utilizing the biomolecule/nanosystems interface. In: Chen EY, Liu WF, Megido L, Diez P, Fuentes M, Fager C, Uskoković DP, editors. Nanotechnologies in preventive and regenerative medicine. Elsevier; 2018. p. 207–97.

[6] Aravamudhan A, Ramos DM, Nada AA, Kumbar AG. Natural polymers: polysaccharides and their derivatives for biomedical applications. In: Kumbar SG, Laurencin CT, Deng M, editors. Natural and synthetic biomedical polymers. Elsevier Science; 2014. p. 67–89.

[7] Suman K, Deepak V, Banik SP. Carbohydrates. In: Kankara M, Sharma NC, Sharma PC, Somani BL, Misra PC, editors. Biomolecules: (introduction, structure & function). National Science Digital Library; 2008. p. 1–93.

[8] Saravanakumar G, Jo DG, Park JH. Polysaccharide based nanoparticles: a versatile platform for drug delivery and biomedical imaging. Curr Med Chem 2012;19:3212–9.

[9] Maji B. Introduction to natural polysaccharides. In: Maiti S, Jana S, editors. Functional polysaccharides for biomedical applications. Woodhead Publishing; 2019. p. 1–31.

[10] Liu Z, Jiao Y, Wang Y, Zhou C, Zhang Z. Polysaccharides-based nanoparticles as drug delivery systems. Adv Drug Deliv Rev 2008;60:1650–62.

[11] Giri TK, Thakur D, Alexander A, Ajazuddin, Badwaik H, Tripathi DK. Alginate based hydrogel as a potential biopolymeric carrier for drug delivery and cell delivery systems: present status and applications. Curr Drug Deliv 2012;9:539–55.

[12] Giri TK, Verma S, Ajazuddin, Alexander A, Badwaik H, Tripathi DK. Prospective and new findings of hydroxypropyl methylcellulose (HPMC) as a potential carrier for gastrorent"ive drug delivery systems. Drug Deliv Lett 2012;2:98–107.

[13] Dey M, Ghosh B, Giri TK. Enhanced intestinal stability and pH sensitive release of quercetin in GIT through gellan gum hydrogels. Colloids Surf B Biointerfaces 2020;196:111341.

[14] Ajazuddin, Alexander A, Khan J, Giri TK, Tripathi DK, Saraf S, Saraf S. Advancement in stimuli triggered in situ gelling delivery for local and systemic route. Expert Opin Drug Deliv 2012;9(12):1573–92.

[15] Satturwar PM, Fulzele SV, Dorle AK. Biodegradation and in vivo biocompatibility of rosin: a natural film-forming polymer. AAPS Pharm Sci Tech 2003;4(4):1–6.

[16] Ajazuddin, Alexander A, Khichariya A, Gupta S, Patel RJ, Giri TK, Tripathi DK. Recent expansions in an emergent novel drug delivery technology: emulgel. J Control Release 2013;171:122–32.

[17] Giri TK, Choudhary C, Alexander A, Ajazuddin, Badwaik H, Tripathy M, Tripathi DK. Sustained release of diltiazem hydrochloride from cross-linked biodegradable IPN hydrogel beads based on pectin and modified xanthan gum. Indian J Pharm Sci 2013;75:619–27.

[18] Shariatinia Z. Pharmaceutical applications of natural polysaccharides. In: Hasnain MS, Nayak AK, editors. Natural polysaccharides in drug delivery and biomedical applications. Academic Press; 2019. p. 15–57.

[19] Kaushik K, Sharma RB, Agarwal S. Natural polymers and their applications. Int J Pharm Sci Rev Res 2016;37(2):30–6.

[20] Kulkarni VS, Butte KD, Rathod SS. Natural polymers–a comprehensive review. Int J Res Pharmaceut Biomed Sci 2012;3(4):1597–613.

[21] Saha S, Giri TK. Breaking the barrier of cancer through papaya extract and their formulation. Anticancer Agents Med Chem 2019;19:1577–87.

[22] Mondal R, Bobde Y, Ghosh B, Giri TK. Development and characterization of a phospholipid complex for effective delivery of capsaicin. Indian J Pharm Sci 2019;81(6):1011–9.

[23] Giri TK. Breaking the barrier of cancer through liposome loaded with phytochemicals. Curr Drug Deliv 2019;16(1):3–17.

[24] Zhu T, Mao J, Cheng Y, Liu H, Lv L, Ge M, Li S, Huang J, Chen Z, Li H, Yang L, Lai Y. Recent progress of polysaccharide-based hydrogel interfaces for wound healing and tissue engineering. Adv Mater Interfaces 2019;6(17):1900761.

[25] Coviello T, Matricardi P, Marianecci C, Alhaique F. Polysaccharide hydrogels for modified release formulations. J Control Release 2007;119:5–24.

[26] Leone G, Barbucci R. Polysaccharide based hydrogels for biomedical applications. In: Hydrogels. Milano: Springer; 2009. p. 25–41.

[27] Thomas F, Hehemann JH, Rebuffet E, Czjzek M, Michel G. Environmental and gut bacteroidetes: the food connection. Front Microbiol 2011;2:93.

[28] Goldfarb KC, Karaoz U, Hanson CA, Santee CA, Bradford MA, Treseder KK, Wallenstein MD, Brodie EL. Differential growth responses of soil bacterial taxa to carbon substrates of varying chemical recalcitrance. Front Microbiol 2011;2:94.

[29] Johnson DR, Goldschmidt F, Lilja EE, Ackermann M. Metabolic specialization and the assembly of microbial communities. ISME J 2012;6:1985–91.

[30] Haichar FZ, Achouak W, Christen R, Heulin T, Marol C, Marais CF, Mougel C, Ranjard L, Balesdent J, Berge O. Identification of cellulolytic bacteria in soil by stable isotope probing. Environ Microbiol 2007;9:625–34.

[31] Wilson DB. Microbial diversity of cellulose hydrolysis. Curr Opin Microbiol 2011;14:259–63.

[32] Anderson I, Abt B, Lykidis A, Klenk HP, Kyrpides N, Ivanova N. Genomics of aerobic cellulose utilization systems in actinobacteria. PLoS One 2012;7, e39331.

[33] Chen J, Lolivret L. The determining role of bolus rheology in triggering a swallowing. Food Hydrocoll 2011;25:325–32.

[34] Hehre EJ. A fresh understanding of the stereochemical behavior of glycosylases: structural distinction of "inverting" (2-MCO-type) versus "retaining" (1-MCO-type) enzymes. Adv Carbohydr Chem Biochem 2000;55:265–310.

[35] Hehre EJ, Okada G, Genghof DS. Glycosylation as the paradigm of carbohydrase action: evidence from the actions of amylases. Adv Chem Ser 1973;117:309–33.

[36] Kean T, Thanou M. Biodegradation, biodistribution and toxicity of chitosan. Adv Drug Deliv Rev 2010;62:3–11.

[37] Ley RE, Peterson DA, Gordon JI. Ecological and evolutionary forces shaping microbial diversity in the human intestine. Cell 2006;124:837–48.

[38] Round JL, Mazmanian SK. The gut microbiota shapes intestinal immune responses during health and disease. Nat Rev Immunol 2009;9:313–23.

[39] Atarashi K, Honda K. Microbiota in autoimmunity and tolerance. Curr Opin Immunol 2011;23:761–8.

[40] Khanna S, Tosh PK. A clinician's primer on the role of the microbiome in human health and disease. Mayo Clin Proc 2014;89:107–14.

[41] Guarner F, Malagelada JR. Gut flora in health and disease. Lancet 2003;361:512–9.

[42] Beaugerie L, Petit JC. Antibiotic-associated diarrhea. Best Pract Res Clin Gastroenterol 2004;18:337–52.

[43] Brandwein M, Katz I, Katz I, Kohen R. Beyond the gut: skin microbiome compositional changes are associated with BMI. Hum Microb J 2019;7:100063.

[44] Xu J, Bjursell MK, Himrod J, Deng S, Carmichael SK, Chiang HC, Hooper LV, Gordon JI. A genomic view of the human-Bacteroides thetaiotaomicron symbiosis. Science 2003;299:2074–6.

[45] Sonnenburg L, Xu J, Leip DD, Chen CH, Westover BP, Weatherford J, Buhler JD, Gordon JI. Glycan foraging in vivo by an intestine-adapted bacterial symbiont. Science 2005;307:1955–9.

[46] Ravcheev DA, Godzik A, Osterman AL, Rodionov DA. Polysaccharides utilization in human gut bacterium Bacteroides thetaiotaomicron: comparative genomics reconstruction of metabolic and regulatory networks. BMC Genomics 2013;14:873–90.

[47] Linhardt RJ, Galliher PM, Cooney CL. Polysaccharide lyases. Appl Biochem Biotechnol 1986;12:135–76.

[48] Zhanga F, Zhangb Z, Linhardt RJ. Handbook of glycomics. Academic Press; 2010. p. 59–80.

[49] Cummings JH, Macfarlane GT. The control and consequences of bacterial fermentation in the human colon. J Appl Bacteriol 1991;70:443–59.

[50] Silvester KR, Englyst HN, Cummings JH. Ileal recovery of starch from whole diets containing resistant starch measured in vitro and fermentation of ileal effluent. Am J Clin Nutr 1995;62:403–11.

[51] Hooper LV, Midtvedt T, Gordon JI. How host-microbial interactions shape the nutrient environment of the mammalian intestine. Annu Rev Nutr 2002;4:283–307.

[52] D'Elia JN, Salyers AA. Effect of regulatory protein levels on utilization of starch by Bacteroides thetaiotaomicron. J Bacteriol 1996;14:7180–6.

[53] Anderson KL, Salyers AA. Biochemical evidence that starch breakdown by Bacteroides thetaiotaomicron involves outer membrane starch-binding sites and periplasmic starch-degrading enzymes. J Bacteriol 1989;171:3192–8.

[54] Reeves AR, Wang GR, Salyers AA. Characterization of four outer membrane proteins that play a role in utilization of starch by Bacteroides thetaiotaomicron. J Bacteriol 1997;179:643–9.

[55] Martens EC, Koropatkin NM, Smith TJ, Gordon JI. Complex glycan catabolism by the human gut microbiota: the Bacteroidetes Sus-like paradigm. J Biol Chem 2009;284:24673–7.

[56] Shipman JA, Berleman JE, Salyers AA. Characterization of four outer membrane proteins involved in binding starch to the cell surface of Bacteroides thetaiotaomicron. J Bacteriol 2000;182:5365–72.

[57] Shipman JA, Cho KH, Siegel HA, Salyers AA. Physiological characterization of SusG, an outer membrane protein essential for starch utilization by Bacteroides thetaiotaomicron. J Bacteriol 1999;181:7206–11.

[58] Tancula E, Feldhaus MJ, Bedzyk LA, Salyers AA. Location and characterization of genes involved in binding of starch to the surface of Bacteroides thetaiotaomicron. J Bacteriol 1992;174:5609–16.

[59] D'Elia JN, Salyers AA. Contribution of a neopullulanase, a pullulanase and an α-glucosidase to growth of Bacteroides thetaiotaomicron on starch. J Bacteriol 1996;178:7173–9.

[60] Cho KH, Cho D, Wang GR, Salyers AA. New regulatory gene that contributes to control of Bacteroides thetaiotaomicron starch utilization genes. J Bacteriol 2001;183:7198–205.

[61] Tester RF, Karkalas J. Carbohydrates-interactions with other food components. In: Caballero B, Finglas P, Toldra F, editors. Encyclopedia of food sciences and nutrition. 2nd ed. Academic Press; 2003. p. 875–81.

[62] Khosravi C, Benocci T, Battaglia E, Benoit I, Vries RP. Sugar catabolism in aspergillus and other fungi related to the utilization of plant biomass. Adv Appl Microbiol 2015;90:1–28.

[63] Giri TK, Vishwas S, Tripathi DK. Synthesis of grafted locust bean gum using vinyl monomer and studies of physicochemical properties and acute toxicity. Nat Prod J 2016;6:1–9.

[64] Giri TK, Pure S, Tripathi DK. Synthesis of graft copolymers of acrylamide for locust bean gum using microwave energy: swelling behavior, flocculation characteristics and acute toxicity study. Polimeros 2015;25:168–74.

[65] Alcázar-Alay SC, Meireles MAA. Physicochemical properties, modifications and applications of starches from different botanical sources. Food Sci Technol 2015;35(2):215–36.

[66] Carvalho AJF. Starch: major sources, properties and applications as thermoplastic materials. In: Belgacem MN, Gandini A, editors. Monomers, polymers and composites from renewable resources. Elsevier Science; 2008. p. 321–42.

[67] Shogren RL. Starch: properties and materials applications. In: Kaplan DL, editor. Biopolymers from renewable resources. Berlin Heidelberg: Springer, Verlag; 1998. p. 30–46.

[68] Stephen MA, Phillips GO, Williams PA. Food polysaccharides and their applications. 2nd ed. CRC Press; 2006. p. 1–712.

[69] Busi MV, Gomez-Casati DF, Martin M, Barchiesi J, Grisolia MJ, Hedin N, Carrillo JB. Starch metabolism in green plants. In: Ramawat K, Mérillon JM, editors. Polysaccharides. Cham: Springer; 2014. p. 329–76.

[70] Talaat HA, Sorour MH, Aboulnour AG, Shaalan HF, Ahmed Enas M, Awad AM, et al. Development of a multicomponent fertilizing hydrogel with relevant techno-economic indicators. Am-Euras J Agric Environ Sci 2008;3:764–70.

[71] Qunyia T, Ganweib Z. Rapid synthesis of a superabsorbent from a saponified starch and acrylonitrile/AMPS graft copolymers. Carbohydr Polym 2005;62:74–9.

[72] Izydorczyk M, Cui SW, Qi W. Polysaccharide gums: structures, functional properties, and applications. In: Cui SW, editor. Food carbohydrates: chemistry, physical properties and applications. CRC Press; 2005.

[73] Shukla RK, Tiwari A. Carbohydrate polymers: applications and recent advances in delivering drugs to the colon. Carbohydr Polym 2012;88:399–416.

[74] Aspinall GO. Cellulose. In: Polysaccharides. 1st ed. Pergamon; 1970. p. 43–53.

[75] Lovegrove A, Edwards CH, Noni I, Patel H, El SN, Grassby T, Zielke C, Ulmius M, Nilsson L, Butterworth PJ, Ellis PR, Shewry PR. Role of polysaccharides in food, digestion, and health. Crit Rev Food Sci Nutr 2017;57(2):237–53.

[76] Sudhakar YN, Selvakumar M, KrishnaBhat D. Biopolymer electrolytes for solar cells and electrochemical cells. In: Biopolymer electrolytes fundamentals and applications in energy storage. Elsevier; 2018. p. 117–49.

[77] Sahin HT, Arslan MB. A study on physical and chemical properties of cellulose paper immersed in various solvent mixtures. Int J Mol Sci 2008;9:78–88.

[78] Brunner G. Processing of biomass with hydrothermal and supercritical water. Supercrit Fluid Sci Technol 2014;5:395–509.

[79] Machmudah S, Wahyudiono, Kanda H, Goto M. Hydrolysis of biopolymers in near-critical and subcritical water. In: González HD, MJG M, editors. Water extraction of bioactive compounds. Elsevier; 2017. p. 69–107.

[80] Ollvelra W, Glasser WG. Hydrogels from polysaccharides. I. Cellulose beads for chromatographic support. J Appl Polym Sci 1996;60:63–73.

[81] Huang W, Wang Y, McMullen LM, McDermott MT, Deng H, Du Y, Zhang L. Stretchable, tough, self-recoverable, and cyto compatible chitosan/cellulose nanocrystals/polyacrylamide hybrid hydrogels. Carbohydr Polym 2019;222:114977.

[82] Chang C, Han K, Zhang L. Structure and properties of cellulose/poly(N-isopropylacrylamide) hydrogels prepared by IPN strategy. Polym Adv Technol 2011;22(9):1329–34.

[83] Lin F, Lu X, Wang Z, Lu Q, Lin G, Huang B, Lu B. In situ polymerization approach to cellulose–polyacrylamide interpenetrating network hydrogel with high strength and pH-responsive properties. Cellul 2019;26(3):1825–39.

[84] Niu L, Zhang D, Liu Y, Zhou X, Wang J, Wang C, Chu F. Combination of acid treatment and dual network fabrication to stretchable cellulose based hydrogels with tunable properties. Int J Biol Macromol 2020;147:1–9.

[85] Pauly M, Gille S, Liu L, Mansoori N, Souza A, Schultink A, Xiong G. Hemicellulose biosynthesis. Planta 2013;238:627–42.

[86] Held MA, Jiang N, Basu D, Showalter AM, Faik A. Plant cell wall polysaccharides: structure and biosynthesis. In: Ramawat K, Mérillon JM, editors. Polysaccharides. Cham: Springer; 2015. p. 3–54.

[87] Arruda IRS, Albuquerque PBS, Santos GRC, Silva AG, Mourão PAS, Correia MTS, et al. Structure and rheological properties of a xyloglucan extracted from Hymenaea courbaril var. courbaril seeds. Int J Biol Macromol 2015;73:31–8.

[88] Kong W, Dai Q, Gao C, Ren J, Liu C, Sun R. Hemicellulose-based hydrogels and their potential application. In: Thakur V, Thakur M, editors. Polymer gels. gels horizons: from science to smart materials. Singapore: Springer; 2008. p. 87–127.

[89] Silva JAL, Rao MA. Pectins: structure, functionality, and uses. In: Stephen MA, Phillips GO, Williams PA, editors. Food polysaccharides and their applications. CRC Press; 2006. p. 353–412.

[90] Giannouli P, Richardson RK, Morris ER. Effect of polymeric cosolutes on calcium pectinate gelation. Part 3. Gum arabic and overview. Carbohydr Polym 2004;55:367–77.

[91] Rehman A, Ahmad T, Aadil RM, Spotti MJ, Bakry AM, Khan IM, Zhao L, Riaz T, Tong Q. Pectin polymers as wall materials for the nano-encapsulation of bioactive compounds. Trends Food Sci Technol 2019;90:35–46.

[92] Sarioglu E, Kocaaga BA, Turan D, Batirel S, Guner FS. Theophylline-loaded pectin-based hydrogel II effect of concentration of initial pectin solution, crosslinker type and cation concentration of external solution on drug release profile. J Appl Polym Sci 2019;48155:1–15.

[93] Jani GK, Shah DP, Prajapati VD, Jain VC. Gums and mucilages: versatile excipients for pharmaceutical formulations. Asian J Pharm Sci 2009;4(5):309–23.

[94] Verbeken D, Dierckx S, Dewettinck K. Exudate gums: occurrence, production, and applications. Appl Microbiol Biotechnol 2003;63:10–21.

[95] Whistler RL. Exudate gums. In: Whistler RL, Bemiller JN, editors. Industrial gums polysaccharides and their derivatives. Academic Press; 1993. p. 309–39.

[96] Nussinovitch A. Exudate gums. In: Hydrocolloid applications. Boston, MA: Springer; 1997. p. 125–39.

[97] Ahmad S, Ahmad M, Manzoor K, Purwar R, Ikram S. A review on latest innovations in natural gums based hydrogels: preparations & applications. Int J Biol Macromol 2019;136:870–90.

[98] Chandini SK, Ganesan P, Bhaskar N. In vitro antioxidant activities of three selected brown seaweeds of India. Food Chem 2008;107:707–13.

[99] Murata M, Nakazoe JI. Production and use of marine algae in Japan. Jpn Agric Res Q 2001;35:281–90.

[100] Kraan S. Algal polysaccharides, novel applications and outlook. In: Chang CF, editor. Carbohydrates: comprehensive studies on glycobiology and glycotechnology. Rijeka, Croatia: InTech; 2012. p. 489–532.

[101] Giri TK, Verma D, Badwaik HR. Effect of aluminium chloride concentration on diltiazem hydrochloride release from pH-sensitive hydrogel beads composed of hydrolyzed grafted k-carrageenan and sodium alginate. Curr Chem Biol 2017;11:44–9.

[102] Giri TK, Verma D, Tripathi DK. Effect of adsorption parameters on biosorption of Pb++ ions from aqueous solution by poly (acrylamide)-grafted kappa-carrageenan. Polym Bull 2015;72:1625–46.

[103] Giri TK, Pradhan M, Tripathi DK. Synthesis of graft copolymer of kappa-carrageenan using microwave energy and studies of swelling capacity, flocculation properties, and preliminary acute toxicity. Turk J Chem 2016;40:283–95.

[104] Holdt SL, Kraan S. Bioactive compounds in seaweed: functional food applications and legislation. J Appl Physiol 2011;23:543–97.

[105] Smidsrod O, Skjak-Bræk G. Alginate as immobilization matrix for cells. Trends Biotechnol 1990;8:71–8.

[106] Arasaki S, Arasaki T. Low calorie, high nutrition vegetables from the sea to help you look and feel better. vol. 60. Tokyo: Japan Publications; 1983.

[107] Rasmussen RS, Morrissey MT. Marine biotechnology for production of food ingredients. Adv Food Nutr Res 2007;52:237–92.

[108] Clark DE, Green HC. Alginic acid and process of making same. US Patent 2036922; 1936.

[109] Draget KI, Taylor C. Chemical, physical and biological properties of alginates and their biomedical implications. Food Hydrocoll 2011;25:251–6.

[110] Usman A, Khalid S, Usman A, Hussain Z, Wang Y. Algal polysaccharides, novel application, and outlook. In: Zia MK, Zuber M, Ali M, editors. Algae based polymers, blends, and composites chemistry, biotechnology and materials science. Elsevier; 2017. p. 115–53.

[111] Lee KY, Mooney DJ. Alginate: properties and biomedical applications. Prog Polym Sci 2012;37:106–26.

[112] Kuo CK, Ma PX. Ionically crosslinked alginate hydrogels as scaffolds for tissue engineering: part 1. Structure, gelation rate and mechanical properties. Biomaterials 2001;22:511–21.

[113] Augst AD, Kong HJ, Mooney DJ. Alginate hydrogels as biomaterials. Macromol Biosci 2006;6:623–33.

[114] Drury JL, Dennis RG, Mooney DJ. The tensile properties of alginate hydrogels. Biomaterials 2004;25:3187–99.

[115] Zhao XH, Huebsch N, Mooney DJ, Suo ZG. Stress-relaxation behavior in gels with ionic and covalent crosslinks. J Appl Phys 2010;107, 063509.

[116] Bazban-shotorbani S, Hasani-sadrabadi MM, Karkhaneh A, Serpooshan V, Jacob KI, Moshaverinia A, Mahmoudi M. Revisiting structure-property relationship of pH-responsive polymers for drug delivery applications. J Control Release 2017;253:46–63.

[117] Alboofetileh M, Rezaei M, Hosseini H, Abdollahi M. Effect of montmorillonite clay and biopolymer concentration on the physical and mechanical properties of alginate nanocomposite films. J Food Eng 2013;117:26–33.

[118] Sharma S, Sanpui P, Chattopadhyay A, Ghosh SS. Fabrication of antibacterial silver nanoparticle-sodium alginate–chitosan. RSC Adv 2012;2:5837–43.

[119] Shah SB, Patel CP, Trivedi HC. Ceric-induced grafting of ethyl-acrylate onto sodium alginate. Angew Makromol Chem 1994;214:75–89.

[120] Radhakrishnan N, Lakshminarayana Y, Devi SU, Srinivasan KSV. Studies on the graft copolymerization of acrylonitrile onto sodium alginate. J Macromol Sci A 1994;31:581–91.

[121] Wu GS, Hou SZ, Chen YQ. Graft copolymerization of methyl methacrylate onto alginic acid using potassium persulfate-urea as initiation system. Chin J Appl Chem 1993;10:51–3.

[122] Wu GS, Li SZ, Wu ZP. ASP-TU initiated graft copolymerization of acrylate monomer onto sodium alginate. Petrochem Technol 1995;24:793–8.

[123] Blair HS, Lai KM. Graft copolymers of polysaccharides: 1. Graft copolymers of alginic acid. Polymers 1982;23:1838–41.

[124] Yang M, Wang L, Xia Y. Ammonium persulphate induced synthesis of polymethyl methacrylate grafted sodium alginate composite films with high strength for food packaging. Int J Biol Macromol 2019;124:1238–45.

[125] Lee SB, Seo SM, Lim YM, Cho SK, Lee YM. Preparation of alginate/poly(N-isopropylacrylamide) hydrogels using gamma-ray irradiation grafting. Macromol Res 2004;12:269–75.

[126] Lahaye M, Kaeffer B. Seaweed dietary fibres: structure, physico-chemical and biological properties relevant to intestinal physiology. Sci Aliment 1997;17:563–84.

[127] Lahaye M. NMR spectroscopic characterisation of oligosaccharides from two Ulva rigida ulvan samples (Ulvales, Chlorophyta) degraded by a lyase. Carbohydr Res 1998;314:1–12.

[128] Lahaye M, Ray B. Cell-wall polysaccharides from the marine green alga Ulva "rigida" (Ulvales, Chlorophyta)dNMR analysis of ulvan oligosaccharides. Carbohydr Res 1996;283:161–73.

[129] Percival VE, McDowell RH. Chemistry and enzymology of marine algal polysaccharides. London, New York: Academic Press; 1967.

[130] Cunha L, Grenha A. Sulfated seaweed polysaccharides as multifunctional materials in drug delivery applications. Mar Drugs 2016;14:42.

[131] Lahaye M, Robic A. Structure and functional properties of ulvan, a polysaccharide from green seaweeds. Biomacromolecules 2007;8:1765–74.

[132] Mišurcová L, Škrovánková S, Samek D, Ambrožová J, Machů L. Health benefits of algal polysaccharides in human nutrition. In: Henry J, editor. Advances in food and nutrition research, vol. 66. Academic press; 2012. p. 75–145.

[133] Robic A, Gaillard C, Sassi JF, Lerat Y, Lahaye M. Ultrastructure of ulvan: a polysaccharide from green seaweeds. Biopolymers 2009;91:652–64.

[134] Morelli A, Chiellini F. Ulvan as a new type of biomaterial from renewable resources: functionalization and hydrogel preparation. Macromol Chem Phys 2020;211:821–32.

[135] Estevez JM, Ciancia M, Cerezo AS. The system of low-molecular-weight carrageenans and agaroids from the room-temperature-extracted fraction of Kappaphycus alvarezii. Carbohydr Res 2000;325:287–99.

[136] De Ruiter GA, Rudolph B. Carrageenan biotechnology. Trends Food Sci Technol 1997;8:389–95.

[137] Funami T, Hiroe M, Noda S, Asai I, Ikeda S, Nishinari K. Influence of molecular structure imaged with atomic force microscopy on the rheological behavior of carrageenan aqueous systems in the presence or absence of cations. Food Hydrocoll 2007;21:617–29.

[138] Hoffman AS. Hydrogel for biomedical applications. Adv Drug Deliv Rev 2002;43:3–12.

[139] Gerlach G, Guenther M, Sorber J, Suchaneck G, Arndt K, Richter A. Chemical and pH sensors based on the swelling behavior of hydrogels. Sens Actuators B 2005;111–112:555–61.

[140] Kylin H. Zur biochemie der meeresalgen. Z Physiol Chem 1913;83:171–97.

[141] Yegappan R, Selvaprithiviraj V, Amirthalingam S. Carrageenan based hydrogels for drug delivery, tissue engineering and wound healing. Carbohydr Polym 2018;198:385–400.

[142] Feng W, Feng S, Tang K, He X, Jing A, Liang G. A novel composite of collagen-hydroxyapatite/kappa-carrageenan. J Alloys Compd 2017;693:482–9.

[143] Sharma A, Bhat S, Vishnoi T, Nayak V, Kumar A. Three-dimensional supermacroporous carrageenan-gelatin cryogel matrix for tissue engineering applications. Biomed Res Int 2013;2013:478279.

[144] Yegappan R, Selvaprithiviraj V, Amirthalingam S, Mohandas A, Hwang NS, Jayakumar R. Injectable angiogenic and osteogenic carrageenan nanocomposite hydrogel for bone tissue engineering. Int J Biol Macromol 2019;122:320–8.

[145] Berteau O, Mulloy B. Sulfated fucans, fresh perspectives: structures, functions, and biological properties of sulfated fucans and an overview of enzymes active toward this class of polysaccharide. Glycobiology 2003;13:29R–40R.

[146] Chollet L, Saboural P, Chauvierre C, Villemin JN, Letourneur D, Chaubet F. Fucoidans in nanomedicine. Mar Drugs 2016;14:145.

[147] Citkowska A, Szekalska M, Winnicka K. Possibilities of fucoidan utilization in the development of pharmaceutical dosage forms. Mar Drugs 2019;17:458–78.

[148] Fitton JH, Stringer DN, Karpiniec SS. Therapies from fucoidan: an update. Mar Drugs 2015;13:5920–46.

[149] Cardoso MJ, Costa RR, Mano JF. Marine origin polysaccharides in drug delivery systems. Mar Drugs 2016;14:34.

[150] Ale MT, Meyer AS. Fucoidans from brown seaweeds: an update on structures, extraction techniques and use of enzymes as tools for structural elucidation. RSC Adv 2013;3:8131–41.

[151] Sezer AD, Cevher E, Hatipoğlu F, Oğurtan Z, Baş AL, Akbuğa J. Preparation of fucoidan-chitosan hydrogel and its application as burn healing accelerator on rabbits. Biol Pharm Bull 2008;31:2326–33.

[152] Chowhan A, Giri TK. Polysaccharide as renewable responsive biopolymer for in situ gel in the delivery of drug through ocular route. Int J Biol Macromol 2020;150:559–72.

[153] Han X, Liu HC, Wang D, Su F, El L, Wu X. Effects of injectable chitosan thermo sensitive hydrogel on dog bone marrow stromal cells in vitro. Shanghai J Stomatol 2011;20:113–8.

[154] Tan YL, Liu CG. Preparation and characterization of self-assembles nanoparticles based on folic acid modified carboxy-methyl chitosan. J Mater Sci Mater Med 2011;22:1213–20.

[155] Zhao L, Zhu L, Liu F, Liu C, Shan-Dan, Wang Q. pH triggered injectable amphiphilic hydrogel containing doxorubicin and paclitaxel. Int J Pharm 2011;410:83–91.

[156] Ranjha NM, Ayub G, Naseem S, Ansari MT. Preparation and characterization of hybrid pH-sensitive hydrogels of chitosan-coacrylic acid for controlled release of verapamil. J Mater Sci Mater Med 2011;21:2805–16.

[157] Synowiecki J, Al-Khateeb NA. Production, properties, and some new applications of chitin and its derivatives. Crit Rev Food Sci Nutr 2003;43:145–71.

[158] Leceta I, Etxabide A, Cabezudo S, De La Caba K, Guerrero P. Bio-based films prepared with by-products and wastes: environmental assessment. J Clean Prod 2014;64:218–27.

[159] Philibert T, Lee BH, Fabien N. Current status and new perspectives on chitin and chitosan as functional biopolymers. Appl Biochem Biotechnol 2017;181:1314–37.

[160] Younes I, Rinaudo M. Chitin and chitosan preparation from marine sources. Structure, properties and applications. Mar Drugs 2015;13:1133–74.

[161] Vilar Junior JC, Ribeaux DR, Alves da Silva CA, De Campos-Takaki GM, De Campos-Takaki GM. Physicochemical and antibacterial properties of chitosan extracted from waste shrimp shells. Int J Microbiol 2016;1–7.

[162] Muzzarelli RAA. Chitin. Oxford, New York: Pergamon Press; 1977.

[163] Rinaudo M. Chitin and chitosan: properties and applications. Prog Polym Sci 2006;31:603–32.

[164] Muzzarelli R. Natural chelating polymers. Oxford: Pergamon Press; 1973. p. 144–76.

[165] Raafat D, Sahl H. Chitosan and its antimicrobial potential—a critical literature survey. Microb Biotechnol 2009;2:186–201.

[166] Vachoud L, Pochat-Bohatier C, Chakrabandhu Y, Bouyer D, David L. Preparation and characterization of chitin hydrogels by water vapor induced gelation route. Int J Biol Macromol 2012;51:431–9.

[167] Elieh-Ali-Komi D, Hamblin MR. Chitin and chitosan: production and application of versatile biomedical nanomaterials. Int J Adv Res 2016;4:411–27.

[168] Majeti NV, Kumar R. A review of chitin and chitosan applications. React Funct Polym 2000;46:1–27.

[169] Giri TK, Thakur A, Alexander A, Ajazuddin, Badwaik H, Tripathi DK. Modified chitosan hydrogels as drug delivery and tissue engineering systems: present status and applications. Acta Pharm Sin B 2012;2:439–49.

[170] Lin Y, Chen Q, Luo H. Preparation and characterization of N-(2-carboxybenzyl)chitosan as a potential pH-sensitive hydrogel for drug delivery. Carbohydr Res 2007;342:87–95.

[171] Mclean J. The discovery of heparin. Circulation 1959;19:75–8.

[172] Casu B. Structure and biological activity of heparin. Adv Carbohydr Chem Biochem 1985;43:51–134.

[173] Albert B, Bray D, Lewis J, Raff M, Roberts K, Watson JD. Molecular biology of the cell. 3rd ed. New York: Garland Publishing; 1994.

[174] Liang OD, Rosenblatt S, Chhatwal GS, Preissner KT. Identification of novel heparin-binding domains of vitronectin. FEBS Lett 1997;407:169–72.

[175] Cole G, Glaser L. A heparin-binding domain from N-CAM is involved in neural cell-substratum adhesion. J Cell Biol 1986;102:403–12.

[176] Seal BL, Panitch A. Physical polymer matrices based on affinity interactions between peptides and polysaccharides. Biomacromolecules 2003;4:1572–82.

[177] Tae G, Scatena M, Stayton PS, Hoffman AS. PEG- cross-linked heparin is an affinity hydrogels for sustained release of vascular endothelial growth factor. J Biomater Sci Polym Ed 2006;17:187–97.

[178] Huffman FG. Uronic acids. In: Caballero B, Finglas P, Toldra F, editors. Encyclopedia of food sciences and nutrition. 2nd ed. Academic Press; 2003. p. 5890–6.

[179] Nurunnabi M, Revuri V, Huh KM, Lee YK. Polysaccharide based nano/microformulation: an effective and versatile oral drug delivery system. In: Andronescu E, Grumezescu AM, editors. Nanostructures for oral medicine micro and nano technologies. Elsevier; 2017. p. 409–33.

[180] Santos MA, Grenha A. Polysaccharide nanoparticles for protein and peptide delivery: exploring less-known materials. Adv Protein Chem Struct Biol 2015;98:223–61.

[181] Lim YZ, Hussain SM, Cicuttini FM, Wang Y. Nutrients and dietary supplements for osteoarthritis. In: Watson RR, Preedy VR, editors. Bioactive food as dietary interventions for arthritis and related inflammatory diseases. 2nd ed. Academic Press; 2019. p. 97–137.

[182] Lamari FN, Karamanos NK. Structure of chondroitin sulfate. Adv Pharmacol 2006;53:33–48.

[183] Barkat K, Ahmad M, Minhas MU, Khalid I, Malik NS. Chondroitin sulfate-based smart hydrogels for targeted delivery of oxaliplatin in colorectal cancer: preparation, characterization and toxicity evaluation. Polym Bull 2019;77:6271–97.

[184] Simão AR, Fragal VH, Lima AMO, Pellá MCG, Garcia FP, Nakamura CV, Tambourgi EB, Rubira AF. pH-responsive hybrid hydrogels: chondroitin sulfate/casein trapped silica nanospheres for controlled drug release. Int J Biol Macromol 2020;148:302–15.

[185] Necas J, Bartosikova L, Brauner P, Kolar J. Hyaluronic acid (hyaluronan): a review. Vet Med 2008;53(8):397–411.

[186] Ho MH, Bhatia NN. Lower urinary tract disorders in postmenopausal women. In: Lobo RA, editor. Treatment of the postmenopausal woman- basic and clinical aspects. Academic Press; 2007. p. 693–737.

[187] Burdick JA, Stevens MM. Biomedical hydrogels. In: Hench LL, Jones JR, editors. Biomaterials, artificial organs and tissue engineering. Woodhead Publishing; 2005. p. 107–15.

[188] Atkins ED, Sheehan JK. The molecular structure of hyaluronic acid. Biochem J 1971;125(4):92.

[189] Xu X, Jha AK, Harrington DA, Farach-Carson MC, Jia X. Hyaluronic acid-based hydrogels: from a natural polysaccharide to complex networks. Soft Matter 2012;8(12):3280.

[190] Borzacchiello A, Russo L, Malle BM, Schwach-Abdellaoui K, Ambrosio L. Hyaluronic acid based hydrogels for regenerative medicine applications. Biomed Res Int 2015;871218:1–12.

[191] Luo J, Wu Z, Lu Y, Xiong K, Wen Q, Zhao L, Wang B, Gui Y, Fu S. Intraperitoneal administration of biocompatible hyaluronic acid hydrogel containing multi-chemotherapeutic agents for treatment of colorectal peritoneal carcinomatosis. Int J Biol Macromol 2020;152:718–26.

Prospect of plant and algal polysaccharides-based hydrogels

Tapan Kumar Giri[a], Dhanabal Kumarasamy[b], Shubham Mukherjee[c], and Madhurima Das[c]

[a]Department of Pharmaceutical Technology, Jadavpur University, Kolkata, West Bengal, India, [b]NSHM Knowledge Campus, Kolkata Group of Institutions, Kolkata, West Bengal, India, [c]Central Drugs Laboratory, Kolkata, West Bengal, India

2.1 Background

Hydrogels are unique three-dimensional (3D) polymeric network structures that absorb a huge amount of water or body fluids and then swell [1–3]. Hydrogels have a soft consistency similar to that of living tissue due to the presence of a large amount of water [4, 5]. In comparison to other synthetic biomaterials, hydrogels are more biocompatible, therefore they are extensively used in tissue regeneration and drug delivery. Today, synthetic hydrogels are becoming more popular because they can achieve high gel strength and their enhanced capability in absorbing a large amount of water [6]. In addition, hydrogels that are prepared using artificial components demonstrated prominent temperature or acid/base stability [7]. Though the synthetic hydrogels are known to possess some desirable properties, they have some drawbacks, for example, the use of reactive or nonbiocompatible materials in the synthesis may be the toxic or carcinogenic even if they are present in trace amounts in the final hydrogel formulation [8]. To overcome this negativity, at present, natural polysaccharides are extensively used owing to their high biocompatibility, low production cost, and self-healing properties [9–13]. Numerous studies found that natural polysaccharides are degraded in the body and act as outstanding materials for biomedical applications.

Plant and Algal Hydrogels for Drug Delivery and Regenerative Medicine
https://doi.org/10.1016/B978-0-12-821649-1.00009-X

Polysaccharides are obtained from various sources such as plants, crawfish or shrimp exoskeletons, and connective tissues of animals [14]. Recently, polysaccharides obtained from plant and algal sources received greater attention in numerous fields. Polysaccharides acquired from plant and algal sources have numerous therapeutic properties including wound healing, antioxidant, immunostimulatory, and anticancer. Among the plant polysaccharides, cellulose, hemicelluloses, pectins, oligosaccharides, guar gum, locust bean gum (LBG), xyloglucan, inulin, and cyclodextrin are widely used, whereas agar, carrageenan, furcellaran, alginate, and fucoidan are widely used as algal polysaccharides.

2.2 History

Hydrogels are extensively used in numerous applications as efficient 3D polymeric materials. They are ideal biomaterials since their hydrated structure is similar to that of living tissue. From the inception of studies on hydrogels, they can be placed into three generations. Recently, research is focused in developing smart hydrogels.

2.2.1 First-generation hydrogels

In the beginning of hydrogel research, studies reported on simple straight networks that provide a soft, water-swollen, elastic, and clear hydrogel instead of brittle gels. For the last two decades, constant research has been performed on remodeling the properties of hydrogels to find better hydrogel composition. In 1894, hydrogel first appeared in scientific literature as an inorganic salt of a natural polymer [15]. In 1958, polyvinyl alcohol (PVA) hydrogel was developed via gamma radiation [16]. Chemical modification was done for the development of the good swelling and good mechanical property-encompassing materials. In 1960, poly-2-hydroxyethyl methacrylate hydrogel was developed that was used in contact lens preparation [17]. The developments of the first generation of hydrogels are represented in Fig. 2.1.

2.2.2 Second-generation hydrogels

In the early 1970s, research studies of hydrogels shifted from simple water-swollen network systems to environment-responsive hydrogel systems. These newer hydrogels were responsive to pH, temperature, and concentration of macromolecules [18]. Extensively studied environmental-sensitive hydrogels pertain to temperature-sensitive systems, also known as thermogels. The cross-linked network structures of polymers are created due to hydrogen bonding, hydrophobic interactions,

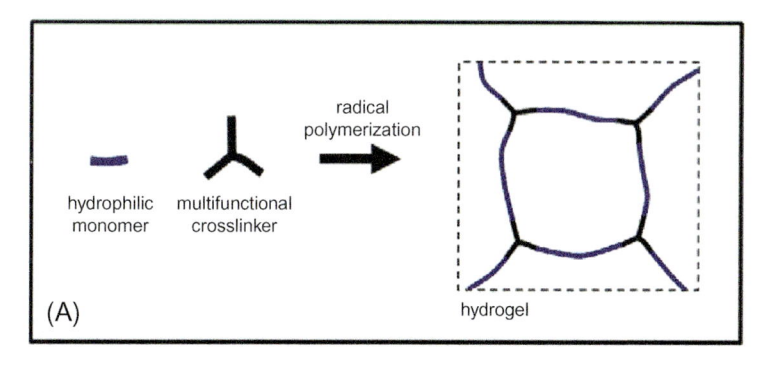

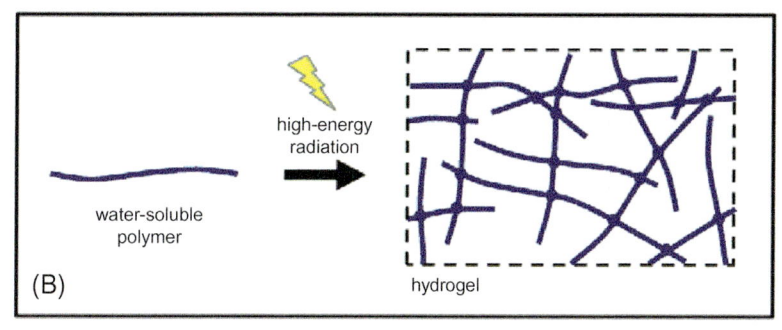

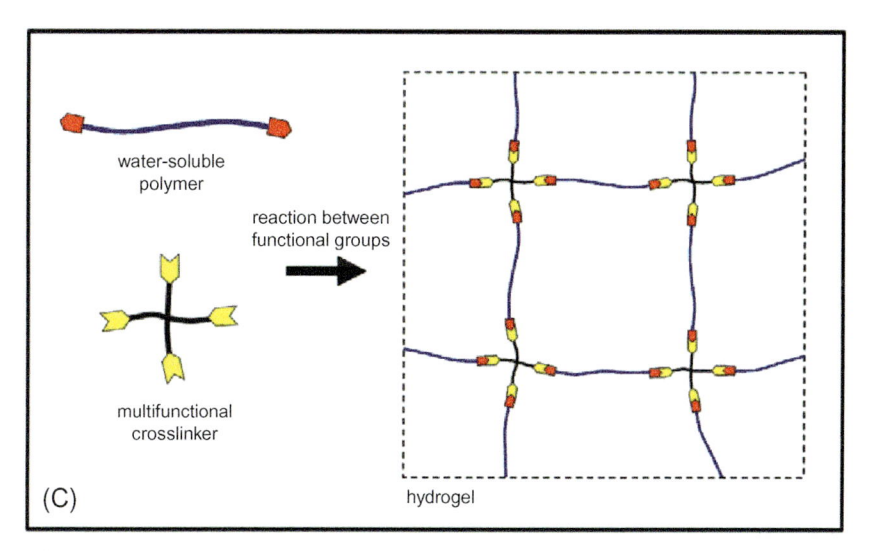

FIG. 2.1   Synthesis of first-generation hydrogels. (A) Polymerization of hydrophilic monomers in the existence of a multifunctional cross-linker; (B) cross-linking of water-soluble polymers by radiation; and (C) cross-linking of water-soluble polymers by reaction between complementary groups. *Reproduced from Buwalda SJ, Boere KWM, Dijkstra PJ, Feijenc J, Vermonden T, Hennink WE. Hydrogels in a historical perspective: from simple networks to smart materials. J Control Release 2014;190:254–273, Copyright (2014), with permission from Elsevier.*

and physical entanglements. A temperature-sensitive property of polymer was utilized for the development of in situ gel hydrogels. These are formulated as solutions and are transformed into gel after administration into the desired body site (in vivo) of application [19, 20]. Poly (N-(2-hydroxypropyl) acrylamide), poly (N-isopropylacrylamide), and poly (ethylene glycol)-polyester are polymers of this type. In the 1970s, Pluronic hydrogels appeared for the controlled delivery of antimicrobials and anesthetics [21, 22]. Recently, Pluronic hydrogels were used in the delivery of ophthalmic drugs [23, 24].

2.2.3 Third-generation hydrogels

In the mid-1990s, another type of hydrogels was developed by a physical cross-linking method that helped enhance the mechanical, thermal, and degradation properties of hydrogels. The in situ gel formation, stereocomplexation, inclusion complex formation methods were invented in this generation of hydrogel development [25]. Poly-N-isopropylacrylamide hydrogels are cross-linked via redox-mediated radical polymerization that results in a responsive hydrogel with reference to pH and temperature [26–28]. Hydrogels based on polylactic acid (PLA) and polyethylene glycol (PEG) copolymers were developed in 1993 via photopolymerization process [29]. In 1994, cross-linked supramolecular PEG hydrogels were developed through the formation of inclusion phenomena [30]. In 1995, hydrogels were developed by blending synthetic and natural polymers to enhance mechanical strength [31]. From 2000 onward, researchers synthesized stereocomplexed enantiomeric poly-L-lactic acid (PLLA)- and poly-D-lactic acid (PDLA)-based injectable hydrogels. In 2000, novel stereocomplex hydrogels were developed through self-assembly of lactic acid grafted to dextran [32]. Stereocomplexes were created between opposite chirality of lactic acid oligomers, confirmed by Fourier-transform infrared spectroscopy (FTIR)-photoacoustic analysis. In 2001, a new PEG hydrogel cross-linked through Michael addition were developed for protein delivery [33]. The zero-order release of protein for 4 days was observed by changing cross-linker functionality. In 2006, novel PVA hydrogels were synthesized by using click chemistry [34]. Initially, alkyne-modified PVA component and azide-modified PVA component were synthesized independently. Then these two parts were cross-linked in the presence of a Cu(I) catalyst through click chemistry.

2.2.4 Smart hydrogels

Numerous chemically cross-linked hydrogels known as smart hydrogels were developed using the knowledge of chemistry of the polymers. The in situ-forming hydrogels, double-network hydrogels, and composite hydrogels are known as smart hydrogels. They showed enhanced mechanical strength and drug release properties. Enzymes such as tyrosinase, peroxidase, and transglutaminase were used to catalyze hydrogel formation [35–37]. This type of hydrogel was used as adhesive material in tissue engineering applications [38]. However, limited stability of some enzymes is the drawback of enzymatically cross-linkable hydrogels. Hydrogel preparations based on merely physical interactions are weak and impede their application in load-bearing tissues [39]. Alternatively, hydrogels cross-linked chemically have slow gelation with early dissolution properties. These drawbacks can be overcome through the preparation of combined pH- and temperature-responsive hydrogel. These types of dual-responsive hydrogels were used in the delivery of indomethacin, insulin, and co-enzyme A (CoA) [40–43]. Synthetic polymers are blended with natural polymers to obtain both bioactive and mechanically strong hydrogels [44, 45]. PEG cross-linked with chitosan, gelatin methacrylamide-PEG, and fibrin-polyurethane are examples of blended hydrogels [46–48].

2.3 Classification of hydrogel

An ideal gel should contain a gelling agent and fluid. Polymers present in the simple gel are not cross-linked, whereas in hydrogels the polymers are cross-linked. Hydrogels are hydrophilic and composed of an aqueous phase and polymer matrix that absorb water [49]. The hydrogel's classification may depend on their structure variation, physical properties, swelling behavior, and preparation method. Morphologically, hydrogels may be amorphous, semicrystalline, and interact with water molecules, which are considered an integral part of hydrogel structure [50].

2.3.1 According to cross-linking mechanism

Cross-linking between the two different polymer chains produces a complex material that shows viscoelastic or pure elastic behavior. There are two categories of hydrogels based on the cross-linking mechanism involved; they are physical hydrogel, which involves physical linkages such as a hydrogen bond, and chemically cross-linked hydrogel, where new covalent bonds are randomly incorporated.

2.3.1.1 Physical cross-linking

The cross-linking process, such as ionic or hydrogen bonding with the water-soluble polymers, is involved in this type of hydrogel synthesis [51, 52]. Physically cross-linked hydrogels are generally known to display pH-dependent swelling, because cross-linking is formed due to the protonation state of carboxylic acid functional groups present in the polymer.

PVAs, PEG, pullulan, and polyacrylamide are generally used polymers in this type of hydrogel. Furthermore, the cross-linking mechanism of these physical hydrogels are characterized by three different ways involving ionic cross-linking, cross-linking by hydrogen bonding, and thermoreversible hydrogels.

Cross-linking by ionic interactions

Hydrogels prepared by this method are used to entrap drugs, living cells, and proteins. Natural algal polysaccharides like alginate cross-linked with divalent or trivalent cations is a well-known example involving this type of cross-linking mechanism. These gels can be destabilized through the removal of cations by employing chelating agents [8].

Cross-linking by hydrogen bonding

Hydrogen-bonded cross-linking was created by a freeze-thawing method, and the resulting hydrogel was strong and elastic owing to entangled polymer chains. The aqueous solution of PVA can form a stronger gel by subjecting the solution to a freeze-thawing method. This type of physically cross-linked gel is stable at optimized conditions for 6 months at 37°C [53].

Thermoreversible hydrogels

The cross-linking method of this type of hydrogel is not formed by covalent bond. They exhibit a solution to gel transformation in response to temperature instead of swelling-shrinking transition. Hydrophobic polymer was cross-linked in an aqueous medium and, with increase in temperature, aggregates their domain to minimize their surface area [54]. Thermoreversible gel was produced when xyloglucan was reduced in the presence of β-galactosidase [55]. The solution to gel conversion temperature of xyloglucan depends on the extent of galactose removal by the enzyme.

2.3.1.2 *Chemically cross-linking hydrogel*

The desirable mechanical strength is achieved through chemically cross-linking hydrogel; today, chemical cross-linking is a priority subject of investigation by hydrogel researchers. Because they have more water content capability of swollen polymeric networks, these hydrogels have wide biomedical applications. This cross-linking method is further divided into categories such as grafting, radical polymerization, condensation, and enzymatic reactions.

Through radical polymerization

In this method, the free radicals are produced at the polymer backbone through the exposure of polymers to X-ray or gamma radiation. The radiolysis of water produces hydroxyl radicals that attack the polymer backbone to form macroradicals. The whole process is performed in an inert atmosphere. The natural and synthetic polymer has been used for the designing of these types of radically cross-linked hydrogels [56].

Through condensation reactions

In their research work, most researchers synthesized hydrogels by condensation reactions. The polymers that are soluble in water are cross-linked through the creation of amide bonds. One of the highly efficient cross-linking agents used in this reaction is N,N-(3-dimethylaminopropyl)-N-ethyl carbodiimide. Numerous hydrogels based on polysaccharides are prepared using this method [57, 58].

Through enzymatic reaction

This type of hydrogel was produced by using enzymes. The most common example of this type of hydrogel was PEG-based hydrogel [59]. The cross-linked hydrogel was prepared using PEG and a lysine-containing polypeptide by utilizing transglutaminase enzyme [60]. The concentration of the macromers determines the gelation and nature of the gel. Clear gels were formed, and the final composition contains 90% water. The developed gels were known to form highly hydrated networks around living cells.

Through grafting

Grafting is a method where polymer branches are connected to the backbone polymer. It improves the functional properties of the backbone polymer [61]. Gelling behavior and aqueous solubility of the polysaccharides can be enhanced through grafting [62]. Grafting of polymer also improves the drug release behavior [63, 64]. Grafted material was obtained in two ways: chemical and radiation grafting. The extent of grafting depends on the duration of activation exposure and concentration of the cross-linker.

Chemical grafting In this grafting method, the chemical reagents are used to activate the polymer backbones. The chemical method of grafting can be initiated through the creation of free radicals, creation of ions, and through living polymerization. Grafting by a free radical method is initiated by a chemical initiator that reacts with the polymer to form a graft copolymer. The ionic generation method of grafting involves creating new type of ions. The N,N-dimethyl acrylamide (DMAAm)-grafted plant polysaccharide LBG was developed by free radical in situ polymerization technique. The cross-linking agent used was N,N'-methylene bis (acrylamide) (MBA) [65]. Fig. 2.2 represents the schematic mechanism for the creation of hydrogel. Initially, an initiator (ammonium persulfate) generates sulfate anion radicals, followed by the formation of alkoxy radicals, which initiates grafting in the existence of monomers and cross-linking agents.

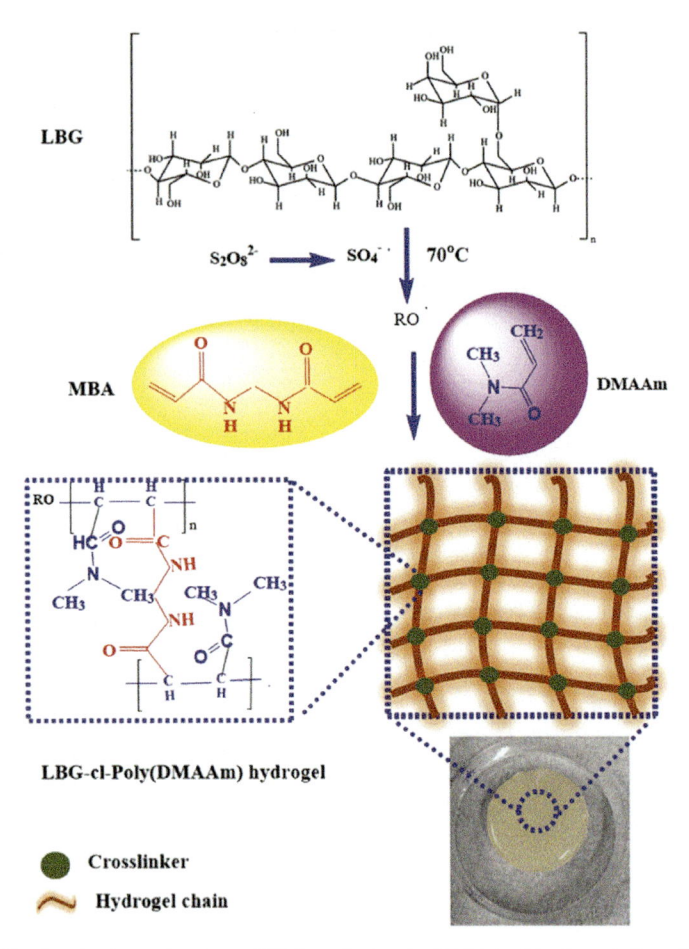

FIG. 2.2   Synthesis mechanism of LBG-grafted poly (DMAAm) hydrogel. *Reproduced from Pandey S, Do JY, Kim J, Kang M. Fast and highly efficient removal of dye from aqueous solution using natural locust bean gum based hydrogels as adsorbent. Int J Biol Macromol 2020;143:60–75, Copyright (2020), with permission from Elsevier.*

Radiation grafting   Gamma and electron beam radiations were used in the radiation grafting technique. The irradiation of the polymer results in homolytic fission and creates free radical-induced cross-polymerization. Radiation grafting method is accurate, simple, and easy to control. The free radicals are created owing to the absorption of energy by the polymer [66–68].

2.3.2 Stimuli-responsive hydrogels

With increasing interest in hydrogel chemistry, a new type of cross-linked hydrogel has been developed, which are known as smart hydrogels [69]. These types of polymer contain complementary functional groups, and depending upon the environment, these hydrogels change their permeability, sol-gel transition properties, mechanical strength, and network structure. At some critical points, the intermolecular interactions depend upon physical stimuli, such as electrical fields, pressure, temperature, etc. The interaction between polymer chains also depends on chemical stimuli like pH and presence or absence of ions/molecules. The swelling and deswelling process of these hydrogels depends on their surrounding environment. Temperature- and pH-sensitive hydrogels were extensively investigated since these two physiological conditions are the most significantly influencing environments inside the body. In a multiresponsive system, multiple responsive mechanisms were present in the same hydrogel system. The biochemical agents, such as ligands, enzymes, and antigens, also act as a biochemical stimulus in responsive hydrogels. These types of hydrogels are extensively used in biomedical fields. Also, these types of hydrogel have a particular interest on the control of cell adhesion and for the formation of in situ gel [70].

2.3.2.1 pH-sensitive hydrogels

Under the stimuli-sensitive systems, pH-sensitive hydrogels are a subset that depends upon the environmental pH. The ionization degree and release of drug are dramatically changed in specific pH environments. The change in pH at different body parts including GIT, inflamed tissue, blood vessels, tumor environment, and intracellular vesicles can induce pH-responsive behavior of the hydrogel system. The anionic and cationic hydrogels are the two distinct groups of pH-sensitive hydrogels. Anionic hydrogels containing sulfonic or carboxylic acid groups are ionized at a pH environment above their pK_a, whereas the cationic hydrogels contain amine groups and are ionized at a pH environment below their pK_b and respond to the environmental pH (Fig. 2.3). At higher pH, polyacrylic acid (anionic) swells more, whereas at lower pH, polymethacrylate (cationic polymer) swells more.

The hydrogel network swelled through electrostatic repulsion when the solution pH was higher or lower than the isoelectric point. The degree of swelling depends mainly upon the polymer's concentration, cross-link density, ionic charge, ionization degree, pH, and ionic strength.

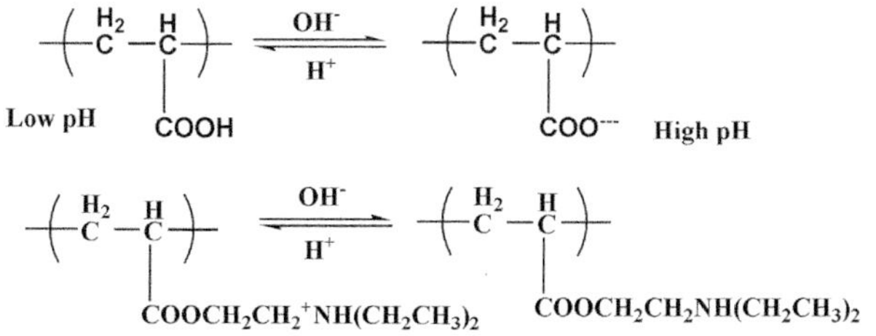

FIG. 2.3 pH-dependent ionization of polyelectrolyte.

Bortezomib-loaded, alginate-conjugated, polydopamine pH-sensitive hydrogels were synthesized for targeting drug molecules to cancer cells [71]. Polydopamine contains catechol moiety that binds to the boronic acid group of bortezomib. The developed hydrogel releases the drug in a pH-dependent manner. The bortezomib dissociates at the acidic environment of cancer tissue and is released from hydrogels. The released drug inhibits proteasome function resulting in cancer cell death (Fig. 2.4).

The dissolution study was performed at pH 5, 6.5, and 7.4 phosphate buffer solution over 7 days (Fig. 2.5). The release of drug was initially burst then in a controlled manner, and 22%, 33%, and 45% of loaded drug was released from the developed hydrogel beads within 12 h at pH 7.4, 6.5, and 5.0, respectively. Conversely, 84%, 51.2%, and 27% of loaded drug was released from the hydrogel beads after 72 h at pH 5, 6.5, and 7.4, respectively. These results clearly demonstrate a pH-dependent drug release pattern from this hydrogel system.

Anionic hydrogel networks

The anionic hydrogels have ionizable acidic functional groups bound to the polymer network. When the pH augments above the pK_a of polymer, it swells owing to the ionization of the acidic functional groups and repulsion among the anions present in the polymer. This type of hydrogel network can work from 1 to 8 pH. The various composition of polymer networks demonstrated a high swelling in the upper part of GIT. A hydrogel system encompassing methacrylate acid copolymer undergoes protonation or complexation with the hydrogel base at low pH, thus it produces collapsed configuration. The ratio of methacrylate in the hydrogel system influences the ratio of hydrogen bonding of the system, thus methacrylate acid assists in tuning the swelling properties of hydrogels. This type of hydrogel system was used to deliver proteins and hormones since the acid labile payload is protected at harsh acidic environment by a collapsed configuration of the hydrogel. The hydrophobic anticancer molecules were not partitioned into the hydrophilic milieu. Thus, if coated with anionic hydrogel, the polymer gives the best results for therapeutic activity.

Cationic hydrogel networks

The ionizable basic functional groups are present at the polymer network in cationic hydrogels. This type of hydrogel undergoes collapsed configuration at a pH environment that is higher than the pK_a of the polymer and swells only at a pH lower than pK_a. Therefore, lower pH triggers the swelling behavior of the cationic hydrogel. These types of hydrogel are basically targeted for the gastrointestinal delivery of drugs since it remains contracted at basic pH and swells only at the stomach and facilitates drug release. The swelling of cationic hydrogels are opposite to the

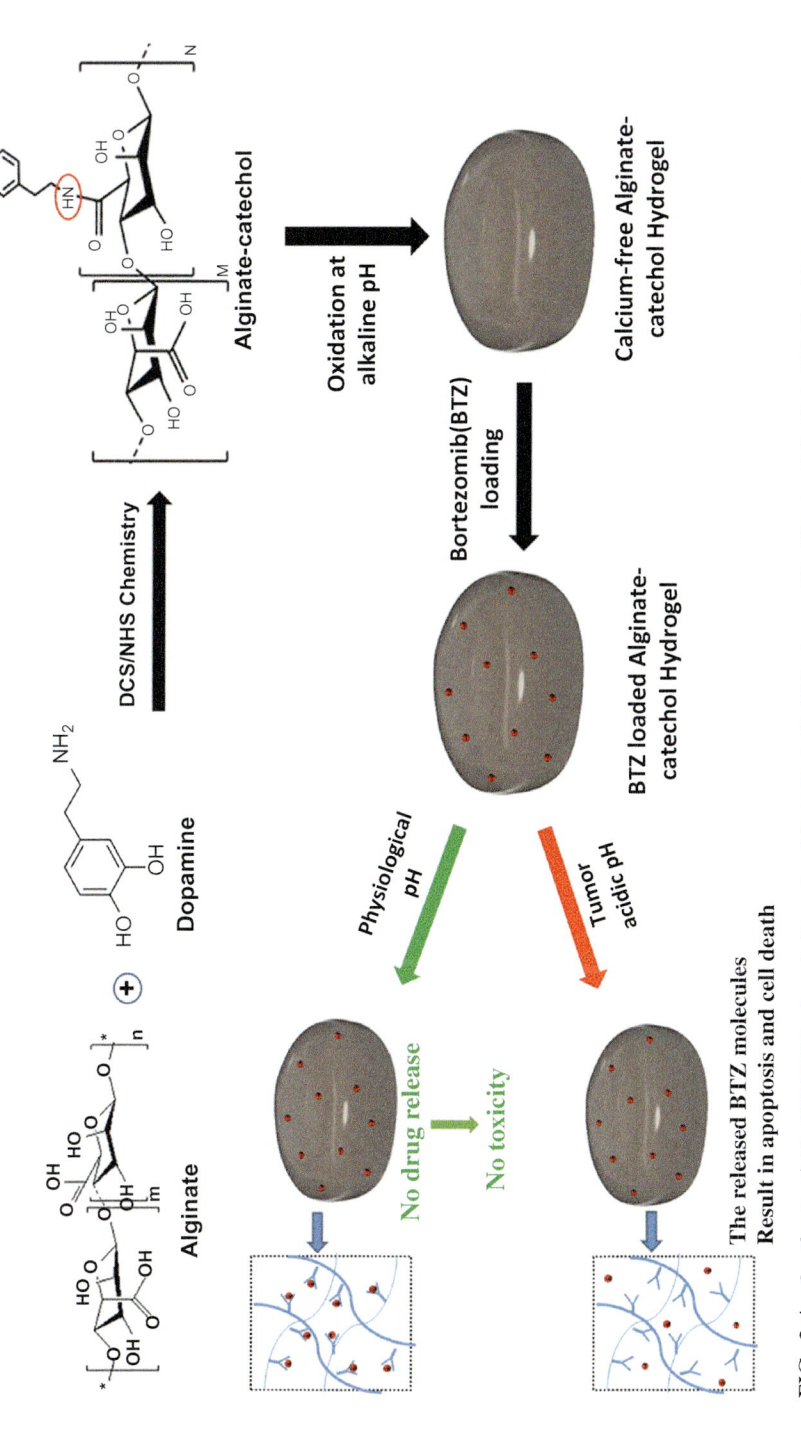

FIG. 2.4 Synthesis of Alg-PD-BTZ hydrogel. *Reproduced from Rezk AI, Obiweluozor FO, Choukrani G, Park CH, Kim CS. Drug release and kinetic models of anticancer drug (BTZ) from a pH-responsive alginate polydopamine hydrogel: towards cancer chemotherapy. Int J Biol Macromol 2019;141:388–400, Copyright (2019), with permission from Elsevier.*

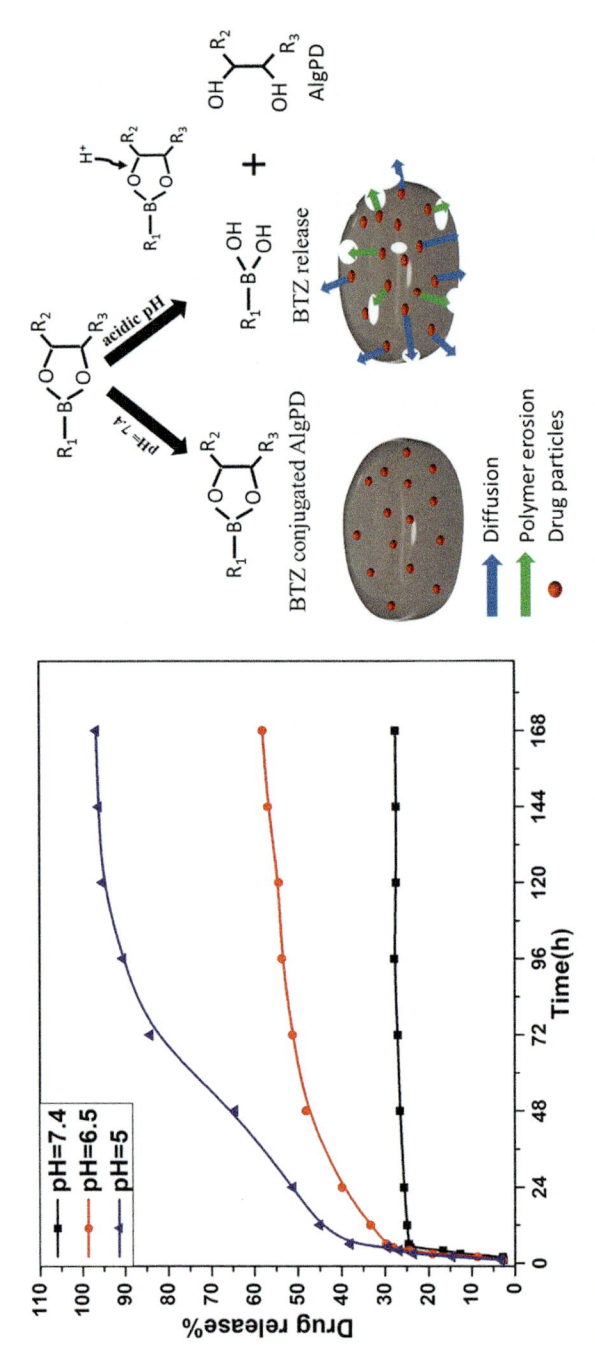

FIG. 2.5 Release of drug from the developed hydrogel. *Reproduced from Rezk AI, Obiweluozor FO, Choukrani G, Park CH, Kim CS. Drug release and kinetic models of anticancer drug (BTZ) from a pH-responsive alginate polydopamine hydrogel: towards cancer chemotherapy. Int J Biol Macromol 2019;141:388–400, Copyright (2019), with permission from Elsevier.*

anionic hydrogel's swelling behavior. Cationic hydrogels have the ability to make a complex with anionic groups of payloads, such as anionic biomacromolecules and nucleic acids. This unique property of the cationic polymers has been extensively exploited in targeted gene delivery systems. The addition of cationic hydrogel forming natural polymers in the hydrogel system influences the transfection efficiency and at the same time ensues the biodegradability of the hydrogel. Moreover, this type of hydrogel was used in the preparation of hydrogel scaffold in tissue engineering. Chitosan, protamine, poly (4-vinyl pyridine), poly (L-arginine), etc. are used as cationic polymers in a hydrogel network. Natural and synthetic cationic hydrogels are both used in the treatment of cancer for delivering chemotherapeutic drugs into cancerous cells [72].

2.3.2.2 Temperature-responsive hydrogels

The thermoresponsive materials have an ability to manipulate and control the gel-forming ability in response to physiological temperature in vivo, and the hydrogel system developed from these materials are widely used in biomedical applications. Swelling and shrinking behavior of this type of hydrogel depends on the changes in the surrounding fluid temperature. The temperature-sensitive hydrogels are primarily categorized as positively sensitive systems and negatively sensitive systems. The thermoresponse of these systems depends on their upper critical or lower critical solution temperature (UCST or LCST) [73]. The hydrogel containing acrylamide and acrylic acid is an example of UCST hydrogel. Hydrogen bond between the acrylamide and acrylic acid networks allows the hydration of the polymer networks at UCST, whereas it shrinks at low temperature. Some random copolymers of acrylic acid-based monomers were also demonstrated to have some unique UCST properties. The UCST systems have ionic species sensitivity so they can be modified with lyophobic or lyophilic comonomers for shifting the critical temperature.

Lower critical solution temperature hydrogels are known as negative temperature hydrogels because the swelling properties of this hydrogel are inversely proportional to the increasing temperature. It was proven that hydrophobicity has a vast effect on swelling responses by these lower critical solution temperature polymers and makes an appropriate biomaterial where drug release is crucial.

2.3.2.3 Glucose-sensitive hydrogels

This type of hydrogel was used to treat diabetes. It is susceptible to the varying concentration of glucose. There are three types, including concanavalin A, phenylboronic acid, and glucose oxidase, that were reported in the literature [74–76]. Phenyl boronic acids are glucose-sensitive compounds and they specifically interact with glucose molecules. Glucose oxidase catalyze the glucose-related reaction and bring changes in the

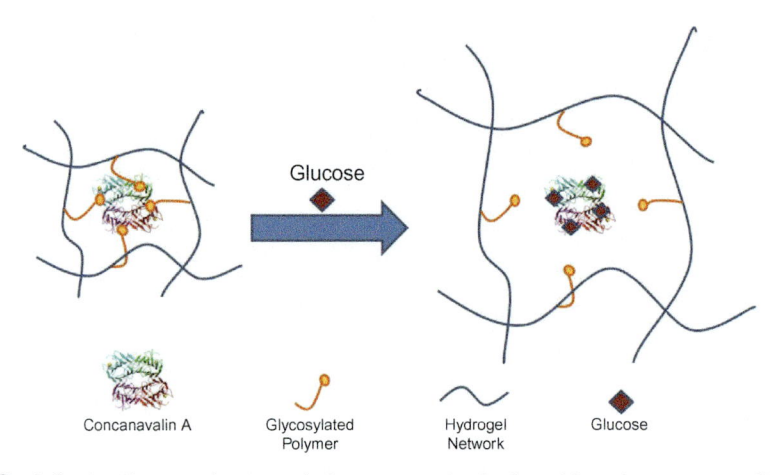

FIG. 2.6 Swelling mechanism of glucose-sensitive hydrogel based on concanvalin A. *Reproduced from Koetting MC, Peters JT, Steichen SD, Peppas NA. Stimulus-responsive hydrogels: theory, modern advances, and applications. Mater Sci Eng R Rep 2015;93:1–49, Copyright (2015), with permission from Elsevier.*

hydrogel. Concanavalin A is a glucose-binding lectin obtained from plants. Insulin-loaded hydrogels were developed where concanavalin A binds with glycosylated portion of the hydrogel. The entry of glucose into the hydrogel matrix is a concentration-dependent process, and it competitively binds with concanavalin A. This is due to the greater affinity of concanavalin A for glucose when compared with the glycosylated portion of hydrogel. Thus, glucose molecules displace the glycosylated portion of hydrogel from concanavalin A and that results in insulin release from the hydrogel [77]. The mechanism of insulin release is represented in Fig. 2.6. Insulin-loaded, glucose-sensitive, glycidyl methacrylate-modified, dextran microgels were developed based on the sugar affinity of concanavalin A [78]. The insulin was released from the hydrogel in response to different concentration of glucose. Moreover, the developed hydrogel is devoid of any in vitro cytotoxicity and releases insulin that was hormonally active. Glucose-responsive hydrogels were also developed by incorporating 3-acrylamidophenylboronic acid [79]. The interaction of phenylboronic acid moieties with glucose resulted in dissolution of the hydrogel that led to the release of payload.

2.3.2.4 Enzyme-sensitive hydrogels

Enzymes play a significant role in numerous biological and chemical processes within and outside the cells as biological catalysts. These types of reactions are extremely specific and demand milder conditions. Enzyme dysregulation is connected with many diseases including cancer, osteoarthritis, cardiovascular disease, Alzheimer's disease, and inflammation [80–83].

Therefore, altered levels of enzyme expression can be exploited as a strategy to design an enzyme-responsive hydrogel for biomedical applications. The enzyme-mediated controlled degradation of matrix becomes a main feature in the design of enzyme-responsive hydrogel prepared using natural and synthetic polymer. The enzyme reactions can occur at neutral or low alkaline or acidic conditions at ambient temperature. Drugs such as doxorubicin, insulin, and ampicillin are incorporated as a payload in enzyme-responsive hydrogel systems to form supramolecular structures [84].

Peptide chains act as linkers for the preparation of enzyme-responsive hydrogels. The peptide cross-linker was used since it releases the molecule in the lysosome of the target cell. For the self-assembly of peptide derivative groups, the three most common enzymes are employed: phosphatases, esterase, and proteases [85]. These three enzymes act as hydrogelators and are able to create supramolecular hydrogel network structures.

Nitric oxide is a biological regulator and cellular signaling molecule that regulates vascular functions, tumor progression, neurological functions, wound healing, and immune responses [86, 87]. Nitric oxide has short half-life, dose-dependent therapeutic effect, and it diffuses in short distance [88]. Therefore, on-demand site-specific delivery of nitric oxide is a prerequisite for effective nitric oxide therapy. Numerous researchers developed hydrogels that release nitric oxide through a β-galactosidase-mediated reaction [89, 90]. The β-galactosidase-sensitive injectable chitosan hydrogel was synthesized for nitric oxide delivery [91]. The developed hydrogel showed outstanding stability and no decomposition of nitric oxide reserve during 6-month storage at room temperature. β-galactosidase hydrolyzed the glycosidic bonds and releases the nitric oxide in micromolar concentrations in a controlled manner (Fig. 2.7). The in vivo studies revealed the enhanced angiogenesis stimulation and endothelial cell proliferation effect of nitric oxide hydrogel.

2.3.2.5 Photoresponsive hydrogels

The light-responsive hydrogels are prospective candidates used in delivery of drugs/genes and in microlenses and sensors. Light stimulation has a capability to finely control the properties of biomaterial by means of adjusting the intensity and wavelength of the light. The hydrogel comprising of β-cyclodextrin derivative and polyacrylic acid copolymer helps to change gel to solution with the irradiation of light at 355 nm wavelength, and in a similar fashion this hydrogel can change solution to gel with light at 450 nm wavelength. This reversible transition ability makes a photoresponsive hydrogel useful in the field of bioengineering applications. Photoresponsive hydrogels were developed in combination with chromophore and thermosensitive hydrogel-forming polymers [92].

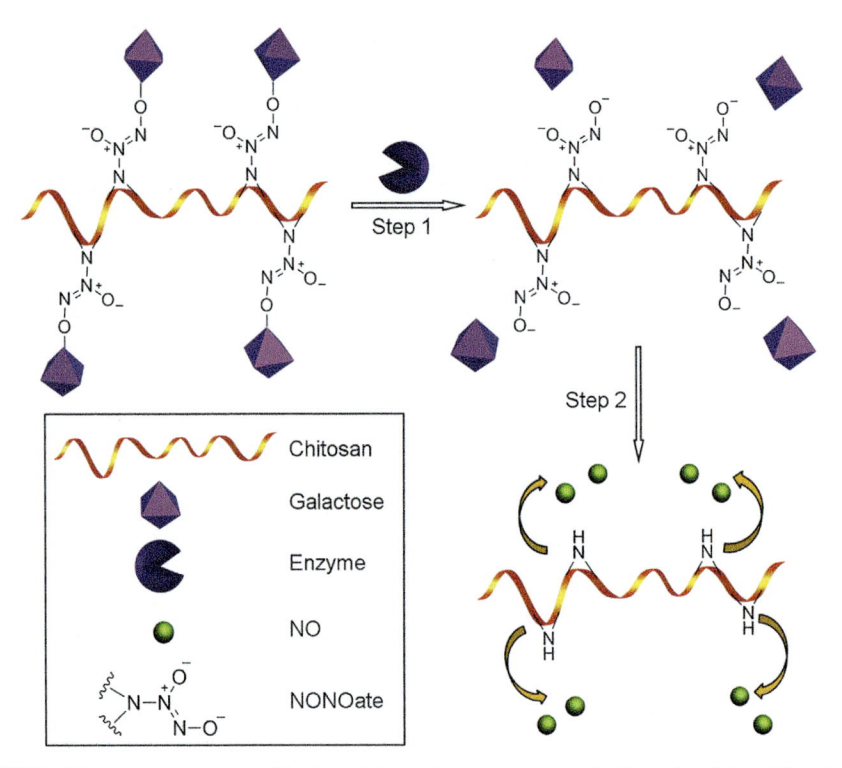

FIG. 2.7   Decomposition of hydrogel through enzyme catalysis. *Reproduced from Zhao Q, Zhang J, Song L, Ji Q, Yao Y, Cui Y, Shen J, Wang PG, Kong D. Polysaccharide-based biomaterials with on-demand nitric oxide releasing property regulated by enzyme catalysis. Biomaterials 2013;34:8450–8458, Copyright (2013), with permission from Elsevier.*

Chromophores can absorb light and dissipate the energy as heat, which increases the local temperature resulting in phase transition of a hydrogel network [93, 94]. Several research groups developed photoresponsive dextran hydrogels modified with cyclodextrin for the delivery of a poorly water-soluble drug [95, 96].

2.4 Biodegradability and biocompatibility of hydrogel

Biocompatibility is a property of a material that estimates how it is compatible with living tissue. Basically, biomaterial is a naturally modified material that does not produce any toxicity or induce any immunological response when exposed to the body or body fluid. Biocompatibility is different from nontoxicity, but in some cases nontoxicity is a match to biocompatibility. Biomaterials also have good bioabsorption. Nontoxic materials cause less acute inflammation and allergy, whereas biocompatible materials cause the least unwanted reactions, least abnormal growth, and in some cases, it may strongly adhere with the organs.

On the other hand, biodegradation is the degradation of materials into simpler substances. Biodegradable polymer-based hydrogels show beneficial properties such as stability, biocompatibility, and more swelling ability to suit specific application purposes. Mechanical strength and the rate of degradation of a hydrogel must depend upon the tissue growth and natural extracellular matrix. The biodegradability depends on the degradation mechanism and the target site [97].

The degradation of hydrogels are predominantly three types, which include degradation of polymer backbones, degradation of cross-linking agents, and separation of pendant chains from the polymer backbone. In the case of hydrogel preparation, generally both polymers (synthetic and natural) are used in combination, and in such cases, the polymer backbone chains are degraded by chemical hydrolysis and produce a lower molecular weight product. Albumin, gelatin, and dextran are the proteins and polysaccharides that are mostly used for biodegradable delivery systems. Unlike the degradable polymer backbone, some oligopeptides containing protein molecules are generally used as degradable cross-linking agents. The macromolecular cross-linkers show early degradation by giving the marginal steric hindrance for the specific enzyme-substrate complexes. In the case of degradable pendent chain containing polymer, the drug molecules were attached to copolymeric complexes, and the degradation rate is dependent upon the rate of drug release [98]. This type of hydrogel system shows some special advantages, such as providing better flexibility in the stability and improving diffusion properties of the drugs.

Nawaz et al. prepared a cross-linked pH-responsive hydrogel based on PVP/gelatin to investigate the polymer biocompatibility and degree of cross-linking [99]. PVP is a synthetic polymer that acts as a biomaterial and shows a film-forming property. Gelatin is a natural polypeptide, obtained from animal sources, and is widely used for its nontoxic and biocompatible properties. A compatibility property was checked by FTIR and differential scanning calorimetry (DSC) studies. The water retention property of a hydrogel network plays a significant role in biomaterial sciences and in ensuring the biocompatible potentiality.

Tehrani et al. prepared teofilin-loaded, pH-responsive hydrogel using PVA and polyacrylic acid by changing maximum cross-linking densities [100]. Blending of PVA and polyacrylic acid by heat treatment provides a stable hydrogel. Then the hydrogel blends were boiled with different concentration of NaOH solutions to increase the pH sensitivity of the gels. Physical compatibility of the hydrogels was tested by FTIR and DSC, and it confirmed the miscibility of the polymer blend. The cytotoxicity test and absence of any toxic leaching compounds approves the cytocompatibility of the hydrogel blends. The developed biocompatible and pH-sensitive hydrogels have been proven to be an appropriate candidate for teofilin oral delivery.

Montesanoa et al. synthesized cellulose-based, biodegradable, super-absorbent hydrogels used for the agriculture field [101]. They used sodium carboxymethylcellulose and hydroxyethylcellulose superabsorbent polymers with a cross-linking agent (citric acid) to reduce their toxicity. Osmotic potentiality test confirms that the hydrogel improved water retention ability, enhanced plant growth promotion, and reduced the detrimental effects of water stress. Prepared hydrogel system demonstrated its potential application in the agriculture field as being biocompatible and biodegradable. Silva et al. reviewed the research performed on the sulfated polysaccharides from numerous algae species found in a marine environment [102]. They have found that the polysaccharides obtained from algae are biocompatible. Morelli et al. synthesized and characterized ulvan-based hydrogels from the waste algal biomass for applications in the biomedical field [103]. Ulvan-acrylate conjugate was prepared through esterification between acryloyl chloride and the hydroxyl group of ulvan molecules. The developed hydrogel provides an advantageous strategy for achieving shorter times of degradation and can be deployed as a prospective candidate in the application of the biomedical field.

2.5 Techniques to prepare hydrogels

Generally, hydrogels are prepared using natural and synthetic polymers. Synthetic polymers are hydrophobic and stronger in comparison to natural ones. Synthetic polymers exhibit long durability and slow rate of degradation since they have higher mechanical strength compared with natural polymer. These contrasting properties can be desirably composed through an optimal formulation design [104]. Natural polymers, having appropriate functional groups, are utilized in the preparation of hydrogels [105]. There are numerous techniques reported for hydrogel preparation. The monomer, cross-linker, and initiators are the three integral parts for hydrogel preparation. The preparation of a hydrogel mass was followed by copious washing steps to remove residual impurities such as unreacted cross-linkers, monomers, and chemical initiators present in the system. The acrylic monomer-based hydrogels were prepared by different techniques such as inverse suspension, diluted solution, and concentrated solution polymerization techniques [106–108].

2.5.1 Physical cross-linking

Physical cross-link gel has gained interest owing to ease of production and devoid of chemical cross-linking agents. When present, these agents may destroy entrapped cells and proteins inside the hydrogels. A wide range of gel textures can be accomplished by careful selection of pH, combination of polymers, and by varying their relative concentrations.

2.5.1.1 *Heating or cooling of polymer solution*

The hydrogel was prepared by cooling hot carrageenan or gelatin solution at different rates. The gel formation is owing to the creation of helix or alliance of the helix and junction zone formation [109]. The carrageenan polymer chains present as random coils in hot solution, and it can change to stiff helical rods upon cooling (Fig. 2.8). The presence of sodium and potassium salts led to stable gel formation owing to further aggregation of double helices. The other example of hydrogel preparation based on heating or cooling of polymer solutions are polypropylene oxide-polyethylene oxide and PLA-PEG hydrogels [110, 111].

2.5.1.2 *Ionic interaction*

Hydrogel was prepared through ionic interaction between a polymer and cross-linking agent. The alginate hydrogels were developed using calcium ion (Ca^{2+}) as an ionic cross-linking agent [112]. The alginate hydrogels were successfully used in applications that involve encapsulation of living cells and proteins [113–116].

2.5.1.3 *Complex coacervation*

The complex coacervate gel was produced when the polyanionic and polycationic polymers are mixed. The fundamental principle of this method involves strong ionic interaction of polymers with opposite charges to form complexes (Fig. 2.9). Complex formation depends on the pH of the solution and polymer concentration. Hydrogels based on chitosan and hyaluronic acid were prepared by coacervation technique [117].

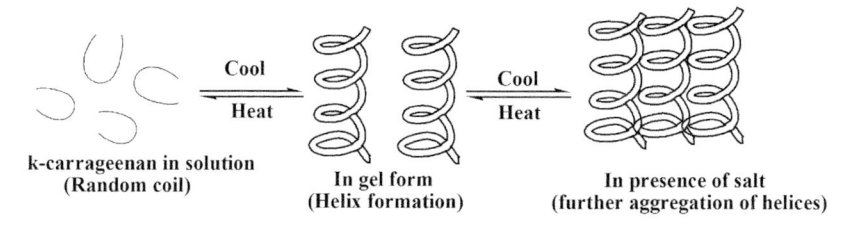

FIG. 2.8   Formation of gel through cooling of hot carrageenan solution.

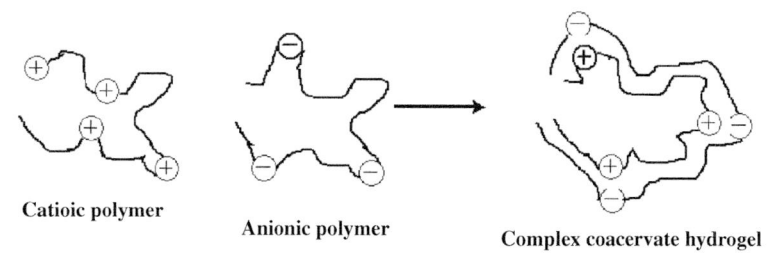

FIG. 2.9   Formation of hydrogel through interaction between polyanion and a polycation.

The developed hydrogel exhibited tunable strength and elasticity. Positively charged (below their isoelectric point) proteins are expected to couple with anionic polymers to form hydrogels [118].

2.5.1.4 Hydrogen bonding

Polymers with carboxylic acid groups can be used to prepare hydrogel through hydrogen bonding by lowering the solution pH. The hydrogen-bonded carboxymethyl cellulose network was formed when sodium carboxymethyl cellulose was dispersed into hydrochloric acid (0.1 M) [119]. The hydrogen bond was established in acidic solution due to displacement of sodium ion by the proton in carboxymethyl cellulose. The solubility of the carboxymethyl cellulose was decreased and formed a rigid hydrogel. The hydrogen-bonded hydrogels were prepared using poly (methacrylic acid), poly (acrylic acid), and PEG [120]. Hydrogen bonds were formed between carboxylic groups, respectively acid and oxygen of PEG. Other polymers were also used in the hydrogel preparation through hydrogen-bonding interaction [121, 122].

2.5.1.5 Heat-induced aggregation

Gum arabic is comprised of 2%–3% proteins. Fractionations by hydrophobic interaction led to three major fractions with varying protein content and molecular weights [123]. The application of heat results in aggregation of proteinaceous components, and this accumulation increases the molecular weight resulting in a hydrogel with improved water binding capacity and mechanical properties [124, 125].

2.5.1.6 Freeze-thawing

The hydrogels were prepared by freeze-thawing, which involves the creation of microcrystals. A tough and elastic gel was produced when aqueous PVA solution undergoes a freeze-thawing cycle [126]. The molecular weight, concentration of PVA, freezing time, freezing cycles, and temperature influenced the properties of gel. Bovine serum albumin-loaded PVA gels were developed by adding protein to the solution of polymer followed by freeze-thawing. The protein was released from the developed hydrogel by Fickian diffusion mechanism [127]. The gel properties could be modulated by adding alginate to the PVA solution before freeze-thawing. The resulting hydrogel showed decreased drug release, and the mechanical strength was improved by augmenting the alginate concentration [128].

2.5.2 Chemical cross-linking

Hydrogels were prepared using a chemical cross-linking agent. The natural and synthetic polymers contain numerous chemically reactive functional groups like primary and secondary hydroxyl, carboxyl, sulfonyl, and amine. These groups are responsible for the cross-linking reaction. Numerous techniques are available in the literature for the preparation of this type of hydrogel.

2.5.2.1 Chemical cross-linker

This type of hydrogel was prepared using cross-linking agents such as glutaraldehyde, epichlorohydrin, etc. Sodium alginate and PVA-based hydrogels were prepared using glutaraldehyde for transdermal delivery of alpha-adrenergic blocker prazocin hydrochloride [129]. The development of hydrogel formulations is represented in Fig. 2.10. When sodium alginate and PVA blends were cross-linked with glutaraldehyde, it forms a new acetal function in random between aldehyde group of glutaraldehyde and hydroxyl groups of polymers resulting in the formation of an interpenetrating polymer network (IPN) structure. The developed hydrogel extends the release of drug up to 24 h, and the drug release correlates with the concentration of glutaraldehyde employed in cross-linking the polymers.

Water-soluble polymer PVA contains hydroxyl groups that are variably cross-linked with glutaraldehyde [130, 131]. Moreover, the polymers containing an amine group can also be cross-linked with the glutaraldehyde [132–134].

2.5.2.2 Grafting

Grafting is a process in which monomers are chemically attached to the polymer backbone. The high-energy radiation or chemical reagents were used to activate the polymer chains and facilitate grafting. There are many polymers that are widely used in the preparation of hydrogels by grafting methods [135, 136]. The hydrogel preparations by bulk polymerization techniques lead to weak structures. These hydrogels need stronger support in the form of surface coating to improve their mechanical properties [137, 138].

Chemical grafting

Activation of polymer backbone using a chemical reagent is practiced in this type of hydrogel system preparation. There are numerous reports of hydrogels made by a chemical grafting method. The pectin-grafted N,N-diethylacrylamide was synthesized by microwave irradiation technique [139]. The synthesized graft copolymer was thermosensitive and is used as a biomaterial. Poly (acrylamide)-grafted carboxymethyl cellulose was synthesized by conventional method [140]. Fig. 2.11 represents the diagram of synthetic assembly. It was observed that the carboxymethyl cellulose and acrylamide were effectively grafted. Moreover, the thermal stability of the developed hydrogel was found to be enhanced by this method of preparation. There are a number of published works on grafted

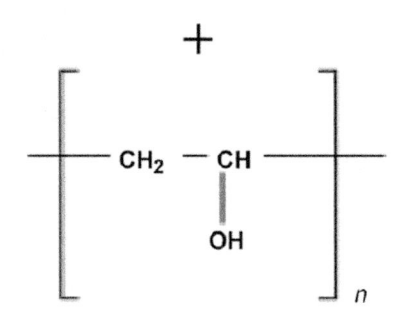

Sodium Alginate

$+$

Poly(vinyl alcohol)

$$OHC-(CH_2)_3-CHO$$
GA

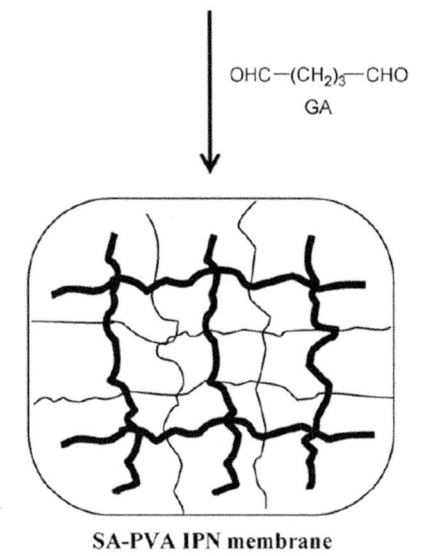

SA-PVA IPN membrane

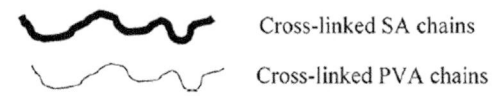

Cross-linked SA chains

Cross-linked PVA chains

FIG. 2.10 Preparation of IPN membrane. *Reproduced from Kulkarni RV, Sreedhar V, Mutalik S, Setty CM, Sa B. Interpenetrating network hydrogel membranes of sodium alginate and poly (vinyl alcohol) for controlled release of prazosin hydrochloride through skin. Int J Biol Macromol 2010;47(4):520–527, Copyright (2010), with permission from Elsevier.*

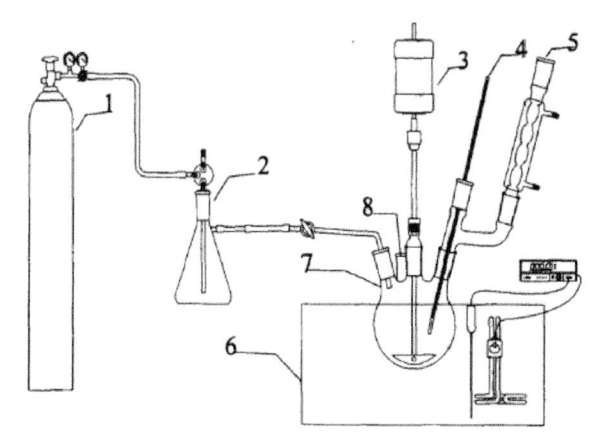

FIG. 2.11   The device diagram of copolymerization: (1)-Nitrogen cylinder; (2)-buffer bottle; (3)-electric mixer; (4)-thermometer; (5)-condensation tube; (6)-thermostat water bath; (7)-reaction flask; (8)-feeding port. *Reproduced from Feng X, Wan J, Deng J, Qin W, Zhao N, Luo X, He M, Chen X. Preparation of acrylamide and carboxymethyl cellulose graft copolymers and the effect of molecular weight on the flocculation properties in simulated dyeing wastewater under different pH condition. Int J Biol Macromol 2020;155:1142–1156, Copyright (2020), with permission from Elsevier.*

acrylamide with starch, carboxymethyl cellulose, and chitosan to enhance the physicochemical properties of polysaccharides [141–145].

Radiation grafting

High-energy radiation, such as electron beam and gamma radiation, were used for the synthesis of grafted hydrogels. An example is moringa gum-grafted N-vinyl imidazole hydrogels, which was prepared by radiation-induced grafting technique [146]. This hydrogel showed slow release of drug without a burst effect. The mechanism of drug release followed non-Fickian diffusion.

2.6 Evaluation of hydrogel

The interlocking network system gives an idea about the internal structure of hydrogel and its physicochemical characteristics. The target application determines the requirement of a number of techniques to be applied in the characterization of hydrogel.

2.6.1 Swelling study

Swelling ability of hydrogels are thoroughly characterized to understand their suitability in drug delivery. Hydrogels are cross-linked polymers and are linked by covalent or noncovalent bonds. Swelling property depends on the cross-link density of the polymer chain [147]. The term "swelling" is used to mean that the hydrogel uptakes water molecules until an equilibrium state is reached, and at the same time the osmotic pressure is balanced by preventing structural deformations [148]. The following equation was used to calculate the swelling ratio: swelling ratio = (swelled sample weight-dry sample weight)/swelled sample weight [149, 150]. Grafted polysaccharide affects the swelling behavior of hydrogels [151]. The swelling of hydrogel was augmented with grafting yield since grafting reduces the crystallinity and converts the polymer into an amorphous from [152].

2.6.2 Rheology

Structural variations in the hydrogel systems, such as cross-links, association, and entanglement, have noticeable effects on the rheological characteristics of hydrogels [153–156]. The rheological tests of gels obtained from the natural glue sourced from *Bletilla striata* showed improved physical strength and viscoelasticity when compared with synthetic carbopol gel [157]. The sol-gel transition of hydrogel prepared by these groups occurred near the body temperature within 20 s [158]. The stiffness of hydrogel prepared from a blend of polysaccharides, such as agarose, methyl cellulose, and chitosan, were augmented when chitosan was cross-linked with an increasing amount of genipine [159].

2.6.3 Scanning electron microscopy

This study has been performed to understand the structure and properties of hydrogel. The surface morphology of hydrogels were extensively examined by scanning electron microscopy. This study helps to see the surface and interior morphology of polysaccharide hydrogels, and it denotes the pore structure [160]. On the basis of pore size determined by scanning electron microscopy, it is possible to differentiate the gel networks between chemically and enzymatically synthesized dextran hydrogels [161]. It has been noticed that an enzymatically prepared hydrogel network gives a homogeneous pore size compared with hydrogels prepared by chemical means. These types of microscopic images are beneficial to visualize and understand the network variations arising due to acetone and air-dried cellulose-based hydrogels. Microscopic structures show that air-dried hydrogel has a dense and smooth surface, but acetone-dried hydrogel showed voids in space with a rough surface. The existence of chemical modifications such as grafting in the hydrogel was shown by scanning electron microscopy. Therefore, this technique was extensively used in the characterization of hydrogel's network structure [162–165].

2.6.4 Porosity and density characterization

Porosity is determined by solvent replacement technique. The preweighed dry hydrogel was placed in absolute ethanol overnight. Then the excess ethanol was blotted and weighed [166, 167]. The following equation was used to calculate hydrogel porosity: porosity $= (m1 - m2)/\rho v$; where $m1 =$ mass of hydrogel before dipping, $m2 =$ mass of hydrogel after dipping, v is hydrogel volume, and ρ is the density of absolute ethanol.

The densities (apparent densities) of dried hydrogels were determined using solvent displacement technique. The preweighed quantity of hydrogels were immersed in hexane and the volume augment was determined [168]. This was the polymer volume. The following equation was used to determine the density of the hydrogel: density $=$ mass of hydrogel/volume of solvent displaced by hydrogel.

2.6.5 In vitro weight loss

Dried hydrogel was immersed in a swelling medium for a predetermined time. Then at specified time intervals, the hydrogels were taken and dried to a constant weight [169]. The weight loss percentage can be determined by using the following equation: % weight loss $=$ (hydrogel initial weight-hydrogel final weight)/hydrogel initial weight $\times 100$.

2.6.6 Mechanical characterization

The structure and composition of a hydrogel affects its mechanical strength. The cross-linking density, polymerization condition, swelling degree, and monomer composition are the parameters that affect the mechanical properties of hydrogel [170]. Hydrogels in a swollen state possess weak mechanical strength owing to high water content [171]. Mechanical ability of hydrogel was measured by bench compactor [172], and tensile strength testing is commonly used for the determination of mechanical ability of hydrogel. Composite hydrogel scaffolds were developed using collagen, chondroitin sulfate, and hyaluronic acid [173]. Genipin was used to cross-link the hydrogel to improve physical and chemical properties. The results showed that compressive modulus improved with augment in the concentration of genipin.

2.6.7 Chemical/physical characterization

The presence of a functional group on hydrogel backbone affects the water holding capacity. The physicochemical characteristics of the hydrogels are tuned through functional group modification. The presence of functional group on hydrogel backbone was characterized by UV-VIS spectroscopy, nuclear magnetic resonance (NMR), infrared spectrophotometry (IR), and mass spectrophotometry (MS) [174].

2.6.8 Determination of void fraction

The fraction of void is the ratio of void volume to total volume of hydrogel [175]. The fraction of void was determined by soaking the hydrogel in the medium; deducting the dry hydrogel weight from the swollen one gives a measure of the volumes of the pores [176].

2.7 Drug release mechanism from hydrogel

Hydrogels are capable of releasing an entrapped drug in a release medium. The release of drug from the hydrogel was controlled through cross-link density and rate of swelling in the release medium. Water-soluble drug release from a matrix is a swelling-controlled diffusion mechanism through concurrent water absorption and drug desorption [177, 178]. When the concentration of solvent overcomes a threshold level, polymeric chains unfold, and a glass-rubbery transformation occurs resulting in the formation of a gel layer. The moving front where swelling process is observed is known as a swelling front. The swelling front separates the non-swelling matrix to the swelling matrix [179]. The dissolved drug in the swollen region diffuses to the outer dissolution medium. In the swollen portion, there is one region where the drug is present as a soluble form, and in the other region, the drug is present as an insoluble and dispersed form [180]. The contact zone between swollen polymer and dissolution medium is called the erosion front through which polymer chains disentangle resulting in matrix erosion [181].

The drug release mechanism consists of an interior and exterior diffusion process. The diffusion of drug from the surface of hydrogel to bulk liquid is called exterior diffusion. Hydrogel systems are of two types: reservoir and matrix systems [182]. In a reservoir system, the inner bulk of the dissolved or suspended drug is bound by a polymer membrane, and diffusion of the drug through this membrane is the rate-limiting step [183, 184]. Polymer membrane absorbs the drug from the reservoir and diffuses it into the surrounding medium. Fick's first law describes the release of a drug from the reservoir system [185, 186].

The drug is homogeneously dispersed or soluble in the polymer matrix system. Higuchi developed an equation to envisage the release rate of a drug from a matrix system [187, 188]. Peppas and coworkers generalized the equation proposed by Higuchi as $M_t/M\alpha = kt^n$ [181, 189], where $M_t/M\alpha$ = fraction of drug release, k = geometric constant, and n = release exponent representing release mechanism. The drug release mechanism is a controlled diffusion when the n values are 0.5 (slab), 0.45 (cylinder), and 0.43 (sphere). The release mechanism is anomalous when the n values are $0.5 < n < 1$ (slab), $0.45 < n < 0.89$ (cylinder), and $0.43 < n < 0.85$ (sphere).

The drug release mechanism is a controlled swelling when the n values are 1 (slab), 0.89 (cylinder), and 0.85 (sphere). The hydrogel's shape can change during the drug release process due to chain cleavage.

2.7.1 Chain cleavage

The drug is covalently bonded to the chain of a polymer in a prodrug hydrogel system, and the release of drug depends on the splitting of the labile covalent bond that links the drug and polymer, not the diffusion process. The therapeutic efficacy of the drug is improved through the prodrug system. Generally, the release of bound drug depends on the rate of degradation of the drug-polymer link. These released free drugs are dissolved by water, and the release of drug follows first order kinetics.

2.7.2 Matrix swelling

After absorption of water, the glass transition temperature (GTT) is lowered due to swelling of polymer chains. The dissolved drug passes through the swollen region of hydrogel to the outer part of the matrix, and such release of drugs does not follow Fickian rules. Absorption of water in the hydrogels showed anomalous drug release mechanisms. When the experimental temperature is higher than the GTT, then the thermodynamic compatibility is favorable resulting in hydrogel swelling with substantial volume expansion. The process of swelling and release of drug displaying Fickian or non-Fickian mechanism depends on the polymer relaxation rate.

2.7.3 Matrix erosion

Generally, two types of matrix erosions (surface and bulk) are known. In surface erosion, the release of a drug is due to polymer surface degradation, whereas, in a bulk erosion system, the whole matrix is quickly hydrated and breaks the polymer chains. Bera et al. prepared an alginate-gum ghatti-coated composite hydrogel matrix containing alginate and gum arabic for intragastric delivery of flurbiprofen [190]. The uncoated composite hydrogels exhibited anomalous diffusion of drugs and indicates both erosion of matrix and diffusion of drug. The absorption of water into the polymer matrix ensued the reduction in the polymer GTT. This leads to a drastic change of the polymer from a glassy state to a rubbery state [191]. The attractive forces between polymers were reduced, which increased the mobility of molecules resulting in drug diffusion. The release mechanism of the coated hydrogel matrix was shifted from anomalous to case-II transport. The rate and extent of water absorption relaxes the macromolecular structure, and this is the rate-controlling step for the release of drug from matrix.

2.8 Conclusion

Plant and algal polysaccharide-based hydrogels are endowed with distinguishing properties such as biodegradability, biocompatibility, high water holding ability, and nontoxicity. These polymers have many advantages owing to their tissue-compatible network morphology and tunable structures that can be explored to facilitate environment sensitivity of the hydrogels and control the rate and extent of drug diffusion. Moreover, the preparation of hydrogels by blending two or more polysaccharides led to the achievement of desirable and tunable properties, and therefore it is found to have wider applications. However, to achieve large-scale commercial applications, further research is required to overcome the limitations and challenges. Moreover, further attention should be paid to advance the green synthesis of plant and algal polysaccharide-based hydrogels for superior physical and biomedical properties that are suitable for biomedical application.

References

[1] Chirani N, Yahia LH, Gritsch L, Motta FL, Chirani S, Fare S. History and applications of hydrogels. J Biomed Sci 2015;4:13.
[2] Giri TK, Adhikary T, Maity S. Development of capsaicin loaded hydrogel beads for in vivo lipid lowering activities of hyperlipidemic rats. Drug Deliv Lett 2019;9:108–15.
[3] Dey M, Das M, Chowhan A, Giri TK. Breaking the barricade of oral chemotherapy through polysaccharide nanocarrier. Int J Biol Macromol 2019;130:34–49.
[4] Ullah F, Othman MBH, Javed F, Ahmada Z, Akil HM. Classification, processing and application of hydrogels: a review. Mater Sci Eng C 2015;57:414–33.
[5] Giri TK, Bhowmick S, Maity S. Entrapment of capsaicin loaded nanoliposome in pH responsive hydrogel beads for colonic delivery. J Drug Deliv Sci Technol 2017;39:417–22.
[6] Kokkarachedu V, Raghavendra GM, Tippabattini J, Mohan YM, Rotimi S. A mini review on hydrogels classification and recent developments in miscellaneous applications. Mater Sci Eng C 2017;79:958–71.
[7] Qinyuan C, Yang J, Xinjun Y. Hydrogels for biomedical applications: their characteristics and the mechanisms behind them. Gels 2017;3:6.
[8] Sood N, Bhardwaj A, Mehta S, Mehta A. Stimuli-responsive hydrogels in drug delivery and tissue engineering. Drug Deliv 2016;23:758–80.
[9] Giri TK, Verma U, Tripathi DK. Effect of adsorption parameters on biosorption of Zn++ ions from aqueous solution by graft copolymer of locust bean gum and polyacrylamide. Indian J Chem Technol 2016;23:93–103.
[10] Badwaik HR, Thakur D, Sakure K, Giri TK, Nakhate KT, Tripathi DK. Microwave assisted synthesis of polyacrylamide grafted guar gum and its application as flocculent for waste water treatment. Res J Pharm Technol 2014;7:401–7.
[11] Giri TK, Thakur D, Alexander A, Ajazuddin, Badwaik H, Tripathy M, Tripathi DK. Biodegradable IPN hydrogel beads of pectin and grafted alginate for controlled delivery of diclofenac sodium. J Mater Sci Mater Med 2013;24:1179–90.
[12] Giri TK, Verma S, Alexander A, Ajazuddin, Badwaik H, Tripathy M, Tripathi DK. Crosslinked biodegradable hydrogel floating beads for stomach site specific controlled delivery of metronidazole. Farmacia 2013;61:533–50.

[13] Badwaik H, Giri TK, Nakhate KT, Kashyap P, Tripathi DK. Xanthan gum and its derivatives as a potential bio-polymeric carrier for drug delivery system. Curr Drug Deliv 2013;10:587–600.

[14] Daniela P, Milena DC, Rolando B. Polysaccharide-based hydrogels: the key role of water in affecting mechanical properties. Polymers 2012;4:1517–34.

[15] Buwalda SJ, Boere KWM, Dijkstra PJ, Feijenc J, Vermonden T, Hennink WE. Hydrogels in a historical perspective: from simple networks to smart materials. J Control Release 2014;190:254–73.

[16] Danno A. Gel formation of aqueous solution of polyvinyl alcohol irradiated by gamma rays from cobalt-60. J Physical Soc Japan 1958;13:722–7.

[17] Wichterle O, Lím D. Hydrophilic gels for biological use. Nature 1960;185:117–8.

[18] Kopecek J. Hydrogels: from soft contact lenses and implants to self-assembled nanomaterials. J Polym Sci A Polym Chem 2009;47:5929–46.

[19] Ruel-Gariépy E, Leroux JC. In situ-forming hydrogels—review of temperature sensitive systems. Eur J Pharm Biopharm 2004;58:409–26.

[20] Ward MA, Georgiou TK. Thermo responsive polymers for biomedical applications. Polymers 2011;3:1215–42.

[21] Chen-Chow PC, Frank SG. In vitro release of lidocaine from pluronic F-127 gels. Int J Pharm 1981;8:89–99.

[22] Nalbandian RM, Henry RL, Wilks HS. Artificial skin. II. Pluronic F-127 silver nitrate or silver lactate gel in the treatment of thermal burns. J Biomed Mater Res 1972;6:583–90.

[23] Desai SD, Blanchard J. In vitro evaluation of pluronic F127-based controlled release ocular delivery systems for pilocarpine. J Pharm Sci 1998;87:226–30.

[24] Katakam M, Ravis WR, Banga AK. Controlled release of human growth hormone in rats following parenteral administration of poloxamer gels. J Control Release 1997;49:21–6.

[25] Rizwan M, Yahya R, Hassan A, Yar M, Azzahari AD, Selvanathan V, Sonsudin F, Abouloula CN. pH sensitive hydrogels in drug delivery: brief history, properties, swelling, and release mechanism, material selection and applications. Polymers 2017;9:137.

[26] Otake K, Inomata H, Konno M, Saito S. Thermal analysis of the volume phase transition with N-isopropylacrylamide gels. Macromolecules 1990;23:283–9.

[27] Inomata H, Goto S, Saito S. Phase transition of N-substituted acrylamide gels. Macromolecules 1990;23:4887–8.

[28] Liang-chang D, Qi Y, Hoffman AS. Controlled release of amylase from a thermal and pH-sensitive, macroporous hydrogel. J Control Release 1992;19:171–7.

[29] Sawhney AS, Pathak CP, Hubbell JA. Bioerodible hydrogels based on photopolymerized poly (ethylene glycol)–co-poly (α-hydroxy acid) diacrylate macromers. Macromolecules 1993;26:581–7.

[30] Li J, Harada A, Kamachi M. Sol–gel transition during inclusion complex formation between a-cyclodextrin and high molecular weight poly(ethylene glycol)s in aqueous solution. Polym J 1994;26:1019–26.

[31] Cascone MG, Sim B, Sandra D. Blends of synthetic and natural polymers as drug delivery systems for growth hormone. Biomaterials 1995;16:569–74.

[32] De Jong SJ, De Smedt SC, Wahls MWC, Demeester J, Kettenes-van Den Bosch JJ, Hennink WE. Novel self-assembled hydrogels by stereocomplex formation in aqueous solution of enantiomeric lactic acid oligomers grafted to dextran. Macromolecules 2000;33:3680–6.

[33] Elbert DL, Pratt AB, Lutolf MP, Halstenberg S, Hubbell JA. Protein delivery from materials formed by self-selective conjugate addition reactions. J Control Release 2001;76:11–25.

[34] Ossipov DA, Hilborn J. Poly(vinyl alcohol)-based hydrogels formed by "click chemistry". Macromolecules 2006;39:1709–18.

[35] Kurisawa M, Chung JE, Yang YY, Gao SJ, Uyama H. Injectable biodegradable hydrogels composed of hyaluronic acid-tyramine conjugates for drug delivery and tissue engineering. Chem Commun 2005;34:4312–4.

[36] Hu BH, Messersmith PB. Enzymatically cross-linked hydrogels and their adhesive strength to biosurfaces. Orthod Craniofac Res 2005;8:145–9.

[37] Chen T, Embree HD, Brown EM, Taylor MM, Payne GF. Enzyme-catalyzed gel formation of gelatin and chitosan: potential for in situ applications. Biomaterials 2003;24:2831–41.

[38] Moreira Teixeira LS, Feijen J, van Blitterswijk CA, Dijkstra PJ, Karperien M. Enzyme-catalyzed crosslinkable hydrogels: emerging strategies for tissue engineering. Biomaterials 2012;33:1281–90.

[39] Drury JL, Mooney DJ. Hydrogels for tissue engineering: scaffold design variables and applications. Biomaterials 2003;24:4337–51.

[40] Park TG. Temperature modulated protein release from pH/temperature-sensitive hydrogels. Biomaterials 1999;20:517–21.

[41] Yong-Hee K, You Han B, Sung WK. pH/temperature-sensitive polymers for macromolecular drug loading and release. J Control Release 1994;28:143–52.

[42] Guo BL, Gao QY. Preparation and properties of a pH/temperature-responsive carboxymethyl chitosan/poly(N-isopropylacrylamide)semi-IPN hydrogel for oral delivery of drugs. Carbohydr Res 2007;342:2416–22.

[43] Shi J, Alves NM, Mano JF. Drug release of pH/temperature-responsive calcium alginate/poly (N-isopropylacrylamide) semi-IPN beads. Macromol Biosci 2006;6:358–63.

[44] Langer R, Tirrell DA. Designing materials for biology and medicine. Nature 2004;428:487–92.

[45] Sionkowska A. Current research on the blends of natural and synthetic polymers as new biomaterials: review. Prog Polym Sci 2011;36:1254–76.

[46] Daniele MA, Adams AA, Naciri J, North SH, Ligler FS. Interpenetrating networks based on gelatin methacrylamide and PEG formed using concurrent thiol click chemistries for hydrogel tissue engineering scaffolds. Biomaterials 2014;35:1845–56.

[47] Huang Y, Zhang B, Xu G, Hao W. Swelling behaviours and mechanical properties of silk fibroin–polyurethane composite hydrogels. Compos Sci Technol 2013;84:15–22.

[48] Tan H, Luan H, Hu Y, Hu X. Covalently crosslinked chitosan–poly(ethylene glycol) hybrid hydrogels to deliver insulin for adipose-derived stem cells encapsulation. Macromol Res 2013;21:392–9.

[49] Garg S, Garg A. Hydrogel: classification, properties, preparation and technical features. Asian J Biomater Res 2016;2(6):163–70.

[50] Parhi R. Cross linked hydrogel for pharmaceutical applications: a review. Adv Pharm Bull 2017;7(4):515–30.

[51] Berger J, Reist M, Mayer JM, Felt O, Gurny R. Structure and interactions in chitosan hydrogels formed by complexation or aggregation for biomedical applications. Eur J Pharm Biopharm 2004;57(1):35–52.

[52] Boucard N, Viton C, Domard A. New aspects of the formation of physical hydrogels of chitosan in a hydroalcoholic medium. Biomacromolecules 2005;6(6):3227–37.

[53] Gibas I, Janik H. Review: synthetic polymer hydrogels for biomedical applications. Chem Chem Technol 2010;4:297–304.

[54] Hu W, Wang Z, Xiao Y, Zhang S, Wang J. Advances in cross-linking strategies of biomedical hydrogels. Biomater Sci 2019;7:843–55.

[55] Miyazaki S, Kawasaki N. Comparison of in situ gelling formulations for the oral delivery of cimetidine. Int J Pharm 2001;220:161–8.

[56] Akhtar MF, Hanif M, Ranjha NM. Methods of synthesis of hydrogels: a review. Saudi Pharm J 2016;24:554–9.

[57] de Nooy AE, Capitani D, Masci G, Crescenzi V. Ionic polysaccharide hydrogels via the Passerini and Ugi multicomponent condensations: synthesis, behavior and solid-state NMR characterization. Biomacromolecules 2000;1:259–67.

[58] Tan H, Chu CR, Payne KA, Marra KG. Injectable in situ forming biodegradable chitosan-hyaluronic acid based hydrogels for cartilage tissue engineering. Biomaterials 2009;30:2499–506.

[59] Sperinde JJ, Griffith LG. Control and predication of gelation kinetics in enzymatically cross-linked poly-(ethylene glycol) hydrogels. Macromolecules 2000;33:5467–80.

[60] Sperinde JJ, Griffith LG. Synthesis and characterization of enzymatically-crosslinked-poly (ethylene glycol) hydrogels. Macromolecules 1997;30:5255–64.

[61] Kagimura FY, da Cunha TTV, Malfatti CRM, Dekker R, Barbosa A, Teixeira S, Salome K. Carboxymethylation of (16)-β-glucan (lasiodiplodan): preparation, characterization and antioxidant evaluation. Carbohydr Polym 2015;127:390–9.

[62] Ahuja M, Singh S, Kumar A. Evaluation of carboxymethyl gellan gum as a mucoadhesive polymer. Int J Biol Macromol 2013;53:114–21.

[63] Ahuja M, Kumar A, Singh K. Synthesis, characterization and in vitro release behavior of carboxymethyl xanthan. Int J Biol Macromol 2012;51:1086–90.

[64] Thakur K, Ahuja M, Kumar A. Carboxymethyl functionalization of amylopectin and its evaluation as a nanometric drug carrier. Int J Biol Macromol 2013;62:25–9.

[65] Pandey S, Do JY, Kim J, Kang M. Fast and highly efficient removal of dye from aqueous solution using natural locust bean gum based hydrogels as adsorbent. Int J Biol Macromol 2020;143:60–75.

[66] Bhattacharya A, Das A, De A. Structural influence on grafting of acrylamide based monomers on cellulose acetate. Indian J Chem Technol 1998;5:135–8.

[67] Chen J, Iwata H, Maekawa Y, Yoshida M, Tsubokawa N. Grafting of polyethylene by g-radiation grafting onto conductive carbon black and application as novel gas and solute sensors. Radiat Phys Chem 2003;67(3–4):397–401.

[68] Yamaki T, Asano M, Maekawa Y, Morita Y, Suwa T, Chen J, Tsubokawa N, Kobayashi K, Kubota H, Yoshida M. Radiation grafting of styrene into cross-linked PTFE films and subsequent sulfonation for fuel cell applications. Radiat Phys Chem 2003;67:403–7.

[69] Ferreira NN, Ferreira LMB, Cardoso VMO, Boni FI, Souza ALR, Gremião MPD. Recent advances in smart hydrogels for biomedical applications: from self-assembly to functional approaches. Eur Polym J 2018;99:117–33.

[70] Mantha S, Pillai S, Khayambashi P, Upadhyay A, Zhang Y, Tao O, Pham HM, Tran SD. Smart hydrogels in tissue engineering and regenerative medicine. Materials 2019;12:3323.

[71] Rezk AI, Obiweluozor FO, Choukrani G, Park CH, Kim CS. Drug release and kinetic models of anticancer drug (BTZ) from a pH-responsive alginate polydopamine hydrogel: towards cancer chemotherapy. Int J Biol Macromol 2019;141:388–400.

[72] Deen GR, Loh XJ. Stimuli responsive cationic hydrogels in drug delivery applications. Gels 2018;4(1):13.

[73] Sanchez IC, Stone MT. Statistical thermodynamics of polymer solutions and blends. In: Paul DR, Bucknall CB, editors. Polymer blends volume 1: formulation. New York: John Wiley & Sons, Inc; 2000.

[74] Qi W, Yan X, Duan L, Cui Y, Yang Y, Li J. Glucose-sensitive microcapsules from glutaraldehyde cross-linked hemoglobin and glucose oxidase. Biomacromolecules 2009;10:1212–6.

[75] Kim JJ, Park K. Modulated insulin delivery from glucose-sensitive hydrogel dosage forms. J Control Release 2001;77:39–47.

[76] Jin X, Zhang X, Wu Z, Teng D, Zhang X, Wang Y, Wang Z, Li C. Amphiphilic random glycopolymer based on phenylboronic acid: synthesis, characterization, and potential as glucose-sensitive matrix. Biomacromolecules 2009;10:1337–45.

[77] Koetting MC, Peters JT, Steichen SD, Peppas NA. Stimulus-responsive hydrogels: theory, modern advances, and applications. Mater Sci Eng R Rep 2015;93:1–49.

[78] Yin R, Bai M, He J, Nie J, Zhang W. Concanavalin A-sugar affinity based system: binding interactions, principle of glucose-responsiveness, and modulated insulin release for diabetes care. Int J Biol Macromol 2019;124:724–32.

[79] Dong Y, Wang W, Veiseh O, Appel EA, Xue K, Webber MJ, Tang BC, Yang XW, Weir GC, Langer R. Injectable and glucose-responsive hydrogels based on boronic acid–glucose complexation. Langmuir 2016;32:8743–7.

[80] Inestrosa NC, Alvarez A, Pérez CA, Moreno RD, Vicente M, Linker C, Casanueva OI, Soto C, Garrido J. Acetylcholinesterase accelerates assembly of amyloid-β-peptides into Alzheimer's fibrils: possible role of the peripheral site of the enzyme. Neuron 1996;16:881–91.

[81] Roy R, Yang J, Moses MA. Matrix metalloproteinases as novel biomarkers and potential therapeutic targets in human cancer. J Clin Oncol 2009;27:5287–97.

[82] Park J, Yun HS, Lee KH, Lee KT, Lee JK, Lee S-Y. Discovery and validation of biomarkers that distinguish mucinous and nonmucinous pancreatic cysts. Cancer Res 2015;75:3227–35.

[83] Murphy G, Nagase H. Progress in matrix metalloproteinase research. Mol Aspects Med 2008;29:290–308.

[84] Abul-Haija YM, Ulijn RV. Enzyme responsive hydrogels for biomedical applications. In: Connon CJ, Hamley IW, editors. Hydrogels in cell-based therapies. The Royal Society of Chemistry; 2014. p. 112–20.

[85] Chandrawati R. Enzyme-responsive polymer hydrogels for therapeutic delivery. Exp Biol Med (Maywood) 2016;241(9):972–9.

[86] Fukumura D, Kashiwagi S, Jain RK. The role of nitric oxide in tumour progression. Nat Rev Cancer 2006;6:521–34.

[87] Carpenter AW, Schoenfisch MH. Nitric oxide release: part II. Therapeutic applications. Chem Soc Rev 2012;41:3742–52.

[88] Mocellin S, Bronte V, Nitti D. Nitric oxide, a double edged sword in cancer biology: searching for therapeutic opportunities. Med Res Rev 2007;27:317–52.

[89] Gao J, Zheng W, Zhang J, Guan D, Yang Z, Kong D, Zhao Q. Enzyme-controllable delivery of nitric oxide from a molecular hydrogel. Chem Commun 2013;49:9173–5.

[90] Yao X, Liu Y, Gao J, Yang L, Mao D, Stefanitsch C, Li Y, Zhang J, Ou L, Kong D, Zhao Q, Li Z. Nitric oxide releasing hydrogel enhances the therapeutic efficacy of mesenchymal stem cells for myocardial infarction. Biomaterials 2015;60:130–40.

[91] Zhao Q, Zhang J, Song L, Ji Q, Yao Y, Cui Y, Shen J, Wang PG, Kong D. Polysaccharide-based biomaterials with on-demand nitric oxide releasing property regulated by enzyme catalysis. Biomaterials 2013;34:8450–8.

[92] Suzuki A, Tanaka T. Phase-transition in polymer gels induced by visible-light. Nature 1990;346:345–7.

[93] Suzuki A, Ishii T, Maruyama Y. Optical switching in polymer gels. J Appl Phys 1996;80:131–6.

[94] Nayak S, Lyon LA. Photoinduced phase transitions inpoly(N-isopropylacrylamide) microgels. Chem Mater 2004;16:2623–7.

[95] Peng K, Cui C, Tomatsu I, Porta F, Meijer AH, Spaink HP, Kros A. Cyclodextrin/dextran based drug carriers for a controlled release of hydrophobic drugs in zebrafish embryos. Soft Matter 2010;6:3778–83.

[96] Peng K, Tomatsu I, Korobko AV, Kros A. Cyclodextrin-dextran based in situ hydrogel formation: a carrier for hydrophobic drugs. Soft Matter 2010;6:85–7.

[97] Naahidi S, Mousa J, Logan M, Wang Y, Yuan Y, Bae H, Dixon B, Chen P. Biocompatibility of hydrogel-based scaffolds for tissue engineering applications. Biotechnol Adv 2017;35:530–44.

[98] Kamath KR, Park K. Biodegradable hydrogels in drug delivery. Adv Drug Deliv Rev 1993;11:59–84.

[99] Nawaz S, Khan S, Farooq U, Haider MS, Ranjha NM, Rasul A, Arshad N, Hameed R. Biocompatible hydrogels for the controlled delivery of anti-hypertensive agent: development, characterization and in vitro evaluation. Des Monomers Polym 2018;21:18–32.

[100] Fahimi Z, Parviz M, Manavitehrani I. Preparation, characterization and controlled release investigation of biocompatible pH-sensitive PVA/PAA hydrogels. Macromol Symp 2010;296:457–65.

[101] Montesanoa FF, Parentea A, Santamaria P, Sannino A, Serio F. Biodegradable superabsorbent hydrogel increases water retention properties of growing media and plant growth. Agric Agric Sci Procedia 2015;4:451–8.

[102] Silva TH, Alves A, Popa EG, Reys LL, Gomes ME, Sousa RA, Silva SS, Mano JF, Reis RL. Marine algae sulfated polysaccharides for tissue engineering and drug delivery approaches. Biomatter 2012;2:278–89.

[103] Morelli A, Betti M, Puppi D, Chiellini F. Design, preparation and characterization of ulvan based thermos-sensitive hydrogels. Carbohydr Polym 2016;136:1108–17.

[104] Tabata Y. Biomaterial technology for tissue engineering applications. J R Soc Interface 2009;6:S311–24.

[105] Shantha KL, Harding DRK. Synthesis and evaluation of sucrose-containing polymeric hydrogels for oral drug delivery. J Appl Polym Sci 2002;84:2597.

[106] Raju KM, Raju MP. Synthesis of novel super absorbing copolymers for agricultural and horticultural applications. Polym Int 2001;50:946–51.

[107] Takeda H, Taniguchi Y. Production process for highly water absorbable polymer. US Patent; 4; 1985. p. 525–7.

[108] Chen J, Zhao Y. Relation between water absorbency and reaction conditions in aqueous solution polymerization of polyacrylate superabsorbent polymers. J Appl Polym Sci 2000;75:808–14.

[109] Funami T, Hiroe M, Noda S, Asai I, Ikeda S, Nishimari K. Influence of molecular structure imaged with atomic force microscopy on the rheological behavior of carrageenan aqueous systems in the presence or absence of cations. Food Hydrocoll 2007;21:617–29.

[110] Hoffman AS. Hydrogels for biomedical applications. Adv Drug Deliv Rev 2002;43:3–12.

[111] Hennink WE, Nostrum CF. Novel crosslinking methods to design hydrogels. Adv Drug Deliv Rev 2002;54:13–36.

[112] Gacesa P. Alginates. Carbohydr Polym 1988;8:161–82.

[113] Goosen MFA, O'Shea GM, Gharapetian HM, Chou S, Sun AM. Optimization of microencapsulation parameters: semipermeable microcapsules as a bioartificial pancreas. Biotechnol Bioeng 1985;27:146–50.

[114] Gombotz WR, Wee SF. Protein release from alginate matrices. Adv Drug Deliv Rev 1998;31:267–85.

[115] Polk A, Amsden B, de Yao K, Peng T, Goosen MFA. Controlled release of albumin from chitosan-alginate microcapsules. J Pharm Sci 1994;83:178–85.

[116] Liu LS, Liu SQ, Ng SY, Froix M, Ohno T, Heller J. Controlled release of interleukin 2 for tumour immunotherapy using alginate/chitosan porous microspheres. J Control Release 1997;43:65–74.

[117] Lalevée G, David L, Montembault A, Blanchard K, Meadows J, Malaise S, Crépet A, Grillo I, Morfin I, Delair T, Sudre G. Highly stretchable hydrogels from complex coacervation of natural polyelectrolytes. Soft Matter 2017;13:6594–605.

[118] Magnin D, Lefebvre J, Chornet E, Dumitriu S. Physicochemical and structural characterization of a polyionic matrix of interest in biotechnology, in the pharmaceutical and biomedical fields. Carbohydr Polym 2004;55:437–53.

[119] Takigami M, Amada H, Nagasawa N, Yagi T, Kasahara T, Takigami S, Tamada M. Preparation and properties of CMC gel. Trans Mater Res Soc Jpn 2007;32:713–6.

[120] Eagland D, Crowther NJ, Butler CJ. Complexation between polyoxyethylene and polymethacrylic acid-the importance of the molar mass of polyethylene. Eur Polym J 1994;30:767–73.

[121] Bell CL, Peppas NA. Modulation of drug permeation through interpolymer complexed hydrogels for drug delivery applications. J Control Release 1996;39:201–7.

[122] Mathur AM, Hammonds KF, Klier J, Scanton AB. Equilibrium swelling of poly (methacrylic acid-g-ethylene glycol) hydrogels. J Control Release 1998;54:177–84.

[123] Islam AM, Phillips GO, Sljivo A, Snowden MJ, Williams PA. A review of recent developments on the regulatory, structural and functional aspects of gum arabic. Food Hydrocoll 1997;11:493–505.

[124] Aoki H, Al-Assaf S, Katayama T, Phillips GO. Characterization and properties of *Acacia senegal* (L.) Willd. var. senegal with enhanced properties (Acacia (sen) SUPER GUM(TM)): part 2—mechanism of the maturation process. Food Hydrocoll 2007;21:329–37.

[125] Aoki H, Katayama T, Ogasawara T, Sasaki Y, Al-Assaf S, Phillips GO. Characterization and properties of *Acacia senegal* (L.) Willd. var. Senegal with enhanced properties (Acacia (sen) SUPER GUM(TM)): part 5. Factors affecting the emulsification of *Acacia senegal* and Acacia (sen) SUPER GUM(TM). Food Hydrocoll 2007;21:353–8.

[126] Yokoyama F, Masada I, Shimamura K, Ikawa T, Monobe K. Morphology and structure of highly elastic poly-(vinyl alcohol) hydrogel prepared by repeated freezing-and-melting. Colloid Polym Sci 1986;264:595–601.

[127] Peppas NA, Scott JE. Controlled release from poly (vinyl alcohol) gels prepared by freeze-thawing processes. J Control Release 1992;18:95–100.

[128] Takamura A, Ishii F, Hidaka H. Drug release from poly (vinyl alcohol) gel prepared by freeze–thaw procedure. J Control Release 1992;20:21–7.

[129] Kulkarni RV, Sreedhar V, Mutalik S, Setty CM, Sa B. Interpenetrating network hydrogel membranes of sodium alginate and poly (vinyl alcohol) for controlled release of prazosin hydrochloride through skin. Int J Biol Macromol 2010;47(4):520–7.

[130] Peppas NA, Benner RE. Proposed method of intracordal injection and gelation of poly(vinyl alcohol) solution in vocal cords: polymer considerations. Biomaterials 1980;1:158–62.

[131] Dai WS, Barbari TA. Hydrogel membranes with mesh size asymmetry based on the gradient crosslinking of poly(vinyl alcohol). J Membr Sci 1999;156:67–79.

[132] Willmott N, Kamel HMH, Cummings J, Stuart JFB, Florence AT. Adriamycin loaded albumin microspheres: lung entrapment and fate in the rat. In: Davies SS, Illum L, Vie JG, Tomlinson E, editors. Microspheres and drug therapy. Pharmaceutical, immunological and medical aspects. Amsterdam: Elsevier; 1984. p. 189–205.

[133] Tabata Y, Ikada Y. Synthesis of gelatin microspheres containing interferon. Pharm Res 1989;6:422–7.

[134] Yamamoto M, Tabata Y, Hong L, Miyamoto S, Hashimoto N, Ikada Y. Bone regeneration by transforming growth factor $\beta1$ released from a biodegradable hydrogel. J Control Release 2000;64:133–42.

[135] Talaat HA, Sorour MH, Aboulnour AG, Shaalan HF, Ahmed Enas M, Awad AM, Ahmed MA. Development of a multicomponent fertilizing hydrogel with relevant techno economic indicators. Am Eurasian J Agric Environ Sci 2008;3(5):764–70.

[136] Tong Q, Zhang G. Rapid synthesis of a superabsorbent from a saponified starch and acrylonitrile/AMPS graft copolymers. Carbohydr Polym 2005;62:74–9.

[137] Das N. Preparation methods and properties of hydrogel: a review. Int J Pharm Pharm Sci 2013;5(3):1–2.

[138] Ratner BD, Weathersby PK, Hoffman AS, Kelly MA, Scharpen LH. Radiation-grafted hydrogels for biomaterial applications as studied by the ESCA technique. J Appl Polym Sci 1978;22:643–64.

[139] Işıklan N, Tokmak S. Microwave based synthesis and spectral characterization of thermo-sensitive poly(N,N-diethylacrylamide) grafted pectin copolymer. Int J Biol Macromol 2018;113:669–80.

[140] Feng X, Wan J, Deng J, Qin W, Zhao N, Luo X, He M, Chen X. Preparation of acrylamide and carboxymethyl cellulose graft copolymers and the effect of molecular weight on the flocculation properties in simulated dyeing wastewater under different pH conditions. Int J Biol Macromol 2020;155:1142–56.

[141] Biswal DR, Singh RP. Characterisation of carboxymethyl cellulose and polyacrylamide graft copolymer. Carbohydr Polym 2004;57:379–87.

[142] Mishra S, Usha Rani G, Sen G. Microwave initiated synthesis and application of polyacrylic acid grafted carboxymethyl cellulose. Carbohydr Polym 2012;87:2255–62.

[143] Shogren RL, Willett JL, Biswas A. HRP-mediated synthesis of starch polyacrylamide graft copolymers. Carbohydr Polym 2009;75:189–91.

[144] Alharbi K, Ghoneim A, Ebid A, El-Hamshary H, El-Newehy MH. Controlled release of phosphorous fertilizer bound to carboxymethyl starch-g-polyacrylamide and maintaining a hydration level for the plant. Int J Biol Macromol 2018;116:224–31.

[145] Singh V, Tiwari A, Tripathi DN, Sanghi R. Microwave enhanced synthesis of chitosan-graft-polyacrylamide. Polymer 2006;47:254–60.

[146] Singh B, Kumar A. Radiation-induced graft copolymerization of N-vinyl imidazole onto moringa gum polysaccharide for making hydrogels for biomedical applications. Int J Biol Macromol 2018;120(Pt B):1369–78.

[147] Omidian H, Hasherni SA, Askari F, Nafisi S. Swelling and cross-link density measurements for hydrogels. Iran J Polym Sci Technol 1994;3:115–9.

[148] Ganji F, Farahani SV, Farahani EV. Theoretical description of hydrogel swelling: a review. Iran Polym J 2010;19:375–98.

[149] Laftah WA, Hashim S, Ibrahim AN. Polymer hydrogels: a review. Polym Plast Technol Eng 2011;50:1475–86.

[150] Abdel-Halim ES, Al-Deya SS. Electrically conducting silver/guar gum/poly (acrylic acid) nanocomposite. Int J Biol Macromol 2014;69:456–63.

[151] Vimala K, Sivudu KS, Mohan YM, Sreedhar B, Raju KM. Controlled silver nanoparticles synthesis in semi-hydrogel networks of poly(acrylamide) and carbohydrates: a rational methodology for antibacterial application. Carbohydr Polym 2009;75:463–71.

[152] Mittal H, Ray SS, Okamoto M. Recent progress on the design and applications of polysaccharide-based graft copolymer hydrogels as adsorbents for wastewater purification. Macromol Mater Eng 2016;301:496–522.

[153] Coviello T, Coluzzi G, Palleschi A, Grassi M, Santucci E, Alhaique F. Structural and rheological characterization of Scleroglucan/borax hydrogel for drug delivery. Int J Biol Macromol 2003;32:83–92.

[154] Kempe S, Metz H, Bastrop M, Hvilsom A, Contri RV, Mäder K. Characterization of thermosensitive chitosan-based hydrogels by rheology and electron paramagnetic resonance spectroscopy. Eur J Pharm Biopharm 2008;68:26–33.

[155] Sahiner N, Singh M, De Kee D, John VT, McPherson GL. Rheological characterization of a charged cationic hydrogel network across the gelation boundary. Polymer 2006;47:1124–31.

[156] Al-Assaf S, Phillips GO, Williams PA. Controlling the molecular structure of food hydrocolloids. Food Hydrocoll 2006;20:369–77.

[157] Cui X, Zhang X, Yang Y, Wang C, Zhang C, Peng G. Preparation and evaluation of novel hydrogel based on polysaccharide isolated from *Bletilla striata*. Pharm Dev Technol 2017;22:1001–11.

[158] Oliveira JT, Santos TC, Martins L, Picciochi R, Marques AP, Castro AG, Neves NM, Mano JF, Reis RL. Gellan gum injectable hydrogels for cartilage tissue engineering applications: in vitro studies and preliminary in vivo evaluation. Tissue Eng Part A 2010;16:343–53.

[159] Pandit V, Zuidema JM, Venuto KN, Macione J, Dai G, Gilbert RJ, Kotha SP. Evaluation of multifunctional polysaccharide hydrogels with varying stiffness for bone tissue engineering. Tissue Eng Part A 2013;19(21–22):2452–63.

[160] Donald AM. The use of environmental scanning electron microscopy for imaging wet and insulating materials. Nat Mater 2003;2:511–6.

[161] Ahmed EM. Polysaccharide hydrogels: synthesis, characterization, and applications. J Adv Res 2015;6:105–21.

[162] Aikawa K, Matsumoto K, Uda H, Tanaka S, Shimamura H, Aramaki Y, Tsuchiya S. Hydrogel formation of the pH response polymer polyvinylacetal diethylaminoacetate (AEA). Int J Pharm 1998;167:97–104.

[163] Aouada FA, de Moura MR, Fernandes PRG, Rubira AF, Muniz EC. Optical and morphological characterization of polyacrylamide hydrogel and liquid crystal systems. Eur Polym J 2005;41:2134–41.

[164] El Fray M, Pilaszkiewicz A, Swieszkowski W, Kurzydlowski KJ. Morphology assessment of chemically modified cryostructured poly (vinyl alcohol) hydrogel. Eur Polym J 2007;43:2035–40.

[165] Pourjavadi A, Kurdtabar M. Collagen-based highly porous hydrogel without any porogen: synthesis and characteristics. Eur Polym J 2007;43:877–89.

[166] Shi GX, Cai Q, Wang CY, Lu N, Wang S, Bei J. Fabrication and biocompatibility of cell scaffolds of poly (L-lactic acid) and poly (L-lactic-co-glycolic acid). Polym Adv Technol 2002;13:227.

[167] Polnok A, Verhoef JC, Borchard G, Sarisuta N, Junginger HE. In vitro evaluation of intestinal absorption of desmopressin using drug-delivery systems based on superporous hydrogels. Int J Pharm 2004;269:303–10.

[168] Chang CS. Measuring density and porosity of grain kernels using a gas pycnometer. Cereal Chem 1988;65:13–5.

[169] Chiu YC, Kocagoz S, Larson JC, Brey EM. Evaluation of physical and mechanical properties of porous poly (ethylene glycol)-co-(L-lactic acid) hydrogels during degradation. PLoS One 2013;9:607–28.

[170] Mauck RL, Yuan X, Tuan RS. Chondrogenic differentiation and functional maturation of bovine mesenchymal stem cells in long-term agarose culture. Osteoarthr Cartil 2006;14:179–89.

[171] Nicodemus GD, Bryant SJ. Cell encapsulation in biodegradable hydrogels for tissue engineering applications. Tissue Eng Part B Rev 2008;14:149–65.

[172] Jaiswal M, Koul V. Assessment of multicomponent hydrogel scaffolds of poly(acrylic acid-2-hydroxy ethyl methacrylate)/gelatin for tissue engineering applications. J Biomater Appl 2011;1:1–14.

[173] Zhang L, Li K, Xiao W, Zheng L, Xiao Y, Fan H, Zhang X. Preparation of collagen–chondroitin sulfate–hyaluronic acid hybrid hydrogel scaffolds and cell compatibility in vitro. Carbohydr Polym 2011;84:118–25.

[174] Mansur HS, Sadahira CM, Souza AN, Mansur AP. FTIR spectroscopy characterization of poly (vinyl alcohol) hydrogel with different hydrolysis degree and chemically cross-linked with glutaraldehyde. Mater Sci Eng 2008;28:539–48.

[175] Chen J, Blevins WE, Park H, Park K. Gastric retention properties of superporous hydrogel composites. J Control Release 2000;55:12–5.

[176] Gorgieva S, Kokol V. Preparation, characterization and in-vitro enzymatic degradation of chitosan-gelatine hydrogel scaffolds as potential biomaterials. J Biomed Mater Res A 2012;100:1655–67.

[177] Lee PI. Novel approach to zero-order drug delivery via immobilized nonuniform drug distribution in glassy hydrogels. J Pharm Sci 1984;73:1344–7.

[178] Lee PI. Dimensional changes during drug release from a glassy hydrogel matrix. Polym Comm 1983;24:45–7.

[179] Colombo P, Bettini R, Peppas NA. Observation of swelling process and diffusion front position during swelling in hydroxypropyl methyl cellulose (HPMC) matrices containing a soluble drug. J Control Release 1999;61:83–91.

[180] Grassi G, Hasa D, Voinovich D, Perissutti B, Dapas B, Farra R, Franceschinis E, Grassi M. Simultaneous release and adme processes of poorly water-soluble drugs: mathematical modeling. Mol Pharm 2010;7:1488–97.

[181] Siepmann J, Siepmann F. Mathematical modeling of drug delivery. Int J Pharm 2008;364:328–43.

[182] Caló E, Khutoryanskiy VV. Biomedical applications of hydrogels: a review of patents and commercial products. Eur Polym J 2015;65:252–67.

[183] Arifin DY, Lee LY, Wang CH. Mathematical modeling and simulation of drug release from microspheres: implications to drug delivery systems. Adv Drug Deliv Rev 2006;58:1247–325.

[184] Bajpai AK, Shukla SK, Bhanu S, Kankane S. Responsive polymers in controlled drug delivery. Prog Polym Sci 2008;33:1088–118.

[185] Li H, Luo R, Lam KY. Modeling of environmentally sensitive hydrogels for drug delivery: an overview and recent developments. Front Drug Des Discovery 2006;2:295–331.

[186] Lin CC, Metters AT. Hydrogels in controlled release formulations: network design and mathematical modeling. Adv Drug Deliv Rev 2006;58:1379–408.

[187] Cooke NE, Chen C. A contribution to a mathematical theory for polymer-based controlled release devices. Int J Pharm 1995;115:17–27.

[188] Grassi M, Grassi G. Mathematical modelling and controlled drug delivery: matrix systems. Curr Drug Deliv 2005;2:97–116.

[189] Peppas NA, Bures P, Leobandung W, Ichikawa H. Hydrogels in pharmaceutical formulations. Eur J Pharm Biopharm 2000;50:27–46.

[190] Bera H, Ippagunta SR, Kumar S, Vangala P. Core-shell alginate-ghatti gum modified montmorillonite composite matrices for stomach-specific flurbiprofen delivery. Korean J Couns Psychother 2017;76:715–26.

[191] Bera H, Boddupalli S, Nayak AK. Mucoadhesive-floating zinc-pectinate-sterculia gum interpenetrating polymer network beads encapsulating ziprasidone HCl. Carbohydr Polym 2015;131:108–18.

3

Starch-based hydrogels

Jyoti Shrivastava and A.K. Bajpai

Bose Memorial Research Lab, Department of Chemistry, Government Science College, Jabalpur, Madhya Pradesh, India

3.1 Introduction

Starch is a known biopolymer and is abundantly found in the plant kingdom on the Earth including various trees, leaves, stems, and roots and different types of seeds, flowers, fruits, and various agricultural crops. The major function of starch is that it supplies carbon and energy to the plants through photosynthesis and, in some way, serves as an energy reservoir of the sun. In plants, the starch is mainly present in the form of granules [1], which are mainly found in seeds, particularly the cereal grains and tubers. The macromolecules of starch undergo breakdown thus converting to glucose, which is responsible for nourishing the plants. In plants, the starch molecules synthesize glucose molecules due to photosynthesis. The starch is produced in the chloroplast part of the green leaves and amyloplasts, which contribute greatly to the reservoir of starch in cereals and tubers [2]. As far as the formation of starch is concerned, it is known that in the chloroplast part, the formation of starch takes place quite speedily, whereas the starch reservoirs found in the amyloplasts take several days or sometimes even several weeks. During the processes of seed germination, fruit maturation, and sprouting of tubers, starch is stored and cyclically mobilized. However, in cereals, the starch is mainly located in the endosperm. From compositional point of view, the fruits such as bananas and mangos contain nearly 70% of starch (by weight), whereas tubers contain 65%–85%, cereals 40%–90%, and roots 30%–70% [3].

Apart from the occurrence of starch in plants, a large amount of starch is present in different food crops such as rice, wheat, maize, potatoes, beans, peas, and sorghum. As a misconception, it is thought that the potatoes are the most starch-containing vegetables, but in comparison with 15% of starch content in potatoes, wheat contains 55%, corn 65%, and rice 75%. Apart from the significance of starch as food component in food

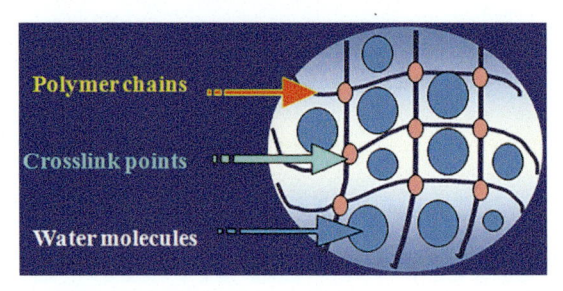

FIG. 3.1   Schematic presentation of a typical hydrogel composed of cross-linked polymer chains accommodating water molecules.

technology and food processing, starch is recognized as one of the important naturally occurring biopolymers in the preparation of hydrogels. Basically, the hydrogels are the three-dimensional networks comprising polymer chains entangled to one another through physical and/or chemical cross-links. The image of a typical hydrogel is shown in Fig. 3.1.

Hydrogels may be prepared from synthetic or naturally occurring polymers and have certain unusual biophysical characteristics such as extraordinary capacity of imbibing water; living tissue-like resemblance, and ability to encapsulate a variety of bioactive compounds such as drugs, enzymes, and genes and retain their biological activity. These are some properties of hydrogels that enable them to emerge as one of the most deserving candidates for biomedical applications such as controlled drug delivery, artificial implants, and wound healing dressings.

3.2 Starch-based hydrogels

Although hydrogels may be composed of both synthetic and natural polymers, the hydrogels prepared from later class of polymers, especially polysaccharides, have attracted great attention worldwide because of peculiar properties of hydrogels. These hydrogels are nontoxic, are blood compatible, and have biodegradable properties and excellent capability to accommodate water and biologically active molecules [4]. The hydrogels prepared from starch have been extensively prepared by joining starch chains through physical, chemical, or noncovalent interactions by using physical conditions, chemical cross-linking agents, grafting other synthetic polymers onto starch backbone by graft copolymerization, or blending starch with other synthetic or naturally occurring polymers.

Although various other biopolymers such as carboxymethyl cellulose (CMC), cellulose, gelatin, alginate, and chitosan have been comprehensively used in the preparation of hydrogels, the hydrogels produced from starch are superior to other hydrogels in some respects. The hydrogels of starch demonstrate superior blood compatibility, controlled degradation rates, economical viability, ease of functionalization and grafting by other polymers, and high capacity to absorb water and other biological fluids. Furthermore, starch-based hydrogels are prone to degradation in various environments and, therefore, have been widely studied in various biomedical and industrial applications such as tissue engineering, food packaging materials, agricultural uses, personal care products, food preservatives, and burn dressings [5]. The starch obtained from different sources such as rice, potato, corn, and other soluble starches have been successfully used in the preparation of hydrogels [6]. Fig. 3.2 depicts a typical photograph of hydrogel prepared form potato starch. The prepared hydrogel seems soft, flexible, and has fairly good capacity of absorbing water into its internal molecular structure. It is worth mentioning here that the accommodation of large amounts of water does not affect the integrity of the hydrogel, thus network enabling them to remain intact even in the swollen state.

The preparation of hydrogels from starch consists of two steps. In the first step, the crystalline structure of starch is disrupted by heating it in water, which is known as gelatinization. The process of gelatinization results in establishing interactions between the starch chains, which leads to solubilization of starch in water. Once the starch is made soluble, it is followed by cross-linking of starch chains to form a three-dimensional structure by a process coined as retrogradation [7]. The cross-linking of

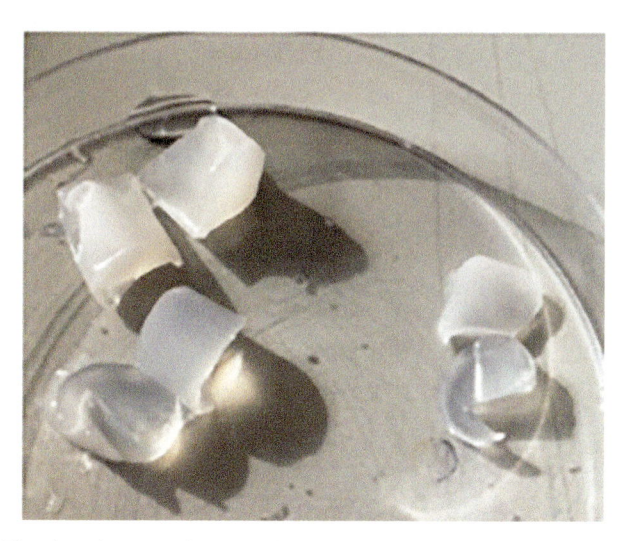

FIG. 3.2   The digital image showing the hydrogel pieces prepared from potato starch. *Reproduced from Rokhade AP, Patil SA, Aminabhavi TM, Synthesis and characterization of semi-interpenetrating polymer network microspheres of acrylamide grafted dextran and chitosan for controlled release of acyclovir. Carbohydr Polym 2007;67:605–613, Copyright (2007), with permission from Elsevier.*

starch chains is normally conducted with the help of some chemical cross-linking agents such as epichlorohydrin that reacts with starch molecules at terminals and produces a three-dimensional structure.

Besides heating starch in water for gelatinization, this step can also be accomplished chemically also using an alkaline solution. The fundamental principle lying behind the cross-linking process is the association of polymer chains to each other through physical or chemical forces using either predetermined experimental conditions or multifunctional chemical compounds that on cross-linking forms hydrogel. From mechanistic viewpoints, the gelatinization process is accompanied by structural changes in starch granules [8]. The gelatinization occurs under certain experimental conditions that depend on the source of starch. The process of gelatinization involves a phase transformation from well-ordered crystalline phase to randomly disordered state. The dissolution of starch comprises hydration of starch granules due to its hydrophilic nature, which is followed by leaching of amylose and disintegration of granules to yield a clear solution of starch. Once the solution of starch is formed, the starch undergoes retrogradation stage, which encompasses recrystallization of starch and reorganization of starch chains to produce polysaccharide hydrogel. The process of gelatinization of starch has been well studied by using analytical techniques such as differential scanning calorimetry (DSC), Fourier transform infrared spectroscopy (FTIR), optical microscopy, and rheology to look into the ongoing processes of phase transformation, structural changes, and mechanical properties [9].

The starch-based hydrogels are highly hydrophilic in nature, and they normally use either native starch or its derivatives. These hydrogels exhibit enormous water sorption capacity, excellent biodegradability, and biocompatibility that ensure their nontoxic nature. The chemically cross-linked hydrogels of starch normally involve free radical-initiated polymerization comprising one-step and two-step synthesis processes, chemical reactions-enabled cross-linking of starch chains, or high-energy radiation-induced polymerization using gamma rays or electron beams. However, for preparing physically cross-linked hydrogels, methods such as self-assembly method and freeze-thawing method are usually used.

3.3 One-step synthesis by free radical polymerization

This is one of the simplest methods to produce starch-based hydrogels, which involves graft copolymerization of a variety of synthetic polymers onto the backbone of starch macromolecules using the principle of free radical copolymerization reaction. For this purpose, low-molecular weight monomers such as acrylamide, acrylic acid, and methacrylic acid are grafted onto starch molecules using free radical initiators such as ammonium persulfate, potassium peroxydiphosphate, and azobisisobu-tyl peroxide (AIBN). The literature is richly documented with this kind of graft copolymerization onto starch. In a typical experiment, Huang et al. studied cellulose laurate, starch nanocrystals acetate (SAN), and solvent chloroform by casting/evaporation technique to prepare bionanocom-posite films. The fabricated films showed notable improvement in tensile strength and permeability on adding SAN [10].

3.4 Two-step syntheses by free radical polymerization

For preparing starch-based hydrogels by two-step synthesis, first of all starch is functionalized with reactive double bonds and then cross-linked using some free radical polymerization initiator in aqueous medium. In a recent study, free radical polymerization method was used to synthe-size pH-sensitive and thermo-responsive hydrogels that could exhibit appreciable swelling characteristics for colon-targeted drug delivery. The hydrogels were prepared by copolymerizing starch with methyl 3-amino crotonate [11]. In addition to this cited example, a number of studies have been accomplished for producing starch-based hydrogels.

3.5 Cross-linking by chemical reaction of complementary groups

It is a recognized fact that polymer molecules may react with one an-other if they contain some specific complimentary functional groups with fair chemical reactivity. Because starch molecules contain hydroxyl and carboxyl functional groups ($-OH$, $-COOH$) in their molecule, it is likely to perform their cross-linking and condensation reactions with other poly-functional carboxylic acids. In a study, starch-based hydrogels were pre-pared by performing cross-linking reaction between karaya gum starch and polyacrylic acid, as reported by Sethi et al. The hydrogels were found to show better hemocompatibility and noncytotoxicity [12].

3.6 Radiation-induced polymerization and cross-linking

High-energy radiation-induced cross-linking and polymerization are very versatile techniques to prepare starch-based hydrogels, and they normally use electron beams or gamma rays for this purpose. When these high-energy radiations pass through aqueous starch solutions, the C–H bonds undergo hemolytic fission, thus producing free radicals along the starch chains. It is also likely that water molecules undergo radiolysis and generate hydroxyl radicals that can abstract a proton from C–H bond of starch, thus producing macroradicals. These macroradicals interact with each other and form a three-dimensional cross-linked network structure. In radiation-induced synthesis, it normally happens that the macroradicals react with oxygen and form peroxide radicals that are quite inert species. It is, therefore, suggested to perform radiation-induced synthesis in an inert atmosphere.

Mohdy and coworkers irradiated ethylene glycol with methacrylic acid onto starch using high-energy gamma rays. It was reported that the resulting hydrogels on irradiation showed remarkably good swelling properties and improvement in thermal stability of starch and find use in various applications [13].

3.7 Physical self-assembly

Another type of hydrogels is made from amphiphilic polysaccharides, which are normally prepared by imparting hydrophobicity to water-soluble polysaccharide that undergo self-association to form micelles-like structures having hydrophilic polar groups orienting toward outside and a hydrophobic core. Following the strategy of self-association, Seon-Min Oh et al. reviewed the starch nanoparticles that were self-assembled by incorporating soluble short chain glucans. The structural characterization, properties, and mechanism of formation were examined. The authors also compared these SNPs (starch nanoparticles) with total hydrolysates SNPs [14].

The as-prepared self-associated hydrogels, however, have some limitations. What actually happens is that because the polysaccharides dissolve in water, stable hydrogels cannot be prepared. An effective remedy of this problem is the judicious combination of synthetic and natural polymers, which nowadays has become an area of immense academic, technological, and industrial interest. The hydrogels prepared as above offer significantly different physicochemical properties from those of their counterpart polymers. The properties of hydrogels can be desirably modulated by adopting different type of physical or chemical methods.

Thus attempting graft copolymerization of starch with ionic polymer such as methacrylic acid (MAAc), a series of hydrogels of different compositions were prepared using radiation-initiated polymerization. It was also tried to prepare potato starch-based hydrogels using the technique of high hydrostatic pressure (HHP), adopting easy and controllable process conditions to synthesize stable hydrogels cross-linked with different cross-linkers, which were further characterized for their structural and mechanical characteristics [15].

Starch has also been combined with other naturally occurring polymers such as alginate, chitosan, and gelatin, and their hydrogels have been fabricated, characterized, and studied.

The hydrogel films of methacrylamide-modified gelatin and starch-pentenoate were also prepared and studied. The superabsorbents are one of the forms of hydrogels and have tremendous applications in healthcare areas. A superabsorbent composed of CMC and starch was prepared following gamma irradiation technique. It was found that the addition of starch as a partial replacement of CMC could improve the gel fraction of starch accompanied by a slight increase in water sorption capacity [16].

Starch-based hydrogels were prepared by Sunarti et al. following chemical cross-linking method. The study included mixing of chitosan with sago and cassava starches cross-linked by methacrylic acid. It was found that the prepared hydrogels had good water absorption capacity and could be used as absorbents in pharmacy and industry [17].

The ionic hydrogels of starch carrying different charges were also reported by Wang et al. who adopted etherification reactions and introduced ionic and solvation groups and hydrogen bonding to a single molecule [18]. Starch was also modified by acrylates, and the prepared hydrogels were found to exhibit special advanced characteristics such as pH sensitivity, extraordinary swelling behavior, desirable kinetics, improved degradation, and superabsorbent properties. It was also found that carboxymethyl sago starch (CMSS) was able to prepare smart hydrogels by adding acetic acid to CMSS as a cross-linker. It is also reported that the smart hydrogels have numerous advantages, particularly, pertaining to swelling behavior in aqueous and different physiological media [19]. Starch-based hydrogels have the characteristic property to imbibe plenty of water. This property of starch hydrogels was used to prepare hydrogel materials of starch oleic acid inclusion complexes that forbid the retrogradation of starch [20].

3.8 Starch-based polymer blends

The concept of fabricating a blend has attracted great attention due to the reason that the properties of a blend are often superior and different from those of their constituent components. An ideal polymer blend may be defined as a homogenous mixture of two or more polymers of different molecular weights and chemical composition in any ratio. In practice, a blend may range from completely miscible to completely miscible mixture. The morphology of a blend is quite sensitive to a number of experimental factors such as mutual compatibility, experimental conditions, presence of additives, annealing temperature, and shear application during processing.

Polymer blends are versatile materials and have wide applications in significant fields such as biomedical, agricultural, industrial, domestic, and defense, and their versatility rests on the fact that the polymer blends have the ability to exploit beneficial properties of their constituent polymers that enable them a tailor-made material. The extreme biocompatibility, economic viability, and controlled biodegradability are some of the properties that make starch-based blends as the first choice materials in especially biomedical community and have been extensively fabricated and used for numerous applications [21].

The history of starch-based synthetic polymer blends dates back to 1973. The literature is richly documented with research work pertaining to the binary blends of starch with a variety of polymers; some of the remarkable polymer blends are with polyurethane (PU), poly(vinyl alcohol) (PVOH), poly(3-hydroxybutyrete) (PHB), polyethylene, poly(lactic acid) (PLA), polyesters, etc. The most common blend of starch was with polyethylene [22]. The blends of hydrophobic polyethylene and hydrophilic starch have been mainly applied for agricultural mulch and food packaging applications [23]. These blends have different phases that can be used to create tailor-made materials.

The increasing pollution due to plastic wastes has forced to use blends of starch with polyethylene and polypropylene, which imparts degradable property to the blends, and on the other hand, the synthetic polymers provide mechanical strength to the blend. The as-prepared starch blends have been used as degradable packaging materials [24].

The naturally occurring polymers cellulose and chitosan have also been blended with starch and are richly documented in literature. These two biopolymers are biodegradable, nontoxic, abundant, renewable, and low-cost materials. Although both these biopolymers are completely miscible with starch, still the poor mechanical behavior remains as an issue, and it also depends on the ratios of starch and these two materials. Apart from these, the process ability also leaves behind a problem due to poor thermal resistance of these biopolymers. A biodegradable blend of chitosan and corn starch was prepared by extrusion process [25]. In another study, the starch was blended with agar-agar, and their films were prepared by solution cast method. The as-prepared films were characterized by differential scanning calorimetric (DSC) technique [26].

Native starch is associated with several well-known limitations such as its poor mechanical strength, fragile thermal stability, and prone to water or moisture absorption [27]. These limitations have been often overcome by blending other suitable materials to starch, which tend to reduce water absorption, improve barrier properties, enhance dimensional stability and biodegradability, and cut off production and process costs. It is also reported that starch blends are normally a little bit brittle in nature, which poses difficulties in processing. This has been quite successfully resolved by addition of low-molecular weight substances, coined as plasticizers, such as glycerol, glucose, sorbitol, urea, and ethylene glycol [28]. The plasticizer when added to starch results in destructuring of starch crystallites and formation of hydrogen bonds between the starch macromolecules and plasticizer molecules [29]. The addition of plasticizer imparts softness and flexibility to starch-based blends and, thus, improves their processibility.

It is important to mention here that the ultimate properties of the blends depend on the nature of the plasticizer used. In general, the added plasticizer provides extensibility to the blend, thus improving the rheology of the blend. This obviously helps in the processibility of the blend and, consequently, improves the end properties. The plasticizer also affects biodegradation profile of the ultimate blend. The field of plasticizer has recently gained tremendous interest due to the efforts devoted in the development of starch-based mechanically strong materials. It has been mentioned in literature that TPS (thermoplastic starch) on blending with biodegradable polymers can become suitable for food packaging applications [30].

3.8.1 Starch/PVA

One of the most popular hydrophilic synthetic polymers that have been used tremendously in preparing polymer-based blends is PVA, which has so many interesting and useful properties such as good film-forming properties, strong conglutination, good barrier properties, and greater thermal stability. Furthermore, the addition of PVA to starch also results in the improvement in mechanical properties, water resistance, and weather resistance of the blend. Because the thermal properties of starch and PVA are quite different from each other, their blends can be best prepared using gelatinization process, which makes use of the fact that both the starch and PVA are soluble in hot water [31]. Because both are hydrophilic, their blending results in compatibility of PVA and starch, which is accompanied by the formation of a continuous phase. Sometimes what happens, when the two polymers are blended perfectly, their properties may be compromised, which is often resolved by the addition of some suitable plasticizers such as glycerol and water, filler materials, and compatibilizers used in blend preparation [32]. The solution cast method is the mostly used method of preparation of starch/PVA blend, which is thermoplastic in nature and prepared by addition of glycerol as plasticizer. It is known that both the PVA and starch undergo biodegradation in microbial environments, and the rate and extent of biodegradation greatly depend on the experimental conditions, chemical composition of the blend, and, most importantly, on the molecular weight of the PVA and degree of hydrolysis [33]. It is also reported that PVA/starch blend has high modulus and adequate biodegradability property that makes this blend a suitable material for food packaging applications. Bagri et al. [34] prepared a cryogel of PVA/starch and reinforced the as-prepared blend with silver hydroxyapatite nanoparticles. The formation of silver hydroxyapatite/PVA/starch nanocomposite is shown in Fig. 3.3.

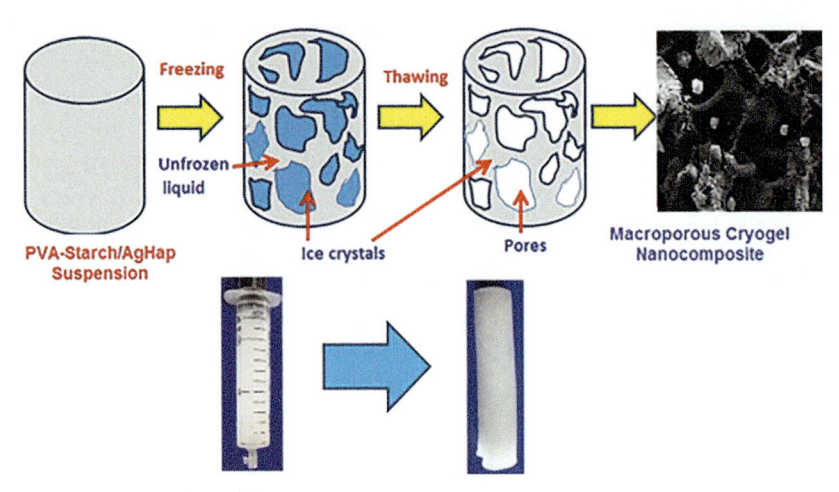

FIG. 3.3 Diagrammatic presentation of formation of nanocomposite of silver hydroxyapatite/PVA/starch under cryogenic conditions. *Reproduced from Bagri L, Saini R, Bajpai AK, Choubey R, Silver hydroxyapatite reinforced poly(vinyl alcohol)—starch cryogel nanocomposites and study of biodegradation, compressive strength and antibacterial activity. Polym Eng Sci 2019;59:254–263, Copyright (2019), with permission from Wiley.*

3.8.2 Starch/PLA

Among the listed polymers, the PLA occupies a prime position due to its biodegradable nature and good mechanical behavior. The biodegradable characteristics of PLA make this polymer as special candidate for biomedical applications. There are available a variety of grades of PLA such as copolymers of poly(L-lactic acid) and poly(D, L-lactic acid) [35].

However, its high cost restricts its universal acceptance.

There are some demerits of PLA, such as poor flexibility, high ductility, and impact resistance, which reduce the overall performance of this polymer.

An excellent solution to this limitation may be a proper and proportionate combination of starch and PLA to give a blend that may exhibit adequate biodegradability and good mechanical behavior. Because PLA also has extremely good biocompatibility, the blends of starch and PLA find significant applications in biomedical fields. However, another serious limitation to this blending of starch and PLA is poor compatibility and adhesion of PLA and starch due to their hydrophobic and hydrophilic nature, respectively. The mutual compatibility may be enhanced with the use of compatibilizers such as methylene diphenyl diisocyanate (MDI), dioctylmaleate, PVA, and poly(hydroxyester-ether). It is, however, known that the addition of TPS to PLA/starch blend is quite beneficial regarding production cost, end properties and performance, and biodegradability [36].

Various studies have revealed that when PLA and starch are added in the ratio of 1:9 (percent by weight), the resulting blend offers quite good miscibility [37]. Because starch is hydrophilic and PLA is hydrophobic in nature, their miscibility during preparation creates problems, and, therefore, compatibilizers are always added to ensure favorable interactions between the starch and PLA molecules. Various compatibilizers used in the fabrication of starch/PLA blends include poly(hydroxyester-ether), (MDI), PLA-graft-(maleic anhydride), PLA-graft-(acrylic acid), and PLA-graft-starch and poly(vinyl alcohol [38]. Besides PLA, chitin has also been used in the preparation of blends with starch [39].

3.8.3 Starch/PCL

Various other polymers that have been tried with starch for preparation of their blends include poly(ε-caprolactone) (PCL), which is a semicrystalline aliphatic polyester often prepared by performing ring-opening polymerization of ε-caprolactone. This polymer is hydrophobic in nature and bears a low melting temperature in the range of 60–65°C. The low temperature poses experimental difficulties in its fabrication, and the solutions for this kind of problem may be either radiation-induced cross-linking of polymers or preparing blend of PCL with other polymers [40]. The degradation rate of PCL intimately depends on its molecular weight and the extent of crystallinity. Thus it is always desirable to copolymerize PCL with other aliphatic polyesters so that its biodegradation property could be improved. It has also been found that the presence of starch always tends to enhance the degradation rate of PCL due to the reason that starch molecules intensified the rate of hydrolysis of PCL.

Another problem in preparation of PCL and starch blend is the occurrence of phase separation that results from the hydrophilic nature of starch and hydrophobic nature of PCL. The interaction between the PCL and starch macromolecules may further be enhanced by using some interfacial agent or compatibilizers that tend to enhance the compatibility of starch and PCL. Iqbal et al. used the interfacial agent polycaprolactone-g-glycidyl methyl acrylate (PCL-g-GMA) made in supercritical carbon dioxide to prepare starch PCL blends. These blends exhibited good mechanical strength [41]. In another study, melt blending technique was used by Su et al. to synthesize starch PCL blends, with methylene diphenyl isocyanate as compatibilizer. The blends marked appreciable increase in mechanical as well as interfacial properties and prospects for biomedical applications [42].

It has also been observed that when PCL is added to starch, it improves the mechanical strength of starch, and at the same time, crystallinity of PCL is reduced, which results in an increased biodegradation of the blend. A series of blends of PCL and starch have been prepared in the recent past; however, high fabrication cost and remarkable variations in properties and performance of the resulting blends have also been noticed [43].

3.8.4 Starch/PHB-HV

Poly(hydroxybutyrate-hydroxyvalerate) (PHB-HV) is another biodegradable polymer and has also been used in preparing blends with starch and its derivatives. Vanovcanova et al. fabricated the blends of starch, PLA, and PHB to study the effect of concentration of PHB and rheological and mechanical properties of the blend. This combination of polymers in the blend enhanced the mechanical and processing properties, thereby making it suitable for industrial purposes [44].

3.8.5 Starch/PBS and starch/PBSA

PBS is known to be a valuable thermoplastic polymer with a high degree of crystallinity. However, due to its highly crystalline nature, the degradation rate of this polymer and its blends is quite low. However, interestingly, the low degradation rate also results in excellent mechanical properties such as impact strength, high thermal stability, and good chemical resistance [45]. When starch is added to PBS, the flexibility and biodegradation of the blend are improved significantly, and the biodegradation time also increases. These properties make this blend an attractive candidate for its applications as packaging material and flushable hygiene products [46]. PBSA (poly(butylene succinate-co-butylene adipate) is another aliphatic thermoplastic copolymer that can be easily prepared by performing polycondensation of 1,4-butanediol with succinic and aliphatic acids. This copolymer is known for its good melt processability, fairly good mechanical properties, controlled biodegradability, and improved thermal and chemical resistance. In a novel study by Lesego et al., butyl-etherified starch/PBSA blends were prepared by melt processing technique, and it was observed that highly branched amylopectin facilitated better chemical interactions with polymer chains when compared with linear amylopectin, which established only feeble interactions with polymer chains [47].

3.9 Ternary blends

In ternary blends, the three polymer components are intimately present in the blend matrix, and the fabrication of ternary blends offers greater chances of variation, and, therefore, a wide variety of blends of different properties can be prepared. The constituent polymers may be either native polymers or grafted ones. The study by Carmona et al. outlined the usage of combinational properties of ductile PCL rigid PLA and low-cost

TPS with compatibilizers such as citric acid, maleic acid, and MDI to prepare the ternary blends. The displayed results showed the crystallization of PCL and PLA in the blend with the increase in tensile strength as well as ductility [48].

In another study, Bella et al. prepared PVA, starch, and CMC ternary blends in the presence of H_2O_2. The resulting ternary blends showed improved thermal stability due to addition of CMC when compared with PVA starch blends [49].

There have also been increased number of investigations in preparing ternary blends of PHB, EVA, and starch, which are altogether different polymers regarding chemical nature and properties. Because the level of compatibility is the key factor that determines the ultimate properties and end use of the product, it was found that the compatibility between PHB and EVA was improved by the presence of vinyl acid content. Thus EVA copolymers can be frequently used as modifiers for preparing PHB/starch blends [50].

3.10 Grafted starch hydrogels

One of the most successful strategies to alter properties of the constituent polymers is graft copolymerization, which has emerged as a vital tool to combine natural and synthetic polymers, thus improving the properties drastically. The central idea of graft copolymerization involves a large change in the properties of the host polymer by grafting a suitable polymer onto the backbone of the host polymer. The grafted copolymer so prepared exhibits significant changes in the properties of the end copolymer when compared with the corresponding properties of host polymer and grafting polymer.

From experimental point of view, the graft copolymerization is a very efficient and easy way to change the properties of the natural and synthetic polymers. This method is more effective in altering the properties than the blending and normally results in a product with entirely different desired properties. From mechanistic considerations, the process of grafting involves creation of active centers on the host macromolecule of natural polymer, which is subsequently followed by sequential addition of monomer molecules, thus developing a polymer molecule that has been grafted onto backbone of natural polymer. The grafting process is often accompanied by cross-linking and branching of the end product, which results in an increase in physical properties of the host polymer. The technique has been frequently applied in the case of chemical modification of edible polymers that results in a grafted polymer with improved shelf life and reduction in microbial infections. In a broad classification, the grafting may be divided into two categories namely, chemical grafting and radiation grafting, which depends on how the host polymer molecule has been activated. In chemical-induced grafting, the initiation is done with the help of some chemical initiators such as potassium persulfate, peroxydiphosphate, benzoyl peroxide, and AIBN, whereas in radiation-induced grafting method, the host polymer and monomer molecules are exposed to high-energy radiations such as gamma rays and electron beam.

Thus the technique of grafting is an efficient way to improve and modify the properties of starch in desired way. For instance, the characteristics such as elasticity, water sorption capacity, ion exchange property, thermal behavior, and resistance to microbial invasion may be significantly improved by conducting graft copolymerization of relevant monomers onto backbone of starch molecules. Starch can be considered as a model substrate for graft copolymerization due to its water solubility, ease of availability, economic viability, and its compatibility to a variety of hydrophilic monomers of ionic or nonionic nature [51]. The modified starch grafted with a variety of polymers has become a material of potential interest, and innumerable applications in food, industry, medicine, technology, and agriculture have been cited in literature [52]. Grafted starch has also been used in paper and textile industry, as superabsorbents in making diapers and sanitary napkins, as soil stabilizers in agriculture, and as a biodegradable material in packaging industry and plastic industry [53]. An easier way of performing graft copolymerization of starch is through free radical initiation using a number of initiators as previously mentioned.

The chemical modification of naturally occurring polymers such as starch, cellulose, chitin, and gelatin has gained immense interest due to their wide applications in various fields. The grafting of synthetic polymers onto natural polymers have opened up new avenues for researchers and given rise to a large number of grafted molecules with distinct and improved properties. In the case of starch, the grafting of vinyl polymers onto its backbone produces modified starch, which due to its low cost, biodegradability, ease of functionalization, nontoxic nature, and water solubility finds a large number of applications in various areas. The starch itself is a versatile material, and it offers a number of chemical transformations such as oxidation, hydrolysis, esterification, and etherification and, therefore, may be modified into the desired useful forms. A large number of studies pertaining to grafting of vinyl and acrylic monomers such as acrylic acid, acrylamide, acrylonitrile, allyl methacrylates, and vinyl ketones have been reported that describe the synthesis, characterization, and various studies of the resulting products [54].

In a drug delivery study by Bardajee et al., a novel poly(acrylic acid) grafted starch/iron oxide magnetic nanocomposite was synthesized, and the drug release profiles of entrapped drug were investigated [55]. The ratio of amylase and amylopectin present in the corn starches was found to exert a significant impact on the rheological properties of concentrated solutions of polyacrylamide-grafted hydrogels, and the problems in extrusion process were examined. It was found that on increasing the amount of amylase content, the viscoelastic moduli of starch melts also increased, which resulted in a decrease in the rheokinetic rate of the starch melts [56].

The use of hydrogels to achieve enhanced oil recovery was examined by grafting polyacrylamide onto starch and preparing its nanocomposites with clay using chromium (III) acetate as a cross-linking agent [57]. A novel study was also undertaken that made use of anionic polymers such as poly(methacrylic acid) for grafting onto gelatinized wheat starch. The as-polymer grafted gelatinized hydrogels also contained montmorillonite, and the resulting nanocomposites have mucoadhesive properties [58]. Some other anionic polymers such as poly acrylamide and 2-acrylamido-2-methylpropane sulfonic acid (AMPS) were also grafted onto food grade native starch taking starch and ionic monomer in the ratio of 1:3. The processing of hydrogel was done using an economically viable technique such as twin-screw extrusion technology [59].

Among various clays, bentonite has been found to affect the water sorption capacity, swelling and temperature responsiveness, and viscosity behavior of polyacrylic acid-grafted starch hydrogel solutions. In this study, polyacrylic acid was grafted onto starch backbone through free radical polymerization of acrylic acid in the immediate presence of cross-linking [60]. Riyajan et al. prepared a pH-sensitive graft copolymer hydrogel by grafting maleated PVA onto cassava starch using potassium persulfate as polymerization initiator [61]. The superabsorbent hydrogels are normally prepared by performing graft copolymerization of acrylic acid and acrylamide monomers onto starch macromolecule using some conventional polymerization initiator or radiation-initiated polymerization. For instance, in a ceric ion-initiated polymerization study, polyacrylic acid chains were grafted onto maize starch to make the grafted hydrogel as pH sensitive. The mechanism of graft copolymerization is depicted in Fig. 3.4 [62].

As far as water sorption capacity of these grafted hydrogels is concerned, they are matchless; however, their poor mechanical strength limits their wide applications, particularly, where the hydrogels have to withstand mechanical forces. The drawback of poor mechanical strength has been resolved by preparing new classes of materials that are known as interpenetrating polymer networks (IPNs) which possess superior mechanical and thermal properties. Some of the notable semi-IPN includes starch-graft-poly (acrylic acid-coacrylamide)/polyvinyl alcohol/clinoptilolite (starch-g-p(AA-co-AAm)/PVA/clino), which was synthesized by free radical graft copolymerization technique in an aqueous solution [63]. Diana Soto synthesized itaconic acid-grafted starch hydrogels by redox-initiated polymerization comprising a redox couple of potassium permanganate/sodium metabisulfite in the presence of a cross-linking agent. The use of itaconic acid checked the hydrolysis of starch, and the

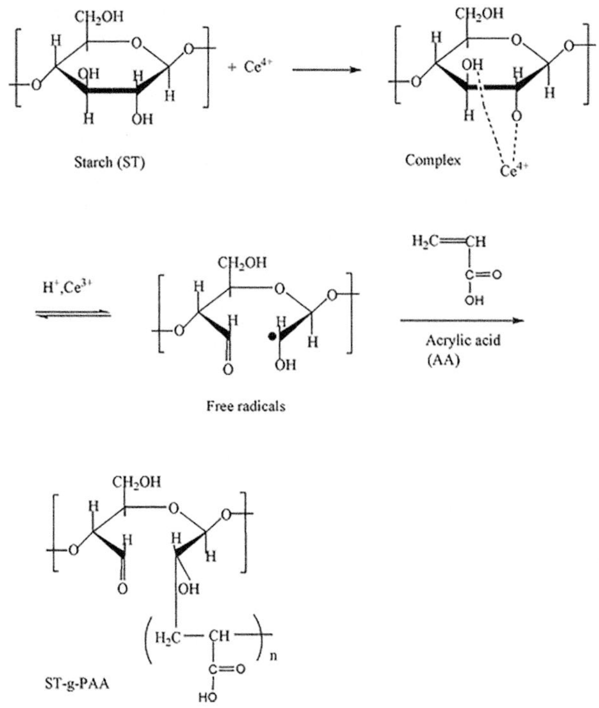

FIG. 3.4 The mechanism of graft copolymerization of acrylic acid onto starch initiated by ceric ions.*Reproduced from Dragan ES, Apopei DF, Synthesis and swelling behavior of pH-sensitive semi-interpenetrating polymer network composite hydrogels based on native and modified potatoes starch as potential sorbent for cationic dyes. Chem Eng J 2011;178:252–263, Copyright (2011), with permission from Elsevier.*

prepared grafted hydrogel was used for the removal of metal ions from their aqueous solutions [64]. Polyacrylic acid was grafted onto cassava starch, and the grafted hydrogel was evaluated for water sorption capacity and water retention characteristics, as published elsewhere [65].

The starch grafted hydrogels have also been sued for the removal of toxic metal ions and other contaminants. This was achieved by conducting graft copolymerization of two functional monomers onto starch using some polymerization initiation technique. For instance, radiation-induced polymerization was used to graft the monomers 2-acrylamido-2-methylpropane-1-sulfonic acid (AMPS) and dimethylaminoethyl methacrylate (DMAEMA) onto starch, and the as-obtained hydrogels were further modified chemically with benzyl chloride [66]. Polyacrylamide was grafted onto starch in the presence of grapheme, and the grafted hydrogel was used for the removal of malachite green dye from aqueous solution [67]. In a study, polycaprolactone was grafted onto starch, and biodegradation of the grafted hydrogel was studied [68].

The grafting of PCL onto starch was confirmed by FTIR spectroscopy, as evident from the appearance of carbonyl group in the FTIR spectra of the product hydrogels. The diameter of the hydrogels was also found to increase due to grafting of PCL.

3.11 Functionalized starch hydrogels

In the present scenario, materials with better physicochemical properties are desirable to achieve quality life and sustainability. Since the past century, polysaccharide-based hydrophilic systems have revolutionized all sectors namely, biomedical, drug delivery, environmental and advanced industrial sectors due to their unique characteristics such as hydrophilicity, swelling ability, biodegradability, nontoxicity, and biocompatibility. Apart from these properties, they possess certain demerits such as uncontrolled swelling profile, poor mechanical and tensile strength, and poor stability, which limit their use for advanced applications where such behavior is desirable. From time to time, different strategies have been adopted to overcome such drawbacks. In literature, various polysaccharides such as alginate, chitosan, carrageenan, cellulose and modified cellulose, gum acacia, guar gum, xanthan gum, starch and modified starch, tragacanth gum, and gum karaya have been modified using diverse class of reinforcing materials [69].

Starch is one of the most abundant biopolymers; it is biodegradable and inexpensive and possesses both primary and secondary hydroxyl groups suitable for being reacted to add specific functionality [6]. Irrespective of the actual microstructure of the starch molecules and their relatively high molar mass disparity, the hydroxyl groups present in these molecules serve as a great platform to append functionalities. Starch is water soluble, and that makes it an easy object for the controlled modification to incorporate active functional groups to improve its application spectrum.

A key to successfully create hydrogels in vitro as well as in vivo with defined biological properties is a well-defined and biologically sustainable synthetic chemistry. It has to allow the modification of polysaccharide backbones for controlled cross-linking and functionalization. The second functionalization step is an important issue when it is planned to introduce an additional bioactive ligand such as adhesion factors, antibiotics, and others.

Recently, the concept of click chemistry has become quite popular, and as a result, bioorthogonal reactions have been studied that very well qualify the requirements of click chemistry, as coined by Sharpless [70]. With this novel synthetic strategy, it is easy to functionalize polysaccharide backbones with greater flexibility to design hydrogels of diversified properties and end use.

Gonzalez et al. modified starch by DA (Dies-Alder) click cross-linking reaction to prepare starch NC (nanocomposite) hydrogels. The reaction involved cross-linking furan-functionalized starch using tetra functional maleimide and CNC nanoreinforcement, thus exhibiting stiffness, porosity, and nontoxicity in the hydrogels [71]. The resulting hydrogels were solid and robust and were able to maintain their shapes even in swollen state.

Although there are a number of techniques to synthesize polymer compounds, however, designing a polymer with well-defined structure is usually not met, and some discrepancies are always present. In the recent past, reversible addition-fragmentation chain transfer (RAFT) polymerization has emerged as a versatile tool to synthesize functionalized polymers with tailor-made and controlled architectures [72]. This is an effective and efficient technique to integrate the advantages of starch and PVA to yield a grafted polymer with controlled macromolecular structure. A large number of studies have been reported that make use of RAFT polymerization. In the case of starch and various grafted polymers and co-polymers, this method of polymerization has resulted in useful materials with well-defined architecture [73].

One of the most striking aspects of starch-based functional polymer materials is their huge role in water/environment management technologies. The basic requirement for such kind of applications is the presence of some specific reactive functional groups such as amino, carboxyl, and amide, which interact with metal ions and other toxicants when the graft polymer has to be used in water remediation [74]. Recent past has witnessed a huge variety of monomers that were having functional groups such as COOH, –OH, –CONH$_2$, –SO$_3$H, or –R$_4$N$^+$, and their respective grafted polymers showed potential in removing toxic metal ions from aqueous solutions. For efficient removal of metal ions, poly(acrylic acid)-based hydrogels have been extensively used either alone or in the form of grafted hydrogels of starch. Besides acrylic- and methacrylic-based grafted polymers, polymers of 2-acrylamido-2-methyl-1-propanesulfonic acid (AMPS) have also been used for the removal of toxic metal ions due to their nontoxic nature, stability in aqueous systems, and low cost. Various starch derivatives containing amide groups were synthesized, and metal ions were removed from aqueous solutions. The removal involves complexation between metal ions and nitrogen of the amide group present in the starch derivative hydrogels [75]. In a novel study by Baghbadorani et al. [76], poly(acrylic acid) chains were grafted onto starch molecule that was treated with cellulose nanofibers. The authors studied the adsorption of copper (II) ions with this ionic adsorbent and proposed the binding mechanism of metal ions with the adsorbent, as depicted in Fig. 3.5.

It has been reported that when starch is oxidized, then it exerts a positive effect on the removal of metal ions because the oxidized starch generates functional groups such as –COOH, –OH, or –COO– groups

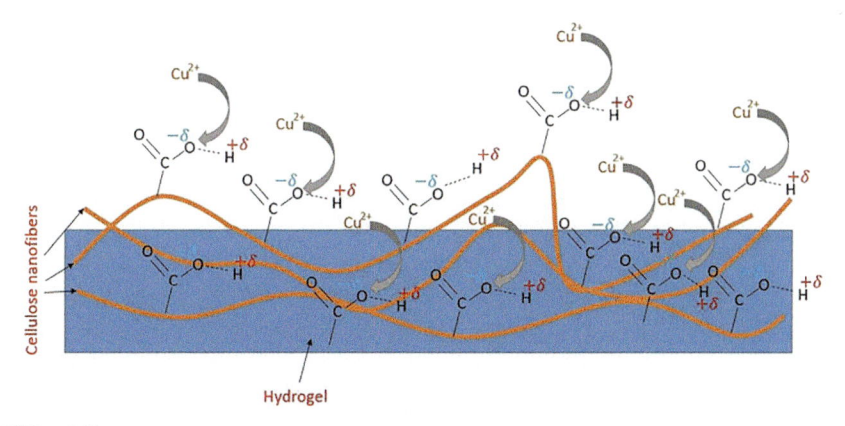

FIG. 3.5 Interaction of Cu (II) ions with starch. *Reproduced from Nooshin Bahadoran Baghbadorani NB, Behzad T, Etesami N, Heidarian P. Removal of Cu2+ ions by cellulose nanofibers-assisted starch-g-poly (acrylic acid) superadsorbent hydrogels. Compos B Eng 2019;176, Copyright (2010), with permission from Elsevier.*

in the starch molecule, and the metal ions have options for coordinating with any of these functional groups of the hydrogel. The literature is richly documented with several excellent articles on functionalization of starch. A semi-IPN composed of grafted chains of poly(acrylic acid) and poly(AMPS) onto starch was prepared by Ganguly et al. by Michael type addition of these two monomers onto starch [77]. The grafted hydrogel was found to exhibit high water swelling capacity, which significantly depended on pH of the swelling in bath in ambient conditions.

Some other chemical synthesis strategies have also been adopted for preparing starch-based hydrogels. In a novel study, Diels-Alder cross-linking reaction was conducted between furan-modified starch and water-soluble bismaleimide. The resulting hydrogel was made conductive by adding graphene layers as a filler material. The conductive hydrogels were characterized by analytical techniques that confirmed that the adopted synthesis method of Diels-Alder reaction was quite appropriate and successful [78]. Synthesis and evaluation of acryloylated starch-g-poly (acrylamide/vinylmethacrylate/1-vinyl-2-pyrrolidone) cross-linked terpolymer was functionalized by dimethylphenylvinylsilane derivative as a novel polymer-flooding agent [79]. In an interesting study, starch was modified with 4-pentenoic anhydride, which results in the formation of 4-pentenoic anhydride, thus yielding starch-pentenoate (SP) having a degree of substitution of 32% [80]. The degree of substitution (DS) is normally determined quantitatively by 1H-NMR spectroscopy and commonly expressed as the amount of modified repeating saccharide units. The literature cites some other chemical methods such as Schiff"s base reaction that was used to functionalize starch with oxidative cleavage to synthesize corresponding dialdehyde derivatives, as reported elsewhere [81]. Fully amorphous nanoparticles of starch were used by Markus Bleuel as building blocks for preparation of functional hydrogels. The as-prepared starch nanoparticles were subjected to methacrylation to yield photopolymerized hydrogel [82].

The application of modified starch in drug delivery technology has also been demonstrated in literature. In a novel study, starch micro/nanohydrogels were integrated with thermoresponsive graphene to yield composite materials that were used as controlled drug delivery systems [83]. Surface modification was used to design chitosan-co-starch-based nanohydrogels that were prepared through surface modification approach using phthalic-anhydride and hexamethylenetetramine through EDC catalyzed carbodiimide coupling reaction. It was observed that functionalization resulted in an increase in density and porosity of the hydrogel, whereas a decrease in cross-linking density was noticed because of hydrophilic contacts developed in aqueous environment under physiological conditions [84].

3.12 Applications of starch-based hydrogels

Starch-based hydrogels are quite cheaper but attractive materials and have been widely used in the synthesis of biodegradable polymers that find numerous applications in medicine, industry, technology, and pharmacy. Some significant applications of starch-based hydrogels have been discussed further.

3.12.1 In food industry

The two prominent applications where starch and starch-based biodegradable hydrogels are primarily used are food packaging materials and edible films. The major prerequisites for food, these applications include reduced food losses, retaining freshness in the foods, and maintaining appearance, flavor, and odor of the packaged food stuffs. The traditional packaging materials such as low-density polyethylene (PDPE) have been and are being used for packaging, but the environmental pollution and the ultimate disposal of these materials have produced a huge problem before the society [85]. It is, therefore, desirable to have a packaging material that is biodegradable in nature and may fulfill the other requirements also such as inertness, good mechanical strength, and barrier properties. In this regard, the starch-based hydrogels are neither completely unreactive nor inhibit the passage of gases into the food stuff; as a consequence, the food may not be preserved safely for longer times. Thus use of starch-based materials containing pertinent filler material may be a good option that may provide better mechanical strength to the packaging material as well as lower the migration of gases or vapors to the food material.

Starch-based edible films are superior in many respects because they are nontoxic, biodegradable, colorless, and tasteless. Moreover, they allow very low permeation of oxygen at low humidity and, therefore, may be proposed as food packaging materials. They are also known to enhance shelf life, thus providing better protection without impairing consumer acceptability. The photographs of some partially biodegradable and edible starch-based products are shown in Fig. 3.6 [86].

Polystyrene, which has a long history to be used in packaging material, has now been replaced by starch by treating with steam to yield foam-like material. The foamed starch is quite soft and can easily be pressed into any desired shape of cups, dishes, trays, etc. These disposables are dissolved in water to give a nontoxic solution, which is further consumed by microbes in the environment [87]. It is, therefore, expected that these starch-based biodegradable disposals may open up new avenues to save the environment and, thus, may record great progress in future.

3.12.2 Sorption of dyes

The increasing use of dyes in the textile industries has posed a serious threat to environmental pollution because the dye containing discharges have developed a variety of diseases in the nearby areas and in the affected population. Not only the textile industry but the paper and plastic industries have also been using synthetic dyes and contributing to the existing problems of water pollution. Although there are numerous methods available for the removal of toxic metal ions namely coagulation, floatation, biological treatment, and adsorption, the adsorption is the most simple and widely used technique because of its simplicity, low cost, and high removal efficiency. The success of this method depends on the nature of the adsorbent and experimental conditions such as surface area of the adsorbent, dye-adsorbent interaction, pH, temperature, and contact time.

A large number and kind of adsorbents such as biological polymers, metallic oxides, clays, and polymers are available as adsorbents for the removal of toxic metal ions; however, the hydrogels based on

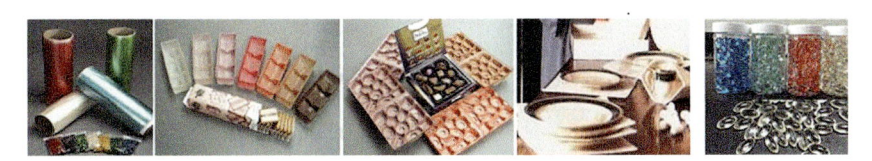

FIG. 3.6 Images of commercialized starch-based products. *Reproduced from Jiang T, Duan Q, Zhu J, Liu H, Yu L. Starch based biodegradable materials: challenges and opportunities. Adv Indus Eng Polym Res 2020;3:8–18, Copyright (2020), with permission from Elsevier.*

polysaccharides have emerged as promising materials for the removal of different toxicants. Recently, polysaccharide-based adsorbents such as starch, alginate, and chitosan have been extensively researched for the removal of toxic metal ions [88]. In an attempt to remove cationic dye from effluents, semi-IPN composite hydrogels were prepared by Dragan et al., which comprised polyacrylamide as a matrix and either native potatoes starch or hydrolyzed potatoes starch with grafted polyacrylonitrile as guest polymers. The guest polymers were prepared in the presence of N'-methylenebisacrylamide (BAAm) as a cross-linker and potassium persulfate as a polymerization initiator. The as-synthesized polymer materials were used for the removal of cationic dye methylene blue, and the removal of dye was optimized under varying experimental conditions [62].

3.12.3 Removal of metal ions

Water remediation using low-cost adsorbents have gained wide interest due to the reason that these adsorbents are collected from waste materials, and therefore this technique contributes to reuse of waste materials and, of course, lowers the cost of removal process. Wang et al. successfully removed Cu (II) ions using hydrogels that were prepared by grafting polyacrylic acid chains onto starch and sodium humate. The adsorption was further confirmed by FTIR spectral analysis, and the adsorption mechanism was found to follow complexation and obeyed Langmuir model [89]. Superabsorbent nanocomposite hydrogels comprising iron oxide, starch, and poly(acrylic acid) were synthesized by free radical polymerization method. The adsorbents were proved to be a good adsorbent for removal of dyes and heavy metal ions such as Cu (Ii) and Pb (II), and the adsorption data fitted well to Langmuir model [90].

Use of ceric ammonium nitrate as an oxidant is widely studied in the synthesis of starch-grafted hydrogels. In a novel study, polyacrylic acid was grafted onto starch using ceric ammonium nitrate as an oxidant, N,N'-methylene bisacrylamide as a cross-linking agent, and montmorrilonite was dispersed into the grafted hydrogel matrix. The as-prepared hydrogels were applied as adsorbents for the removal of Cu (II) and Pb (II) ions from aqueous solutions. The results indicated that Cu (II) ions had adsorbed to a greater extent than Pb (II) ions. The adsorption data were applied to various adsorption models, and it was found that the adsorption process obeyed Freundlich isotherm model more than the Langmuir model [91].

3.12.4 Agriculture

There are three major applications of starch-based biodegradable polymers in agriculture namely, controlled release of fertilizers, coverage of greenhouse, and mulch films. Another thrust area in agricultural and environmental sciences is the excessive use of fertilizers that not only harms the soil quality but also affects the water bodies in the nearby areas. The heavy irrigation and rains lead to leaching of excess fertilizers, and therefore it is desirable to develop controlled release systems for application of fertilizers and other agrochemicals. The starch-based hydrogels have shown promise in providing controlled release of fertilizers, and their biodegradation leads to controlled delivery of agrochemicals into the agricultural field. This obviously results in reduced environmental pollution and, consequently, improves the water quality [92]. Another advantage of starch-based hydrogels is the nontoxic nature of the biodegradation products that maintains the quality of the soil.

After using, starch-based films can be ploughed into soil and disposed directly. Moreover, no toxic residues are formed after the degradation of starch-based biodegradable polymers. Thus the development of starch-based materials for agriculture applications is being continued. Azeem et al. used rotatory fluidized bed equipment for controlled release of urea by using tapioca starch, PVA, and citric acid in the form of coating material. The coated urea was further coated by a geopolymer so as to increase its properties of controlled release and productivity of CRU (controlled release urea) [93].

Water and fertilizers are the two main factors that limit the agricultural products, so it is important to enhance the use of fertilizer nutrients and water resources. Approximately 40%–70% of nitrogen of the applied normal fertilizers is released into the environment and cannot be absorbed by plants, which can cause serious environmental pollution. Studies have exhibited that slow or controlled release technology could be an alternative to decrease such problems and reduce the loss of normal fertilizers.

Studies have shown that superabsorbent hydrogels help to decrease irrigation water consumption, enhance fertilizer retention in the soil, decline the death rate of plants, and increase plant growth rates [94]. In a relevant study, controlled release of herbicides could be achieved by the starch-agar-based hydrogels. It was observed that the soil conditioning property of both starch and agar polymers led to the increase in the plant growth as well as improvement in soil health [95].

The absorption capacity of general hydrogels in water is less than 100% ($1\,g = g$), but the superabsorbent hydrogels have absorption capacity in water of about 1000%–100,000% (10–$1000\,g = g$) [96].

Peidayesh reported the preparation of baked hydrogels from corn starch and chitosan blends cross-linked by CA by a semidry method without solvent, which could be used for water maintaining at large areas, so that it could be considered to be applied for more efficient watering of fields in agriculture. This effort is required as an innovative approach toward a friendly environment [97].

Another hydrogel use for agricultural application is in controlled pesticide formulations. Pesticides have been widely used in agriculture, and the utilization of pesticides can increase food production significantly. However, this causes serious environmental pollution and ecological problems because a huge amount of applied pesticides cannot totally reach their intended target because of volatilization, degradation, and leaching.

Some of the advantages of utilization of controlled pesticide formulations include decreasing leaching, degradation, and volatilization, reduction of residues on food stuffs, and reducing dermal toxicity [98]. Some recent advances in agricultural using starch-based hydrogels are presented here. Abd El-Mohdy et al. reported the preparation of starch = (ethylene glycol-co-methacrylic acid) [Starch = (EG-co-MAA)] hydrogels using gamma irradiation for controlled release of three types of pesticides including thiophanate methyl (TF), fluometuron (FH), and trifluralin (TI) [99].

3.12.5 Electrical uses

Another very interesting application of hydrogels is their application as external cable to safeguard the electrical cables by preventing diffusion of water molecules into cables. These polymer materials are used as water blocking tapes and wrapped over the electrical and transmission cables that are normally buried under the earth. These tapes function by absorbing water into their structure without permitting water to enter the cable if any how the coating of the cable is lost. These water-blocking tapes are fabricated by dispersing superabsorbent polymers into fabrics [100].

Willfahrt fabricated hydrogels based on corn starch and citric acid, which could be printed by screen printing technique and further used in electronics application. These hydrogels were also used as printable gel for fully printed supercapacitors. These printable hydrogels can be easily prepared and do not make use of any toxic substances [101].

3.12.6 Construction of buildings

It is a normal practice to demolish concrete robust buildings by using explosives such as dynamite. However, the use of explosives is not a routine method for demolition because there are certain complications such as destruction of surrounding architecture also. It is, therefore, recommended to use certain tools such as impact steel balls and hammers, which also pose noise and problems with dust contaminations. It has, therefore, been thought to develop such hydrogels-based demolishing agent, which facilitates the process of demolition. These intended materials are nothing but superabsorbents of starch-based polymers.

Kobayashi et al. developed a graft copolymer composed of polyacrylonitrile-grafted starch and lime particles as demolition-facilitating agent. For the purpose of demolition, the substances are put inside the holes created in the demolishing building, and water is sprayed. The water reacts with quick lime, which expands and demolishes the structure [102].

3.12.7 Personal care products

The property of water sorption and retention of water molecules within the hydrogel network without undergoing any disruption has been well used in making personal daily care products such as diapers and sanitary napkins. Carboxylated cassava starch-based hydrogels of biodegradable nature were used for making sanitary pads, as reported by Afolabi [103]. The hydrogels exhibited good water and saline retention behavior and, therefore, were found to be well suited for pads and napkins.

3.12.8 Tissue engineering

The emergence of porous, soft, and biocompatible hydrogels has opened up new areas of biomedical applications, and tissue engineering is obviously one of them. Tissue engineering is an excellent biological technique to repair cartilage and bone tissue reconstruction and regeneration [104]. Since 1990s, various attempts have been made to test different biomaterials for testing cartilage- and bone tissue engineering applications [105]. Although different kinds of biomaterials such as ceramics, composites, and metallic implants have been used and judged for their performance, polymer-based hydrogels owe a prime position because of their special biophysical properties and tissue-like resemblance. The hydrogels also have similarity to extracellular matrix regarding internal structure and porous morphology, which facilitates cell transplantation and proliferation [106].

The frequent use of injectable hydrogels for cartilage- and bone tissue-engineering applications has gained immense interest because they can replace implantation surgery and form any desired shape to match irregular defects [107]. The schematic presentation of mechanism of application of injectable hydrogels for cartilage- and bone tissue-engineering is depicted in Fig. 3.7

Natural polymer-based hydrogels such as starch, chitosan, alginate, cellulose, and gelatin have been frequently used in tissue engineering applications because of the reason that these hydrogels can gain any shape such as beads, particles, films, sheets, and fibers and, therefore, can be used conveniently and desirably without any adverse side effects. Viyoch et al. blended chitosan and starch and fabricated an injectable thermosensitive hydrogel for chondrocyte delivery. The researchers noted that starch was able to enhance the pore sizes of the hydrogels, which is mandatory for cartilage tissue engineering [108]. In another study, Sá-Lima et al. designed thermoresponsive chitosan-starch hydrogel as an injectable vehicle for cell delivery [109].

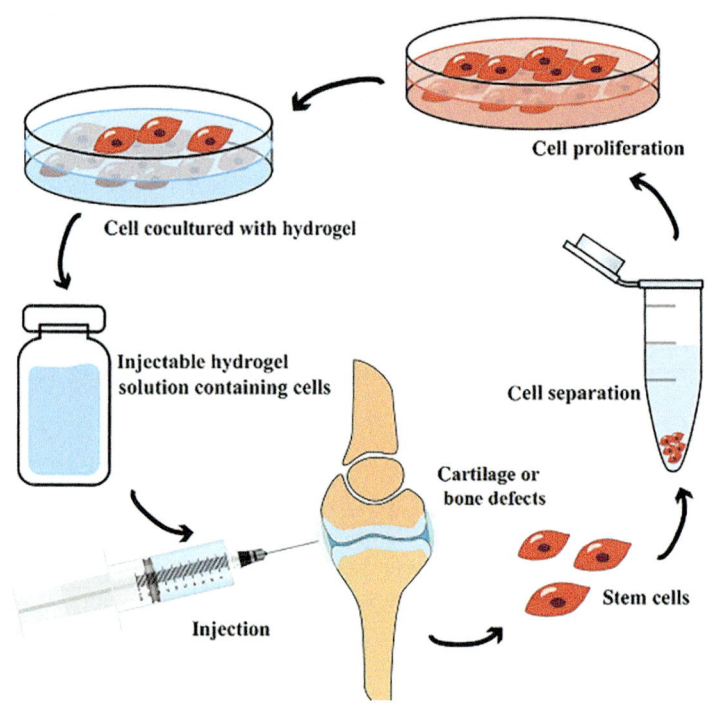

FIG. 3.7 Scheme showing approaches to make injectable hydrogels for bone-tissue engineering applications. *Reproduced from Liu M, Zeng X, Ma C, et al. Injectable hydrogels for cartilage and bone tissue engineering. Bone Res 2017;5:17014, Copyright (2017), with permission from Wiley.*

The heart is an engineered architecture of the nature. The heart functions such that the cardiac muscles undergo frequent and regular contraction, enabling a continuous supply of oxygen and micronutrients enriched blood to different parts of the body. The blood is supplied to cardiac muscles by the coronary arteries (CAs) muscle [110]. When the CA becomes narrow or the blood clogs due to some or other reasons, the blood supply is restrained, thus causing death of the heart cells, leading to myocardial infarction (MI). This consequently adversely affects the heart functions. Once the phenomenon of MI occurs, the collagen-containing scar tissue fill up the infracted area, experiencing a higher pressure during the contraction cycle (systole). When the scar tissues get thin, there is a further fall in the heart function, which ultimately results in congestive heart failure (CHF) [111]. The starch-based hydrogels have also been used in tissue engineering to correct various physiological disorders. In a study by Nieuwenhovea et al., various hydrogels were prepared, which comprised poly(methacrylamide)-grafted gelatin and starch pentenoate that excellently mimic extracellular matrix (ECM) to be used in tissue engineering [112].

Marrella et al. [113] reviewed the role of different types of hydrogels in skeletal bone engineering and discussed their functional mechanisms. Mao et al. [114] fabricated starch-based adhesive hydrogels and evaluated their potential to be used for wound healing and hemostats. The authors also studied the viscoelastic behavior of the as-prepared hydrogels. Ounkaew et al. [115] prepared ternary hydrogels composed of carboxymethylated starch/poly(vinyl alcohol)/nanosilver and examined their suitability as wound healing matrices. The authors observed that impregnation of silver improved the storage modulus and swelling index of the hydrogels. Nieuwenhove et al. [116] prepared gelatin and starch-based hydrogels and studied in vitro mesenchymal stem cell behavior of the hydrogels. The gelatin was methacrylated, and different hydrogels of varying composition were prepared by varying the ratio of gelatin to starch. It was found that the hydrogels did not exhibit any adverse response on the adipose tissue derived from stem cells, which were cultured on the hydrogels. Deepa et al. [117] prepared an IPN composed of poly(N-isopropylacrylamide) and starch, which was impregnated with silica nanoparticles. The formation of IPN is schematically presented in Fig. 3.8. The temperature-sensitive poly(N-isopropylacrylamide) enabled the hydrogel to respond to external stimuli and exhibited remarkable tensile properties. The IPN films were found to be suitable for biomedical applications.

Bakrudeen et al. prepared starch nanocrystals that were further impregnated into different polymers and loaded with various antiviral drugs. The drug-loaded polymer matrices were characterized by different techniques and evaluated for transdermal applications. Batool et al. [118] prepared a binary blend of PVA and starch and impregnated silver nanoparticles to design antibacterial nanocomposite membranes that

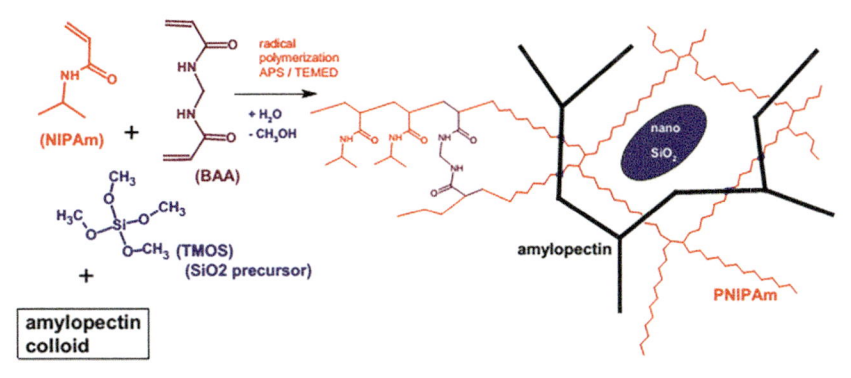

FIG. 3.8 Schematic presentation of fabrication of poly (N-isopropylacrylamide-silica-starch IPN hydrogels. *Reproduced from Deepa K, Strachota A, Slouf M, Brus J. Poly (N-isopropylacrylamide)-SiO₂ nanocomposites interpenetrated by starch: stimuli-responsive hydrogels with attractive tensile properties. Eur Polym J 2017;88:349–372, Copyright (2017), with permission from Elsevier.*

were further evaluated for wound dressing applications. Bagri et al. [119] prepared starch/PVA blends using successive freeze-thaw method, which enables the formation of crystallites of starch and PVA chains due to imposed cryogenic conditions. The hydrogels were porous in nature and suggested as good materials for tissue engineering applications. The formation of crystalline regions due to freeze-thaw process is schematically shown in Fig. 3.9.

Both natural and synthetic hydrogels are suitable for cardiac tissue engineering because their soft and viscoelastic nature mimic the native tissue. Collagen, gelatin, laminin, matrigel, hyaluronic acid (hyaluronan), alginate, and chitosan are typical natural hydrogels. They have similar or even identical structures to the molecules in biological organisms, thereby reducing the possibility of immune response when implanted in vivo.

3.12.9 Drug delivery systems

Starch-based hydrogels have some peculiar advantages over other natural polymers such as:

(1) Fair biocompatibility;
(2) Biodegradable and nontoxic nature of the end products after biodegradation;
(3) Good mechanical behavior; and
(4) Controlled degradation.

The drug delivery technique aims at delivering controlled amount of drug at the desires sites, thus minimizing exposure of other healthy tissues to administered drug. Furthermore, the manipulation of chemical composition of drug delivery systems enables to control the amount of the delivered drug. The porosity, size of pores, pore size distribution, and morphology also have impact on the performance of the drug-carrying device.

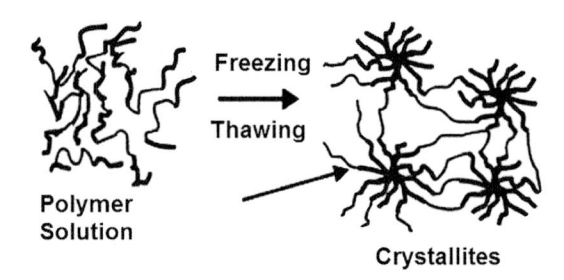

FIG. 3.9 Schematic presentation of cryogel of starch and PVA by freeze-thaw method. *Reproduced from Bagri LP, Bajpai J, Bajpai AK. Cryogenic designing of biocompatible blends of polyvinyl alcohol and starch with macroporous architecture. J Macromol Sci Pure Appl Chem A 2009;46:1060–1068, Copyright (2009), with permission from Taylor and Francis.*

The hydrogels of polysaccharides such as starch, chitosan, and cellulose have been largely used as drug delivery systems. Likhitkar and Bajpai [120] fabricated iron oxide-impregnated starch nanoparticles and loaded them with anticancer drug cisplatin. The authors confirmed the superparamagnetic nature of the particles and studied the controlled release of cisplatin under applied magnetic field, as depicted in Fig. 3.10.

The delivery of drugs to the colon has been successfully achieved by using starch-based hydrogels, as reported elsewhere [120, 121]. It is important to see that for formulating a colon drug delivery system, the drug entrapped in the hydrogel must be preserved in the highly acidic environment of the stomach and delivered to colon where medium is slightly alkaline. For this purpose, the polymeric systems need to swell in the basic intestinal medium but minimally in acidic medium [121, 122].

Budianto used starch as an encapsulation material to fabricate a drug delivery system [122]. However, the degradation of starch hydrogel occurs quite rapidly during metabolism in human stomach. Thus it is required to modify starch regarding its degradation property especially for gastrointestinal drug. In this research, three modified starch-based hydrogels were synthesized, that is, cross-linked starch hydrogel, semi-IPN, and full-IPN starch hydrogel using poly(N-vinyl-pyrrolidone). Semi-IPN and cross-linked starch hydrogel have required properties and, consequently, will not be degraded easily during metabolism.

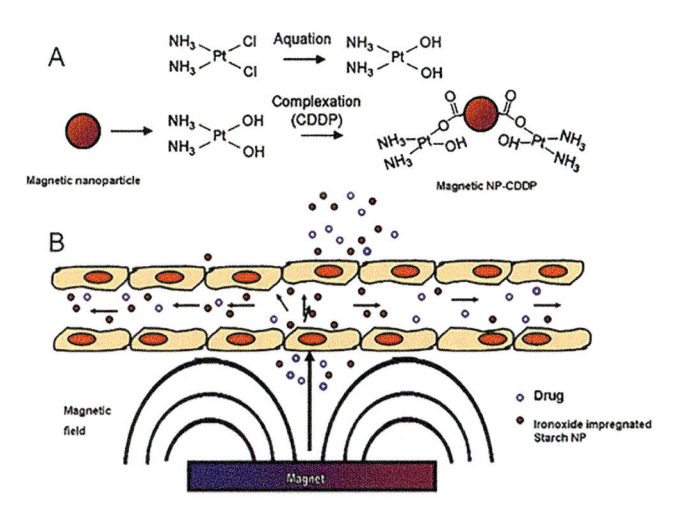

FIG. 3.10 Schematic presentation of (A) binding of cisplatin drug molecules to the iron oxide-impregnated starch nanoparticles and (B) possible targeting of cells by the released drug due to applied magnetic field. *Reproduced from Likhitkar S, Bajpai AK. Magnetically controlled release of cisplatin from superparamagnetic starch nanoparticles. Carbohydr Polym 2012;87:300–308, Copyright (2012), with permission from Elsevier.*

Relatively stiff and touch monolithic (nonporous) centimeter-sized hydrogels were prepared, which offered very fast and extensive deswelling (and volume shrinkage) in response to temperature and to pH jumps. The materials of these types were primarily composed of poly (N isopropyl acrylamide-co-sodium methacrylate) intercalated by starch. The release of theophylline was successfully tested, and it was found that the release kinetics is governed by deswelling kinetics and that the drug was released nearly quantitatively [123].

Starch-based hydrogels have been largely prepared by various researchers. Biodegradable hydroxyl methacrylate starch hydrogel shows the sustained release properties for the in vitro FITC-antihuman antibodies and in vivo IgG-FITC [124]. The in situ hydrogels of starch-based nanoparticle and polyvinylamine prepared by Schiff's base reaction was used to study controlled release of doxorubicin [125].

Mohammad Reza Saboktakin prepared carboxymethyl starch (CMS) hydrogel using dextran sulfate (DS) as polyanionic polymer to achieve complex coacervation for the incorporation and controlled release of an antiangiogenesis hexapeptide; this was the first report describing the use of DS to formulate CMS-based hydrogels. Hydrogels for photodynamic treatment of cancer have also been tried [126]. Kleawkla prepared hydrogels from deprotonated natural rubber latex (DNRL) with gelatinized starch. Hydrogels from DNRL with gelatinized starch are able for use as wound dressing in medical application [127]. Biodegradability and thermal properties of polycaprolactone/starch nanocomposite as a biopolymer was studied by Al-Mulla [128]. Researchers have successfully prepared hydrogels from cassava starch for tablet superdisintegrant. Cassava starch is a favorable material because it is abundant in nature, it is highly pure, and it has the ability to undergo the chemical modification to alter the structures and improve the properties. The process makes use of chemical reactions using citric acid, an edible organic acid, as a cross-linking agent [129]. Soe et al. [130] prepared glutinous rice starch-chitosan composite films for buccal drug delivery of hydrophilic drugs such as lidocaine hydrochloride. The authors characterized the blend film and studied its mechanical properties and evaluated the effect of experimental conditions on the released amount of the drug.

3.13 Current challenges and future prospects

The starch-based hydrogel materials are quite promising materials and have quite a good number of useful properties. However, in spite of its wide acceptance, some of its properties hinder its performance, especially in biomedical applications. The poor mechanical strength, its rapid biodegradable nature, inert nature of the molecules, and difficulty in functionalization are some of its limitation, which needs modification and improvements. Furthermore, the cross-linking of starch by epichlorohydrin is also questionable because epichlorohydrin is quite toxic and must be recommended for cross-linking. Thus an efficient and eco-friendly cross-linking agent is needed for cross-linking of starch and its derivatives.

On the other hand, the biodegradability of starch enables it for food packaging applications because the problems with disposal of plastic wastes are at the top. The synthetic chemistry has to find some solution to substantially enhance the mechanical properties of starch without compromising with its biodegradation nature. The starch and its derivatives such as grafted starch, functionalized starch, and blended starch could be excellent materials for food and other packaging purposes. If the said properties are improved, then considering the economic viability of starch, this material may prove to be a game changer in the future.

3.14 Conclusions

Starch-based hydrogels are very promising materials and owe a wide spectrum of applications, including agriculture, medicine, biomedical, pharmacy, edible products, etc. This natural polymer and its modified forms have attractive properties such as occurrence in abundance, biodegradable nature, nontoxicity, blood compatibility, water solubility, prone to biodegradation etc. Starch can be easily transformed into several useful forms such as blends with other polymers, grafting of vinyl polymers onto starch backbone, and functionalization to more reactive species. Apart from food and other technological applications of starch, it is more applied in agriculture, drug delivery system, tissue engineering, removal of dyes and toxic metal ions, electrical appliances, and building construction materials.

References

[1] Smith AM. Starch and starch granules. In: Encyclopedia of Life Sciences (ELS). Chichester: John Wiley & Sons, Ltd; 2010.

[2] Malinova I, Qasim AM, Brust H, Fettke J. Parameters of starch granule genesis in chloroplasts of arabidopsis thaliana. Front Plant Sci 2018. https://doi.org/10.3389/fpls.2018.00761.

[3] Santana AL, Meireles MAA. New starches are the trend for industry applications: a review. Food Public Health 2014;4:229–41.

[4] Nagam SP, Jyothi AN, Poojitha J, Aruna S, Nadendla RR. A comprehensive review on hydrogels. Int J Curr Pharm Res 2016;8:19–23.

[5] Ismail H, Irani M, Ahmad Z. Starch-based hydrogels: present status and applications. Int J Polym Mater Polym 2013;62:411–20.

[6] Xiao C. Current advances of chemical and physical starch-based hydrogels. Starch-Stärke 2013;65:82–8.

[7] Biduski B, Ferreira-Da Silva WM, Colussi R, El-Halal SLM, Loong-Tak L, Guerra-Dias AR, Zavareze ER. Starch hydrogels: the influence of the amylose content and gelatinization method. Int J Biol Macromol 2018;113:443–9.

[8] Schirmer M, Jekle M, Becker T. Starch gelatinization and its complexity for analysis. Starch-Starke 2015;67:30–41.

[9] Carlstedt J, Wojtasz J, Fyhr P, Kocherbitov V. Understanding starch gelatinization: the phase diagram approach. Carbohydr Polym 2015;129:62–9.

[10] Huang F-Y, Wu X-J, Yu Y, Yan-Hua L. Preparation and properties of cellulose laurate (CL)/starch nanocrystals acetate (SNA) bio-nanocomposites. Polymers 2015;7:1331–45.

[11] Malana MA, Aftab F, Batool SR. Synthesis and characterization of stimuli-responsive hydrogel based on starch and methyl-3-aminocrotonate: swelling and degradation kinetics. Polym Bull 2019;6.

[12] Sethi S, Kaith BS, Kaur M, Sharma N, Khullar S. Study of a cross-linked hydrogel of karayagum and starch as a controlled drug delivery system. J Biomater Sci Polym Ed 2019;30:1687–708.

[13] Abd El-Mohdy HL, Hegazy EA, El-Nesr EM, El-Wahab MA. Synthesis, characterization and properties of radiation-induced starch/(EG-co-MAA) hydrogels. Arab J Chem 2016;9:S1627–35.

[14] Seon-Min O, Lee B-H, Seo D-H, Choi H-W, Kim B-Y, Bai M-Y. Starch nanoparticles prepared by enzymatic hydrolysis and self assembly of short-chain glucans. Food Sci Biotechnol 2020;29:585–98.

[15] Larrea-Wachtendor D, Tabilo-Munizaga G, Ferrari G. Potato starch hydrogels produced by high hydrostatic pressure (HHP): a first approach. Polymers 2019;11. 1673.1-18.

[16] Fekete T, Borsa J, Takács E, Wojnárovits L. Synthesis of carboxymethylcellulose/starch superabsorbent hydrogels by gamma irradiation. Chem Cent J 2017;11:46.1–10.

[17] Sunarti TC, Febrian MI, Ruriani E, Yuliasih I. Some properties of chemical cross-linking biohydrogel from starch and chitosan. Int J Biomater 2019;1–6.

[18] Wang J, Sun H, Li J, Dong D, Zhang Y, Yao F. Ionic starch-based hydrogels for the prevention of nonspecific protein adsorption. Carbohydr Polym 2015;117:384–91.

[19] Al-Zahara NF, Mohamood T, Zainuddin N, Ahmad@Ayob M, Tan SW. Preparation, optimization and swelling study of carboxymethyl sago starch (CMSS)–acid hydrogel. Chem Cent J 2018;12. 133. 1-10.

[20] Intan SN, Rachmawati R. Inclusion complexes between starch and oleic acid as hydrogel materials. Key Eng Mater 2019;811:8–13.

[21] Encalada K, Aldá MB, Proaño E, Valle V. An overview of starch-based biopolymers and their biodegradability. Ciencia e Ingeniería 2018;39:3.245–258.

[22] Hammache Y, Serier A, Chaoui S. The effect of thermoplastic starch on the properties of polypropylene/high density polyethylene blend reinforced by nano-clay. Mater Res Express 2020;7. 025308.1-12.

[23] Berber-Yamak H. Thermal, mechanical and water resistance properties of LDPE/Starch bio-based polymer blends for food packing applications. J Turkish Chem Soc Sect Chem 2016;3:637–58.

[24] Amin AMM, Sauid SM, Ku Hamid KH. Polymer-starch blend biodegradable plastics: an overview. Adv Mater Res 2015;1113:93–8.

[25] Mendes JF, Paschoalinb RT, Carmona VB, Sena Neto AR, Marques ACP, Marconcini JM, Mattoso LHC, Medeiros ES, Oliveira JE. Biodegradable polymers blends based on corn starch and thermoplastic chitosan processed by extrusion. Carbohydr Polym 2016;137:452–8.

[26] Mujaheddin, Jagadish RL, Sheshappa Rai K, Guru GS. Miscibility studies of agar-agar/starch blends using various techniques. Int J Res Pharm Chem 2012;2(4):2231–781.

[27] Teixeira E, Curvelo A, Corrêa A, Marconcini J, Glenn G, Mattoso L. Properties of thermoplastic starch from cassava bagasse and cassava starch and their blends with poly (lactic acid). Ind Crop Prod 2012;37:61–8.

[28] Bhanu P, Gupta V, Pathania D, Singha A. Synthesis, characterization and antibacterial activity of biodegradable starch/PVA composite films reinforced with cellulosic fibre. Carbohydr Polym 2014;109:171–9.

[29] Amine B, Chalamet Y. Effects of relative humidity and ionic liquids on the water content and glass transition of plasticized starch. Carbohydr Polym 2013;97:665–7.

[30] Muller IDJ, González-Martínez C, Chiralt A. Combination of poly(lactic) acid and starch for biodegradable food packaging. Materials 2017;10:952.1–22.

[31] Wang J-l, Cheng F, Zhu P-x. Structure and properties of urea-plasticized starch **films** with different urea contents. Carbohydr Polym 2014;101:1109–15.

[32] Tang X, Alavi S. Recent advances in starch, polyvinyl alcohol based polymer blends, nanocomposites and their biodegradability. Carbohydr Polym 2011;85:7–16.

[33] Azahari N, Othman N, Ismail H. Biodegradation Studies of polyvinyl alcohol/corn starch blend films in solid and solution media. J Phys Sci 2011;22:15–31.

[34] Bagri L, Saini R, Bajpai AK, Choubey R. Silver hydroxyapatite reinforced poly(vinyl alcohol)—starch cryogel nanocomposites and study of biodegradation, compressive strength and antibacterial activity. Polym Eng Sci 2019;59:254–63.

[35] Murariu M, Dubois P. PLA composites: from production to properties. Adv Drug Deliv Rev 2016;107:17–46.

[36] Soares F, Yamashita F, Müller C, Pires A. Effect of cooling and coating on thermoplastic starch/poly (lactic acid) blend sheets. Polym Test 2014;33:34–9.

[37] Zuo Y, Gu J, Cao J, Wei S, Tan H, Zhang Y. Effect of starch/polylactic acid ratio on the interdependence of two-phase and the properties of composites. J Wuhan Univ Technol Mater Sci Ed 2015;30:1108–14.

[38] Luciana B, Fabían V, Inês BM, Pedro S. Molecular dynamic evaluation of starch-PLA blends nanocomposite with organoclay by proton NMR relaxometry. Polym Test 2013;32:1181–5.

[39] Olaiya NG, Surya I, Oke PK, Rizal S, Sadiku ER, Ray SS, Farayibi PK, Hossain MS, Abdul Khalil HPS. Properties and characterization of a PLA–chitin–starch biodegradable polymer composite. Polymers 2019;11. 1656.1-16.

[40] Ortega-Toro R, Muñoz A, Talens P, Chiralt A. Improvement of properties of glycerol plasticized starch films by blending with a low ratio of polycaprolactone and/or polyethylene glycol. Food Hydrocoll 2016;56:9–19.

[41] Iqbal M, Mensen C, Qian X, Picchioni F. Green processes for green products: the use of supercritical CO_2 as green solvent for compatibilized polymer blends. Polymers 2018;10:1285.

[42] Su J, Chen L, Li L. Characterization of polycaprolactone and starch blends for potential application within the biomaterials field. Afr J Biotechnol 2012;11(3):694–701.

[43] Mahieu A, Terrié C, Agoulon A, Leblanc N, Youssef B. Thermoplastic starch and poly(ε-caprolactone) blends: morphology and mechanical properties as a function of relative humidity. J Polym Res 2013;20:229.1–13.

[44] Vanovčanova Z, Alexy P, Feranc J, Plavec R, Bočkaj J, Kaliňakova L, Tomanova K, Perďochova D, Šarisky D, Galisova I. Effect of PHB on the properties of biodegradable PLA blends. Chem Pap 2016;70(10):1408–15.

[45] Kanitporn SI, Koombhongse P, Chirachanchai S. Starch grafted poly(butylene succinate) via conjugating reaction and its role on enhancing the compatibility. Carbohydr Polym 2013;102:95–102.

[46] Ramesh B, Kevin O'C, Ramakrishna S. Current progress on bio-based polymers and their future trends. Prog Biomater 2013;2:1–16.

[47] Lesego M, Sinha S, Jalama K. The effect of starch amylose content on the morphology and properties of melt-processed butyl-etherified starch/poly [(butylene succinate)-co-adipate] blends. Carbohydr Polym 2017;155:89–100.

[48] Carmona VB, Corrêa AN, Marconcini JM, Henrique L, Mattoso C. Properties of a biodegradable ternary blend of thermoplastic starch (TPS), poly(e-caprolactone) (PCL) and poly(lactic Acid) (PLA). J Polym Environ 2014. https://doi.org/10.1007/s10924-014-0666-7.

[49] Bella GR, Jeba Jeevitha RS, Avila Thanga Booshan S. Polyvinyl alcohol/starch/carboxymethyl cellulose ternary polymer blends: Synthesis, characterization and thermal properties. Int J Curr Res Chem Pharm Sci 2016;3:43–50.

[50] Ma P, Xu P, Chen M, Dong W, Cai X, Schmit P, Spoelstra A, Lemstra P. Structure–property relationships of reactively compatibilized PHB/EVA/starch blends. Carbohydr Polym 2014;108:299–306.

[51] Moharami S, Jalali M. Removal of phosphorus from aqueous solution by Iranian natural adsorbents. Chem Eng J 2013;223:328–39.

[52] Yan H, Li H, Yang H, Li A, Cheng R. Removal of various cationic dyes from aqueous solutions using a kind of fully biodegradable magnetic composite microsphere. Chem Eng J 2013;223:402–11.

[53] Jyothi AN. Starch graft copolymers: novel applications in industry. Compos Interfaces 2010;17:165–74.

[54] Bhuyan MM, Dafader NC, Hara K, Okabe H, Hidaka Y, Rahman MM, Khan MMR, Rahman N. Synthesis of potato starch-acrylic-acid hydrogels by gamma radiation and their application in dye adsorption. Int J Polym Sci 2016;1–11.

[55] Bardajee GR, Hooshyar Z. A novel biocompatible magnetic iron oxide nanoparticles/hydrogel based on poly (acrylic acid) grafted onto starch for controlled drug release. J Polym Res 2013;20:298.1–13.

[56] Bao X, Yu L, Shen S, Simon GP, Liu H, Chen L. How rheological behaviors of concentrated starch affect graft copolymerization of acrylamide and resultant hydrogel. Carbohydr Polym 2019;219:395–404.

[57] Singh R, Mahto V. Synthesis, characterization and evaluation of polyacrylamide graft starch/clay nanocomposite hydrogel system for enhanced oil recovery. Pet Sci 2017;14:765–77.

[58] Güler MA, Gök MK, Figen AK, Özgümüş S. Swelling, mechanical and mucoadhesion properties of Mt/starch-g-PMAA nanocomposite hydrogels. Appl Clay Sci 2015;112–113:44–5.

[59] Siyamak S, Luckman P, Laycock B. Rapid and solvent-free synthesis of pH-responsive graft-copolymers based on wheat starch and their properties as potential ammonium sorbents. Int J Biol Macromol 2020;149:477–86.

[60] Chaudhuri SD, Mandal A, Dey A, Chakrabarty D. Tuning the swelling and rheological attributes of bentonite clay modified starch grafted polyacrylic acid based hydrogel. Appl Clay Sci 2020;185:105405.

[61] Riyajan SA, Sukhlaaied W, Keawmanga W. Preparation and properties of a hydrogel of maleated poly(vinylalcohol) (PVAM) grafted with cassava starch. Carbohydr Polym 2015;122:301–7.

[62] Dragan ES, Apopei DF. Synthesis and swelling behavior of pH-sensitive semi-interpenetrating polymer network composite hydrogels based on native and modified potatoes starch as potential sorbent for cationic dyes. Chem Eng J 2011;178:252–63.

[63] Olad A, Doustdar F, Gharekhani H. Starch-based semi-IPN hydrogel nanocomposite integrated with clinoptilolite: preparation and swelling kinetic study. Carbohydr Polym 2018;200:516–28.

[64] Soto D, Urdaneta J, Pernia K, Leon O, Munoz-Bonilla A, Fernandez-Garcı M. Itaconic acid grafted starch hydrogels as metal remover: capacity, selectivity and adsorption kinetics. J Polym Environ 2016;24:343–55.

[65] Witono JR, Noordergraaf IW, Heeres HJ, Janssen LPBM. Water absorption, retention and the swelling characteristics of cassava starch grafted with polyacrylic acid. Carbohydr Polym 2014;103:325–32.

[66] Farag AM, Sokker HH, Zayed EM, Nour Eldien FA, Alrahman NMA. Removal of hazardous pollutants using bifunctional hydrogel obtained from modified starch by grafting copolymerization. Int J Biol Macromol 2018;120:2188–99.

[67] Hosseinzadeh H, Ramin S. Fabrication of starch-graft-poly(acrylamide)/graphene oxide/hydroxyapatite nanocomposite hydrogel adsorbent for removal of malachite green dye from aqueous solution. Int J Biol Macromol 2018;106:101–15.

[68] Cuevas-Carballo B, Duarte-Aranda S, Canché-Escamilla G. Properties and biodegradability of thermoplastic starch obtained from granular starches grafted with polycaprolactone. Int J Polym Sci 2017;1–13.

[69] Sharma N, Rana VS. A review on polysaccharide based nanocomposite hydrogel systems fabrication using diverse reinforcing materials. J Polym Compos 2020;8:6–17.

[70] Kolb HC, Finn MG, Sharpless KB. Click chemistry: diverse chemical reactions from a few good reactions. Angew Chem Int Ed 2001;40:2004–21.

[71] González K, Guarest O, Palomares T, Alonso-Varona A, Eceiza A, Gabilondo N. The role of cellulose nanocrystals in biocompatible starch based clicked nanocomposite hydrogels. Int J Biol Macromol 2020;143:265–72.

[72] Xu JT, Tao L, Boyer C, Lowe AB, Davis TP. Combining thio-bromo 'click' chemistry and RAFT polymerization: a powerful tool for preparing functionalized multiblock and hyperbranched polymers. Macromolecules 2010;43:20–4.

[73] Lu DR, Xiao CM, Xu SJ, Ye YF. Tailor-made starch-based conjugates containing well-defined poly (vinyl acetate) and its derivative poly (vinyl alcohol). Express Polym Lett 2011;5:535–44.

[74] Xie G, Shang X, Liu R, Hu J, Liao S. Synthesis and characterization of a novel amino modified starch and its adsorption properties for Cd(II) ions from aqueous solution. Carbohydr Polym 2011;84:430–8.

[75] Singh PN, Tiwary D, Sinha I. Starch-functionalized magnetite nanoparticles for hexavalent chromium removal from aqueous solutions. Desalin Water Treat 2016;57:12608–19.

[76] Nooshin Bahadoran Baghbadorani NB, Behzad T, Etesami N, Heidarian P. Removal of Cu^{2+} ions by cellulose nanofibers-assisted starch-g-poly (acrylic acid) superadsorbent hydrogels. Compos B Eng 2019;176.

[77] Ganguly S, Maity T, Mondal S, Das P, Das NC. Starch functionalized biodegradable semi-IPN as a pH-tunable controlled release platform for memantine. Int J Biol Macromol 2017;95:185–98.

[78] González K, García-Astrain C, Santamaria-Echart A, Ugarte L, Avérous L, Eceiza A, Gabilondo N. Starch/graphene hydrogels via click chemistry with relevant electrical and antibacterial properties. Carbohydr Polym 2018;202:372–81.

[79] El-hoshoudy AN, Desouky SM. Synthesis and evaluation of acryloylated starch-g-poly (acrylamide/vinylmethacrylate/1-vinyl-2-pyrrolidone) cross-linked terpolymer functionalized by dimethylphenylvinylsilane derivative as a novel polymer-flooding agent. Int J Biol Macromol 2018;116:434–42.

[80] Nieuwenhove IV, Salamon A, Peters K, Graulus GJ, Martins JC, Frankel D, Kersemans K, De Vos F, Vlierberghe SV, Dubruel P. Gelatin- and starch-based hydrogels. Part A: hydrogel development, characterization and coating. Carbohydr Polym 2016;152:129–39.

[81] Nada AA, Soliman AAF, Aly AA, Abou-Okeil A. Stimuli-free and biocompatible hydrogel via hydrazone chemistry: synthesis, characterization, and bioassessment. Starch-Stärke 2019;71. 1800243.1-9.

[82] Majcher MJ, McInnis CL, Himbert S, Alsop RJ, Kinio D, Bleuel M, Rheinstadter MC, Smeets NMB, Hoare T. Photopolymerized starch nanoparticle (SNP) network hydrogels. Carbohydr Polym 2020;236. 115998.1-10.

[83] Sattari M, Fathi M, Daei M, Erfan-Niya H, Barar J, Entezami AA. Thermoresponsive graphene oxide–starch micro/nanohydrogel composite as biocompatible drug delivery system. BioImpacts 2017;7:167–75.

[84] Ullah F, Javed F, Zakaria MR, Jamila N, Khattak R. Determining the molecular-weight and interfacial properties of chitosan built nanohydrogel for controlled drug delivery applications. Biointerface Res Appl Chem 2019;9:4452–7.

[85] Ali SS, Qazi IA, Arshad M, Khan Z, Voice TC, Mehmood CT. Photocatalytic degradation of low density polyethylene (LDPE) films using titania nanotubes. Environ Nanotechnol Monit Manag 2016. https://doi.org/10.1016/j.enmm.2016.01.001.

[86] Jiang T, Duan Q, Zhu J, Liu H, Yu L. Starch based biodegradable materials: challenges and opportunities. Adv Indus Eng Polym Res 2020;3:8–18.

[87] Meng L, Liu H, Yu L, Duan Q, Chen L, Liu F, Shao Z, Shi K, Lin X. How water acting as both blowing agent and plasticizer affect on starch-based foam. Ind Crop Prod 2019;134:43–9.

[88] Al-Aidy H, Amdeha A. Green adsorbents based on polyacrylic acid-acrylamide grafted starch hydrogels: the new approach for enhanced adsorption of malachite green dye from aqueous solution. Int J Environ Anal Chem 2020. https://doi.org/10.1080/03067319.2020.1711896.

[89] Zheng Y, Hua S, Wang A. Adsorption behavior of Cu^{2+} from aqueous solutions onto starch-g-poly (acrylic acid)/sodium humate hydrogels. Desalination 2010;263:170–5.

[90] Saberi A, Alipour E, Sadeghi M. Superabsorbent magnetic Fe_3O_4-based starch-poly (acrylic acid) nanocomposite hydrogel for efficient removal of dyes and heavy metal ions from water. J Polym Res 2019;26:271.

[91] Güçlü G, Al E, Emik S, İyim TB, Özgümüş S, et al. Removal of Cu^{2+} and Pb^{2+} ions from aqueous solutions by starch-graft-acrylic acid/montmorillonite superabsorbent nanocomposite hydrogels. Polym Bull 2010;65:347–62.

[92] Perez JJ, Francois N. J. Chitosan-starch beads prepared by ionotropic gelation as potential matrices for controlled release of fertilizers. Carbohydr Polym 2016;148:134–42.

[93] Azeem B, KuShaari K, Naqvi M, Keong LK, Almesfer MK, Al-Qodah Z, Naqvi SR, Elboughdiri N. Production and characterization of controlled release urea using biopolymer and geopolymer as coating materials. Polymers 2020;12:400.1–29.

[94] Behera S, Mahanwar PA. Superabsorbent polymers in agriculture and other applications: a review. Polym-Plast Technol Mater 2019. https://doi.org/10.1080/25740881.2019.1647239.

[95] Singh B, Sharma DK, Negi S, Dhiman A. Synthesis and characterization of agar-starch based hydrogels for slow herbicide delivery applications. Int J Plast Technol 2015;19:263–74.

[96] Zohuriaan-Mehr M, Omidian H, Doroudiani S, Kabiri K. Advances in non-hygienic applications of superabsorbent hydrogel materials. J Mater Sci 2010;45:5711–35.

[97] Peidayesh H, Ahmadi Z, Khonakdar HA, Abdouss M, Chodák I. Baked hydrogel from corn starch and chitosan blends cross-linked by citric acid: preparation and properties. Polym Adv Technol 2020;1–14.

[98] Chevillard A, Angellier-Coussy H, Guillard V, Gontard N, Gastaldi E. Controlling pesticide release via structuring agropolymer and nanoclays based materials. J Hazard Mater 2012;205–206:32–9.

[99] Abd El-Mohdy HL, Hegazy EA, El-Nesr EM, El-Wahab MA. Control release of some pesticides from starch/(ethylene glycol-co-methacrylic acid) copolymers prepared by γ-irradiation. J Appl Polym Sci 2011;122:1500–9.

[100] Norris R, Weimann PA. US Patent 6631229; 2003.

[101] Willfahrt A, Steiner E, Hoetzel J, Crispin X. Printable acid-modified corn starch as non-toxic, disposable hydrogel-polymer electrolyte in supercapacitors. Appl Phys A 2019;125:474.

[102] Kobayashi W, Otaka S, Nagai M. US Patent 1990; 4:952:243.

[103] Afolabi TA. Synthesis of biodegradable superabsorbent hydrogel from carboxymetylated cassava starch for use in sanitary pads. J Chem Soc Nigeria 2019;44:433–52.

[104] Kim TG, Shin H, Lim DW. Biomimetic scaffolds for tissue engineering. Adv Funct Mater 2012;22:2446–68.

[105] Shin SR, Li YC, Jang HL, et al. Graphene-based materials for tissue engineering. Adv Drug Deliv Rev 2016;105:255–74.

[106] Mantha S, Pillai S, Khayambashi P, Upadhyay A, Zhang Y, Tao O, Pham HM, Tran SD. Smart hydrogels in tissue engineering and regenerative medicine. Materials (Basel) 2019;12:3323.1–33.

[107] Liu M, Zeng X, Ma C, et al. Injectable hydrogels for cartilage and bone tissue engineering. Bone Res 2017;5:17014.

[108] Ngoenkam J, Faikrua A, Yasothornsrikul S, Viyoch J. Potential of an injectable chitosan/starch/beta-glycerol phosphate hydrogel for sustaining normal chondrocyte function. Int J Pharm 2010;391:115–24.

[109] Sá-Lima H, Caridade SG, Mano JF, et al. Stimuli-responsive chitosan starch injectable hydrogels combined with encapsulated adipose derived stromal cells for articular cartilage regeneration. Soft Matter 2010;6:5184–95.

[110] Li Z, Guan J. Hydrogels for cardiac tissue engineering. Polymers 2011;3:740–61.

[111] Wang F, Guan J. Cellular cardiomyoplasty and cardiac tissue engineering for myocardial therapy. Adv Drug Deliv Rev 2010;62:784–97.

[112] Van Nieuwenhovea I, Salamonb A, Petersb K, Graulusa GJ, Martinsc JC, Frankeld D, et al. Gelatin- and starch-based hydrogels. Part A: hydrogel development, characterization and coating. Carbohydr Polym 2016;152:129–39.

[113] Marrella A, Lee TY, Lee DH, Karuthedom S, Syla D, Chawla A, Khademhosseini A, Jang HL. Engineering vascularized and innervated bone biomaterials for improved skeletal tissue regineratin. Mater Today 2018;21:362–76.

[114] Mao Y, Li P, Yin J, Bai Y, Zhou H, Lin X, Yang H, Yang L. Starch-based adhesive hydrogel with gel-point viscoelastic behavior and its application in wound sealing and hemostasis. Mater Sci Technol 2021;63:228–35. https://doi.org/10.1016/j.jmst.2020.02.071.

[115] Ounkaew A, Kasemsiri P, Jetsrisuparb K, Uyama H, Hsu Y-I, Boonmars T, Artchayasawat A, Knijnenburg JTN, Chindaprasirt P. Synthesis of nanocomposite hydrogel based carboxymethylstarch/polyvinyl alcohol/nanosilver for biomedical materials. Carbohydr Polym 2020;248. https://doi.org/10.1016/j.carbpol.2020.116767.

[116] Nieuwenhove IV, Salamon A, Adam S, Dubruel P, Vlierberghe SVF, Peterse K. Gelatin- and starch-based hydrogels. Part B: in vitro mesenchymal stem cell behavior on the hydrogels. Carbohydr Polym 2017;161:295–305. https://doi.org/10.1016/j.carbpol.2017.01.010.

[117] Deepa K, Strachota A, Slouf M, Brus J. Poly (N-isopropylacrylamide)-SiO$_2$ nanocomposites interpenetrated by starch: stimuli-responsive hydrogels with attractive tensile properties. Eur Polym J 2017;88:349–72.

[118] Batool S, Hussain Z, Niazi MBK, Liaqat U, Afzal M. Biogenic synthesis of silver nanoparticles and evaluation of physical and antimicrobial properties of Ag/PVA/starch nanocomposites hydrogel membranes for wound dressing application. J Drug Del Sci Technol 2019;52:403–14.

[119] Bagri LP, Bajpai J, Bajpai AK. Cryogenic designing of biocompatible blends of polyvinyl alcohol and starch with macroporous architecture. J Macromol Sci Pure Appl Chem A 2009;46:1060–8.

[120] Likhitkar S, Bajpai AK. Magnetically controlled release of cisplatin from superparamagnetic starch nanoparticles. Carbohydr Polym 2012;87:300–8.

[121] Mahkam M. Modified chitosan cross-linked starch polymers for oral insulin delivery. J Bioact Compat Polym 2010;25:406–18.

[122] Rositaningsih N, Budianto E. Synthesis and characterisation of starch-PVP as encapsulation material for drug delivery system. World Acad Sci Eng Technol Int J Mater Metall Eng 2017;11:1.

[123] Strachota B, Strachota A, Slouf M, Brus J, Cimrova V. Monolithic intercalated PNIPAm/starch hydrogels with very fast and extensive one-way volume and swelling responses to temperature and pH: prospective actuators and drug release systems. Soft Matter 2019. https://doi.org/10.1039/c8sm02153h. The Royal Society of Chemistry.

[124] Wohl-Bruhn S, Badar M, Bertz A, et al. Comparison of in vitro and in vivo protein release from hydrogel systems. J Control Release 2012;162:127–33.

[125] Li Y, Liu C, Tan Y, et al. In situ hydrogel constructed by starch based nanoparticles via a Schiff base reaction. Carbohydr Polym 2014;110:87–94.

[126] Saboktakin MR. Synthesis and characterization of modified starch hydrogels for photodynamic treatment of cancer. J Cancer Sci Ther 2013;5:10.

[127] Kleawkla A, Srivipak S, Threenet E, Wongputtisin P. Effect of crosslinking agent and starch contents on hydrogel from deproteinized natural rubber latex and starch. J Sci Technol 2018;10:13–8.

[128] Emad A, Jaffar Al-Mulla J. Biodegradability and thermal properties of polycaprolactone/starch nanocomposite as a biopolymer. Int J Bioeng Life Sci 2014;8:5.

[129] Thai petty patent (Patent No. 10517) BIOTEC. Kasetsart University and Chiang Mai University, Biotec News; 2018.

[130] Soe MT, Pongjanyakul T, Limpongsa E, Jaipakdeeb N. Modified glutinous rice starch-chitosan composite films for buccal delivery of hydrophilic drug. Carbohydr Polym 2020;245. 116556 Available online 18 July 2019 1359-8368/© 2019 Elsevier Ltd. All rights reserved.

4

Cyclodextrins-based hydrogel

Eva Pinho

National Institute for Agrarian and Veterinarian Research (INIAV),
Vila do Conde, Portugal

4.1 Introduction

Current pharmaceutical research, both academia and industrial, are experiencing difficulties on the discovery and development of new drugs, mainly due to the demanding, time-consuming, and expensive tasks required to put a new molecule on the market. Thus, optimization of existing formulations by enhancing their therapeutic effectiveness has been used as a viable and less costly alternative. This strategic improvement of drug delivery systems has been widely used for challenging molecules, such as hormonal, gene, or cancer therapies [1].

Cyclodextrins, truncated-shaped oligosaccharides, have taken an active role in the development of new delivery systems capable of meeting the specific needs necessary to enhance molecules' therapeutic effectiveness. Typically, they have been used as drug carriers to improve solubility, stability, and bioavailability of bioactive molecules [2]. Moreover, cyclodextrins can modulate the release of a wide range of drugs through the inclusion complex formation [3, 4]. Such versatility is augmented by their high level of biocompatibility as approved by U.S. Food and Drug Administration (FDA) for food and drug applications [5]. In recent years, the growing utilization of these molecules in pharmaceutical products has been boosted by biotechnological advances that improved the production process of cyclodextrins and their derivatives. Currently, the molecules are chemically synthesized on a large scale with high purity and reduced production costs. In fact, more than 56 medicines with cyclodextrins in their formulation are currently available on the market [6]. Most of those products are for oral, ocular, and parental administration routes, but nasal and topical products are also accessible [7, 8].

In recent years, the use of hydrogels—three-dimensional networks able to absorb high water content— as drug delivery systems has increased as a consequence of their versatility and viscoelastic properties [9]. Hydrogels' size—macro-, micro-, or nanostructures—can be tailored through chemical synthesis to meet the challenging demands of today's drug delivery systems [1]. Cyclodextrins-based hydrogels have been developed to overcome hydrogels' limitations with regard to poor loading and controlled release of drugs, especially hydrophobic molecules. Moreover, cyclodextrins can improve hydrogels' swelling capacity and benefit from the network protection, avoiding rapid inclusion complex dissolution when in contact with the physiological environment [10].

Thus, this chapter summarizes the latest research and development regarding cyclodextrins-based hydrogels for drug delivery purposes. This chapter simultaneously explores the utility of cyclodextrin as carriers and hydrogel formation as a unique approach for the development of drug delivery system. Literature concerning cyclodextrins-based hydrogels is quite extensive and highly specialized, thus cyclodextrins/cellulose hydrogels will be described with more detail. Most relevant data on the applications of cyclodextrins-based hydrogels, published in the period from 2010 to 2020, are summarized in the following sections. However, some works published before this period are also mentioned if considered fundamental.

4.2 Cyclodextrins

Cyclodextrins were described for the first time by Schardinger in 1903, but their structure and physicochemical properties were only fully detailed later in the 1940s [3]. Cyclodextrins, structurally related natural oligosaccharides, are secondary products of cellulose bacterial digestion. These cyclic oligosaccharides are composed of six, seven, or eight glucose residues linked by a (1-4) glycosidic bond, assuming a glucopyranoside units chair conformation [11]. Such a unique chemical structure results of molecules with a truncated cone shape and a microheterogeneous environment [12] (Fig. 4.1). Cyclodextrins' outer surface exhibits a hydrophilic character since the hydroxyl groups are orientated to the exterior with the primary hydroxyl groups of the sugar residues at the narrow edge and the secondary hydroxyl groups at the wider edge. The molecule's interior has a lipophilic behavior, mainly due to the skeleton of carbon and oxygen orientation (Fig. 4.1) [2].

In nature, it is possible to find cyclodextrins comprising six (α), seven (β), and eight (γ) glucopyranose units with a molecular weight range from 1000 to 2000 Da (Fig. 4.2). All three molecules share the same cavity height but have a distinguished volume and diameter. The β-cyclodextrin is the

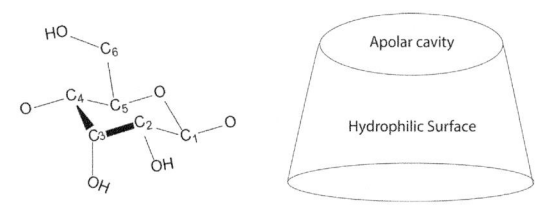

FIG. 4.1 Schematic representation of the cyclodextrin chemical structure (right) and truncated aspect (left).

most used for drug delivery purposes since it has the lowest cost production, higher availability, and enhanced inclusion complex-forming properties [6]. By chemical synthesis, other cyclodextrins can be produced at a laboratory scale with less than six and more than eight units. Indeed, depending on the transferase used during enzymatic starch degradation, starch origin, and reaction conditions, different types of cyclodextrins may be synthetized [13].

Aqueous solubility has been described as the major limitation of cyclodextrins, especially for the β-cyclodextrins (Fig. 4.2). Precipitation of solid cyclodextrins complexes occur above solubility limit. In fact, cyclodextrins in an aqueous environment are classified as homogenous molecular

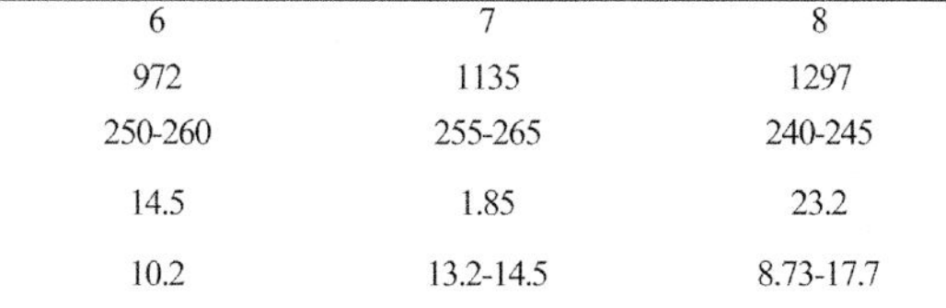

	α - cyclodextrin	β - cyclodextrin	γ - cyclodextrin
Glucose Units	6	7	8
Molecular weight	972	1135	1297
Melting Range	250-260	255-265	240-245
Water Solubility (g 100 mL^{-1}, 25°C)	14.5	1.85	23.2
Crystal water (wt %)	10.2	13.2-14.5	8.73-17.7
Water molecules in Cavity	6	11	17
Diameter (Å)	4.7-5.3	6.0-6.5	7.5-8.3
Torus Height (Å)	7.9	7.9	7.9
Cavity Volume			
Per molecule (Å)	174	252	472
Per gram (mL)	0.10	0.14	0.20
Per mol (mL)	104	157	258
Partial Molar Volume (mL mol^{-1})	611.4	703.8	801.2

FIG. 4.2 The three native cyclodextrins and their main characteristics.

dispersions due to their ability of self-association and aggregates to form micelle-like structures [14, 15]. Cyclodextrins' solubility limit is a consequence of the strong intermolecular hydrogen bonding in the crystal state. To improve cyclodextrins' solubility, several techniques have been described. For example, the addition of polymers (carbamazepine/hydroxypropyl methylcellulose) or salts (sodium acetate/benzalkonium chloride) has been used as enhancers of cyclodextrins' solubility [14, 15]. Another alternative is the use of cyclodextrins derivatives obtained by chemical modification of their hydroxyl groups or lipophilic methoxy groups [14, 15]. Each glucopyranose unit has three reactive hydroxyl groups with different ratios of reactivity and function. For example, the β-cyclodextrin allows the substitution of 21 hydroxyl groups by chemical or enzymatic reaction. Cyclodextrins derivatives can be synthesized through amination, esterification, or etherification of the primary or secondary hydroxyl groups of naturally occurring molecules (Fig. 4.3) [16].

These derivatives can be classified according to their behavior in aqueous systems, i.e., hydrophilic, hydrophobic, or ionizable derivatives (Table 4.1).

For example, hydrophilic derivatives (2,6-dimethyl-β-cyclodextrin; 2,3,6,-trimethyl-β-cyclodextrin; or 2-hydroxypropyl-β-cyclodextrin) have better solubility in water. Thus, they are suitable for inclusion complex formation with poor water-soluble molecules. Otherwise, the hydrophobic

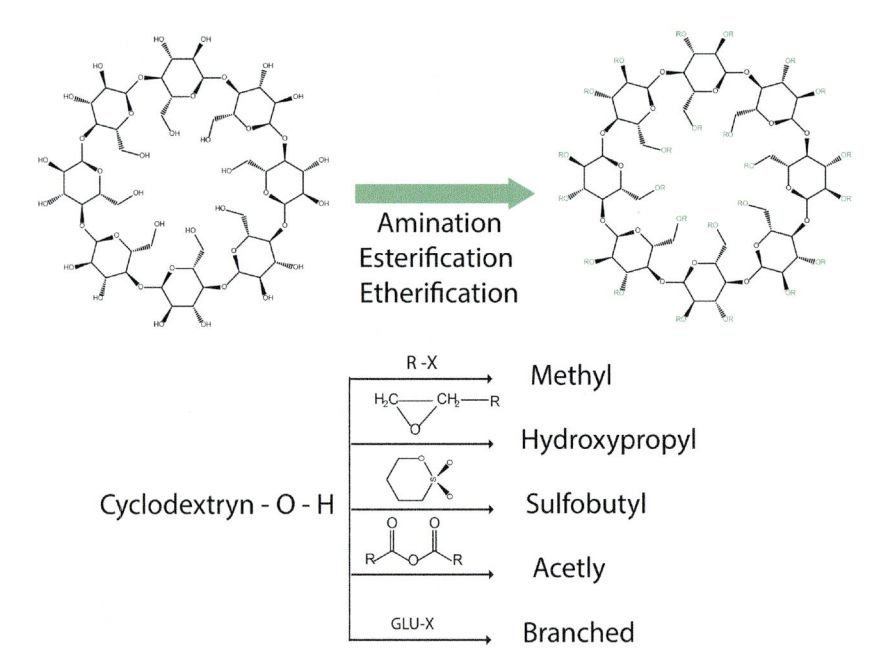

FIG. 4.3   Cyclodextrin points of modification.

TABLE 4.1 Common β-cyclodextrins derivatives used for drug delivery purposes.

CD' derivatives	Characteristic
Hydrophilic derivatives	
M-β-CD	Soluble in cold water and in organic solvents, surface active
DM-β-CD	
TM-β-CD	
DMA-β-CD	Soluble in water
Hydroxyalkylated-β-CD	
2-HE-β-CD	Amorphous mixture with different degrees of substitution, highly water-soluble (> 50%), low toxicity
2-HP-β-CD	
3-HP-β-CD	
3-HP-β-CD	
2,3-DHP-β-CD	
Branched-β-CD	
G_1-β-CD	Highly water-soluble (> 50%), low toxicity
G_2-β-CD	
GUG-β-CD	
Hydrophobic derivatives	
Alkylated-β-CD	Poorly water-soluble, soluble in organic solvents, surface-active
DE-β-CD	
TE-β-CD	
Acylated-β-CD (C2—C18)	
TA-β-CD	Poorly water-soluble, soluble in organic solvents
TV-β-CD	Film formation
Ionizable derivatives	
Anionic-β-CD	pKa = 3 to 4, soluble at pH 4
CME-β-CD	

derivatives, for example, 2,6-diethyl-β-cyclodextrin, can modulate the release rate of molecules with high solubility. The ionizable derivatives (O-carboxymethyl-O-ethyl-β-cyclodextrin, per-o-valeryl-β-cyclodextrin, or sulfate/sulfobutylether-β cyclodextrin) may improve the dissolution rate and inclusion capacity, and reduce the side effects of specific molecules. The derivatives 2-hydroxypropyl-β-cyclodextrin and the sulfobutylether-β-cyclodextrin are the most used cyclodextrin derivatives, being present in several products approved by the FDA. Because of that, their safety and physicochemical properties have been extensively characterized [17]. Otherwise, the remaining cyclodextrin derivatives need further characterization as to their biological properties and toxicity to the human body.

Cyclodextrins' chemical modifications can be beyond solubilization improvement. For example, functional groups capable of molecular recognition can be added to cyclodextrins, enabling their use as enzyme mimics, targeted drug delivery, or analytical chemistry applications [17–22].

4.2.1 Safety and regulatory status

Safety is a deal-breaker regarding molecule or polymer application in pharmaceutical formulations. Cyclodextrins' safety and toxicity profile is directly linked to the route of administration. They are considered nontoxic at low to moderate dosages when administered orally. Cyclodextrins are large hydrophilic molecules with an elevated number of hydrogen donors and acceptors. Thus, they cannot be absorbed by the gastrointestinal tract [17]. Moreover, cyclodextrins α- and β- can only be fermented by the intestinal microbiome. Otherwise, γ-cyclodextrin can be hydrolyzed by human saliva and pancreatic amylase, resembling starch and other linear dextrin metabolisms, thus only small amounts of this cyclodextrin reach the intestine [7, 12].

Regarding intravenous administration, at low dosages cyclodextrins are rapidly metabolized and are excreted intact by the kidney. Hemolytic effects have been associated with the systemic administration of cyclodextrins in several in vitro studies, but toxicological implication on in vivo studies have been considered negligible [12, 21].

Cyclodextrins' regulatory status is in continued actualization, mainly due to the new data available each year. However, regulatory agencies are still skeptical regarding its safety for pharmaceutical applications, and each agency imposes different restrictions. For example, in Japan, native cyclodextrins are classified as natural products, and their use in food or drug formulations have low limitations. In the United States, native cyclodextrins' usage in food products is regulated by the FDA and classified as "Generally Regarded as Safe" (GRAS). α-Cyclodextrin and γ-cyclodextrin can be taken without restrictions, while the oral intake of β-cyclodextrin is limited to $5\,\mathrm{mg\,kg^{-1}\,day^{-1}}$, maximum [23]. Concerning pharmaceutical applications, both the FDA and European Medicines Agency (EMA) have imposed stricter restrictions on the use of cyclodextrins. EMA recommends against the administration of α-cyclodextrin and β-cyclodextrin directly into the bloodstream due to renal toxicity. Such recommendation was made based on in vitro studies results that suggests that native cyclodextrins cause hemolysis and erythrocyte membrane destabilization since they are able to complex with phospholipids and cholesterol [24].

Nevertheless, some cyclodextrin derivatives benefits from less strict restrictions regarding their pharmaceutical application. For example, 2-hydroxypropyl-β-cyclodextrin and 2-hydroxypropyl-γ-cyclodextrin have been approved as excipients by the FDA. The 2-hydroxypropyl-β-cyclodextrin is considered nontoxic when administered in low to moderated doses. It has an improved solubility and consequently a more favorable toxicological profile when compared with the parental cyclodextrin. Moreover, sulfobutylether-β-cyclodextrin, synthetized to overcome the nephrotoxicity of the native cyclodextrin, has FDA approval for several oral and intravenous applications [25]. Otherwise, studies have reported a toxic effect after oral and intravenous administration of methylated cyclodextrin (a lipophilic derivative), mainly due to the high absorption by the gastrointestinal tract and rapid diffusion into the systemic circulation [12, 21]. Heptakis-2,3,6-tris-O-methyl-β-cyclodextrin has the classification of unsafe for humans as consequence of its hemolytic action and renal toxicity. However, heptakis-2,6-di-O-methyl-β-cyclodextrins, which exhibit liver toxicity, can be used on injectable vaccines at low concentrations, according to FDA classification. The safety profile of cyclodextrins' derivatives with random O-methylation substitutions is set by the substitution degree. For example, the EMA recommends against the use of derivatives with 1.8 methoxyl groups per glucose unit for intravenous formulations, based on its hydrolytic action and renal toxicity. In opposition, derivatives with a low degree of substitution (0.568 methoxyl groups per glucose unit) have been classified as biosafe and approved for dermal application [26, 27].

Several pharmaceutical products containing cyclodextrins are currently on the market, and examples are listed in Table 4.2. Cyclodextrins' regulatory status will be improved by the new data available and their beneficial use to treat acute and life-treating diseases, overcoming regulatory agencies' resistance.

4.3 Inclusion complex

4.3.1 Formation and stability

Cyclodextrins' distinctive molecular shape and structure (Fig. 4.1) allow it to accommodate guest molecules inside its cavity, acting as a molecular carrier [17]. Such a feature has been widely explored by the pharmaceutical industry to improve drug solubility, bioavailability, mask odors and flavors, or protect against environmental degradation (temperature, pH, light, oxidation) [6, 28].

The inclusion complex formation, i.e., the acceptance of a molecule (or part of it) into cyclodextrins' inner cavity, results from a dimensional fit between both players. The process is stabilized by no covalent bonds established or broken and by the equilibrium between the molecules in

TABLE 4.2 Pharmaceutical products containing cyclodextrins currently on the market.

Cyclodextrin	Drug	Administration route	Trade name	Market
α-Cyclodextrin	Cefotiam hexetil hydrochloride	Oral	Pansporin T	Japan
β-Cyclodextrin	Benexate hydrochloride	Oral	Ulgut, Lonmiel	Japan
	Omeprazole	Oral	Omebeta	Europe
	Piroxicam	Oral	Brexin	Europe
2-Hydroxypropyl-β-cyclodextrin	Cisapride	Rectal	Propulsid	Europe
	Itraconazole	Oral, Intravenous	Sporanox	Europe, USA
	Mitomycin	Intravenous	Mitozytrex	USA
Randomly methylated β-cyclodextrin	17b-Estradiol	Nasal drops	Aerodiol	Europe
Sulfobutylether-β-cyclodextrin	Voriconazole	Intravenous	Vfend	Europe, USA
	Ziprasidone maleate	Intramuscular	Geodon, Zeldox	Europe, USA
2 - Hydroxypropyl-γ-cyclodextrin	Diclofenac sodium	Eye drops	Voltaren	Europe

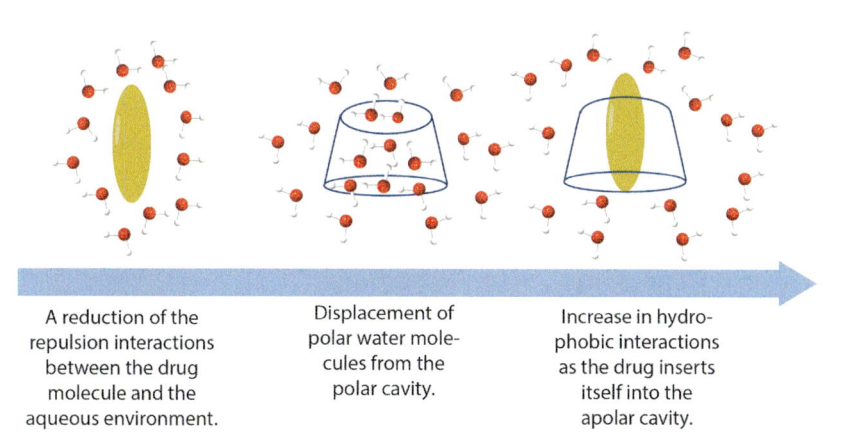

| A reduction of the repulsion interactions between the drug molecule and the aqueous environment. | Displacement of polar water molecules from the polar cavity. | Increase in hydrophobic interactions as the drug inserts itself into the apolar cavity. |

FIG. 4.4   Molecular mechanism of inclusion complex formation.

complex and in solution [29]. Once inside the cavity, the molecules suffer conformational adjustments to maximize the contribution of weak Van der Waal's forces. Other molecular interactions, such as electrostatic, hydrogen bond, or charge-transfer, are also involved in this process [17].

Therefore, the inclusion complex formation process occurs at the molecular level (Fig. 4.4) with the substitution of enthalpy-rich water molecules from the central cavity by the lipophilic molecule or part of it [30]. Two main factors dictated the success of the inclusion complex formation between cyclodextrins and a specific drug molecule. Steric is probably the most important factor since it is limited by the size ratio between cyclodextrins' cavity and molecule/moieties. This factor defines the classes of molecules that will better fit in each cyclodextrin. Although the three natural cyclodextrins have similar size, they differ in the number of glucose units and, consequently, on the cavity diameter (Fig. 4.2) [31, 32]. Hence, α-cyclodextrin is able to accommodate compounds of lower molecular weight or compounds with an aliphatic side chain. β-Cyclodextrin complex preferably with aromatic and heterocyclic molecules, and γ-cyclodextrin can establish inclusion complexes with larger molecules, such as macrocycles or steroids [2, 28].

Thermodynamic stability is the other crucial factor for the complex inclusion formation. Complexation will only occur if the system assumes a favorable energetically state when the molecule is pulled into the inner cyclodextrin hollow. As described earlier, cyclodextrins' most stable structure resembles a truncated cone with most of the hydrophobic chemical groups oriented to the interior, and both openings (larger and smaller) exhibiting hydroxyl groups to the external environment (Fig. 4.1). Four energetic mechanisms are involved in this process: (1) polar water molecules' displacement from the apolar cyclodextrin cavity, (2) increased number of hydrogen bonds formed as the displaced water returns to the larger pool, (3) repulsive interactions reduction between the drug and aqueous environment, and (4) hydrophobic interactions increased as the molecule inserts into the cyclodextrin cavity [33, 34].

Moreover, additional factors such as temperature, pH, and solvents seem to contribute to the inclusion complex formation [34]. The inclusion complex formation is a dynamic process that is stabilized when the drug and cyclodextrin reach equilibrium [2]. In fact, the inclusion complex is very stable and possesses a long shelf-life at ambient temperature and under dry conditions [35, 36]. However, it can be disrupted by a rise in temperature or by exposing the complex to water, which can replace the drug within the cyclodextrin cavity. However, this is helpful when the goal is to achieve a controlled release of the drug [37].

Several techniques have been described for the inclusion complex formation between drugs and cyclodextrins and include physical mixing, kneading method, spray drying, lyophilization, coprecipitation, solvent evaporation, neutralization precipitation, milling, and supercritical antisolvent technique. Nevertheless, the method selection must be based on drug's properties, the facilities available, and the cost involved [30].

4.3.2 Characterization

Inclusion complex formation induces physicochemical changes on the complexed molecule and on the cyclodextrin. Besides the improvement of molecules' important features, such changes are also used to characterize the inclusion complex. Alteration on solubility or chemical reactivity of the drug, after inclusion complex formation, can be determined by ultraviolet/visible spectrum (UV/VIS) absorbance, fluorescence, nuclear magnetic resonance chemical shifts, drug retention, pKa value, or potentiometric measurements. Moreover, models of artificial biological membranes have been used to assess the chemical stability and drug permeability improvement after drug complexation [23]. The aqueous medium where the inclusion complex is dispersed can also be monitored by measuring alterations on conductivity, freezing point, viscosity, or calorimetric titration. Nevertheless, the choice of the suitable method to characterize the inclusion complex formation will always depend both on the drug molecule and the cyclodextrins' physicochemical properties [23, 28].

The results obtained from these experimental measurements allow the determination of the system's stoichiometry and stability constant (K), crucial parameters for inclusion complex characterization. Stoichiometry represents the ratio between the number of drug molecules complexed with one cyclodextrin (Fig. 4.5). Most of the inclusion complexes reported have a 1:1 stoichiometry, meaning that one cyclodextrin can accommodate one drug molecule. However, the same cyclodextrin can interact with two or more drugs molecules (1:2), and one guest can complex with more than

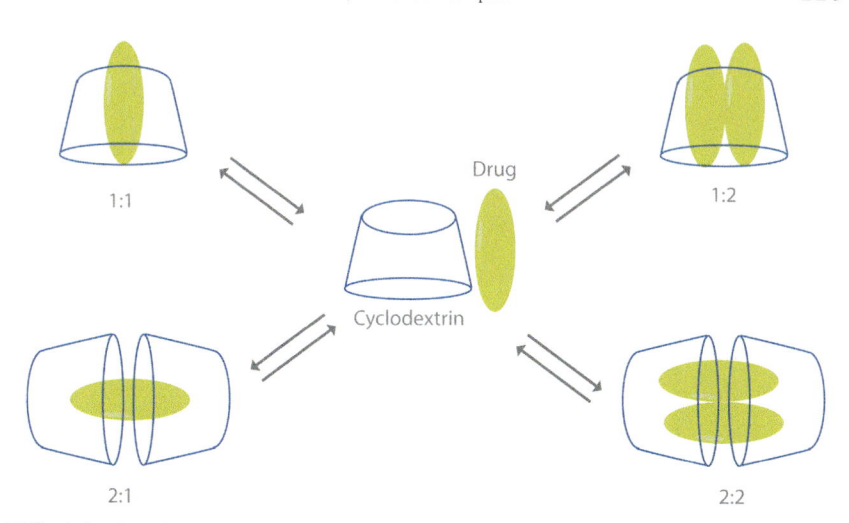

FIG. 4.5 Stoichiometry of the inclusion complexes formation between cyclodextrins and drugs molecules.

one cyclodextrin (2:1). The last case is the least frequent [28]. The stability constant represents the thermodynamic equilibrium between free and complexed molecules. A stable inclusion complex is characterized by a high stability constant. Moreover, thermodynamic parameters (enthalpy, entropy, and free Gibbs energy) must also be considered during complexation process characterization, since the temperature influences cyclodextrins' and drug molecules' interaction [34].

Phase-solubility methodology has been frequently applied to calculated inclusion complexes' stoichiometry and stability constant through plotting drug solubility against cyclodextrin concentration [28]. The methodology developed by Higuchi and Connors described phase-solubility profiles (Fig. 4.6) by establishing a relationship between the effects of the carrier (cyclodextrin) concentration on the solubility of the drug (subtract). Two phase solubility profiles can be obtained: A-type (usually for water-soluble cyclodextrins) and B-type (for natural cyclodextrins, especially β-cyclodextrin). The first is achieved for inclusion complexes where the drug solubility increases with the cyclodextrin concentration. In this situation, the complexes' solubility is greater than the noncomplexed molecules. If the increase in solubility is linear, an A_L subtype profile is obtained. For slopes lower than 1 unit, a 1:1 complex is formed. Otherwise, slopes above 1 unit are characteristic of higher order complexes. If the solubilization is more efficient at higher concentrations of the drug or cyclodextrin, then an isothermal curve with positive divergence from linearity is observed. In this case, the phase solubility profile is characterized as A_P, and a complex with first order with respect to the drug but second or higher order regarding the cyclodextrin is expected. Contrariwise, if the deviation of linearity is negative, then the phase solubility profile is A_N.

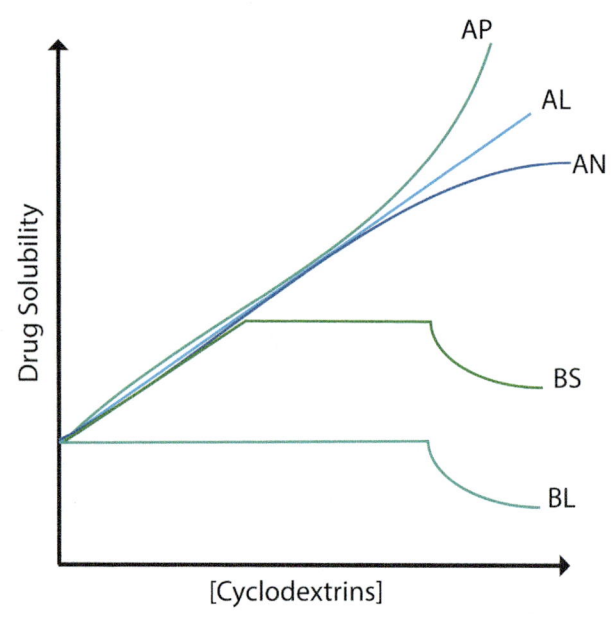

FIG. 4.6 Phase solubility diagrams and their classification according to Higuchi and Connors.

B-type complexes are indicative of inclusion complexes with limited water solubility. Two subtypes have been described. B_S profile is obtained when the cyclodextrin concentration increases and a soluble complex is formed, enhancing the substrate total solubility. The substrate total solubility increases until reaching a point in the solubilization process where the maximum solubility of the drug is achieved. Above this point, solid precipitates are formed because of the solid drug that remains uncomplexed. The B_L type is similar to B_S except that the complexes being formed are so insoluble that they do not give rise to the initial ascending component of the isotherm curve [12].

4.4 Cyclodextrin-based hydrogel

Hydrogels are three-dimensional networks formed by polymers able to absorb large amounts of solvent. Their suitable properties, such as softness, hydrophilicity, superabsorbency, viscoelasticity, biodegradability and biocompatibility, make them a material with high potential for the development of drug delivery systems [2]. Another advantage of hydrogels is the possibility of tailoring their properties through chemical synthesis conditions and the type of polymers. For example, hydrogels can be manufactured to react to different environmental stimuli like pH, temperature, electric field, magnetic field, ionic strength of solution, or biological molecules [9, 38]. Nevertheless, most of the hydrogels need covalent cross-linking or harsh environmental conditions to achieve the gel state. Thus, increasing the complexity of drug adsorption and, ultimately, impairing drug molecules' integrity which restricts their applicability as a drug delivery system [39]. Hence, the research in this area has been focused on the development of hydrogels avoiding the use of cross-linking agents on their synthesis process or the need of extreme pH or temperature granting optimal drug adsorption and delivery properties [2, 40].

Usually, the sustained release of hydrogels depends on hydrophobic interactions that result in poor control over drug loading with low selectivity and specificity. Hydrophobic domains have been integrated into the hydrogels' networks to overcome this drawback. However, it may cause alterations on hydrogels' microstructures and/or swelling properties. Another approach to improve hydrogels' drug delivery capacity is the inclusion of hydrophobic pockets into the network, for example, cyclodextrins [41]. Such structures act as drugs carriers with high specificity, offering more versatility with minor interference on hydrogels' properties. Toward this end, cyclodextrins have been extensively used to improved hydrogels' drug delivery properties [10].

Cyclodextrin-based hydrogels (Fig. 4.7) result from trapping cyclodextrins in parts of long polymers or copolymers with high molecular weights [10]. Cyclodextrins can be incorporated into the hydrogel network by two approaches: (1) as a chemical attached to the polymeric network or (2) by interaction with components of physically cross-linked hydrogels [2, 41, 42].

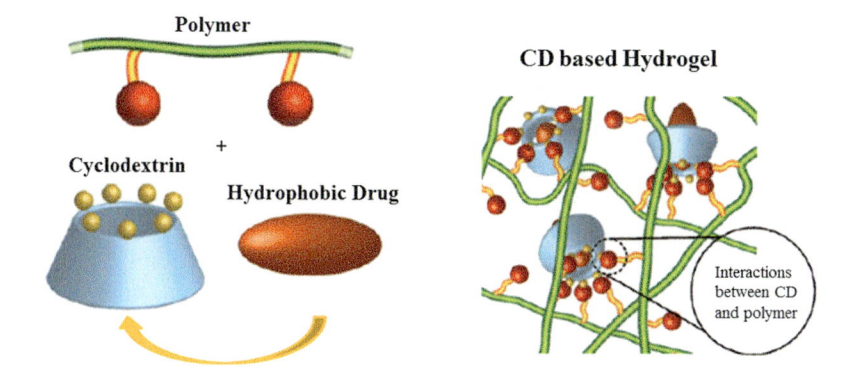

FIG. 4.7 Schematic representation of the CD-based hydrogel, where CD may have two utilities: (1) cross-linker and (2) a drug carrier.Figure adapted from Pinho E, Grootveld M, Soares G, Henriques M. Cyclodextrin-based hydrogels toward improved wound dressings. Crit Rev Biotechnol 2014;34:328–37. https://doi.org/10.3109/07388551.2013.794413.

4.4.1 Chemical hydrogels

Chemical cyclodextrin-based hydrogels are usually formed from polypseudorotaxanes or polyrotaxanes with cyclodextrins covalently attached by cross-linking agents or by modifications on the polymeric backbone [42]. For example, biodegradable polymers with hydrolyzable threads have been developed for drug and gene delivery applications [43]. The first published work describing the method to synthetize this type of supramolecular network reported the chemical cross-linking of three native cyclodextrins (α, β, and γ) with epichlorohydrin, a bifunctional cross-linking agent. It was proven that the cyclodextrins allocated on the hydrogel network were available to form a complex with a variety of poorly water-soluble drugs [2, 43]. Hydrogels' properties, such as swelling and drug-loading capacity, were enhanced and the toxicity of epichlorohydrin was reduced by performing the cross-linking in the presence of cationic or anionic compounds [2, 43]. Li and coworkers [44] synthetized a positively charged network by cross-linking β-cyclodextrin with choline chloride in the presence of epichlorohydrin. Such hydrogel was able to effectively encapsulate and release the anti-inflammatory drug naproxen, with lower toxicity compared with hydrogels without cyclodextrins [44]. Negatively charged epichlorohydrin cross-linking β-cyclodextrin networks containing carboxymethyl groups were also developed [45]. In this case, the hydrogels were loaded with cationic drugs with microbicidal properties against mucosal infections. These hydrogels were developed to be used as wound dressing or chewing gum formulations [45]. Other cross-linking agents were employed on the synthesis of cyclodextrin-based hydrogels, such as diepoxides, alkyleneglycoldi (epoxypropyl) ethers, the diisocyanate hexamethylene diisocyanate, or anhydrides [46].

Cyclodextrins derivatives (methyl-β-cyclodextrin, sulfobutylether-β-cyclodextrin or 2-hydroxypropyl-β-cyclodextrin) have been utilized frequently mainly due to the ability of these cyclodextrins to enhance hydrogels' swelling capacity [2, 46]. Water-soluble polymers have been combined with these cyclodextrins to customize mechanical properties of covalently linked networks. By adding poly(N-isopropylacrylamide) with terminal carboxyl acid groups to precross-linked β-cyclodextrin hydrogel with amine-functionalized epichlorohydrin, Nozaki et al. [47] obtained a material with temperature-dependent behavior [47].

Additionally, chemical cross-linking cyclodextrin-based hydrogels can be obtained through the use of cyclodextrins as a cross-linking agent, resulting in hydrogels with enhanced properties [2, 15, 41]. For example, a network induced by temperature was obtained through the esterification of cyclodextrins hydroxyl groups with poly(acrylic acid)'s carboxylic acid groups, resulting in the generation of an anhydride between poly(acrylic acid) chains [48]. Paradossi and coworkers [49] described the synthesis of a heterogeneous biocatalyst gel system loaded with copper(II) ions by cross-linking chitosan with an oxidized (aldehyde-containing) cyclodextrin via reductive amination [49]. An improvement of this network was reporter later [50, 51]. Taking advantage of click chemistry, a highly selective copper(I)-catalyzed 1,3-dipolar cyclo was added during hydrogel generation between an alkyne-modified cyclodextrin and an azide-functionalized poly(N-isopropylacrylamide)-co-(hydroxyethyl) methacrylate. Such methodology permitted an effective control of the gelation rate and the reaction conditions [50, 51].

Copolymerization and chemical- or radiation-mediated inductions have been frequently employed to synthesize cyclodextrin-based hydrogels [10]. Vinyl- or (meth) acryloyl-modified cyclodextrin monomers with further vinyl monomers (acrylic acid, 2 poly(N-isopropylacrylamide)-co-(hydroxyethyl) methacrylate) are, probably, the most studied combination [2, 15, 41]. For example, γ-cyclodextrin/poly(acrylic acid) systems with pH-dependent swelling properties [52] and β-cyclodextrin/maleic anhydride hydrogels with both temperature- and pH-dependent behavior [53] have been described, showing suitable properties as drug delivery materials. Moreover, maleic anhydride and poly(D,L-lactic acid), maleic anhydride-substituted block copolymer of Pluronic F68 and polycaprolactone have been exploited to produced hydrogels via radical polymerization together with cyclodextrin derivatives with controlled characteristics [43].

Another strategy used to synthesize covalently linked polymer/cyclodextrin is cross-linking cyclodextrins to reactive polymer end-groups. For example, the hydrogel obtained after cross-linking cyclodextrins to end-modified polyethylene glycol chains showed swelling properties depend on the network composition (i.e., polymer:cyclodextrin ratio). The hydrogels gather suitable properties for biomedical applications. The polymer polyethylene glycol contributed to the biocompatibility and non-immunogenicity, and the cyclodextrins add effective loading capacity of hydrophobic drugs [54, 55].

4.4.2 Physical hydrogels

Although the chemical hydrogels gather suitable properties for drug delivery purposes, the use of a cross-linking agents may cause adverse effects, such as toxicity in vivo. Thus, selected systems have been developed in which gelation is induced via complexation between cyclodextrins and polymer chains [39, 41]. Physical hydrogels are characterized by their reversible behavior since the network is stabilized by noncovalent electrostatic or hydrophobic interactions between amphiphilic polymers, by hydrogen bonding, or by stereocomplex formation between polymers with opposite chirality. This synthesis is usually executed in aqueous environments simultaneously with the drug loading, thus avowing harsh environmental conditions and favoring the application of these systems as drug delivery materials [56].

Poly(D,L-lactic acid), polyethylene glycol, and poly(phenylene oxide) are the most common polymers used to produce physical cyclodextrins-based hydrogels [41]. Polyethylene glycol is the most widely employed due to its biocompatibility, biodegradability, and hydrophilicity, properties that render the network suitable for biomedical applications [39]. A α-cyclodextrin/polyethylene glycol and its copolymers have been applied to synthesize hydrogels for the medical field [57]. Moreover, modifications to these materials were made to improve their physicochemical and biocompatible properties [39, 57]. For example, the hydrogel obtained by the triblock polyethylene glycol-poly(phenylene oxide)-polyethylene glycol displayed weak physical interactions between chains in aqueous environments, as a consequence of the hydrophilic behavior of polyethylene glycol. Thus, this copolymer was unsuitable for long-term drug release applications. However, when cyclodextrins were used as a trap to polyethylene glycol segments, the polymer hydrophobicity was modified, and lower polymer concentration was required to achieve the gel state. Also, this cyclodextrin-based hydrogel had thermoreversible behavior [39]. The use of polyhydroxybutyrate, an optically active and biodegradable polyester with high crystallinity and hydrophobic properties, instead of poly(phenylene oxide), improved the biodegradability of the network. Furthermore, an increase in the copolymer stability was observed, mainly due to the complementation of the complexation between the α-cyclodextrin and polyethylene glycol with hydrophobic interactions between the mid-placed polyhydroxybutyrate blocks. Thus, this copolymer (α-cyclodextrin/polyethylene glycol-polyhydroxybutyrate-polyethylene glycol) is a thyrotrophic and reversible supramolecular hydrogel able to sustain the release of macromolecular drugs for long periods without a requirement for postapplication removal since it is biodegradable [39, 41, 43]. Similar results were reported for the copolymer α-cyclodextrin/polyethylene glycol-polycaprolactone [39, 41, 43]. Polycaprolactone is an amphiphilic biodegradable copolymer that competed with the polyethylene glycol complexation with the cyclodextrin. The reversible properties of these physical hydrogels result from the entropically unfavorable inclusion complex between the polymer and the cyclodextrin. Therefore, changes in the environmental conditions, such as temperature or pH values, can induce dissociation of the polymer from the cyclodextrins [43]. Both works sustained the possibility of developing physical hydrogels stabilized by the inclusion complex formation between biopolymers and cyclodextrins for drug delivery applications without compromising their biocompatibility [39, 41, 43].

4.4.3 Mechanisms of drug delivery

Cyclodextrins-based hydrogels drug delivery is highly dependent on the swelling and release properties of the polymeric network and on the inclusion complex stability between cyclodextrins and the drug. These materials' drug delivery capacities are set by the following process: solvent transport into the polymeric matrix, polymer swelling, solute diffusion and erosion/relaxation of the swollen polymer, and inclusion complex dissolution [58–60]. In fact, several studies had proven that the use of cyclodextrins on the polymeric hydrogel benefits their drug delivery properties [39, 58, 61].

Mathematical models, combined with experimental observations, have been used to provide new insights into the release mechanism of cyclodextrins-based hydrogels. This theoretical approach predicts the temporal release of the drug molecules trapped in cyclodextrins' cavity and the hydrogel network [58, 62]. Thus, the mathematical models support the optimal design of pharmaceutical formulations by clarifying the release mechanisms through experimental verification [58, 62]. Most of the existing models are established upon diffusion equations since drugs diffusion is a strong function of the structure through which the release takes place [58, 63, 64].

Korsmeyer-Peppas model (Eq. 4.1) is a simple and semiempirical model that relates drug release with elapsed time [65].

$$\frac{M_t}{M_\infty} = k_{KP} t^n \tag{4.1}$$

where t is the release time (min), M_t is the amount of drug delivered at time t, M_∞ is the total amount of drug delivered, k_{KP} is a kinetic constant, and the diffusional exponent, n, gives an indication of the mechanism of drug release and takes various values depending on the geometry of the release device [66]. The value of n equals 0.5 for the Fickian diffusion, 0.5–1.0 for the anomalous (non-Fickian) transport (i.e., a mixed diffusion and chain relaxation mechanisms), and 1.0 means a Case II transport (zero order), which reflects the influence of polymer relaxation on the drug movement within the matrix. Values of n greater than 1 result in what some authors called Super Case II-transport [65]. To determine these constants, the first 60% of drug release data are fitted to Eq. (4.1), since it has been described that, for Fickian release, the best-fitting corresponds to the first 60% of the fractional release. This simple semiempirical equation can be used to express drug release from swellable polymers [66].

Higuchi developed several theoretical models to study the drug release [67]. In summary, a simplified **Higuchi model** can be expressed as Eq. (4.2):

$$\frac{M_t}{M_\infty} = k_H t^{0.5} \tag{4.2}$$

where k_H is the Higuchi diffusion constant. This model shows good correlation in the release profiles whose predominant mechanism is simple Fickian diffusion. Using the simplified Higuchi model [58], diffusional coefficients can be determined according to Eq. (4.3):

$$q = 2C_0 \left(\frac{Dt}{\pi} \right)^{0.5} \tag{4.3}$$

where q is the amount of drug released into the medium per unit area of exposure ($mg\,cm^{-2}$), C_0 is the amount of drug loaded per unit volume of disc ($mg\,cm^{-3}$), D is the apparent diffusion coefficient of drug ($cm^2\,s^{-1}$), and t represents the time elapsed since the start of drug release.

Zero order kinetic model is expressed as Eq. (4.4):

$$\frac{M_t}{M_\infty} = k_0 t \tag{4.4}$$

where M_t/M_∞ is the fractional drug release, and k_0 is the zero order release constant. The release profiles that present a better fit to this model generally agree with those that show a Case II transport mechanism in the Korsmeyer-Peppas model [58].

A standardized version of the first order kinetic model can be expressed as Eq. (4.5) [58]:

$$\frac{M_t}{M_\infty} = 1 - e^{-k_1 t} \tag{4.5}$$

where k_1 is the first order release constant. This model shows good correlations in the release profiles whose predominant mechanism is simple diffusion anomalous behavior.

The contribution of Fickian and non-Fickian release can be evaluated by using the Peppas-Sahlin model Eq. (4.6) [49]:

$$\frac{M_t}{M_\infty} = k_D t^m + k_R t^{2m} \tag{4.6}$$

where M_t and M_∞ are the absolute cumulative amount of drug released at time (t, minute) and infinite time, and k_D (diffusional constant), k_R, and m are constants [68]. This release kinetics model considers the diffusional and relaxational mechanism associated with the anomalous drug-release process of hydrogels [69]. Considering the right side of Eq. (4.1), the first term calculates the molecular diffusion of the drug as a consequence of the chemical potential gradient, Fickian contribution (F). The second term represents the Case II relaxation contribution (R), set by the stress and state-transition of swelling-controlled drug release [9, 59, 70].

4.5 Cyclodextrin/cellulose hydrogels

Research on hydrogels has taken advantage of the synergetic properties of cyclodextrins and cellulose to develop several drug delivery systems [71–75]. These systems combine the adsorption and wettability properties of cellulose with cyclodextrins' ability to form an inclusion complex with a wide range of molecules [71–75]. Cyclodextrins can be used as monomers of the cellulose hydrogel or as a cross-linking agent; in both cases, cyclodextrins' cavity must be available to interact with the drug molecule [74].

Cellulose and their derivatives, as a sustainable and versatile material for drug delivery, have experienced increased interest by researchers and the pharmaceutical industry [76]. It is a unique polymer with suitable properties for pharmaceutical applications, such as availability, mechanical robustness, stability, hydrophilicity, and biodegradability, yet with low cost [77–81].

4.5.1 Cellulose structure

Cellulose is a natural polymer of glucose with a structural function on plants [82]. This polymer can also be synthetized by some bacteria strains for cell protection or adhesion [83, 84]. Plant and bacteria cellulose share the same chemical structure, diverging on the physical properties and macromolecular structure [85–87]. The cellulose building blocks, β-1,4-D (+)-glucopyranose, are linked by 1,4-glycosidic bonds creating the long cellulose chain. These bonds control the steric events that prevent the free rotation of the anhydroglucose-pyranose. Each building block has three hydroxyl groups, one primary on C6 and two secondaries on C2 and C3. The abundancy of hydroxyl groups and the chain conformation enable a complex hydrogen bond network, between and within the cellulose chains, contributing to the cellulose's excellent mechanical properties as well as to its susceptibility to crystallization [83, 88–90]. This chemical structure is also accountable for the hydrophilic behavior of cellulose and consequently its high surface energy, biodegradability, thermal stability, and chemical reactiveness [91, 92]. According to its origin, isolation, or processing, cellulose assumes different crystallization states being classified as a polymorph material [93].

Modifications on cellulose have been synthetized over the past years to amplify its application in the materials field. The main chemical reactions for cellulose modification are: (1) esterification, (2) etherification, (3) replacement of the hydroxyl groups by amine or halogen groups, (4) replacement of hydrogen molecules by sodium, (5) oxidation, or (6) addition compounds with acids, bases, and salts (Fig. 4.8) [89, 94–96]. These modifications will only affect the terminal groups or individual members without

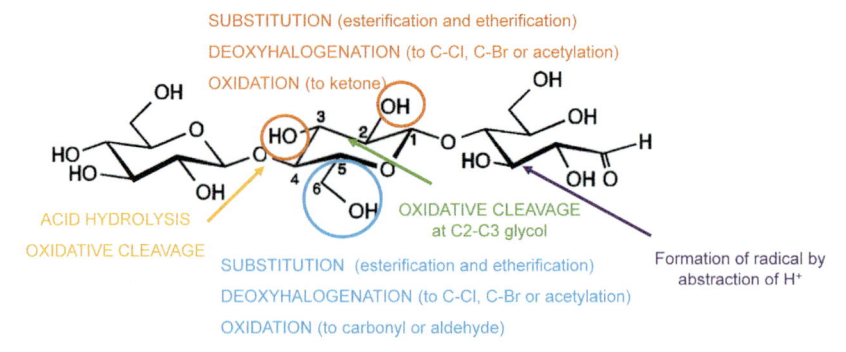

FIG. 4.8   Cellulose chemical structure and chemical reactions sites.Adapted from Pinho E, Soares G. Functionalization of cotton cellulose for improved wound healing. J Mater Chem B 2018;6:1887–98. https://doi.org/10.1039/c8tb00052b.

breaking down the chain. Thus, the effect on cellulose physiochemical properties is minimal [89, 94]. However, chemical reactions targeting the degradation of the main chain (hydrolysis or glycosidic bonds oxidation) have also been applied with the expense of polymer stability [76].

Current research on the application of cellulose for drug delivery comprises several formulations, such as nanoparticles [97], microparticles [98], tablets [99], transdermal drug delivery systems [99], and hydrogels [33, 98, 100–104].

As mentioned earlier, the abundant hydroxyl groups of cellulose are the prime targets for modification, including hydrogel synthetization, given rise to wide range of structures with fascinating properties. Cellulose-based hydrogels can be achieved by the chemical or physical stabilization of cellulosic materials in aqueous solutions. Moreover, cellulose can be combined with synthetic or natural polymers to obtain hydrogels with tailored properties [105]. Such materials gather suitable properties for drug delivery applications such as hydrophilic/hydrophobic character, elasticity, water absorption capacity, adhesive features, adsorption or ion exchange skills, and thermal, optical, and mechanical resistance [106]. Moreover, cellulose and its derivatives-based hydrogels have been developed and optimized to meet the challenging needs of the pharmaceutical industry. For example, stimuli-responsive hydrogels capable of behavior modification (swelling or deswelling, jellification) in response to environmental stimuli, such as temperature and pH, have been developed [107].

4.5.2 Cyclodextrins/cellulose hydrogels on drug delivery

Cellulose and cyclodextrins as pharmaceutical excipients for drug delivery systems have experienced increased interest mainly driven by the consumer demand for natural and friendly materials, as well as their ability of sustained drug release [25, 100]. Hydrogels obtained from the combination of cyclodextrins and cellulose allows modulation of the drug loading and releasing, offering distinct mechanics to regulate the release profiles by controlling the synthesis parameters [25, 100].

Zhang and coworkers developed a method to synthesize β-cyclodextrin/cellulose hydrogels by chemical cross-linking [100]. The hydrogel synthesis was performed in basic solution (sodium hydroxide and urea) using epichlorohydrin as a cross-linking agent [100]. Hydrogels' swelling degree and, consequently, water uptake were inversely proportional to the cyclodextrin concentration. The drug loading and release properties of the developed polymeric network was assessed for 5-fluorouracil, bovine serum albumin, or aniline blue. The inclusion complexation of 5-fluorouracil with β-cyclodextrin prevented its release, and weak interactions were reported between bovine serum albumin and β-cyclodextrin. Otherwise, the complexation of aniline blue induced an increase of fluorescence [100]. A similar hydrogel was prepared by Rodriguez-Tenreiro and coworkers [108]. The cyclodextrin-based hydrogel synthesis was performed with only one step, using condensation with ethylene glycol diglycidyl ether to obtain polymeric networks, under mild environmental conditions, and without previous modification on the cyclodextrins structure. Cyclodextrins-based hydrogels synthesized by this method showed good swelling and mechanical properties, and enhanced ability to load and release bioactive molecules [108–112].

Similar hydrogels were prepared by Pinho and coworkers [33, 101]. β-Cyclodextrin and 2-hydroxypropyl-β-cyclodextrin were used to produce cyclodextrin-based hydrogel using hydroxypropyl methylcellulose and were cross-linked with 1,4-butanediol diglycidyl ether. This cellulose derivative has been used in this type of hydrogel due to its high swelling ability and biocompatibility [59, 113]. Hydrogels produced under alkaline pH and mild temperature avoid toxic by-products from undesirable side reactions associated with high temperatures [101]. The hydrogels obtained combine good physicochemical properties (viscoelasticity, superabsorbency) and high ability to retain and deliver phenolic acids with the preservation of gallic and caffeic acid antibacterial activity and effect on fibroblasts, regardless of the cyclodextrin used (β-cyclodextrin or 2-hydroxypropyl-β-cyclodextrin) [33, 101]. A hydrogel with pH-sensitive swelling behavior was reported by adding chitosan to cyclodextrin-hydroxypropyl methylcellulose hydrogels [9]. Chitosan-based hydrogels show a typical pH-sensitive swelling, being swollen in an acidic medium due to the protonated amine group's repulsion and shrinking in neutral and alkaline medium, influenced by the unprotonated amine groups [9]. The synthetized hydrogels (cyclodextrin-chitosan-cellulose) delivery capacity was pH-dependent and was more efficient at pH 7. Based on the Peppas-Sahlin model, Fickian diffusion was the main mechanism responsible for caffeic acid release [9].

Modified chitosan, combined with hydroxyethyl cellulose and sulfobutylether-β-cyclodextrin, was used in the synthesis of a three-dimensional double-network hydrogel [114]. Phenolphthalein was used as a drug model to assess the adsorption and releasing ability of the developed hydrogel for hydrophobic molecules. It was rapidly absorbed by the hydrogel mainly due to the cyclodextrin inclusion complex formation. Phenolphthalein releases was also fast as a consequence of the ion-exchange interactions of the polymers on the network [114].

Huang and coworkers [115] reported an in situ hydrogel for oral administration with a zero order release kinetic of glipizide used as drug model. The hydrogel network was constituted by hydroxypropyl cellulose and β-cyclodextrin. The gel state was achieved when in contact with the gastrointestinal fluid. In accordance with the other works mentioned before, the inclusion complex formation formed between β-cyclodextrin and glipizide improved the drug solubility at different pH values [115].

Supramolecular hydrogels combining cellulose nanocrystals, β-cyclodextrins, and poly(ethylene oxide)-poly(propylene oxide)-poly(ethylene oxide) were prepared to study the release profile of this network type. Using doxorubicin hydrochloride as a drug model, Lin and Dufreene [116] characterized the release mechanism of poly(ethylene oxide)-poly(propylene oxide)-poly(ethylene oxide)/α-cyclodextrin hydrogels. It was observed a drug release behavior fitting the Fickian diffusion when Ritger-Peppas equation was used [116]. Similar work using modified cellulose nanocrystals and poly(ethylene oxide)-poly(propylene oxide)-poly(ethylene oxide)/β-cyclodextrin hydrogels reported an anomalous release mechanism of doxorubicin hydrochloride [99, 116]. Malik and coworkers [117] optimized the synthesis hydrogels obtained from the combination of β-cyclodextrin, modified cellulose nanocrystals, acrylic acid, and $N'N'$-methylene bis-acrylamide by free radical polymerization. This complex network was able to successfully deliver acyclovir, an antiviral drug. Nevertheless, a better release profile was observed for the polymeric network with highest content of acrylic acid at pH 7.4, a cumulative drug release of 96% was obtained. A pH-dependent swelling was also reported for this hydrogel [117].

Additionally, a supramolecular hydrogel resulting from the physical assembly of poly(ethylene oxide)-poly(propylene oxide)-poly(ethylene oxide), hydroxyethyl cellulose, and α-cyclodextrin was produced to enhance the solubilization and release of griseofulvin, an antifungal drug [118]. The cyclodextrin used was capable of forming supramolecular structures with both polymers, poly(ethylene oxide)-poly(propylene oxide)-poly(ethylene oxide) and hydroxyethyl cellulose. The cyclodextrins present on the polymeric network improved the drug solubilization and avoided phase separation. The rheological and bioadhesive properties of developed complex network could be tailored by changing the ratio of the polymers. Moreover, this ternary supramolecular hydrogel was able to sustain the release of several drugs for long periods of time with enhanced biocompatibility [118].

4.6 Conclusion

Hydrogels provide major benefits as drug delivery systems mainly due to their versatility and viscoelastic properties. However, regarding their drug delivery applications, the trapping of low to moderately hydrophobic bioactive molecules is not very efficient, and their release is rapid and nonlinear over time. Cyclodextrins can form inclusion complexes with a wide range of bioactive molecules and also with polymers. Cyclodextrins can act, simultaneously, as therapeutic agent carriers and as enhancers of favorable hydrogel properties in biosystems. Therefore, cyclodextrin-based hydrogels are a viable option for the development of optimized drug delivery systems.

References

[1] Otero-Espinar FJ, Torres-Labandeira JJ, Alvarez-Lorenzo C, Blanco-Méndez J. Cyclodextrins in drug delivery systems. J Drug Deliv Sci Technol 2010;20:289–301. https://doi.org/10.1016/S1773-2247(10)50046-7.

[2] Pinho E, Grootveld M, Soares G, Henriques M. Cyclodextrin-based hydrogels toward improved wound dressings. Crit Rev Biotechnol 2014;34:328–37. https://doi.org/10.3 109/07388551.2013.794413.

[3] Loftsson T, Brewster ME. Pharmaceutical applications of cyclodextrins: basic science and product development. J Pharm Pharmacol 2010;62:1607–21. https://doi. org/10.1111/j.2042-7158.2010.01030.x.

[4] Popielec A, Loftsson T. Effects of cyclodextrins on the chemical stability of drugs. Int J Pharm 2017;531:532–42. https://doi.org/10.1016/j.ijpharm.2017.06.009.

[5] Shulman M, Cohen M, Soto-Gutierrez A, Yagi H, Wang H, Goldwasser J, et al. Enhancement of naringenin bioavailability by complexation with hydroxypropoyl-β-cyclodextrin. PLoS ONE 2011;6. https://doi.org/10.1371/journal.pone.0018033.

[6] Crini G, Fourmentin S, Fenyvesi É, Torri G, Fourmentin M, Morin-Crini N. Cyclodextrins, from molecules to applications. Environ Chem Lett 2018;16:1361–75. https://doi.org/10.1007/s10311-018-0763-2.

[7] Gidwani B, Vyas A. A comprehensive review on cyclodextrin-based carriers for delivery of chemotherapeutic cytotoxic anticancer drugs. Biomed Res Int 2015;2015. https://doi.org/10.1155/2015/198268.

[8] Muankaew C, Loftsson T. Cyclodextrin-based formulations: a non-invasive platform for targeted drug delivery. Basic Clin Pharmacol Toxicol 2018;122:46–55. https://doi. org/10.1111/bcpt.12917.

[9] Pinho E, Machado S, Soares G. Smart hydrogel for the pH-selective drug delivery of antimicrobial compounds. Macromol Symp 2019;385:1–7. https://doi.org/10.1002/ masy.201800182.

[10] Alvarez-Lorenzo C, Moya-Ortega MD, Loftsson T, Concheiro A, Torres-Labandeira JJ. Cyclodextrin-based hydrogels. Cyclodextrins Pharm Cosmet Biomed Curr Futur Ind Appl 2011;297–321. https://doi.org/10.1002/9780470926819.ch16.

[11] Zhu C, Krumm C, Facas GG, Neurock M, Dauenhauer PJ. Energetics of cellulose and cyclodextrin glycosidic bond cleavage. React Chem Eng 2017;2:201–14. https://doi.org/10.1039/C6RE00176A.

[12] Jambhekar SS, Breen P. Cyclodextrins in pharmaceutical formulations I: structure and physicochemical properties, formation of complexes, and types of complex. Drug Discov Today 2016;21:356–62. https://doi.org/10.1016/j.drudis.2015.11.017.

[13] Crini G, Fourmentinn S, Lichtfouse E. Cyclodextrin fundamentals. React Anal 2018. https://doi.org/10.1007/978-3-319-76159-6.

[14] Zhang X, Zhang C, Sun G, Xu X, Tan Y, Wu H, et al. Cyclodextrins and their derivatives in the resolution of chiral natural products: a review. Instrum Sci Technol 2012;40:194–215. https://doi.org/10.1080/10739149.2011.651675.

[15] Zhang J, Ma PX. Cyclodextrin-based supramolecular systems for drug delivery: recent progress and future perspective. Adv Drug Deliv Rev 2013;65:1215–33. https://doi.org/10.1016/j.addr.2013.05.001.

[16] Loftsson T, Duchêne D. Cyclodextrins and their pharmaceutical applications. Int J Pharm 2007;329:1–11. https://doi.org/10.1016/j.ijpharm.2006.10.044.

[17] Sharma N, Baldi A. Exploring versatile applications of cyclodextrins: an overview. Drug Deliv 2016;23:739–57. https://doi.org/10.3109/10717544.2014.938839.

[18] Del Valle EMM. Cyclodextrins and their uses: a review. Process Biochem 2004;39:1033–46. https://doi.org/10.1016/S0032-9592(03)00258-9.

[19] Duan MS, Zhao N, Össurardóttir ÍB, Thorsteinsson T, Loftsson T. Cyclodextrin solubilization of the antibacterial agents triclosan and triclocarban: formation of aggregates and higher-order complexes. Int J Pharm 2005;297:213–22. https://doi.org/10.1016/j.ijpharm.2005.04.007.

[20] Senti G, Iannaccone R, Graf N, Felder M, Tay F, Kündig T. A randomized, double-blind, placebo-controlled study to test the efficacy of topical 2-hydroxypropyl-beta-cyclodextrin in the prophylaxis of recurrent herpes Labialis. Dermatology 2013;226:247–52. https://doi.org/10.1159/000349991.

[21] Mellet CO, Fernández JMG, Benito JM. Cyclodextrin-based gene delivery systems. Chem Soc Rev 2011;40:1586–608. https://doi.org/10.1039/c0cs00019a.

[22] Liu Y, Song Y, Chen Y, Li XQ, Ding F, Zhong RQ. Biquinolino-modified β-cyclodextrin dimers and their metal complexes as efficient fluorescent sensors for the molecular recognition of steroids. Chem - A Eur J 2004;10:3685–96. https://doi.org/10.1002/chem.200305724.

[23] Braga SS. Cyclodextrins: emerging medicines of the new millennium. Biomol Ther 2019;9. https://doi.org/10.3390/biom9120801.

[24] EMA. Background review for cyclodextrins used as excipients In the context of the revision of the guideline on Excipients in the label and. Ema 2014;44.

[25] Muankaew C, Loftsson T. Cyclodextrin-based formulations: a non-invasive platform for targeted drug delivery. Basic Clin Pharmacol Toxicol 2018;122:46–55. https://doi.org/10.1111/bcpt.12917.

[26] Kiss T, Fenyvesi F, Bácskay I, Váradi J, Fenyvesi É, Iványi R, et al. Evaluation of the cytotoxicity of β-cyclodextrin derivatives: evidence for the role of cholesterol extraction. Eur J Pharm Sci 2010;40:376–80. https://doi.org/10.1016/j.ejps.2010.04.014.

[27] Szente L, Singhal A, Domokos A, Song B. Cyclodextrins: assessing the impact of cavity size, occupancy, and substitutions on cytotoxicity and cholesterol homeostasis. Molecules 2018;23:1–15. https://doi.org/10.3390/molecules23051228.

[28] Pinho E, Grootveld M, Soares G, Henriques M. Cyclodextrins as encapsulation agents for plant bioactive compounds. Carbohydr Polym 2014;101:121–35. https://doi.org/10.1016/j.carbpol.2013.08.078.

[29] Pinho E, Soares G, Henriques M. Evaluation of antibacterial activity of caffeic acid encapsulated by β-cyclodextrins. J Microencapsul 2015;32:804–10. https://doi.org/10.3109/02652048.2015.1094531.

[30] Marques HMC. A review on cyclodextrin encapsulation of essential oils and volatiles. Flavour Fragr J 2010;25:313–26. https://doi.org/10.1002/ffj.2019.

[31] Messner M, Kurkov SV, Jansook P, Loftsson T. Self-assembled cyclodextrin aggregates and nanoparticles. Int J Pharm 2010;387:199–208. https://doi.org/10.1016/j.ijpharm.2009.11.035.

[32] Nardello-Rataj V, Leclercq L. Encapsulation of biocides by cyclodextrins: toward synergistic effects against pathogens. Beilstein J Org Chem 2014;10:2603–22. https://doi.org/10.3762/bjoc.10.273.

[33] Pinho E, Henriques M, Soares G. Caffeic acid loading wound dressing: physicochemical and biological characterization. Ther Deliv 2014;5:1063–75. https://doi.org/10.4155/tde.14.77.

[34] Pinho E, Soares G, Henriques M. Cyclodextrin modulation of gallic acid in vitro antibacterial activity. J Incl Phenom Macrocycl Chem 2015;81:205–14. https://doi.org/10.1007/s10847-014-0449-8.

[35] Gim SY, Jung JY, Kwon YJ, Kim MJ, Kim GH, Lee JH. Application of β-cyclodextrin, chitosan, and collagen on the stability of tocopherols and the oxidative stability in heated oils. Eur J Lipid Sci Technol 2017;119:1–9. https://doi.org/10.1002/ejlt.201700124.

[36] Wadhwa G, Kumar S, Chhabra L, Mahant S, Rao R. Essential oil–cyclodextrin complexes: an updated review. J Incl Phenom Macrocycl Chem 2017;89:39–58. https://doi.org/10.1007/s10847-017-0744-2.

[37] Jug M, Beæireviæ-laæan M. Cyclodextrin-based pharmaceuticals. Med Sci 2008;9–26.

[38] Rizwan M, Yahya R, Hassan A, Yar M, Azzahari AD, Selvanathan V, et al. pH sensitive hydrogels in drug delivery: brief history, properties, swelling, and release mechanism, material selection and applications. Polymers (Basel) 2017;9. https://doi.org/10.3390/polym9040137.

[39] Li J. Self-assembled supramolecular hydrogels based on polymer-cyclodextrin inclusion complexes for drug delivery. NPG Asia Mater 2010;2:112–8. https://doi.org/10.1038/asiamat.2010.84.

[40] Zou H, Guo W, Yuan W. Supramolecular hydrogels from inclusion complexation of α-cyclodextrin with densely grafted chains in micelles for controlled drug and protein release. J Mater Chem B 2013;1:6235. https://doi.org/10.1039/c3tb21181a.

[41] Arslan M, Sanyal R, Sanyal A. Cyclodextrin-containing hydrogel networks. Encycl Biomed Polym Polym Biomater 2016;2243–58. https://doi.org/10.1081/e-ebpp-120050543.

[42] Yao X, Huang P, Nie Z. Cyclodextrin-based polymer materials: from controlled synthesis to applications. Prog Polym Sci 2019;93:1–35. https://doi.org/10.1016/j.progpolymsci.2019.03.004.

[43] Chen G, Jiang M. Cyclodextrin-based inclusion complexation bridging supramolecular chemistry and macromolecular self-assembly. Chem Soc Rev 2011;40:2254–66. https://doi.org/10.1039/c0cs00153h.

[44] Li J, Xiao H, Li J, Zhong Y. Drug carrier systems based on water-soluble cationic β-cyclodextrin polymers. Int J Pharm 2004;278:329–42. https://doi.org/10.1016/j.ijpharm.2004.03.026.

[45] Dos Santos JFR, Torres-Labandeira JJ, Matthijs N, Coenye T, Concheiro A, Alvarez-Lorenzo C. Functionalization of acrylic hydrogels with α-, β- or γ-cyclodextrin modulates protein adsorption and antifungal delivery. Acta Biomater 2010;6:3919–26. https://doi.org/10.1016/j.actbio.2010.04.013.

[46] Van De Manakker F, Vermonden T, Van Nostrum CF, Hennink WE. Cyclodextrin-based polymeric materials: synthesis, properties, and pharmaceutical/biomedical applications. Biomacromolecules 2009;10.

[47] Nozaki T, Maeda Y, Kitano H. Cyclodextrin gels which have a temperature responsiveness. J Polym Sci Part A Polym Chem 1997;35:1535–41. https://doi.org/10.1002/(SICI)1099-0518(199706)35:8<1535::AID-POLA22>3.0.CO;2-7.

[48] Bibby DC, Davies NM, Tucker IG. Investigations into the structure and composition of β-cyclodextrin/poly(acrylic acid) microspheres. Int J Pharm 1999;180:161–8. https://doi.org/10.1016/S0378-5173(99)00004-6.

[49] Paradossi G, Cavalieri F, Crescenzi V. 1H NMR relaxation study of a chitosan-cyclodextrin network. Carbohydr Res 1997;300:77–84. https://doi.org/10.1016/S0008-6215(97)00023-2.

[50] Rostovtsev VV, Green LG, Fokin VV, Sharpless KB. A stepwise huisgen cycloaddition process: copper(I)-catalyzed regioselective "ligation" of azides and terminal alkynes. Angew Chem Int Ed 2002;41:2596–9. https://doi.org/10.1002/1521-3773(20020715)41:14<2596::AID-ANIE2596>3.0.CO;2-4.

[51] Tornøe CW, Christensen C, Meldal M. Peptidotriazoles on solid phase: [1,2,3]-Triazoles by regiospecific copper(I)-catalyzed 1,3-dipolar cycloadditions of terminal alkynes to azides. J Organomet Chem 2002;67:3057–64. https://doi.org/10.1021/jo011148j.

[52] Siemoneit U, Schmitt C, Alvarez-Lorenzo C, Luzardo A, Otero-Espinar F, Concheiro A, et al. Acrylic/cyclodextrin hydrogels with enhanced drug loading and sustained release capability. Int J Pharm 2006;312:66–74. https://doi.org/10.1016/j.ijpharm.2005.12.046.

[53] Liu Y, Fan X. Synthesis, properties and controlled release behaviors of hydrogel networks using cyclodextrin as pendant groups. Biomaterials 2005;26:6367–74. https://doi.org/10.1016/j.biomaterials.2005.04.011.

[54] Cesteros LC, Ramírez CA, Pecina A, Katime I. Synthesis and properties of hydrophilic networks based on poly(ethylene glycol) and β-cyclodextrin. Macromol Chem Phys 2007;208:1764–72. https://doi.org/10.1002/macp.200700109.

[55] Salmaso S, Semenzato A, Bersani S, Matricardi P, Rossi F, Caliceti P. Cyclodextrin/PEG based hydrogels for multi-drug delivery. Int J Pharm 2007;345:42–50. https://doi.org/10.1016/j.ijpharm.2007.05.035.

[56] Ahmed EM. Hydrogel: preparation, characterization, and applications: a review. J Adv Res 2015;6:105–21. https://doi.org/10.1016/j.jare.2013.07.006.

[57] Estévez CA, Isasi JR, Larrañeta E, Vélaz I. Release of β-galactosidase from poloxamine/α-cyclodextrin hydrogels. Beilstein J Org Chem 2014;10:3127–35. https://doi.org/10.3762/bjoc.10.330.

[58] Machín R, Isasi JR, Vélaz I. Hydrogel matrices containing single and mixed natural cyclodextrins. Mechanisms of drug release. Eur Polym J 2013;49:3912–20. https://doi.org/10.1016/j.eurpolymj.2013.08.020.

[59] Siepmann J, Peppas NA. Modeling of drug release from delivery systems based on hydroxypropyl methylcellulose (HPMC). Adv Drug Deliv Rev 2001;48:139–57. https://doi.org/10.1016/S0169-409X(01)00112-0.

[60] Lin CC, Metters AT. Hydrogels in controlled release formulations: network design and mathematical modeling. Adv Drug Deliv Rev 2006;58:1379–408. https://doi.org/10.1016/j.addr.2006.09.004.

[61] Bibby DC, Davies NM, Tucker IG. Mechanisms by which cyclodextrins modify drug release from polymeric drug delivery systems. Int J Pharm 2000;197:1–11. https://doi.org/10.1016/S0378-5173(00)00335-5.

[62] Peppas NA, Narasimhan B. Mathematical models in drug delivery: how modeling has shaped the way we design new drug delivery systems. J Control Release 2014;190:75–81. https://doi.org/10.1016/j.jconrel.2014.06.041.

[63] Larrañeta E, Martínez-Ohárriz C, Vélaz I, Zornoza A, Machín R, Isasi JR. In vitro release from reverse poloxamine/α-cyclodextrin matrices: modelling and comparison of dissolution profiles. J Pharm Sci 2014;103:197–206. https://doi.org/10.1002/jps.23774.

[64] Das S, Subuddhi U. Cyclodextrin mediated controlled release of naproxen from pH-sensitive chitosan/poly(vinyl alcohol) hydrogels for colon targeted delivery. Ind Eng Chem Res 2013;52:14192–200. https://doi.org/10.1021/ie402121f.

[65] Korsmeyer RW, Gurny R, Doelker E, Buri P, Peppas NA. Mechanisms of solute release from porous hydrophilic polymers. Int J Pharm 1983;15:25–35. https://doi.org/10.1016/0378-5173(83)90064-9.

[66] Ritger PL, Peppas NA. A simple equation for description of solute release II. Fickian and anomalous release from swellable devices. J Control Release 1987;5:37–42. https://doi.org/10.1016/0168-3659(87)90035-6.

[67] Higuchi T. Mechanism of sustained-action medication. Theoretical analysis of rate of release of solid drugs dispersed in solid matrices. J Pharm Sci 1963;52:1145–9. https://doi.org/10.1002/jps.2600521210.

[68] Peppas NA, Sahlin JJ. A simple equation for the description of solute release. III. Coupling of diffusion and relaxation. Int J Pharm 1989;57:169–72. https://doi.org/10.1016/0378-5173(89)90306-2.

[69] Siepmann J, Siepmann F. Mathematical modeling of drug delivery. Int J Pharm 2008;364:328–43. https://doi.org/10.1016/j.ijpharm.2008.09.004.

[70] Anon. Mathematical models of drug release. Strateg Modify Drug Release Pharm Syst 2015;63–86. https://doi.org/10.1016/b978-0-08-100092-2.00005-9.

[71] Boztas AO, Karakuzu O, Galante G, Ugur Z, Kocabas F, Altuntas CZ, et al. Synergistic interaction of paclitaxel and curcumin with cyclodextrin polymer complexation in human cancer cells. Mol Pharm 2013;10:2676–83. https://doi.org/10.1021/mp400101k.

[72] Namgung R, Mi Lee Y, Kim J, Jang Y, Lee BH, Kim IS, et al. Poly-cyclodextrin and poly-paclitaxel nano-assembly for anticancer therapy. Nat Commun 2014;5:1–12. https://doi.org/10.1038/ncomms4702.

[73] Brackman G, Garcia-Fernandez MJ, Lenoir J, De Meyer L, Remon JP, De Beer T, et al. Dressings loaded with Cyclodextrin–Hamamelitannin complexes increase Staphylococcus aureus susceptibility toward antibiotics both in single as well as in mixed biofilm communities. Macromol Biosci 2016;859–69. https://doi.org/10.1002/mabi.201500437.

[74] Rivera-Delgado E, Von Recum HA. Using affinity to provide long-term delivery of antiangiogenic drugs in cancer therapy. Mol Pharm 2017;14:899–907. https://doi.org/10.1021/acs.molpharmaceut.6b01109.

[75] Yang JS, Yang L. Preparation and application of cyclodextrin immobilized polysaccharides. J Mater Chem B 2013;1:909–18. https://doi.org/10.1039/c2tb00107a.

[76] Cova TF, Murtinho D, Pais AACC, Valente AJM. Combining cellulose and cyclodextrins: fascinating designs for materials and pharmaceutics. Front Chem 2018;6:1–19. https://doi.org/10.3389/fchem.2018.00271.

[77] Östmark E, Harrison S, Wooley KL, Malmström EE. Comb polymers prepared by ATRP from hydroxypropyl cellulose. Biomacromolecules 2007;8:1138–48. https://doi.org/10.1021/bm061043w.

[78] Hiriart-Ramírez E, Contreras-García A, Garcia-Fernandez MJ, Concheiro A, Alvarez-Lorenzo C, Bucio E. Radiation grafting of glycidyl methacrylate onto cotton gauzes for functionalization with cyclodextrins and elution of antimicrobial agents. Cellul 2012;19:2165–77. https://doi.org/10.1007/s10570-012-9782-5.

[79] Singh B, Dhiman A. Designing bio-mimetic moxifloxacin loaded hydrogel wound dressing to improve antioxidant and pharmacology properties. RSC Adv 2015;5:44666–78. https://doi.org/10.1039/c5ra06857f.

[80] Kalia S, Dufresne A, Cherian BM, Kaith BS, Avérous L, Njuguna J, et al. Cellulose-based bio- and nanocomposites: a review. Int J Polym Sci 2011;2011. https://doi.org/10.1155/2011/837875.

[81] Medronho B, Andrade R, Vivod V, Ostlund A, Miguel MG, Lindman B, et al. Cyclodextrin-grafted cellulose: physico-chemical characterization. Carbohydr Polym 2013;93:324–30. https://doi.org/10.1016/j.carbpol.2012.08.109.

[82] Chang C, Zhang L. Cellulose-based hydrogels: present status and application prospects. Carbohydr Polym 2011;84:40–53. https://doi.org/10.1016/j.carbpol.2010.12.023.

[83] Belgacem MN, Gandini A. Production, chemistry and properties of cellulose-based materials. Biopolym—new mater sustain film coatings. Wiley; 2011. https://doi.org/10.1002/9781119994312.ch8.

[84] Luan J, Wu J, Zheng Y, Song W, Wang G, Guo J, et al. Impregnation of silver sulfadiazine into bacterial cellulose for antimicrobial and biocompatible wound dressing. Biomed Mater 2012;7. https://doi.org/10.1088/1748-6041/7/6/065006.

[85] Sannino A, Demitri C, Madaghiele M. Biodegradable cellulose-based hydrogels: design and applications. Materials (Basel) 2009;2:353–73. https://doi.org/10.3390/ma2020353.

[86] Dahman Y. Nanostructured biomaterials and biocomposites from bacterial cellulose nanofibers. J Nanosci Nanotechnol 2009;9:5105–22. https://doi.org/10.1166/jnn.2009.1466.

[87] Solway DR, Clark WA, Levinson DJ. A parallel open-label trial to evaluate microbial cellulose wound dressing in the treatment of diabetic foot ulcers. Int Wound J 2011;8:69–73. https://doi.org/10.1111/j.1742-481X.2010.00750.x.

[88] Gurdag G, Sarmad S. Cellulose graft copolymers: synthesis, properties, and applications. Polysacch Based Graft Copolym 2013;1–353. https://doi.org/10.1007/978-3-642-36566-9.

[89] Pérez S, Samain D. Structure and engineering of celluloses. vol. 64; 2010. https://doi.org/10.1016/S0065-2318(10)64003-6.

[90] Atalla RH, Isogai A. Celluloses. Compr Nat Prod II Chem Biol 2010;493–539. https://doi.org/10.1016/B978-008045382-8.00691-2.

[91] Gordon S, Hsieh Y-L. Cotton: science and technology. vol. 53; 2013. https://doi.org/10.1017/CBO9781107415324.004.

[92] Carlmark A, Larsson E, Malmström E. Grafting of cellulose by ring-opening polymerisation—a review. Eur Polym J 2012;48:1646–59. https://doi.org/10.1016/j.eurpolymj.2012.06.013.

[93] Pinho E, Soares G. Functionalization of cotton cellulose for improved wound healing. J Mater Chem B 2018;6:1887–98. https://doi.org/10.1039/c8tb00052b.

[94] Granström M, Kilpeläinen PI. Cellulose derivatives: synthesis, properties and applications. PhD; 2009.

[95] Liu J, Willför S, Xu C. A review of bioactive plant polysaccharides: biological activities, functionalization, and biomedical applications. Bioact Carbohydr Diet Fibre 2015;5:31–61. https://doi.org/10.1016/j.bcdf.2014.12.001.

[96] Varshney VK, Naithani S. Chemical functionalization of cellulose derived from nonconventional sources. Cell Fibers Bio-Nano-Polym Compos 2011;43–61. https://doi.org/10.1007/978-3-642-17370-7.

[97] Mohan Yallapu M, Ray Dobberpuhl M, Michele Maher D, Jaggi M, Chand CS. Design of curcumin loaded cellulose nanoparticles for prostate cancer. Curr Drug Metab 2011;13:120–8. https://doi.org/10.2174/138920012798356952.

[98] Li X, Xie S, Pan Y, Qu W, Tao Y, Chen D, et al. Preparation, characterization and pharmacokinetics of doxycycline hydrochloride and florfenicol polyvinylpyrroliddone microparticle entrapped with hydroxypropyl-β-cyclodextrin inclusion complexes suspension. Colloids Surf B Biointerfaces 2016;141:634–42. https://doi.org/10.1016/j.colsurfb.2016.02.027.

[99] Anon. Nanocellulose and nanohydrogel matrices; 2017. https://doi.org/10.1002/9783527803835.

[100] Zhang L, Zhou J, Zhang L. Structure and properties of β-cyclodextrin/cellulose hydrogels prepared in NaOH/urea aqueous solution. Carbohydr Polym 2013;94:386–93. https://doi.org/10.1016/j.carbpol.2012.12.077.

[101] Pinho E, Henriques M, Soares G. Cyclodextrin/cellulose hydrogel with gallic acid to prevent wound infection. Cellul 2014;21:4519–30. https://doi.org/10.1007/s10570-014-0439-4.

[102] Ghorpade VS, Yadav AV, Dias RJ. Citric acid crosslinked cyclodextrin/hydroxypropylmethylcellulose hydrogel films for hydrophobic drug delivery. Int J Biol Macromol 2016;93:75–86. https://doi.org/10.1016/j.ijbiomac.2016.08.072.

[103] Gafitanu CA, Filip D, Cernatescu C, Rusu D, Tuchilus CG, Macocinschi D, et al. Design, preparation and evaluation of HPMC-based PAA or SA freeze-dried scaffolds for vaginal delivery of fluconazole. Pharm Res 2017;34:2185–96. https://doi.org/10.1007/s11095-017-2226-z.

[104] Sun N, Wang T, Yan X. Self-assembled supermolecular hydrogel based on hydroxyethyl cellulose: formation, in vitro release and bacteriostasis application. Carbohydr Polym 2017;172:49–59. https://doi.org/10.1016/j.carbpol.2017.05.026.

[105] Onofrei M, Filimon A. Cellulose-based hydrogels: designing concepts, properties, and perspectives for biomedical and environmental applications. Polym Sci Res Adv Pract Appl Educ Asp 2016;108–20.

[106] Peng N, Wang Y, Ye Q, Liang L, An Y, Li Q, et al. Biocompatible cellulose-based superabsorbent hydrogels with antimicrobial activity. Carbohydr Polym 2016;137:59–64. https://doi.org/10.1016/j.carbpol.2015.10.057.

[107] Liu S, Luo W, Huang H. Characterization and behavior of composite hydrogel prepared from bamboo shoot cellulose and β-cyclodextrin. Int J Biol Macromol 2016;89:527–34. https://doi.org/10.1016/j.ijbiomac.2016.05.023.

[108] Rodriguez-Tenreiro C, Alvarez-Lorenzo C, Rodriguez-Perez A, Concheiro A, Torres-Labandeira JJ. Estradiol sustained release from high affinity cyclodextrin hydrogels. Eur J Pharm Biopharm 2007;66:55–62. https://doi.org/10.1016/j.ejpb.2006.09.003.

[109] Rodriguez-Tenreiro C, Alvarez-Lorenzo C, Rodriguez-Perez A, Concheiro A, Torres-Labandeira JJ. New cyclodextrin hydrogels cross-linked with diglycidylethers with a high drug loading and controlled release ability. Pharm Res 2006;23:121–30. https://doi.org/10.1007/s11095-005-8924-y.

[110] Blanco-Fernandez B, Lopez-Viota M, Concheiro A, Alvarez-Lorenzo C. Synergistic performance of cyclodextrin-agar hydrogels for ciprofloxacin delivery and antimicrobial effect. Carbohydr Polym 2011;85:765–74. https://doi.org/10.1016/j.carbpol.2011.03.042.

[111] Garcia-Fernandez MJ, Brackman G, Coenye T, Concheiro A, Alvarez-Lorenzo C. Antiseptic cyclodextrin-functionalized hydrogels and gauzes for loading and delivery of benzalkonium chloride. Biofouling 2013;29:261–71. https://doi.org/10.1080/08927014.2013.765947.

[112] Lorenzo A, Rodríguez-Tenreiro C, Torres Labandeira JJ, Concheiro Nine A. Method of obtaining hydrogels of cyclodextrins with glycidyl ethers, compositions thus obtained and applications thereof. PCT/ES2006/000096 (87); 2008.

[113] Zugasti ME, Zornoza A, Goñi MDM, Isasi JR, Vélaz I, Martín C, et al. Influence of soluble and insoluble cyclodextrin polymers on drug release from hydroxypropyl methylcellulose tablets. Drug Dev Ind Pharm 2009;35:1264–70. https://doi.org/10.1080/03639040902882306.

[114] Han S, Wang T, Yang L, Li B. Building a bio-based hydrogel via electrostatic and host-guest interactions for realizing dual-controlled release mechanism. Int J Biol Macromol 2017;105:377–84. https://doi.org/10.1016/j.ijbiomac.2017.07.049.

[115] Huang H, Wu Z, Qi X, Zhang H, Chen Q, Xing J, et al. Compression-coated tablets of glipizide using hydroxypropylcellulose for zero-order release: in vitro and in vivo evaluation. Int J Pharm 2013;446:211–8. https://doi.org/10.1016/j.ijpharm.2013.01.039.

[116] Lin N, Dufresne A. Supramolecular hydrogels from in situ host-guest inclusion between chemically modified cellulose nanocrystals and cyclodextrin. Biomacromolecules 2013;14:871–80. https://doi.org/10.1021/bm301955k.

[117] Malik NS, Ahmad M, Minhas MU. Cross-linked β-cyclodextrin and carboxymethyl cellulose hydrogels for controlled drug delivery of acyclovir. PLoS ONE 2017;12:1–17. https://doi.org/10.1371/journal.pone.0172727.

[118] Marcos X, Pérez-Casas S, Llovo J, Concheiro A, Alvarez-Lorenzo C. Poloxamer-hydroxyethyl cellulose-α-cyclodextrin supramolecular gels for sustained release of griseofulvin. Int J Pharm 2016;500:11–9. https://doi.org/10.1016/j.ijpharm.2016.01.015.

5

Potential of guar gum hydrogels in drug delivery

Subhraseema Das[b] and Usharani Subuddhi[a]

[a]Dept. of Chemistry, NIT Rourkela, Rourkela, Odisha, India, [b]Dept. of Chemistry, Ravenshaw University, Cuttack, Odisha, India

5.1 Introduction

Polymers, in general, have become a quintessential part of mankind. Natural polymers, in particular, have demonstrated terrific potential in all aspects. They have blossomed as viable alternatives over their synthetic counterparts in the fields of energy, electronics, and medicine. Owing to their magnificent attributes such as accessibility, biocompatibility and biodegradability, natural polymers have predominantly secured their position as frontline materials in health care. Polysaccharide gums are one of the inexhaustible natural resources for potential applications in biomedicine. The term "gum" generally implies to naturally occurring polysaccharides and their derivatives, which can hydrate in water (hot/cold), either by forming gels or emulsions [1–3]. Gums may be resourced from microbes, weeds, or plants. Microbial gums are mainly produced by fermentation of specific microorganisms and include pullulan, gellan, xanthan, and dextran gums, to name a few [4, 5]. Gums such as arabic, tragacanth, ghatti, and karaya are obtained as natural exudates of different tree species through a process known as gummosis [6,7]. Another class of gums is the seed gums, which are extracted from the seed embryos. Tamarind gum, tara gum, locust bean gum, and guar gum (GG) are a few seed gums that find unparallel applications in medicine.

GG is obtained from the embryo of *Cyamopsis tetragonolobus*, family Leguminosae. It contains about 80% galactomannan, 12% water, 5% protein, 2% acidic insoluble ash, 0.7% ash, and 0.7% fat [8]. In addition to its biomedical applications, GG has profound industrial utilities as a thickener, binder, or viscosifier. The vast spectrum of GG applicability has been illustrated in Fig. 5.1. One of the striking features of GG is its

Plant and Algal Hydrogels for Drug Delivery and Regenerative Medicine
https://doi.org/10.1016/B978-0-12-821649-1.00006-4

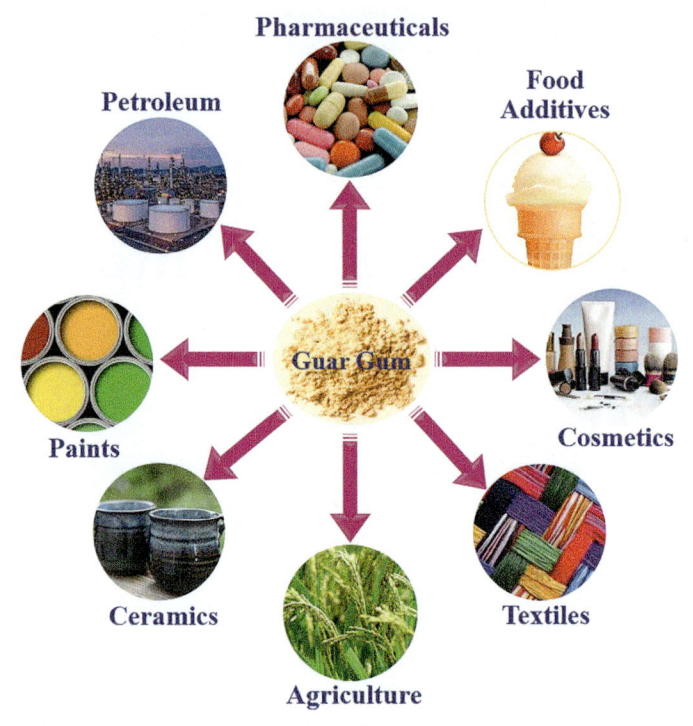

FIG. 5.1   Diverse applications of guar gum.

prompt hydration in aqueous solution. An aqueous GG solution is a viscous pseudoplastic solution having low shear viscosity when compared with other hydrocolloids [9–11]. This gelling characteristic has rendered GG an essential function in pharmaceutics, especially in the delivery of therapeutics. This chapter puts forth a brief overview of GG regarding its extraction and processing, properties and chemistry, and, most importantly, its application as drug delivery systems. As a powerhouse of versatility, the applications of GG toward the delivery of an array of drugs are discussed at length.

5.2 Extraction and processing of GG

5.2.1 Cultivation

Guar cultivation is mostly found in the west and northwestern regions of India, Sudan, Pakistan, semiarid areas of Texas in the United States, South Africa, and Australia. Guar plant has high environmental temperature tolerance ability and is vulnerable to frost [12, 13]. It requires a thirsty climate with sparse but regular rainfall and optimum soil temperature between

25°C and 30°C. Optimal rain is required before plantation and maturation of seeds; however, excess of moisture before growth and after maturation reduces the quality of guar beans [14–16]. The environmental conditions of India and Pakistan are most suitable for guar cultivation, and these two countries contribute up to 90% of the global production of guar seeds [16].

Guar plants grow on an average around 0.6 m tall, and the fruit shells are of 3–13 cm long containing a few spherical and light brown seeds [17–19]. The seed of guar encloses an endosperm that provides nutrition to the embryo during germination. The embryo (germ) is further surrounded by a hull, jointly referred to as guar meal, a source of protein. The embryo, which is the innermost part, approximately constitutes 43%–47% of the total seed weight [17, 20].

5.2.2 Processing

First, the endosperm is separated from the hull and embryo by grinding and sieving. The endosperm is now referred to as guar splits and undergoes further processing to obtain marketable GG. A schematic depiction of the extraction process of GG is presented in Fig. 5.2. The guar meal obtained from husk and germ, which is a major byproduct, is used as cattle fodder. The polished guar splits are crushed into powder by a number of methods and techniques based on the demand of the final products. The prehydrated splits are further grinded in an ultra-fine grinder. Several grades of GG are available depending on particle size, viscosity, color, and hydration rate [11, 16, 17]. A slight variation in solubilization

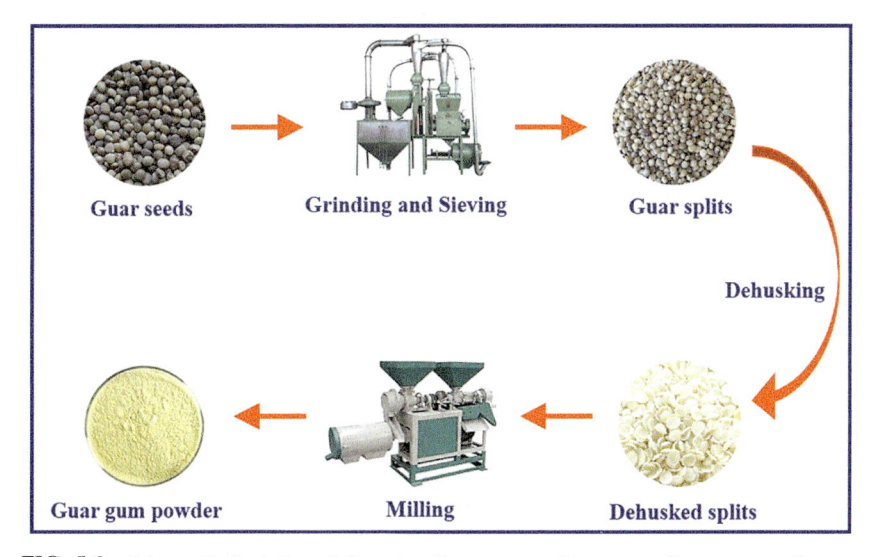

FIG. 5.2 Schematic depiction of the extraction process of guar gum from guar seeds.

rate and viscosity has been observed in different batches of GG because of its source. GG is graded as food grade or industrial grade depending on its viscosity and presence of impurities.

5.3 Chemistry of GG

5.3.1 Composition, structure, and molecular weight

Chemical methods (acid hydrolysis, periodate oxidation, ethylation, etc.), analytical methods, physical methods (optical rotation and X-ray diffraction), and selective enzymatic hydrolysis methods have been used to gain an insight into the structural and behavioral mode of GG [12, 17–19, 21–23]. GG comprises linear chains of (1 → 4)-β-D-mannopyranosyl units with α-D-galactopyranosyl units attached by (1 → 6) linkages (Fig. 5.3). Contemporary studies have indicated the ratio of mannose to galactose units in GG, ranging somewhere between 1.6:1 and 1.8:1, but overall, it has been approximated to 2:1 [24]. GG is particularly different from other plant gums and mucilages due to the absence of uronic acid in its backbone [17]. High-performance size exclusion chromatography and low-angle laser scattering studies have revealed the average molecular weight of GG to be in the order of 10^6 [25, 26].

5.3.2 Viscosity

Viscosity of GG is defined as its rate of hydration in cold water to form a viscous solution [16, 27, 28]. GG exhibits thixotropic behavior when completely hydrated. GG solutions having concentrations less than 1% is less

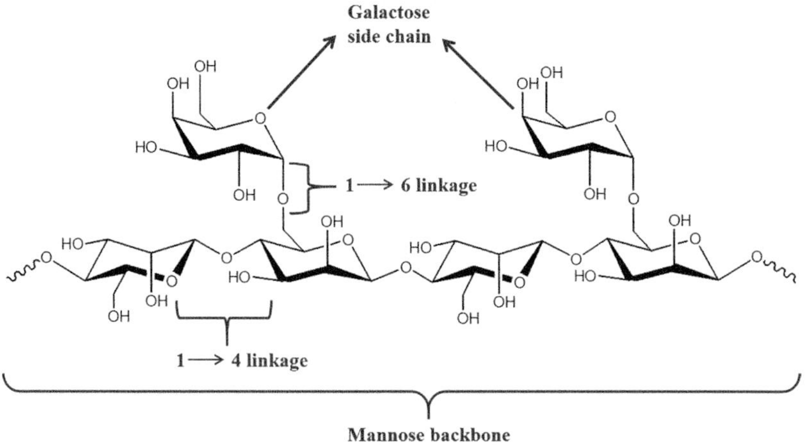

FIG. 5.3   Chemical structure of guar gum.

thixotropic, whereas a high thixotropic nature is seen in solutions having concentrations more than 1% [29, 30]. A good quality GG having an aqueous dispersion of 1% may possess a viscosity of around 10,000 cp [31]. The viscosity of GG is mainly dependent on various parameters namely, concentration, pH, temperature, pressure, time, ionic strength, and quantity of agitation [28, 32].

5.3.3 Rheology

Rheology reveals about the deformation incurred on any material on application of an external force. Aqueous solution of GG is known to demonstrate a pseudoplastic or shear-thinning behavior known as non-Newtonian behavior, which implies a decrease in the viscosity on increase in the shear rate [33, 34]. An increase in the molecular weight and polymer concentration increases the shear-thinning behavior. At lower frequency range, 1% aqueous solution of GG exhibits a distinctive behavior with the dominance of loss modulus (G'') over storage modulus (G'), but in higher frequency range, G' dominates over the G'' [35]. Moreover, both G' and G'' of aqueous GG solution have been evidenced to decrease with storage time [36].

5.3.4 Hydrogen bonding activity

Availability of numerous hydroxyl moieties in GG backbone makes it prone to extensive hydrogen bonding in aqueous solution. H-bonding of GG has also been witnessed with cellulosic materials and hydrated minerals. Addition of even small quantity of GG to any system has been observed to distinctly modify its electrokinetic behavior [29]. The replacement of hydroxyl groups in GG by hydroxypropyl causes steric hindrance, and hence the extent of hydrogen bonding is reduced [16, 17, 37].

5.3.5 Hydration rate

The rate of hydration of GG depends on the size of GG powder. Fine mesh of GG is usually used to obtain a quick viscosity. However, a practical time of 2h is generally warranted to obtain a maximum viscous solution [16, 29]. GG solutions are quite stable in the broad pH range of 1.0–10.5 owing to their uncharged behavior. It has also been evidenced that the presence of salts, and particularly brine, restricts the hydration rate of GG [38, 39].

5.4 Properties of GG making it suitable for drug delivery applications

Of the various natural polysaccharides, GG has garnered substantial attention as a promising biomaterial in targeted delivery of therapeutics

[8, 17, 40]. The main advantages of GG, a natural edible polysaccharide, are its versatility in natural resources, low cost in processing, and the ease of its fabrication with other polymers, making it a very accessible material for use as carriers of therapeutics. Furthermore, GG is highly stable, non-toxic, biocompatible, and biodegradable in nature. GG remains undigested in the stomach and is degraded by the colonic microflora and, therefore, deemed particularly useful in the design of colon-specific delivery systems. In addition, its stability over a wide pH range and compatibility with other polymers makes it an irresistible choice for oral formulations [8, 11, 17, 18, 40]. Moreover, GG has already been approved by the FDA for pharmaceutical applications; an enteric-coated GG-based tablet of ketoprofen (50 and 100 mg) is currently marketed under the tradename (KETOPROFEN-E), produced by AA Pharma Inc., Ontario, Canada [40].

5.5 Limitations of pristine GG and modification strategies

The basic structure and inherent physicochemical properties of GG makes it a potent candidate for diverse applications. Nonetheless, certain shortcomings such as nonuniform rate of hydration, turbidity, and lack of mechanical integrity in aqueous dispersions and a greater vulnerability to microbial invasion hinders its applications and, thus, calls for modification strategies [41, 42].

5.5.1 Chemical modification

Addition of new functional groups to the GG backbone not only enhances the mechanical integrity but also imparts tailorable properties for desired applications [17, 32, 43]. Moreover, chemical modification and derivatizations of GG eradicates or minimizes the limitations associated with pristine GG. Chemical modification mainly aims at grafting, cross-linking, and derivatization of GG. Common examples of chemically modified GG include hydroxypropyl GG [44], hydroxypropylethyl GG [45], carboxymethyl GG [46, 47], acryloyloxy GG [48], methyl and hydroxypropyl methyl GG [49], methacryloyl GG [50], and GG esters [51, 52].

5.5.2 Formulation of GG with other polymers

GG has been assimilated with an array of polymers (natural/synthetic) and used for industrial and pharmaceutical applications. The synergism observed in the resulting formulations further broadens the range of accessible properties. The following section presents a comprehensive overview on the design and applications of GG and its derivatives, particularly in biomedicine.

5.5.2.1 Integration with natural polymers

GG derivatives with other naturally occurring biopolymers such as alginate, cellulose, chitosan, xanthan, starch, whey protein, and others have been explored for various biomedical applications. Table 5.1 collates the diverse pharmaceutical applications of GG and its biopolymer-based derivatives that have been explored in the literature.

5.5.2.2 Integration with synthetic polymers

Integrating synthetic polymers with GG improves the physicochemical properties of the biopolymer and aids in alleviating the shortcomings of the pure GG. Synthetic polymers such as polyvinyl alcohol (PVA), polyacrylic acid, polyacrylamide, poly(N-isopropylacrylamide), and poloxamer have been taken in conjugation with GG to form myriad architectures to cater to an array of pharmaceutical utilities. Table 5.2 enlists the GG derivatives with synthetic polymers that have been explored in the literature for their potential pharmaceutical applications.

5.6 Delivery of therapeutics from GG hydrogel

GG and its derivatives have come a long way in the world of pharmaceutics, in general, and drug delivery, in particular. The versatility of GG as a binding, thickening, suspending, and emulsifying candidate proves its potency in drug delivery systems [17, 18]. Furthermore, the physicochemical properties of GG can be attuned to get the desired solubility, film-forming ability, and swelling. Chemical derivatization has evolved as a promising tool to tailor native GG as per need. GG and its derivatives have been broadly investigated in targeted drug delivery systems owing to the versatile nature to get an appropriate drug release profile (fast/sustained). Polymeric hydrogels are undeniably the most extensive class of biomedical architectures used lately for the same. The adaptability of GG to various chemical reactions yields myriad hydrogel-based formulations in the form of microspheres, microcapsules, tablets, scaffolds, nanogels, etc., which makes it a highly attractive biomaterial for drug delivery purposes. A wide range of strategies have been adopted for the construction of GG-based hydrogels for applications in drug delivery. Such methods commonly include polymeric grafting, cross-linking (physical/chemical), and formation of drug-polymer conjugates (Fig. 5.4). Physically cross-linked GG hydrogels could be achieved by using different triggers such as pH, ionic strength, light, and temperature, as well as through physicochemical interactions (H-bonding, hydrophobic interactions, and supramolecular chemistry). Chemically/covalently cross-linked hydrogels could be rationalized by the use of conventional cross-linkers (glutaraldehyde and ethylene glycol dimethacrylate (EGDMA)) and polymer-polymer cross-linking.

TABLE 5.1 Integration of GG with various natural biopolymers that have been explored in the literature for potential biomedical applications.

Sl. no.	Polymers used	Preparation method	Formulation	Application	Ref.
1.	GG and chitosan	Solution casting	Films	Antimicrobial activity against *Staphylococcus aureus*, *Escherichia coli*	[53]
2.	Chitosan and polyacrylamide-*g*-GG	Emulsion cross-linking; glutaraldehyde as cross-linker	Microsphere	Controlled release of ciprofloxacin	[54]
3.	Sodium alginate and PNIPAAm-*g*-GG	Emulsion cross-linking; glutaraldehyde as cross-linker	Microsphere	Controlled release of isoniazid	[55]
4.	GG and chitosan	Solution casting; glutaraldehyde as cross-linker	Hydrogel	Dermal patch for sustained release of paracetamol	[56]
5.	GG and chitosan-*g*-PCL micelles	Hydrophilic inner and hydrophobic outer core interaction	Hydrogel	Mucoadhesive hydrogels for delivery of rifampicin	[57]
6.	GG and xanthan gum	Solution casting	Bioadhesive films	Improved bioavailability of domperidone	[58]
7.	GG and cellulose nanocrystals	Solution casting using borax	Nanocomposite hydrogel	Self-healing hydrogel	[59]
8.	GG and sago starch	Blending	Films	Antimicrobial activity against *B. cereus*, *E. coli*	[60]

9.	GG, sago starch, and whey protein	Blending	Films	Antimicrobial activity against *Bacillus cereus*, *E. coli*	[61]
10.	GG and sodium alginate	Solution casting; glutaraldehyde as cross-linker	Hydrogel	Controlled delivery of protein (BSA)	[62]
11.	GG and karaya gum	Powdered compression	Matrix tablets	Sustained drug release	[63]
12.	GG and agarose	Solution casting	Membrane	Biosensors	[64]

PNIPAAm, poly(*N*-isopropyl acrylamide); *PCL*, poly(ε-caprolactone).

TABLE 5.2 Integration of GG with synthetic polymers for various pharmaceutical applications.

Sl. no.	Polymers used	Preparation method	Formulation	Application	Ref.
1.	GG-*g*-acrylic acid	In situ free radical polymerization; L-alanine as cross-linker	Hydrogel	Self-healing hydrogels and sustained release of levofloxacin	[65]
2.	GG, polyacrylic acid, β-cyclodextrin	In situ free radical polymerization and TEOS as cross-linker	Hydrogel	Controlled release of dexamethasone	[66]
3.	Cellulose reinforced PNIPAAm-*g*-GG	Free radical polymerization	Nanocomposite hydrogel	Transdermal patch for sustained release of diltiazem	[67]
4.	GG, PVA, and silver nanoparticles	Blending	Nanocomposite hydrogels	Antibacterial and antioxidant activities	[68]
5.	Nanosilica-reinforced polyacrylamide-*g*-GG	Free radical polymerization and solution casting	Nanocomposite hydrogels	Transdermal sustained delivery of diltiazem	[69]
6.	GG, PNIPAAm, and β-cyclodextrin	In situ free radical polymerization and TEOS as cross-linker	Hydrogel	Controlled release of 5-fluorouracil	[70]
7.	GG and PEGDGE	Solution casting	Hydrogel	Biomedical applications	[71]
8.	Gold-cellulose nanofiller-reinforced GG and PVA	Polyelectrolyte complex formation	Film	Transdermal delivery of diltiazem HCl	[72]
9.	Polyacrylamide-*g*-GG	Emulsification	Microgels	Colonic delivery of diltiazem HCl and nifedipine	[73]
10.	GG-*g*-PCL	Microwave-assisted grafting	Nanomicelles	Drug delivery	[74]
11.	GG and glycerol	Solution casting and borax as cross-linker	Hydrogel	Skin-sensitive sensors and injectable hydrogels	[75]
12.	GG and poloxamer-407	In situ gelation	In situ gel	Ophthalmic drug delivery	[76]

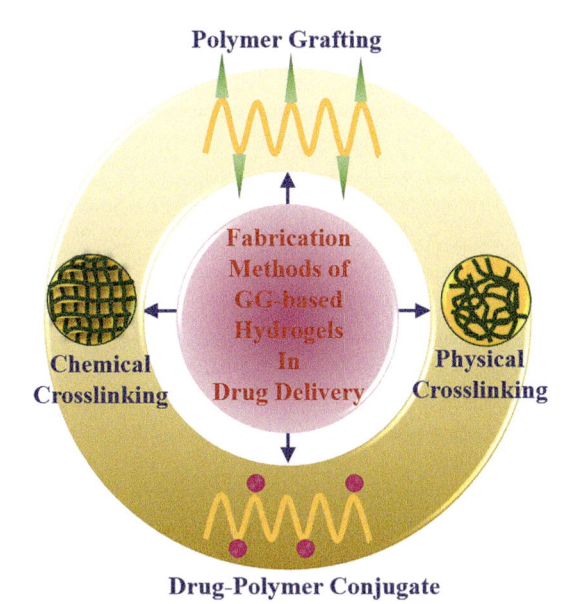

FIG. 5.4 Different approaches for fabrication of GG-based hydrogels in drug delivery.

5.6.1 Delivery of antihypertensive drugs

Antihypertensive drugs are used for the treatment of hypertension. Antihypertensive therapy pursues to prevent the difficulties associated with high blood pressure such as stroke and myocardial infarction [77]. Common antihypertensive drugs are verapamil hydrochloride, metoprolol tartrate, metoprolol succinate, diltiazem hydrochloride, nifedipine, atenolol, carvedilol, propranolol hydrochloride, etc. Although effective, the plasma life of these drugs generally is very short, < 3–4 h. Therefore such medications warrant a sustained delivery. Consequently, GG-based formulations have blossomed as reliable oral sustained delivery platforms of such drugs [40].

Polyacrylamide-*g*-GG hydrogels were loaded with diltiazem (DLT) hydrochloride and compressed into tablets [78]. The authors observed that the tablets were pH-responsive and are particularly suited for intestinal delivery of the drug at a controlled rate. The in vivo sustained release of DLT from GG tablets were performed on healthy human volunteers wherein no adverse effect was witnessed on plasma concentrations [79].

GG-*g*-polyacrylamide copolymer was cross-linked with glutaraldehyde to form hydrogel microspheres and exploited for delivery of verapamil (VPR) and nifedipine (NFD) [80]. A controlled drug release profile was realized for both the drugs whence the release rate was strongly determined by the cross-linker content, drug content, and the drug loading method. VPR-encapsulated GG microspheres were formulated by cross-linking with sodium alginate [81]. An extended release of VPR up to 12 h was observed from the microspheres. In another report; NFD was encapsulated in GG hydrogels processed by supercritical technology [82]. NFD release was prolonged for up to 14 days from the formulations. Interpenetrating polymeric network microspheres of GG and PVA have been prepared by cross-linking with glutaraldehyde [83]. NFD release from the microspheres indicated them as potent carriers of the drug.

An oral GG-based sustained delivery system for metoprolol tartrate was designed in the form of a three-layered matrix tablet [84]. The findings of the study validated the potential of the three-layered GG tablets as oral controlled drug delivery devices. A bilayer tablet of atorvastatin and atenolol was synthesized by Dey et al. [85]. The purpose was to develop bilayer tablets that are characterized by initial fast release of atorvastatin in the stomach followed by a sustained release of atenolol. To achieve this feat, inclusion complexes of atorvastatin with β-cyclodextrin (β-CD) was first used for the fast-release layer to improve the dissolution of atorvastatin. Then xanthan gum and GG were integrated in the sustained release layer. From the drug release studies; it was witnessed that more than 60% atorvastatin was released from the fast-release layer in the initial 2 h, which was then followed by a sustained release of atenolol for 12 h. Furthermore, the pharmacokinetics also affirmed the dual nature of drug release by formulation of such bilayer tablets.

The antihypertensive peptide (AhP) obtained from whey protein hydrolase having sequence KGYGGVSLPEW has potential interest in therapeutic applications. But during passage through the gut, these peptides lose a part of their therapeutic efficacy owing to the acidic pH environment and enzyme-facilitated degradation. The buccal administration of these peptides avoids the degradation in the gut and improves their bioavailability. In a novel approach, the buccal delivery of AhP from composite system (GfNp) comprising integrated PLGA nanoparticles and GG films was reported [86]. The composite system GfNp was found to provide the slowest release of AhP when compared with individual PLGA nanoparticles and GG films. The release kinetics obeyed Higuchi model implying the important contribution from the drug diffusion along with erosion toward the release of the carried peptide. Incorporation of nanoparticles onto a hydrogel matrix is known to minimize the burst release effect of medications. Moreover, the composite system GfNp was found to offer a synergistic and better in vitro permeability of the TR146 cells; thus it has been suggested as a better alternative to conventional per os delivery systems.

In a very recent study, a biphasic pulsed "tablets in capsule" drug release system for losartan potassium was developed using an erodible GG time spacer tablet [87]. The histological evaluation on intestinal cells indicated high cell viability. From the release kinetics study, the drug release occurred because of swelling of the erodible tablet, followed by diffusion and erosion of GG. A good stability was observed for the capsule with a shelf life of 15 months. The developed biphasic pulsed drug release system was indeed potent for chronotherapeutics in hypertension [87].

5.6.2 Delivery of anticancer drugs

The chemotherapeutic agent 5-fluorouracil (5FU) has displayed strong clinical activity against colorectal cancer. Still, 5FU is administered intravenously till date. Thus to obviate patient noncompliances, an oral delivery for 5FU is generally warranted. Naturally occurring polysaccharides such as GG finds massive preference for the same. A plethora of literature reports establish the high efficacy of GG as oral controlled delivery devices for 5FU. In a recent study; magnetic hydrogel microspheres comprising GG, cellulose, and Fe_3O_4 were synthesized and explored for their delivery characteristics of 5FU [88]. The authors observed that 5FU delivery was impacted by GG, cellulose, and Fe_3O_4 content, and a controlled release was evident for 36 h. In another report, pH-responsive microgels composed of chitosan and GG-g-poly[(2-dimethylamino)ethylmethacrylate] copolymer were fabricated by emulsion cross-linking with glutaraldehyde [89]. In vitro 5FU release from the microgels in pH 1.2 and 7.4 revealed a prolonged delivery to the colon. Dual-sensitive composite hydrogel of GG and polyacrylamidoglycolic acid graft copolymer and its silver nanocomposite hydrogel have been successfully explored for oral controlled 5FU delivery [90]. pH-responsive GG/poly(acrylamide-co-acrylamidoglycolicacid) hydrogel matrices loaded with 5FU have been synthesized by Reddy et al. wherein a sustained delivery was achieved in pH 7.4 [91]. A study by Das and Subuddhi concerned with the fabrication of thermoresponsive hydrogels of GG and PNIPAAm for 5FU delivery [70]. To achieve the same, the authors first prepared freeze-dried solid inclusion complexes (ICs) of 5FU in β-CD. The preformed ICs were then loaded onto the GG-PNIPAAm hydrogels. The 5FU release was considerably prolonged from the hydrogels loaded with 5FU-β-CD ICs at 37°C in comparison with hydrogels loaded with free 5FU only. From the kinetics assay, the authors inferred that the cumulative influence of GG content and β-CD was decisive in regulating 5FU delivery.

Doxorubicin (DOX) is a byproduct of actinobacteria *Streptomyces peucetius* var. Casieus and belongs to anthracycline class [92], which is broadly used as a chemotherapeutic agent [93, 94]. Kang et al. reported DOX and metformin HCl–loaded GG microparticles prepared by emulsification cum solidification method. The in vitro release of DOX and metformin HCl in simulated gastric fluid (SGF) and simulated intestinal fluid (SIF) were 9.3% and 9.6%, in 2 h, and 10.8% and 14.7% in the next 3 h, respectively, and the highest release was observed in the SIF (about 68% and 73.3%) [94]. The designed microparticles targeted the drug combination to colon and improved the efficiency. In a study by Mushtaq et al., cobalt ferrite nanoparticles (CFNPs) were coated with GG, gum Arabic, and poly(methacrylic acid) and conjugated with DOX [95]. The authors evidenced that the CFNPs coated with GG exhibited optimal DOX release with upgraded cytocompatibility against Chinese hamster ovary (CHO) cell line. Murali et al. designed an injectable hydrogel that comprised aminated GG (AGG), Fe_3O_4-ZnS core-shell nanoparticles (CSNPs), and DOX hydrochloride. It was reported that approximately 90% of DOX was released from the hydrogel (AGG-CSNP-DOX) over a prolonged period of 20 days (Fig. 5.5) [96].

Methotrexate (MTX) is an anticancer drug that acts by inhibiting folic acid metabolism. Folic acid–conjugated GG nanoparticles and folic acid charged with MTX were synthesized for colonic delivery of MTX [97]. MTX release was protected in the upper part of gut, whereas optimal release took place in pH 6.8. Moreover, an in vivo study recommended the superior uptake of MTX in colon, suggesting their potential in the

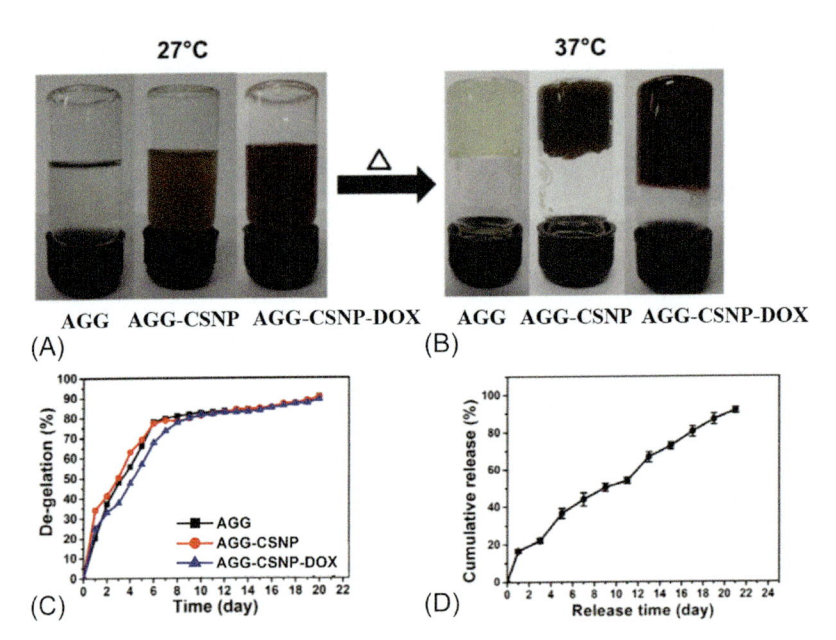

FIG. 5.5   Digital images showing the physical state of aminated guar gum (AGG), AGG-core-shell nanoparticles (AGG-CSNP), and doxorubicin-loaded AGG-CSNP (AGG-CSNP-DOX) systems as a function of temperature at (A) 27°C and (B) 37°C; (C) In vitro degelation patterns of AGG, AGG-CSNP, and AGG-CSNP-DOX hydrogel systems; (D) In-vitro drug release pattern of AGG-CSNP-DOX hydrogel. *Reprinted from Murali R, Vidhya P, Thanikaivelan P. Thermoresponsive magnetic nanoparticle-aminated guar gum hydrogel system for sustained release of doxorubicin hydrochloride. Carbohydr Polym 2014;110:440–5. Copyright (2014) with permission from Elsevier.*

treatment of colorectal carcinoma. Chaurasia et al. synthesized GG microspheres using glutaraldehyde as the cross-linker [98]. MTX release was largely affected by GG and glutaraldehyde content. Optimal release was evidenced in rat cecal content. The in vivo study revealed about 79% of drug release in the colon from the microspheres formulation, whereas plain drug suspension could deliver only 23% to the targeted site.

Curcumin, a diarylheptanoid is potent for the treatment of colon cancer. Its potential application is impeded by poor aqueous solubility and stability. The inability of gut enzymes to digest certain plant polysaccharides can be of advantage toward the development of colon targeting delivery systems for curcumin. Taking a cue from this, researchers have used GG to develop delivery systems for curcumin. Curcumin-loaded GG matrix tablets were evaluated in SGF, SCF, and SIF. [99]. An optimal drug release was witnessed in the SIF for a prolonged period of 24h. In a relatively novel strategy, the formulation of liquisolid tablets for colon delivery of curcumin using GG and Eudragit was inspected by Kumar et al. [100]. The liquisolid tablets restricted curcumin release in the stomach and small intestine. The formulation with Eudragit and GG in a ratio of 10:40 was ascertained the optimal with 86.4% drug release. The authors concluded that coating a liquisolid tablet with GG could blossom as a promising tool for colon-specific delivery of therapeutics.

5.6.3 Delivery of antifungal drugs

Metronidazole (MTZ) is a household name as an antifungal agent. The efficacy of GG-based formulations toward delivery of MTZ is well-documented. Chourasia et al. reported the colon targeted release of MTZ from cross-linked GG microspheres [101]. In vitro release suggested that only 15.27% of MTZ was released in SGF (2h) and SIF (3h). However, the release study in the SCF indicated a higher release of drug. In another report, polyethylene glycol diglycidyl ether (PEGDGE) cross-linked GG hydrogel loaded with MTZ was synthesized by Panariello et al. [102]. A sustained MTZ release profile was achieved from the hydrogel over a period of 10h. Very recently, microwave irradiated synthesis of microporous interpenetrating polymeric networks of carrageenan and GG incorporated with MTZ was reported by Swain and Bal [103]. The results evidenced a target-oriented controlled device for MTZ. Concerning the delivery of another antifungal agent fluconazole, an in situ GG-based gel has been explored for its controlled delivery potential [104]. The developed gels effectively prolonged the release rate of fluconazole. Amphotericin B is another antifungal agent that has been entrapped in enteric-coated GG nanoparticles [105]. Drug release was accomplished in a controlled manner from the formulations.

Vaginal delivery systems represent a crucial class of drug delivery because women of all age groups are affected in some or other way. Vaginal infections are typically featured by irritation or vulvar itching, discharge, and odor. A key feature of a vaginal delivery system lies in the bioadhesion of the formulation. GG has demonstrated tremendous potential as bioadhesive controlled vaginal drug delivery systems in the form of vaginal tablets and gels owing to its ability to bind to epithelial surfaces, thereby increasing the residence time. A series of tablets comprising hydroxypropylmethyl cellulose (HPMC) and GG prepared by direct compression technique were assessed for the delivery of the antifungal agent clotrimazole [106]. The tablets showed a long residence time of more than 12 h and reduced the burst effect of the drug locally. In another study, bioadhesive vaginal tablets containing ornidazole were formulated using pectin and GG [107]. The tablets were assayed for irritational effect on cow vaginal mucosa. The authors observed that the tablets did not induce any adverse effect on the bovine vaginal mucosa and was also endowed with enough bioadhesive characteristics. Furthermore, the tablets also prolonged the delivery of ornidazole, and thus are indeed potent in vaginal delivery. Vaginal tablets containing clotrimazole and MTZ have been developed using various polymers including GG by Alam et al. [108]. The drug-loaded formulations also contained *Lactobacillus acidophilus* spores with an aim to treat mixed vaginal infections. Ex vivo studies revealed prolonged retention of the tablets inside the vaginal tube for more than 24 h. The tablets fared much better regarding spreadability and antimicrobial activity than their marketed counterparts.

5.6.4 Delivery of antibiotics

Ciprofloxacin (CFX) belongs to the class of fluoroquinolone antibiotics family having plasma half-life of 4 h and is commonly used in bacterial infection, typhoid fever, septicemia, and gonorrhea. Kajjari et al. reported the encapsulation of CFX onto microspheres of chitosan and acrylamide-*g*-GG cross-linked with glutaraldehyde [53]. The encapsulation efficiency was found to be 74%, and CFX release was prolonged for 12 h. The controlled release of CFX from bigels comprising GG hydrogel and sorbitan monostearate-sesame oil–based organogel was reported by Singh et al. [109]. The bigels having lower proportion of organogel exhibited higher drug delivery and followed zero-order release kinetics.

Cefadroxil is yet another antibiotic belonging to the class of cephalosporins. Blend microspheres of GG and chitosan were prepared and investigated for controlled delivery of cefadroxil [110]. The release experiments in pH 7.4 indicated a slow delivery for 10 h.

5.6.5 Delivery of antiinflammatory drugs

Ibuprofen (IBF) is a potent nonsteroidal antiinflammatory drug (NSAID) that needs no introduction. It is widely recommended for pain, fever, and inflammation. Development of GG formulations for IBF delivery has been on the rise lately. Blend polymeric films comprising cationic GG and sodium carboxymethyl cellulose have proven themselves as potent sustained delivery carriers for IBF [111]. In addition, glutaraldehyde cross-linked GG disks have been assessed for IBF delivery [112]. The in vitro evaluation of the disks validated them as colon-specific controlled releasing IBF systems. In another study, GG-montmorillonite nanocomposites were explored for IBF delivery [113]. The nanocomposites exhibited slower delivery in pH 7.4, thereby suggesting their potential toward colonic delivery of IBF.

Another member of the NSAID family is ketoprofen (KTF). To encapsulate KTF; polyelectrolyte hydrogel tablets of cationic GG and acrylic acid were constructed by photoinitiated free radical polymerization [114]. KTF-loaded hydrogels were then compressed to tablets. As indicated from the release experiments, the tablets could be efficaciously exploited for the colonic delivery of KTF. Another study pointed the grafting of amphiphilic GG and poly(ε-caprolactone) by microwave irradiation [73]. The graft copolymer was capable of assembling into nanosized micelles and, thus, could effectively encapsulate KTF. The developed system could achieve a prolonged release of KTF over a span of 10–68 h.

Indomethacin (IND) is another NSAID commonly used for the relief of pain. A delivery system for IND was fabricated by coating GG and Eudragit FS30D onto drug-loaded pellets [115]. A retarded release of IND was observed in the colon. Diclofenac is yet another remarkable NSAID widely prescribed for pain relieving. Acrylic-grafted GG-nanosilica membrane were constructed and proved potent for controlled transdermal delivery of diclofenac [116]. Aceclofenac, another well-known NSAID, has also been encapsulated onto glutaraldehyde cross-linked GG microspheres and their release characteristics assayed by Ravi et al. [117]. The results indicated optimal release in rat cecal contents, thereby endorsing their high potential in colonic delivery.

Dexamethasone (DX) is a widely recognized corticosteroid medication, primarily used for its antiinflammatory response. Recently, DX has been hailed as a wonder drug for treatment of novel corona virus (Covid-19); it has been found to reduce the mortality rate of patients with acute respiratory complications. To construct a controlled delivery vehicle for DX, smart hydrogels comprising GG and polyacrylic acid reinforced with β-CD were designed by Das and Subuddhi [66]. It was observed that the hydrogels containing β-CD effectively lowered the rate of DX release in comparison with the hydrogels without β-CD. A strong dependence of

DX release was ascertained to GG content. The higher the GG amount, the slower the DX release. In addition, DX release profiles in SGF and SIF recommended the hydrogels as oral sustained delivery carriers of DX (Fig. 5.6).

5.6.6 Delivery of antiviral drugs

Abacavir is a prominent antiviral drug. Microencapsulation of abacavir has been performed onto carboxymethyl GG microspheres with the sole purpose to accomplish a sustained delivery [118]. It was observed that the microspheres could effectually prevent the drug release

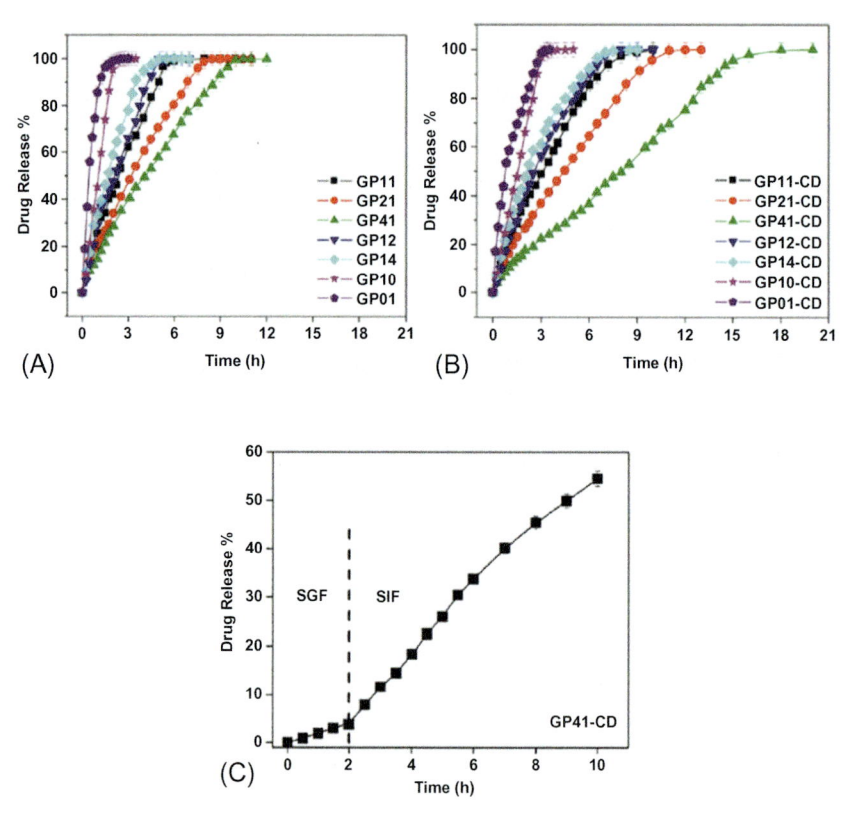

FIG. 5.6   Dexamethasone (DX) release from (A) guar gum-polyacrylic acid (GP) and (B) guar gum-polyacrylic acid-β-cyclodextrin (GP-CD) hydrogels in pH 7.4 at 37°C. (C) DX release profile from GP41-CD hydrogel in SGF and SIF at 37°C. Numerical in the sample designation represent the weight of guar gum (g) and acrylic acid (g) used in the synthesis. 1 implies 0.1 g, 2 for 0.2 g, and 4 for 0.4 g of parent components. *Reprinted from Das S, Subuddhi U. pH-Responsive guar gum hydrogels for controlled delivery of dexamethasone to the intestine. Int J Biol Macromol 2015;79:856–63. Copyright (2015), with permission from Elsevier.*

in stomach and prolong for 28 h in colon. Zidovudine is another widely prescribed antiviral agent. GG matrix tablets have been evaluated for their controlled releasing properties of zidovudine [119]. The tablets were found to retard the release for more than 12 h and were stable for up to 3 months.

5.6.7 Delivery of antitubercular drugs

Tuberculosis (TB) is a chronic disease caused by bacteria of the genus *Mycobacterium* (*M. tuberculosis, M. africanum,* and *M. bovis*). The use of Bacillus Calmette-Guerin (BCG) vaccination and chemoprophylaxis for the treatment and control of tuberculosis has still been not accepted by all [120]. The incapability of delivery of the therapeutics at the specific site, toxic side effects, noncompliance, and lengthy treatment time arouses some limitations for the use of the conventional methods [121–123]. Various strategies have come to the forefront to overcome these hindrances by implicating a selective delivery system to the affected area. Recently, inhalable delivery systems have garnered significant interest for the delivery of tubercular drugs because the local delivery of drugs to the lungs lowers the side effects, improves the bioavailability of drugs, reduces dose frequency, and shortens the treatment time [123, 124]. Of particular interest are two widely used antitubercular drugs: isoniazid (INZ) and rifampicin (RIF). The potential of RIF-INZ-loaded spray dried nanoembedded microparticles of chitosan, GG, mannan, and GG-coated chitosan against TB was evaluated by Goyal et al. [125]. The authors observed that the GG batches demonstrated remarkable flow ability among the lot. The in vivo lung distribution study revealed that the GG-coated chitosan exhibited sustained release of drug at the target site and, hence, enhanced its therapeutic efficacy. A fivefold demotion in the number of bacilli compared with the control was clearly evident. This study highlighted the potential of GG-coated chitosan microparticles for efficient TB therapy.

Another study concerns the development of pH-sensitive hydrogel microspheres of PVA and acrylic acid-*g*-GG for controlled delivery of INZ [126]. The authors also noted that the release time of INZ was significantly increased up to 8 h from its short plasma half-life of 0.5–1.6 h. Encapsulation of INZ onto microspheres of sodium alginate and PNIPAAm-*g*-GG has also been performed [54]. The microspheres were dual responsive, exhibiting both pH- and temperature-sensitivity. INZ delivery was significantly prolonged up to 12 h from these microspheres. In another development, enteric-coated microparticles of chitosan and GG were explored for INZ delivery [127]. The microparticles inhibited the burst release of INZ in the gastric media, but an enhancement was evident in the intestinal media, which further extended for a period of around 50 h.

5.6.8 Delivery of anti-HIV drugs

AIDS is an infectious disease caused by the human immunodeficiency virus (HIV). However, the female population has relatively no control for the prevention of heterosexual HIV transmission and is a primary cause of deaths as per the reports of the WHO. Thus women-centric formulation for the prevention of AIDS is the need of the hour. In this context, vaginal microbicides offer a great many advantages regarding allowing the availability of the drug at the local site and minimizing side effects. Tenofovir (TFV) is an antiretroviral drug widely studied for its inclusion in microbicide systems. Lyophilized bioadhesive vaginal bigels of GG and sesame oil were prepared using Span 60 and Tween 60 and explored for controlled delivery of TFV (Fig. 5.7) [128]. In addition to controlling the

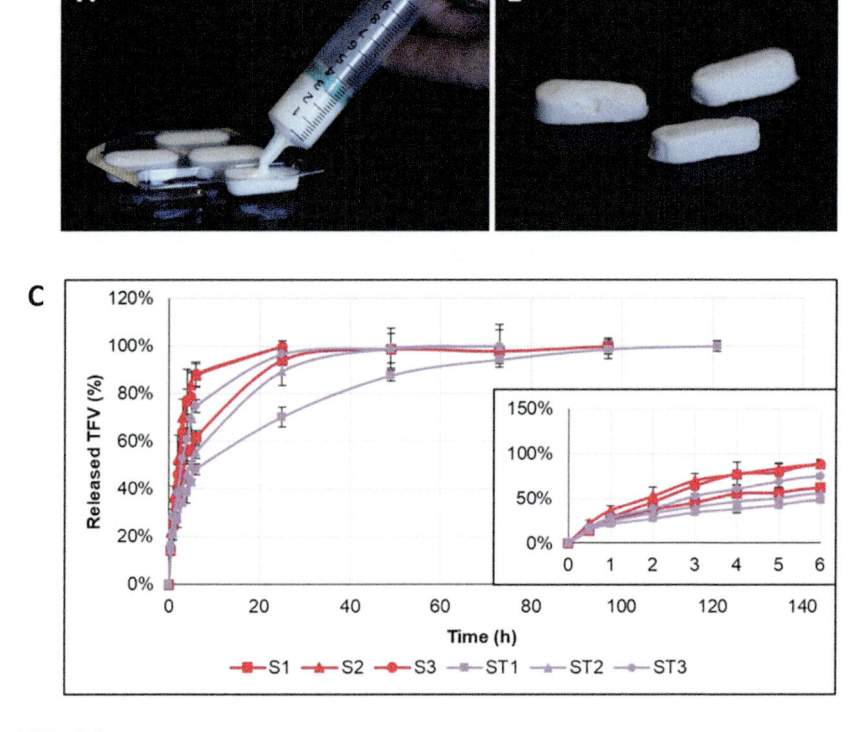

FIG. 5.7 (A) and (B) Physical appearance of freeze-dried bigels of guar gum and sesame oil and (C) sustained release profile of tenofovir from the bigels. S1, S2, and S3 correspond to the formulations prepared using span 60 as surfactant, whereas ST1, ST2, and ST3 indicate those prepared using both span 60 and tween 60. *Reprinted from Martín-Illana A, Cazorla-Luna R, NotarioPérez F, Bedoya LM, Ruiz-Caro R, Veiga M-D. Freeze-dried bioadhesive vaginal bigels for controlled release of tenofovir. Eur J Pharm Sci 2019;127:38–51. Copyright (2019), with permission from Elsevier.*

rate of delivery of TFV; the bigels exhibited higher bioadhesion time, thus ensuring that they can remain at the vaginal site for longer periods without the risk of clearance by vaginal fluids.

Concerning another report, vaginal mucoadhesive tablets were constructed using various polymers such as HPMC, chitosan, GG, and Eudragit for the release of TFV. The formulations served two purposes: first, the vaginal release of TFV was significantly prolonged for 72 h and second, the vaginal residence time was notably increased to 96 h [129]. Similar results are also reported by Notario-Perez et al. in their research paper, where a sustained release of TFV was evident from GG-containing delivery system [130].

Didanosine (DNS), a highly active antiretroviral drug, is also used for the treatment of HIV/AIDS. GG matrix tablets have proved their mettle toward the oral sustained release of DNS. Soumya et al. constructed DNS-encapsulated tablets using different biopolymers such as GG, xanthan gum, and karaya gum by wet granulation method [131]. The tablets were found to be stable and could sustain DNS release for 8 h. Ramesh et al. reported enteric-coated matrix tablets of GG and other polymers for the colon-targeted delivery of DNS [132]. The release of DNS was lower in acidic medium (less than 20%), whereas about 80%–100% of drug was released in pH 7.4 in a controlled manner.

5.6.9 Delivery of antidiabetic drugs

Metformin hydrochloride remains the first-line drug therapy for patients with Type 2 diabetes mellitus (T2DM). An obstacle to an effective metformin therapy is the high incidence of concomitant gastrointestinal symptoms such as abdominal discomfort and nausea. To improve patient compliances, metformin HCl-encapsulated sustained release tablets were developed using GG and HPMC [133]. The drug release evaluations revealed that the HPMC alone could not prevent the burst release. However, when taken in combination with GG, the release was prolonged effectively for 12 h. Hence the role of GG is crucial in the fabrication of sustained release tablets of metformin in T2DM therapy.

Glimepiride is a second good choice to metformin in the monotherapy of T2DM. Glimepiride-loaded polyacrylamide-g-GG pellets have been constructed for colonic delivery [134]. Apart from exhibiting a high stability of 60 days, the pellets demonstrated pH-responsive drug-releasing characteristics. Sustained release drug profile at the colon was obtained from the aforesaid pellets, thereby validating them as potent antidiabetic drug carriers.

Nateglinide (NTG) is an antihyperglycemic agent recommended for noninsulin-dependent diabetes mellitus (NIDDM). Bashir et al. have evaluated sustained release microspheres of NTG using GG and olibanum gum synthesized by calcium chloride/sodium alginate ionic gelation method [135]. The release studies in SIF (pH 7.2) indicated a sustained release of NTG from the microspheres for a period extending up to 12 h. An improved patient compliance was also observed because of lesser dosing frequency.

5.6.10 Delivery of anticonvulsant drugs

Carbamazepine (CBZ) is an anticonvulsant drug primarily used for epilepsy and neuropathic pain. An oral jelly formulation of CBZ was prepared using pectin and GG [136]. The CBZ jellies were stable up to 90 days and exhibited better spreadability than currently available medications. This study indicated that the prepared jellies could be effectually used to improve palatability for use in pediatric, geriatric, and dysphagic patients.

Pregabalin (PRG) is an antiepileptic drug prescribed for the treatment of partial seizures, diabetic neuropathy, and postherpetic neuralgia. However, its short half-life necessitates the need for a sustained release system. In this regard, Kanwar et al. designed floating tablets of PRG encapsulated in xanthan gum and GG matrices [137]. The tablets showed higher floating time (> 24 h with a lag time of about 7 min) with a prolonged PRG release profile. The in vivo pharmacodynamic studies further revealed that the onset of jerks and clonus were significantly delayed.

5.6.11 Delivery of antiasthmatic drugs

Theophylline (THP) is a respiratory medication of high repute for asthma and chronic obstructive pulmonary disease (COPD). Owing to its low oral bioavailability and short half-life (6 h), THP requires frequent dosing [138]. Thus a sustained release of THP is always desirable. GG-based formulations have emerged as viable platforms to aid in prolonged delivery of THP. Phadke et al. chemically modified GG to carboxymethyl GG, which was then emulsified with gelatin solution to obtain microspheres [139]. The microspheres successfully delayed the release up to 26 h. Encapsulation of THP has also been performed in GG matrices to develop sustained release THP tablets wherein a desired slow-release profile was witnessed [140].

5.6.12 Delivery of antiemetic drugs

Antiemetics are used in the treatment of nausea and emesis. Significant research has been devoted toward the delivery of antiemetic drugs through the nasal route because it offers superiorities regarding fast and high drug concentration, thereby improving patient compliances [141]. In this regard, in situ gelling nasal inserts comprising GG and xanthan gum were prepared by freeze-drying technique for the sustained delivery of the common antiemetic drug metoclopramide hydrochloride [142]. The authors concluded that the freeze-dried inserts delayed the drug release in comparison with the pristine polymers. More so, the inserts displayed excellent bioadhesion potential, thus implying an improvement in the nasal residence time.

5.6.13 Delivery of antidepressant drugs

Venlafaxine (VLF) is an antidepressant medication used to treat major depressive disorder, anxiety disorder, panic disorder, and phobia. Multiparticulate granules of xanthan gum and GG were fabricated in different ratios [143]. In comparison with the commercially available VLF tablets; the developed granules sustained VLF release for more than 20 h. The authors concluded that the use of natural polymers played a crucial role in retarding the drug release.

Buproprion (BPR) is another drug prescribed for the treatment of major depressive disorder. Sustained release tables of BPR were formulated using GG, Eudragit, and HPMC at different concentrations [144]. Tablets comprising GG and HPMC were much effective as controlled delivery devices for BPR. Moreover, the synthesized tablets exhibited better sustained release properties than the marketed formulations.

5.6.14 Delivery of anthelmintic drugs

Anthelmintic drugs are a group of medications that expel parasitic worms from the body without harming the host. Mebendazole (MBZ) and albendazole (ABZ) are a couple of commonly used anthelmintic drugs. GG as carrier matrices were developed for MBZ delivery [145]. The tablets released 8%–15% MBZ in the physiological environment of the stomach, but it was significantly improved up to 82% in the SCF. No change in the physical appearance and drug dissolution rate of the tablets was witnessed even after storage for 3 months at 75% humidity. Moreover, the pharmacokinetic evaluations of these tablets against an immediate release tablet were conducted in six healthy human volunteers [146]. The oral administration of the GG tablets revealed that MBZ produced peak plasma concentration (C_{max} of 25.7 ± 2.6 ng/mL) at 9.4 ± 1.7 h (T_{max}). On the other hand; the commercial tablet displayed a C_{max} of 37.2 ± 6.8 ng/mL at 3.4 ± 0.9 h (T_{max}). Hence the findings of the study clearly demonstrated that the GG tablets delayed the T_{max} time and lowered the C_{max}; paving the path for better local action in the colon.

Patients having helminthiasis show the presence of eggs/cysts of parasites in stool samples along with a decreased hemoglobin content. ABZ is the preferred choice for the treatment of human intestinal capillariasis because it is effective against eggs, larvae, and adult worms. However, conventional ABZ doses sometimes release in the stomach and cause systemic side effects. Thus targeting ABZ to colon is not only beneficial to reduce the side-effects but also is a safe way of administration. GG matrix tablets were designed for colonic delivery of ABZ by Krishnaiah et al. [147]. The tablets restricted the release of ABZ in the stomach and intestine but showed a significant improvement in SCF. The tablets exhibited stability for a period of 6 months. To further improve the bioavailability of ABZ; solid ICs of β-CD and ABZ were prepared and then loaded onto GG matrices [148]. A slow drug-release profile to the colon was manifested from the tablets containing the ICs, which ascertained their potency as controlled delivery devices. The aforementioned tablets were also subjected to in vivo pharmacokinetic evaluation and clinical efficacy in human volunteers [149]. The results of the investigation revealed that apart from improving the bioavailability of ABZ on inclusion; the tablets also promoted a controlled delivery because of the presence of β-CD. The clinical studies conducted on patients having helminthiasis showed that the GG colon-targeted tablets reduced eggs/ gram count quicker than the conventional formulations, resulting in an improved hemoglobin content and clinical performance.

5.6.15 Delivery of antihistamine drugs

Antihistamines are a class of drugs that oppose the activity of histamine receptors in the body. H_1- and H_2-antihistamines are the two largest types. H_2-antihistamines, particularly, bind to histamine H_2 receptors primarily in the stomach. Ranitidine (RTD) and famotidine (FTD) are two commonly used H_2 receptor antagonists. Gastroretentive delivery systems have come a long way for controlled release of drugs in the gastric region. Among various gastroretentive systems, floating delivery systems have sparked interest because they enhance the gastric residence time without affecting the gastric emptying time. Hence there is need for the use of nonerodable polymeric systems for treatment of gastric maladies. A gastroretentive floating delivery system for FTD was fabricated using GG and gellan gum [150]. Sodium bicarbonate was chosen as the effervescent-producing agent. The developed system needed a time of 20 ± 0.5 to 25 ± 2 min for self-unfolding and remained buoyant. The cumulative drug release indicated them to be novel delivery devices for FTD. In another report concerning the gastroretentive delivery of RTD, floating delivery systems were constructed using GG and xanthan gum [151]. Addition of citric acid caused faster RTD release in the stomach, whereas the release rate was greatly retarded when stearic acid was added to the formulation. This study emphasized that a desired dissolution profile for RTD could be achieved by choosing a suitable agent wisely.

5.6.16 Delivery of antimuscarinic drugs

Tolterodine is an antimuscarinic drug that is used to treat urinary incontinence. Blend microspheres of GG and soy protein isolates were prepared by cross-linking with calcium chloride [152]. It was observed drug release rate was affected by the GG content. The higher the GG content, the slower the drug release. The microspheres sustained the release for more than 12 h and, thus, could be efficaciously used for delivery of antimuscarinic drugs.

5.6.17 Delivery of antipyretic and analgesic drugs

Paracetamol is one of the widely prescribed antipyretics. In certain cases; oral administration of paracetamol has led to irritation in gastric mucosa due to its acidic nature. In rare cases, it has been reported to impair liver metabolism. Thus designing a transdermal delivery system for paracetamol would be beneficial because the risks of hepatic toxicity could be evaded. In view of this, hydrogels comprising chitosan and GG were fabricated as dermal patches for delivery of paracetamol [56]. The drug release was studied using an avian skin model. In addition to exhibiting a sustained drug releasing behavior, the hydrogel patches also demonstrated good antimicrobial activity and high biocompatibility.

Naproxen (NAP) is a well-known analgesic recommended for the treatment of rheumatoid arthritis. Chronotherapeutic delivery of NAP has proven to be a blessing for the patients. In this context, Hadi et al. evaluated matrix-mini-tablets of NAP for chronotherapy treatment of rheumatism [153]. The mini-tablets of NAP were formulated using different polymers such as GG, sodium alginate, Eudragit, and cellulose. The thickness of the tablets ranged between 2.04 ± 0.01 mm and 2.11 ± 0.01 mm, with a drug encapsulation efficiency of more than 95%. The tablets could effectively prevent the release of NAP in the gastric pH, and an optimal release was evident in the ileo-colonic pH. It was further observed that as the GG content was increased, the lag time (time taken for < 10% NAP release) also increased, thereby decreasing the NAP delivery rate. In another report, chronotherapeutic delivery of NAP was performed using GG and ammonium cross-linked GG tablets [154]. In comparison with pristine GG tablets, the ammonium cross-linked GG tablets displayed a more sustained release feature. The release was minimal in the stomach even after 4 h, but it improved significantly in the cecal medium. The findings of the above two reports clearly put forward the efficacy of GG-based tablets for chronotherapeutic delivery of NAP toward the treatment of arthritis.

5.6.18 Delivery of proteins

One of the most important reasons, which demands intravenous administration of protein drugs, is its instability [8]. Because proteins are largely susceptible to degradation in gastric environment, a successful protein delivery needs to overcome various hindrances associated with the process, which mostly includes prevention of proteolytic breakdown in the gut [8, 155]. Thus pH-sensitive formulations have become an obligatory requirement for protein delivery. George and Abraham synthesized pH-responsive alginate and GG hydrogels cross-linked with glutaraldehyde [62]. Bovine serum albumin (BSA) release from the hydrogels indicated lower amounts (~ 20%) in pH 1.2 and higher amounts (~ 90%) in pH 7.4 medium. Hence the developed hydrogels could be efficaciously used for the delivery of BSA to the intestine through the oral route. Another report focuses on the construction of pH-responsive hydrogel microspheres of GG and methacrylic acid [156]. BSA release extended well beyond 72 h, with higher amounts of drug releasing at pH 6.8. Hydrogels of GG prepared through esterification with 1,2,3,4-butanetetracarboxylic dianhydride were exploited for deliveries of BSA and hen egg white lysozyme [157] (Fig. 5.8). The hydrogels exhibited long-term release properties for both the proteins and, thus, were potent for protein delivery. In slightly modified approaches, metal ion cross-linked carboxymethyl GG microspheres were investigated for BSA delivery [158, 159]. Although negligible release occurred in the medium of pH 1.2, a complete release of BSA was evident in a pH 7.4 medium. These metal ion cross-linked gastric-resistant microbeads are truly potent for protein delivery.

5.6.19 Delivery of genes

To expound the possibilities of GG to deliver nucleic acids in gene delivery applications, Bansal et al. developed a series of gene carriers by conjugating GG with low-molecular weight polyethyleneimine (PEI) [160]. The constructed formulations efficiently carried pDNA into the cells and were endowed with superior transfection efficiency than the standard transfection reagents. Another report concerned the grafting of carboxymethyl GG to PEI as an effective gene delivery vehicle [161].

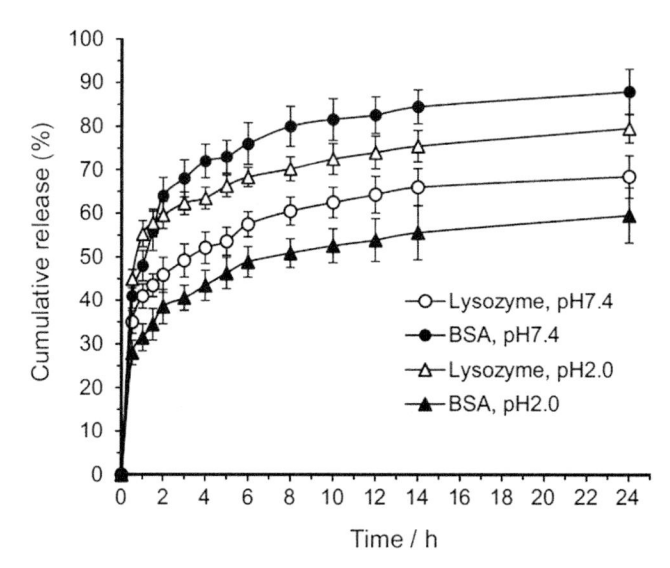

FIG. 5.8 Release profile of lysozyme and BSA from guar gum hydrogels prepared through esterification with 1,2,3,4-butanetetracarboxylic anhydride (BTCA) in pH2.0 and pH7.4. *Reprinted from Kono H, Otaka F, Ozaki M. Preparation and characterization of guar gum hydrogels as carrier materials for controlled protein drug delivery. Carbohydr Polym 2014;111:830–40. Copyright (2014), with permission from Elsevier.*

The results suggested that the copolymer exhibited strong pDNA condensation aptitude by forming positively charged polyplexes. More so, enhanced transfection efficiency was also witnessed from the copolymer. Thus GG-based formulations could be duly explored in viral and nonviral gene delivery therapy.

5.7 GG hydrogels in tissue engineering

Tissue engineering has evolved into a promising line of approach to assemble constructs that restore, maintain, and repair damaged tissues or, in many cases, wholesome organs. Hydrogels of GG and/or its derivatives have been the frontrunners in tissue regeneration owing to their biocompatibility and gel-forming characteristics. In a bid to comply to the current demand in bone diseases, composite scaffolds of GG, gellan gum, and hydroxyapatite were explored as potential bone grafts by Anandan et al. [162]. The high mechanical strength of the scaffolds enabled them to be used as bone scaffolds. Furthermore, the cytotoxic evaluations of the scaffolds on murine fibroblast (L929) and osteosarcoma (MG63) cells revealed them to be nontoxic, cell proliferation supportive, and suitable for bone reconstruction. Another report points to the potency of an injectable guar-based hydrogel for osteoblastic cell growth [163]. In this study, hydroxypropyl guar-*graft*-poly(N-vinylcaprolactam) copolymer performed efficiently as a remarkable scaffold material for osteoblast cell differentiation. In addition, the scaffold exhibited formation of an apatite-like network structure on its surface after being soaked in simulated body fluid (SBF) solution for 7 days. The same research group prepared novel bionanocomposite hydrogels comprising a blend of hydroxypropyl GG, PVA, and nanohydroxyapatite [164]. The cell viability studies in MC3T3 bone cells revealed that the materials supported osteoblastic activity without any adverse effect on the cells. A study by Kundu et al. investigated the possible use of carboxymethyl GG and PVA scaffolds in tissue engineering [165]. The interaction of the developed scaffold with Vero cells displayed no cytotoxicity and promoted cell proliferation. The authors concluded that the developed macroporous scaffolds could be effective in tissue engineering applications. In another instance, carboxymethyl GG nanoscaffolds have been assessed for the growth of RAW 264.7 macrophage cells, NIH3T3 fibroblasts, and bone marrow-mesenchymal stem cells (BM-MSCs) [166]. All the cell types successfully grew and proliferated on the scaffold, even under inflammatory and hypoxic conditions after 48 h. A biodegradable hydrogel based on GG-methacrylate (GG-MA) macromonomers was studied for tissue regeneration efficacy wherein human endothelial cell line EA.hy926 was photoencapsulated into the hydrogel [167]. In this study, GG of varying molecular weights was first modified with glycidyl methacrylate to form a series of GG-MA macromonomers. The GG-MA hydrogels were then synthesized by dissolving the macromonomers in PBS (pH 7.4) and exposing to UV radiation. The hydrogel demonstrated significant endothelial cell proliferation and could be used for in situ tissue engineering (Fig. 5.9).

Collagen-poly(dialdehyde) GG-based hybrid scaffolds have been reported for tissue regeneration by Ragothaman et al. [168]. The developed scaffolds possessed a microporous three-dimensional honeycomb structure with an improved thermal stability. The remarkable increase in NIH 3T3 fibroblast cell density and proliferation on the scaffolds suggested their high potency in tissue engineering applications. Another report from the same research group demonstrated that loading the aforementioned scaffolds with platelet derived growth factor not only promoted rapid tissue regeneration but also provided stronger tissues [169]. A novel attempt incepted on carrageenan-GG scaffolds revealed their good hemocompatibility and platelet adhesion characteristics [170]. The excellent cell proliferation features of the scaffolds were witnessed in mice model. This study validated that the constructed scaffolds are viable candidates for tissue regeneration.

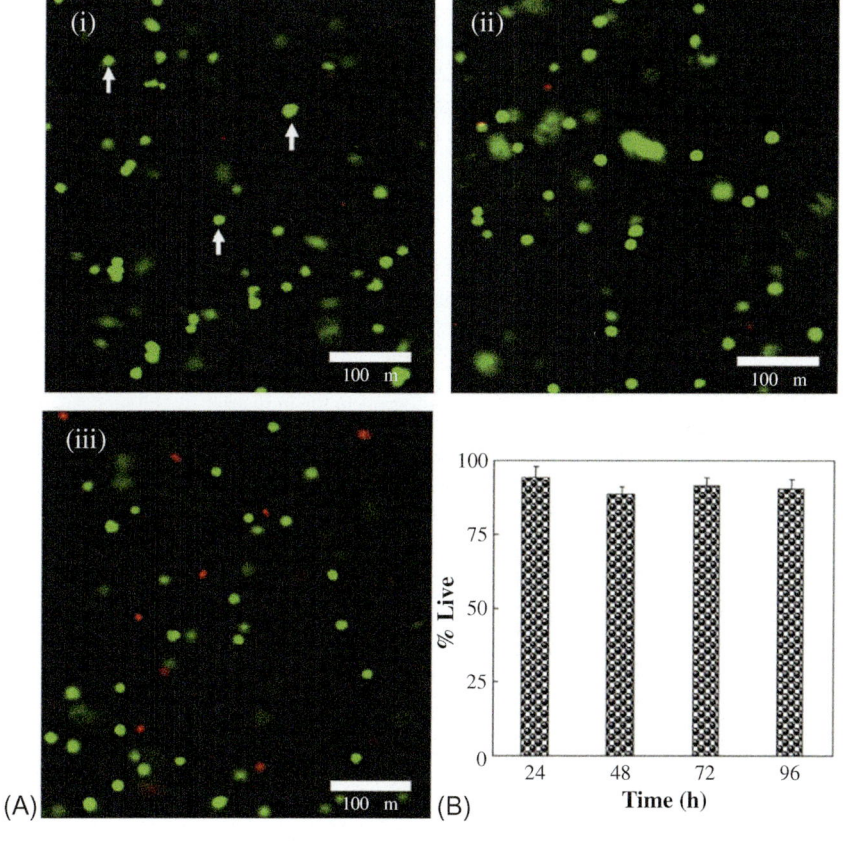

FIG. 5.9 (A) Viability of EA.hy926 cells seeded in GG-methacrylate (GG-MA) hydrogels at (i) 0.05%, (ii) 0.1%, and (iii) 0.15% (w/v) of GG-MA macromonomer concentration after 24 h. (B) Plot depicting the percent of live cells in hydrogels with 0.15% GG-MA macromonomer. *Reprinted from Tiwari A, Grailer JJ, Pilla S, Steeber DA, Gong S. Biodegradable hydrogels based on novel photopolymerizable guar gum–methacrylate macromonomers for in situ fabrication of tissue engineering scaffolds. Acta Biomater 5:3441–52. Copyright (2009), with permission from Elsevier*

5.8 Conclusion and perspectives

GG is undoubtedly a biopolymer *par excellence* in biomedicine. Owing to its versatility, GG has been tailored with a plethora of polymers to yield derivatives endowed with enhanced physicochemical characteristics and functionalities. GG-based biomaterials are promising candidates for delivery of an assortment of medications, including protein drugs and genes. Judicious choice of reagents has helped achieve a drug release profile of choice from GG formulations. The flexibility of GG hydrogel to adapt to various architectures such as tablets, capsules, microspheres, and nanoparticles further enhances its already highly acclaimed stature. Engineering of novel GG-based biomaterials with high precision regarding bioactivities is imperative for targeted and sustained delivery of therapeutics. The design of such biomaterials would undeniably revolutionize the star stature of GG in the world of biomedicine.

References

[1] Rana V, Rai P, Tiwary AK, Singh RS, Kennedy JF, Knill CJ. Modified gums: approaches and applications in drug delivery. Carbohydr Polym 2011;83:1031–47.

[2] Ribeiro AJ, de Souza FRL, Bezerra JMNA, Oliveira C, Nadvorny D, Monica F, et al. Gums' based delivery systems: review on cashew gum and its derivatives. Carbohydr Polym 2016;147:188–200.

[3] Zare EN, Makvandi P, Tay FR. Recent progress in the industrial and biomedical applications of tragacanth gum: a review. Carbohydr Polym 2019;212:450–67.

[4] Giavasis I. Production of microbial polysaccharides for use in food. In: McNeil B, Archer D, Giavasis I, Harvey L, editors. Microbial production of food ingredients, enzymes and neutraceuticals. Cambridge: Woodhead Publishing Ltd.; 2013. p. 413–68.

[5] Linton JD, Ash SG, Huybrechts L. Microbial polysaccharides. In: Byrom D, editor. Biomaterials. London: Palgrave Macmillan; 1991. p. 215–61.

[6] Verbeken D, Dierckx S, Dewettinck K. Exudate gums: occurrence, production and applications. Appl Microbiol Technol 2003;63:10–21.

[7] Barak S, Mudgil D, Taneja S. Exudate gums: chemistry, properties and food applications——a review. J Sci Food Agric 2020;100:2828–35.

[8] Prabaharan M. Prospective of guar gum and its derivatives as controlled drug delivery systems. Int J Biol Macromol 2011;49:117–24.

[9] Cheetham NWH, Mashimba ENM. Conformational aspects of xanthan-galactomannan gelation. Further evidence from optical-rotation studies. Carbohydr Polym 1990;14:17–27.

[10] Brosio E, Dubado A, Verzegnassi B. Pulsed field gradient spin-echo NMR measurement of water diffusion coefficient in thickening and gelling agents: guar galactomannan solutions and pectin gels. Cell Mol Biol 1994;40:569–73.

[11] George A, Shah PA, Shrivastav PS. Guar gum: versatile natural polymer for drug delivery applications. Eur Polym J 2019;112:722–35.

[12] Maier H, Anderson M, Karl C, Magnuson K, Whistler RL. Guar, locust bean, tara and fenugreek gums. In: Whistler RL, Bemiller JN, editors. Industrial gums: polysaccharides and their derivatives. New York: Academic Press; 1993. p. 181–226.

[13] Goldstein AM, Alter EN, Seaman JK. Guar gum. In: Whistler RL, editor. Industrial gums: polysaccharides and their derivatives. New York: Academic Press; 1973. p. 303–22.

[14] Anderson E. Endosperm mucilages of legumes: occurrence and composition. Ind Eng Chem 1949;41:2887–90.

[15] Venkateswarlu B, Raikhy NP, Aggarwal RK. Effect of inoculation and cobalt application on nodulation and nitrogen uptake in guar (Cyamopsis tetragonoloba L.). J Ind Soc Soil Sci 1982;30:550–1.

[16] Mudgil D, Barak S, Khatkar BS. Guar gum: processing, properties and food applications—a review. J Food Sci Technol 2014;51(3):409–18.

[17] Thombare N, Jha U, Mishra S, Siddiqui MZ. Guar gum as a promising starting material for diverse applications: a review. Int J Biol Macromol 2016;88:361–72.

[18] Sharma G, Sharma S, Kumar A, Al-Muhtaseb AH, Naushad M, Ghfar AA, Mola GT, Stadler FJ. Guar gum and its composites as potential materials for diverse applications: a review. Carbohydr Polym 2018;199:534–45.

[19] Chudzikowski RJ. Guar gum and its applications. J Soc Cosmet Chem 1971;22:43–60.

[20] Butt MS, Shahzadi N, Sharif MK, Nasir M. Guar gum: a miracle therapy for hypercholesterolemia, hyperglycemia and obesity. Critic Rev Food Sci Nutr 2007;47:389–96.

[21] McCleary BV. Enzymic hydrolysis, fine structure, and gelling interaction of legume-seed D-galacto-D-mannans. Carbohydr Res 1979;71:205–30.

[22] Grasdalen H, Painter TJ. N.M.R. studies of composition and sequence in legume-seed galactomannans. Carbohydr Res 1980;81:59–66.

[23] Tripathy S, Das MK. Guar gum: present status and applications. J Pharm Sci Innov 2013;2(4):24–8.

[24] Garti N, Leser ME. Emulsification properties of hydrocolloids. Polym Adv Technol 2001;12:123–35.

[25] Barth HG, Smith DA. High-performance size-exclusion chromatography of guar gum. J Chromatogr 1981;206:410–5.

[26] Vijayendran BR, Bone T. Absolute molecular weight and molecular weight distribution of guar by size exclusion chromatography and low-angle laser light scattering. Carbohydr Polym 1984;4:299–311.

[27] Bai L, Liu F, Xu X, Huan S, Gu J, McClements DJ. Impact of polysaccharide molecular characteristics on viscosity enhancement and depletion flocculation. J Food Eng 2017;207:35–45.

[28] Thakur S, Sharma B, Verma A, Chaudhary J, Tamulevicius S, Thakur VK. Recent approaches in guar gum hydrogel synthesis for water purification. Int J Polym Anal Char 2018;23:621–32.

[29] Glicksman M. Gum technology in the food industry. New York: Academic Press; 1969.

[30] Wang T, Zhang M, Fang Z, Liu Y, Gao Z. Rheological, textural and flavour properties of yellow mustard sauce as affected by modified starch, xanthan and guar gum. Food Bioproc Tech 2016;9:849–58.

[31] Parija S, Misra M, Mohanty AK. Studies of natural gum adhesive extracts: an overview. J Macromol Sci C Polym Rev 2001;41:175–97.

[32] Zhang L-M, Zhou J-F, Hui PS. A comparative study on viscosity behavior of water-soluble chemically modified guar gum derivatives with different functional lateral groups. J Sci Food Agric 2005;85:2638–44.

[33] Tantry JS, Mangal NS. Rheological study of guar gum. Ind J Pharm Sci 2001;63:74–6.

[34] Achayuthakan P, Suphantharika M. Pasting and rheological properties of waxy corn starch as affected by guar gum and xanthan gum. Carbohydr Polym 2008;71:9–17.

[35] Shobha MS, Tharanathan RN. Rheological behaviour of pullulanase-treated guar galactomannan on co-gelation with xanthan. Food Hydrocolloid 2009;23:749–54.

[36] Chenlo F, Moreira R, Silva C. Rheological behaviour of aqueous systems of tragacanth and guar gums with storage time. J Food Eng 2010;96:107–13.

[37] Cheng Y, Prud'homme RK. Measurement of forces between galactomannan polymer chains: effect of hydrogen bonding. Macromolecules 2002;35:10155–61.

[38] Carlson WA, Ziegenfuss EM, Overton JD. Compatibility and manipulation of guar gum. Food Technol 1962;16:50–4.

[39] Doyle JP, Giannouli P, Martin EJ, Brooks M, Morris ER. Effect of sugars, galactose content and chain length on freeze-thaw gelation of galactomannans. Carbohydr Polym 2006;64:391–401.

[40] Aminabhavi TM, Nadagouda MN, Joshi SD, More UA. Guar gum as platform for the oral controlled release of therapeutics. Expert Opin Drug Deliv 2014;11(5):753–66.

[41] Dodi G, Hritcu D, Popa MI. Carboxymethylation of guar gum: synthesis and characterization. Cellulose Chem Technol 2011;45:171–6.

[42] Trivedi J, Kalia K, Patel NK, Trivedi HC. Ceric-induced grafting of acrylonitrile onto sodium salt of partially carboxymethylated guar gum. Carbohydr Polym 2005;60:117–25.

[43] Dong C, Tian B. Studies on preparation and emulsifying properties of guar galactomannan ester of palmitic acid. J Appl Polym Sci 1999;72:639–45.

[44] Xiao C, Zhang J, Zhang Z, Zhang L. Study of blend films from chitosan and hydroxypropyl guar gum. J Appl Polym Sci 2003;90:1991–5.

[45] Lapasin R, De Lorenzi L, Pricl S, Torriano G. Flow properties of hydroxypropyl guar gum and its long-chain hydrophobic derivatives. Carbohydr Polym 1995;28:195–202.

[46] Pal S. Carboxymethyl guar: its synthesis and macromolecular characterization. J Appl Polym Sci 2009;111:2630–6.

[47] Gao J, Grady BP. Reaction kinetics and subsequent rheology of carboxymethyl guar gum produced from guar splits. Ind Eng Chem Res 2018;57:7345–54.

[48] Shenoy MA, D'Melo DJ. Synthesis and characterization of acryloyloxy guar gum. J Appl Polym Sci 2010;117:148–54.

[49] Risica D, Barbetta A, Vischetti L, Cametti C, Dentini M. Rheological properties of guar and its methyl, hydroxypropyl and hydroxypropyl-methyl derivatives in semidilute and concentrated aqueous solutions. Polymer 2010;51:1972–82.

[50] Xiao W, Dong L. Studies on methacryloyl guar gum: surface morphology, crystallinity, biodegradability and viscosity behavior of semi-dilute solutions. Adv Mater Res 2011;279:327–32.

[51] Oblonsek M, Sostar-Turk S, Lapasin R. Rheological studies of concentrated guar gum. Rheol Acta 2003;42:491–9.

[52] Sharma BR, Kumar V, Soni PL. Ce(IV)-ion initiated graft copolymerization of methyl methacrylate onto guar gum. J Macromol Sci Part A 2003;40:49–60.

[53] Rao MS, Kanatt SR, Chawla SP, Sharma A. Chitosan and guar gum composite films: preparation, physical, mechanical and antimicrobial properties. Carbohydr Polym 2010;82:1243–7.

[54] Kajjari PB, Manjeshwar LS, Aminabhavi TM. Novel interpenetrating polymer network hydrogel microspheres of chitosan and poly(acrylamide)-*grafted*-guar gum for controlled release of ciprofloxacin. Ind Eng Chem Res 2011;50:13280–7.

[55] Kajjari PB, Manjeshwar LS, Aminabhavi TM. Novel pH- and temperature-responsive blend hydrogel microspheres of sodium alginate and PNIPAAm-g-GG for controlled release of isoniazid. AAPS Pharm Sci Tech 2012;13:1147–57.

[56] Sami AJ, Khalid M, JamilT AS, Mangat SA, Shakoori AR, Iqbal S. Formulation of novel chitosan guargum based hydrogels for sustained drug release of paracetamol. Int J Biol Macromol 2018;108:324–32.

[57] Yuan X, Praphakar RA, Munusamy MA, Alarfaj AA, Kumar SS, Rajan M. Mucoadhesive guar gum hydrogel inter-connected chitosan-g-polycaprolactone micelles for rifampicin delivery. Crabohydr Polym 2019;206:1–10.

[58] Singh M, Tiwary AK, Kaur G. Investigations on interpolymer complexes of cationic guar gum and xanthan gum for formulation of bioadhesive films. Res Pharm Sci 2010;5:79–87.

[59] Fan Q, Jiang C, Wang W, Bai L, Chen H, Yang H, Wei D, Yang L. Eco-friendly extraction of cellulose nanocrystals from grape pomace and construction of self-healing nanocomposite hydrogels. Cellulose 2020;27:2541–53.

[60] Dhumal CV, Ahmed J, Bandara N, Sarkar P. Improvement of antimicrobial activity of sago starch/guar gum bi-phasic edible films by incorporating carvacrol and citral. Food Packag Shelf Life 2019;21:100380.

[61] Dhumal CV, Pal K, Sarkar P. Synthesis, characterization and antimicrobial efficacy of composite films from guar gum/sago starch/whey protein isolate loaded with carvacrol, citral and carvacrol-citral mixture. J Mater Sci Mater Med 2019;30:117.

[62] George M, Abraham TE. pH sensitive alginate–guar gum hydrogel for the controlled delivery of protein drugs. Int J Pharm 2007;335:123–9.

[63] Senapati MK, Srinatha A, Pandit JK. In vitro release characteristics of matrix tablets: studies of karaya gum and guar gum as release modulators. Indian J Pharm Sci 2006;68:824–6.

[64] Bagal D, Karve MS. Entrapment of plant invertase within novel composite of agarose–guar gum biopolymer membrane. Anal Chim Acta 2006;555:316–21.

[65] Sharma S, Afgan S, Deepak, Kumar A, Kumar R. L-Alanine induced thermally stable self-healing guar gum hydrogel as potential drug vehicle for sustained release of hydrophilic drug. Mater Sci Eng C 2019;99:1384–91.

[66] Das S, Subuddhi U. pH-responsive guar gum hydrogels for controlled delivery ofdexamethasone to the intestine. Int J Biol Macromol 2015;79:856–63.

[67] Dutta K, Das B, Orasugh JT, Mondal D, Adhikari A, Rana D, Banerjee R, Mishra R, Kar S, Chattopadhyay D. Bio-derived cellulose nanofibril reinforced poly(N-isopropylacrylamide)-g guar gum nanocomposite: an avant-Garde biomaterial as a transdermal membrane. Polymer 2018;135:85–102.

[68] Das T, Yeasmin S, Khatua S, Acharya K, Bandyopadhyay A. Influence of a blend of guar gum and poly(vinyl alcohol) on long term stability, and antibacterial and antioxidant efficacies of silver nanoparticles. RSC Adv 2015;5:54059–69.

[69] Dutta K, Das B, Mondal D, Adhikari A, Rana D, Chattopadhyay AK, Banerjee R, Mishra R, Chattopadhyay D. An ex situ approach to fabricating nanosilica reinforced polyacrylamide grafted guar gum nanocomposites as an efficient biomaterial for transdermal drug delivery application. New J Chem 2017;41:9461–71.

[70] Das S, Subuddhi U. Guar gum-poly(N-isopropylacrylamide) smart hydrogels for sustained delivery of 5-fluorouracil. Polym Bull 2019;76:2945–63.

[71] Barbucci R, Pasqui D, Favaloro R, Panariello G. A thixotropic hydrogel from chemically cross-linked guar gum: synthesis, characterization and rheological behaviour. Carbohydr Res 2008;343:3058–65.

[72] Anirudhan TS, Nair SS, Sekhar C. Deposition of gold-cellulose hybrid nanofiller on a polyelectrolyte membrane constructed using guar gum and poly(vinyl alcohol) for transdermal drug delivery. J Membrane Sci 2017;539:344–57.

[73] Soppimath KS, Kuklarni AR, Aminabhavi TM. Chemically modified polyacrylamide-g-guar gum-based crosslinked anionic microgels as pH-sensitive drug delivery systems: preparation and characterization. J Control Release 2001;75:331–45.

[74] Tiwari A, Prabhaharan M. An amphiphilic nanocarrier based on guar gum-graft-poly(ε-caprolactone) for potential drug-delivery applications. J Biomater Sci Polym Ed 2010;21:937–49.

[75] Pan X, Wang Q, Ning D, Dai L, Liu K, Ni Y, Chen L, Huang L. Ultraflexible self-healing guar gum-glycerol hydrogel with injectable, antifreeze, and strain-sensitive properties. ACS Biomater Sci Eng 2018;4:3397–404.

[76] Bhowmik M, et al. Effect of xanthan gum and guar gum on in situ gelling ophthalmic drug delivery system based on poloxamer-407. Int J Biol Macromol 2013;62:117–23.

[77] Laurent S. Antihypertensive drugs. Pharmacol Res 2017;124:116–25.

[78] Toti US, Aminabhavi TM. Modified guar gum matrix tablet for controlled release of diltiazem hydrochloride. J Control Release 2004;95:567–77.

[79] Altaf SA, Yu K, Parasrampuria J, Friend DR. Guar gum-based sustained release diltiazem. Pharm Res 1998;15:1196–201.

[80] Soppimath KS, Aminabhavi TM. Water transport and drug release study from cross-linked polyacrylamide grafted guar gum hydrogel microspheres for the controlled release application. Eur J Pharm Biopharm 2002;53:87–98.

[81] Saravankumar K, Thulluru A, Samineni R, Ishwarya M, Nagaveni P, Mahammed N. Effect of sodium alginate in combination with natural and synthetic polymers on the release of verapamil HCl from its floating microspheres. J Pharm Sci Res 2019;11:2028–35.

[82] Horvat G, Pantic M, Knez Z, Novak Z. Encapsulation and drug release of poorly water soluble nifedipine from bio-carriers. J Non Cryst Solid 2018;481:486–93.

[83] Soppimath KS, Kulkarni AR, Aminabhavi TM. Controlled release of antihypertensive drug from the interpenetrating network poly(vinyl alcohol)–guar gum hydrogel microspheres. J Biomater Sci Polym Ed 2000;11:27–43.

[84] Krishnaiah YSR, Karthikeyan RS, Satyanarayana V. A three-layer guar gum matrix tablet for oral controlled delivery of highly soluble metoprolol tartrate. Int J Pharm 2002;241:353–66.

[85] Dey S, Chattopadhyay S, Mazumder B. Formulation and evaluation of fixed-dose combination of bilayer gastroretentive matrix tablet containing atorvastatin as fast-release and atenolol as sustained-release. Biomed Res Int 2014;2014:396106.

[86] Castro PM, Baptista P, Madureira AR, Sarmento B, Pintado ME. Combination of PLGA nanoparticles with mucoadhesive guar-gum films for buccal delivery of antihypertensive peptide. Int J Pharm 2018;547:593–601.

[87] Gangwar G, Kumar A, Pathak K. Utilizing guar gum for development of "tabs in cap" system of losartan potassium for chronotherapeutics. Int J Biol Macromol 2015;72:812–8.

[88] Li Y, Feng Y, Jing J, Yang F. Cellulose/guar gum hydrogel microspheres as a magnetic anticancer drug carrier. Bioresources 2019;14(2):3615–29.

[89] Eswaramma S, Reddy NS, Rao KSVK. Carbohydrate polymer based pH-sensitive IPN microgels: synthesis, characterization and drug release characteristics. Mater Chem Phys 2017;195:176–86.

[90] Palem RR, Shimoga G, Rao KSVK, Lee S-H, Kang TJ. Guar gum graft polymer-based silver nanocomposite hydrogels: synthesis, characterization and its biomedical applications. J Polym Res 2020;27:68.

[91] Reddy GV, Reddy NS, Nagaraja K, Rao KSVK. Synthesis of pH responsive hydrogel matrices from guar gum and poly(acrylamide-co-acrylamidoglycolicacid) for anticancer drug delivery. J Appl Pharm Sci 2018;8(08):084–91.

[92] Westman EL, Canova JM, Radhi IJ, Koteva K, Kireeva I, Waglechner N, Wright GD. Bacterial inactivation of the anticancer drug doxorubicin. Chem Biol 2012;19(10):1255–64.

[93] Elbialy NS, Mady MM. Ehrlich tumor inhibition using doxorubicin containing liposomes. Saudi Pharm J 2015;23(2):182–7.

[94] Kang RK, Mishra N, Rai VK. Guar gum micro-particles for targeted co-delivery of doxorubicin and metformin HCL for improved specificity and efficacy against colon cancer: in vitro and in vivo studies. AAPS Pharm Sci Tech 2020;21:48.

[95] Mushtaq MW, Kanwal F, Batool A, Jamil T, Zia-ul-Haq M, Ijaz B, Huang Q, Ullah Z. Polymer-coated $CoFe_2O_4$ nanoassemblies as biocompatible magnetic nanocarriers for anticancer drug delivery. J Mater Sci 2017;52:9282–93.

[96] Murali R, Vidhya P, Thanikaivelan P. Thermoresponsive magnetic nanoparticle-aminated guar gum hydrogel system for sustained release of doxorubicin hydrochloride. Carbohydr Polym 2014;110:440–5.

[97] Sharma M, Malik R, Verma A, Dwivedi P, Banoth GS, Pandey N, Sarkar J, Mishra PR, Dwivedi AK. Folic acid conjugated guar gum nanoparticles for targeting methotrexate to colon cancer. J Biomed Nanotechnol 2013;9(1):96–106.

[98] Chaurasia M, Chourasia MK, Jain NK, et al. Cross-linked guar gum microspheres: a viable approach for improved delivery of anticancer drugs for the treatment of colorectal cancer. AAPS Pharm Sci Tech 2006;7(3), E143.

[99] Elias EJ, Anil S, Ahmad S, Anwar D. Colon targeted curcumin delivery using guar gum. Nat Prod Commun 2010;5(6):915–8.

[100] Kumar VS, John R, Sabitha M. Guargum and eudragit coated curcumin liquid solid tablets for colon specific drug delivery. Int J Biol Macromol 2018;110:318–27.

[101] Chourasia MK, Jain SK. Potential of guar gum microspheres for target specific drug release to colon. J Drug Target 2004;12(7):435–42.

[102] Panariello G, Favaloro R, Forbicioni M, Caputo E, Barbucci R. Synthesis of a new hydrogel, based on guar gum, for controlled drug release. Macromol Symp 2008;266:68–73.

[103] Swain S, Bal T. Carrageenan-guar gum microwave irradiated micro-porous interpenetrating polymer network: a system for drug delivery. Int J Polym Mater Polym Biomater 2019;68:256–65.

[104] Kumar JR, Muralidhara S, Dhanaraj SA. Development and in vitro evaluation of guar gum based fluconazole in situ gel for oral thrush. J Pharm Sci Res 2012;4:2009–14.

[105] Ray L, Karthik R, Srivastava V, et al. Efficient antileishmanial activity of amphotericin B and piperine entrapped in enteric coated guar gum nanoparticles. Drug Deliv Transl Res 2021. https://doi.org/10.1007/s13346-020-00712-9.

[106] Bhat SR, Shivakumar HG. Bioadhesive controlled release clotrimazole vaginal tablets. Trop J Pharm Res 2010;9:339–46.

[107] Baloglu E, Ozyazici M, et al. Bioadhesive controlled release systems of ornidazole for vaginal delivery. Pharm Dev Technol 2006;11:477–84.

[108] Alam MA, Ahmad FJ, Khan ZI, Khar RK, Ali M. Development and evaluation of acid-buffering bioadhesive vaginal tablet for mixed vaginal infections. AAPS Pharm Sci Tech 2007;8:229.

[109] Singh VK, Banerjee I, Agarwal T, Pramanik K, Bhattacharya MK, Pal K. Guar gum and sesame oil based novel bigels for controlled drug delivery. ColloidSurf B: Biointerface 2014;123:582–92.

[110] Reddy KM, Babu VR, Sairam M, Subha MCS. Development of chitosan-guar gum semi-interpenetrating polymer network microspheres for controlled release of ce-fadroxil. Design Monomer Polym 2006;9:491–501.

[111] Yi J-Z, Zhang L-M. Biodegradable blend films based on two polysaccharide deriva-tives and their use as ibuprofen-releasing matrices. J Appl Polym Sci 2007;103:3553–9.

[112] Das A, Wadhwa S, Srivastava AK. Cross-linked guar gum hydrogel discs for colon-specific delivery of ibuprofen: formulation and in vitro evaluation. Drug Deliv 2006;13:139–42.

[113] Dziadkowiec J, Mansa R, Quintela A, Rocha F, Detellier C. Preparation, characteriza-tion and application in controlled release of ibuprofen-loaded guar gum/ montmoril-lonite bionanocomposites. Appl Clay Sci 2017;135:52–63.

[114] Huang Y, Yu H, Xiao C. pH-sensitive cationic guar gum/poly (acrylic acid) polyelec-trolyte hydrogels: swelling and in vitro drug release. Carbohydr Polym 2007;69:774–83.

[115] Ji C, Xu H, Wu W. *In vitro* evaluation and pharmacokinetics in dogs of guar gum and Eudragit FS30D-coated colon-targeted pellets of indomethacin. J Drug Target 2007;15:123–31.

[116] Giri A, Bhunia T, Mishra SR, et al. Acrylic acid grafted guargum–nanosilica mem-branes for transdermal diclofenac delivery. Carbohydr Polym 2013;91:492–501.

[117] Ravi P, Kusumanchi RMR, Mallikarjun V, Rao BB, Narender R. Formulation and eval-uation of guar gum microspheres of aceclofenac for colon targeted drug delivery. J Pharm Res 2010;3:1510–2.

[118] Sullad AG, Majeshwar LS, Aminabhavi LS. Microspheres of carboxymethyl guar gum for *in vitro* release of abacavir sulfate: preparation and characterization. J Appl Polym Sci 2011;122:452–60.

[119] Yadav AS, et al. Design and evaluation of guar gum based controlled release matrix tablets of zidovudine. J Pharm Sci Technol 2010;2:156–62.

[120] Kaur M, Garg T, Rath G, Goyal AK. Current nanotechnological strategies for effective delivery of bioactive drug molecules in the treatment of tuberculosis. Crit Rev Ther Drug Carrier Syst 2014;31:49–88.

[121] Garg T, Rath G, Goyal AK. Inhalable chitosan nanoparticles as antitubercular drug carriers for an effective treatment of tuberculosis. Artif Cell Nanomed Biotechnol 2016;44:997–1001.

[122] Kaur M, Malik B, Garg T, Rath G, Goyal AK. Development and characterization of guar gum nanoparticles for oral immunization against tuberculosis. Drug Deliv 2015;22:328–34.

[123] Kaur R, Garg T, Gupta UD, Gupta P, Rath G, Goyal AK. Preparation and character-ization of spray-dried inhalable powders containing nanoaggregates for pulmonary delivery of anti-tubercular drugs. Artif Cell Nanomed Biotechnol 2016;44:182–7.

[124] Parida SK, Axelsson-Robertson R, Rao MV, et al. Totally drug-resistant tuberculosis and adjunct therapies. J Intern Med 2015;277(4):388–405.

[125] Goyal AK, Garg T, Rath G, Gupta UD, Gupta P. Development and characterization of nanoembedded microparticles for pulmonary delivery of antitubercular drugs against experimental tuberculosis. Mol Pharm 2015;12(11):3839–50.

[126] Sullad AG, Manjeshwar LS, Aminabhavi TM. Novel pH-sensitive hydrogels prepared from the blends of poly(vinyl alcohol) with acrylic acid-graft-guar gum matrixes for isoniazid delivery. Ind Eng Chem Res 2010;49:7323–9.

[127] Angadi SC, Manjeshwar LS, Aminabhavi TM. Coated interpenetrating blend microparticles of chitosan and guar gum for controlled release of isoniazid. Ind Eng Chem Res 2013;52:6399–409.

[128] Martín-Illana A, Cazorla-Luna R, NotarioPérez F, Bedoya LM, Ruiz-Caro R, Veiga M-D. Freeze-dried bioadhesive vaginal bigels for controlled release of tenofovir. Eur J Pharm Sci 2019;127:38–51.

[129] Notario-Perez F, Martín-Illana A, Cazorla-Luna R, Ruiz-Caro R, Bedoya L-M, Tamayo A, Rubio J, Veiga M-D. Influence of chitosan swelling behaviour on controlled release of tenofovir from mucoadhesive vaginal systems for prevention of sexual transmission of HIV. Mar Drugs 2017;15:50.

[130] Notario-Perez F, Martín-Illana A, Cazorla-Luna R, Ruiz-Caro R, Bedoya L-M, Tamayo A, Rubio J, Veiga M-D. Optimization of Tenofovir release from mucoadhesive vaginal tablets by polymer combination to prevent sexual transmission of HIV. Carbohydr Polym 2018;179:305–16.

[131] Soumya P, Rao NGR, Kistayya C, Reddy BM. Design and development of oral sustained release matrix tablets of didanosine. Asian J Pharm ClinRes 2014;7:38–44.

[132] Ramesh C, Ramu B, Rajkamal B. Formulation of colon specific didanosine enteric coated matrix tablets using ph sensitive polymer. Pharm Chem J 2016;3(2):207–20.

[133] Wadher KJ, Kakde RB, Umekar MJ. Study on sustained-release metformin hydrochloride from matrix tablet: influence of hydrophilic polymers and in vitro evaluation. Int J Pharm Investig 2011;1:157–63.

[134] Gowrav MP, Hani U, Shivkumar HG, Osmani RAM, Srivastava A. Polyacrylamide grafted guar gum based glimepiride loaded pH sensitive pellets for colon specific drug delivery: fabrication and characterization. RSC Adv 2015;5:80005–15.

[135] Bashir S, Nazir I, Khan HU, et al. In vitro evaluation of nateglinide-loaded microspheres formulated with biodegradable polymers. Trop J Pharm Res 2014;13:1047–53.

[136] Prakash K, Satyanarayana VM, Nagiat HW, et al. Formulation development and evaluation of novel oral jellies of carbamazepine using pectin, guar gum, and gellan gum. Asian J Pharm 2014;8:241–9.

[137] Kanwar N, Kumar R, Sarwal A, Sinha VR. Preparation and evaluation of floating tablets of pregabalin. Drug Dev Ind Pharm 2016;42:654–60.

[138] Das S, Maharana J, Mohanty S, Subuddhi U. Spectroscopic and computational insights into theophylline/β-cyclodextrin complexation: inclusion accomplished by diverse methods. J Microencapsul 2018;35:667–79.

[139] Phadke KV, Manjeshwar LS, Aminabhavi TM. Biodegradable polymeric microspheres of gelatin and carboxymethyl guar gum for controlled release of theophylline. Polym Bull 2014;71:1625–43.

[140] Khullar P, Khar RK, Agarwal SP. Evaluation of guar gum in the preparation of sustained-release matrix tablets. Drug Develop Ind Pharm 1998;24:1095–9.

[141] Ozsoy Y, Gungor S. Nasal route: an alternative approach for antiemetic drug delivery. Expert Opin Drug Deliv 2011;8:1439–53.

[142] Dehgan MH, Girase M. Freeze-dried xanthan/guar gum nasal inserts for the delivery of metoclopramide hydrochloride. Iran J Pharm Res 2012;11:513–21.

[143] Jyothi BJ, Doniparthi J. Venlafaxine hydrochloride granules using natural polymers as multiparticulate drug delivery system. Asian J Pharm 2017;11:S810–7.

[144] Paudel A, Shrestha ST, Pandey YR, Shrestha SC. Formulation and in-vitro evaluation of bupropion hydrochloride controlled release tablet. Int J Pharm Sci Res 2014;5:2783–90.

[145] Krishnaiah YSR, Raju PV, Kumar BD, Bhaskar P, Satyanarayana V. Development of colon targeted drug delivery systems for mebendazole. J Control Release 2001;77:87–95.

[146] Krishnaiah YSR, Raju PV, Kumar BD, Satyanarayana V, Karthikeyan RS, Bhaskar P. Pharmacokinetic evaluation of guar gum-based colon-targeted drug delivery systems of mebendazole in healthy volunteers. J Control Release 2003;88:95–103.

[147] Krishnaiah YSR, Latha K, Rao LN, Karthikeyan RS, Bhaskar P, Satyanarayana V. Development of colon targeted oral guar gum matrix tablets of albendazole for the treatment of helminthiasis. Indian J Pharm Sci 2003;65:378–85.

[148] Shyale S, Chowdhury KPR, Krishnaiah YSR. Development of colon-targeted albendazole-β-cyclodextrin-complex drug delivery systems. Drug Dev Res 2005;65:76–83.

[149] Shyale S, Chowdhury KPR, Krishnaiah YSR, Bhat NK. Pharmacokinetic evaluation and studies on the clinical efficacy of guar gum-based oral drug delivery systems of albendazole and albendazole-β-cyclodextrin for colon-targeting in human volunteers. Drug Dev Res 2006;67:154–65.

[150] Koteswari P, et al. Fabrication of a novel device containing famotidine for gastro retentive delivery using carbohydrate polymers. J Pharm Drug Deliv Res 2015;4:1.

[151] Dave BS, Amin AF, Patel MM. Gastroretentive drug delivery system of ranitidine hydrochloride: formulation and in vitro evaluation. AAPS Pharm Sci Tech 2004;5:77–82.

[152] Veerapratap S, Prabhakar MN, Chandrasekhar M, et al. Preparation of biodegradable polymeric blend microspheres of soy protein isolate/guar gum and release studies of tolterodine drug. Int J Adv Chem Sci 2015;3:171–7.

[153] Hadi MA, Rao NGR, Rao AS. Formulation and evaluation of ileo-colonic targeted matrix-mini-tablets of naproxen for chronotherapeutic treatment of rheumatoid arthritis. Saudi Pharm J 2016;24:64–73.

[154] Lakshmi KR, Muzib YI, Voleti VK. Design and evaluation of colon specific drug delivery of naproxen sodium using guar gum and crosslinked guar gum. Int J Pharm Pharm Sci 2011;4:284–8.

[155] Vermonden T, Censi R, Hennink WE. Hydrogels for protein delivery. Chem Rev 2012;112:2853–88.

[156] Sharma S, Kaur J, Sharma G, et al. Preparation and characterization of pH-responsive guar gum microspheres. Int J Biol Macromol 2013;62:636–41.

[157] Kono H, Otaka F, Ozaki M. Preparation and characterization of guar gum hydrogels as carrier materials for controlled protein drug delivery. Carbohydr Polym 2014;111:830–40.

[158] Thimma RT, Tammishetti S. Barium chloride crosslinked carboxymethyl guar gum beads for gastrointestinal drug delivery. J Appl Polym Sci 2001;82:3084–90.

[159] Reddy T, Tammishetti S. Gastric resistant microbeads of metal ion cross-linked carboxymethyl guar gum for oral drug delivery. J Microencapsul 2002;19:311–8.

[160] Bansal R, Singh AK, Gandhi RP, Pant AB, Kumar P, Gupta KC. Galactomannan-PEI based non-viral vectors for targeted delivery of plasmid to macrophages and hepatocytes. Eur J Pharm Biopharm 2014;87:461–71.

[161] Jana P, Sarkar K, Mitra T, Chatterjee A, Gnanamani A, Chakraborti G, Kundu PP. Synthesis of a carboxymethylated guar gum grafted polyethyleneimine copolymer as an efficient gene delivery vehicle. RSC Adv 2016;6:13730–41.

[162] Anandan D, Madhumathi G, Nambiraj NA, Jaiswal AK. Gum based 3D composite scaffolds for bone tissue engineering applications. Carbohydr Polym 2019;214:62–70.

[163] Parameswaran-Thankam A, Parnell CM, Watanabe F, RanguMagar AB, Chhetri BP, Szwedo PK, Biris AS, Ghosh A. Guar-based injectable thermoresponsive hydrogel as a scaffold for bone cell growth and controlled drug delivery. ACS Omega 2018;3:15158–67.

[164] Parameswaran-Thankam A, Al-Ankaby Q, Al-karakooly Z, RanguMagar AB, Chhetri BP, Ali N, Ghosh A. Fabrication and characterization of hydroxypropyl guar-poly (vinyl alcohol)-nano hydroxyapatite composite hydrogels for bone tissue engineering. J Biomater Sci Polym Ed 2018;29:2083–105.

[165] Kundu S, Das A, Basu A, Ghosh D, Datta P, Mukherjee A. Carboxymethyl guar gum synthesis in homogeneous phase and macroporous 3D scaffolds design for tissue engineering. Carbohydr Polym 2018;191:71–8.

[166] Mitra S, Ghosh N, Banerjee ER. Carboxymethyl guar gum nanoscaffold as matrix for cell growth in vitro. J Lung Pulm Respir Res 2018;5, 00156.

[167] Tiwari A, Grailer JJ, Pilla S, Steeber DA, Gong S. Biodegradable hydrogels based on novel photopolymerizable guar gum–methacrylate macromonomers for in situ fabrication of tissue engineering scaffolds. Acta Biomater 2009;5:3441–52.

[168] Ragothaman M, Palanisamy T, Kalirajan C. Collagen–poly(dialdehyde) guar gum based porous 3D scaffolds immobilized with growth factor for tissue engineering applications. Carbohydr Polym 2014;114:399–406.

[169] Ragothaman M, Thangavel P, Kalirajan C, Palanisamy T. Biomimetic hybrid porous scaffolds immobilized with platelet derived growth factor-BB promote cellularization and vascularization in tissue engineering. J Biomed Mater Res Part A 2016;104:388–96.

[170] Swain S, Bal T. Microwave irradiated carrageenan-guar gum micro-porous IPN: a novel material for isotropic tissue scaffolding. Int J Polym Mater Polym Biomater 2019;68:796–804.

6

Hemicelluloses-based hydrogels

Xiao-Feng Sun, Tao Zhang, and Hai-Hong Wang

Xi'an Key Lab of Functional Organic Porous Materials, School of Chemistry and Chemical Engineering, Northwestern Polytechnical University, Xi'an, People's Republic of China

6.1 Introduction

Hydrogels have three-dimensional polymer networks that can swell in some solvents but are insoluble in these solvents. After Wichterle and Lím first reported on hydrogels [1], studies on hydrogels became increasingly active to explore their synthesis methods and applications in biomedicine, agriculture, food, water treatment, etc. After decades of development, hydrogels have been applied successfully to some aspects, such as controllable drug release [2, 3], tissue engineering [4], sensors [5], contact lenses [6], water treatment [7, 8], and so on.

Depending on the difference of cross-linking methods, hydrogels are classified into physical hydrogels, chemical hydrogels, and other hydrogels. Physical hydrogels are produced by weak molecular secondary forces such as hydrogen bonds or ionic interactions, and chemical hydrogels are produced by covalent bonds [9]. On the basis of response to external stimuli, hydrogels are divided into conventional gels and environmentally sensitive gels. The volume of conventional gels does not change or changes little in solvents under environmental conditions while environmentally sensitive hydrogels can change their volumes sharply with slight changes of environmental conditions such as pH or temperature, which attracted more attention for use in sensors, controlled-release switches, etc. [10]. The polymer sources are another classification of hydrogels, and hydrogels are divided into synthetic polymers gels and natural polymers-based gels. Various natural polymers, e.g., alginate [11], chitosan [12, 13], gelatin [14], hyaluronate [15], starch [16], cellulose [17, 18], and hemicelluloses [19], have been widely utilized to fabricate hydrogels due to their biocompatibility, biodegradability, and abundant sources. However, natural

Plant and Algal Hydrogels for Drug Delivery and Regenerative Medicine
https://doi.org/10.1016/B978-0-12-821649-1.00014-3

polymers are generally unstable and easily degradable. Blending with synthetic polymers or other natural polymers has played a significant role in a series of natural hydrogels to improve their mechanical properties. The performances of hydrogels, including mechanical properties, water retentivity, drug delivery, and environmental sensitivity determined by the structure of the hydrogels, are influenced by some important factors, such as polymerization method, monomer(s), cross-linker(s), amount and type of the used surfactants, stirrer reactor geometry, reaction temperature, and the stirring rate [20].

Hemicelluloses or polyoses can be traced back to Schulze in 1891 [21], and they are abundant in the cell walls of plants and comprise roughly one-fourth to one-third of the plant's material. The content will differ in amount according to the plant species, such as fast-growing poplar wood (27.1%), maize stems (28.0%), oil palm frond fiber (30.8%), barley straw (34.9%), rice straw (35.8%), rye straw (36.9%), and wheat straw (38.8%) [22]. In plant cell walls, many different polysaccharides form a highly organized architecture. Woods have a lot of galactans and arabinans in the primary walls and middle lamellae, 4-O-methylglucuronoxylan for hardwood, and glucomannan for softwood in secondary walls [23]. The predominant hemicelluloses in hardwood are acetylated acidic xylans; birchwood contains 35% of these hemicelluloses, but only 13% acidic xylans were found in cottonwood, and hardwood also contains less content of mannan. The predominant hemicelluloses in softwood are galactoglucomannans that are also partially acetylated. In addition to the previously mentioned hemicelluloses, an arabinogalactan was found with 10%–20% of the dry weight of the larch heartwood [24]. Grass has arabinoxylans in secondary walls and xyloglucan in middle lamellae and primary walls. Xylans extracted from cereal straws and grasses were characterized with the same backbone as the xylans found in wood, and straw or grass xylans comprise relatively higher content of L-arabinofuranosyl units, giving rise to being more highly branched and lower content of uronic acids.

Hemicelluloses are heteropolysaccharides and classically defined as the alkali/water-soluble polysaccharides after extractions of the wax, protein, starch, and pectin from plant cell walls. Hemicelluloses are comprised of various monosaccharide units, arranged with diverse amounts and various substituents. The main monosaccharides of hemicelluloses are β-D-xylose, β-D-mannose, α-L-arabinose, α-D-galactose, β-D-glucose, α-D-galacturonic acid, 4-O-methyl-α-D-glucuronic acid, and β-D-glucuronic acid. The general formulae of hemicelluloses are $(C_6H_{10}O_5)_n$ and $(C_5H_8O_4)_n$ that named hexosans and pentosans, respectively [25]. The hemicelluloses of wheat straw, maize straw, and barley straw are comprised of xylans as the predominate polysaccharides, and straw xylans were substituted by α-L-arabinofuranose, α-D-xylose, and acetyl group (DS = 0.1–0.2) at O-3 and/or O-2 of xylose of main chain [26–28].

The acetylated hemicelluloses, like other polysaccharides, are soluble in strong polar solvents such as *N,N*-dimethylformamide/LiCl, dimethyl sulfoxide, and ionic liquids. The cell walls of straws and grasses have some phenolic acid substituents, which are cross-linked to xylans by ester structures, and ferulates and *p*-coumaryl groups are chemically linked at the O-5 position of arabinose substituents of arabinoglucuronoxylans (Fig. 6.1). Xylans with high proportion of side chain substitutions and substituents, such as α-L-arabinofuranose and D-glucopyranosyluronic acid units, are relatively water-soluble and attached less tightly to cellulose, whereas the hemicelluloses with rare side chains are water-insoluble and attached more tightly to cellulose.

Hemicelluloses have been proven to possess some physiological properties, such as innate immunological defense and anticancer effect, promoting cell adhesion and proliferation, and inhibiting cell mutation, which make hemicelluloses-based hydrogels applicable in drug release and biomedical engineering [61]. Compared with crystalline cellulose, the amorphous structure of hemicelluloses makes them open to chemical modification and hydrophilic, and hemicelluloses have become potential polysaccharides for producing high-performance hydrogels, which has

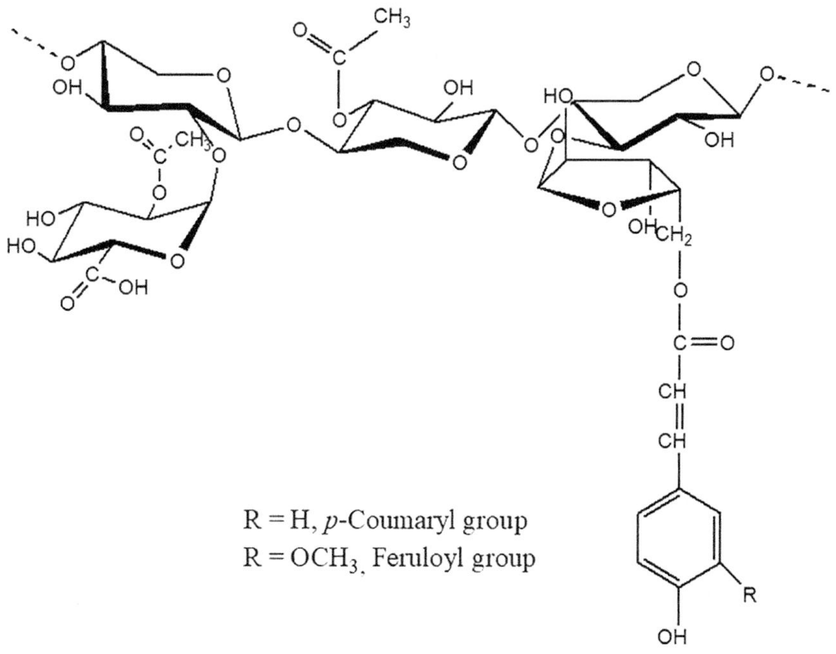

R = H, *p*-Coumaryl group
R = OCH$_3$, Feruloyl group

FIG. 6.1 Structure of 4-O-methylglucuronoarabinoxylan with esterified ferulic acid and acetyl groups. *Reproduced from Sun XF, Fowler P, Zhang GC, Rajaratnam M. Extraction and characterization of hemicelluloses from maize stem. Phytochem Anal 2010;21:406–415, Copyright (2010), with permission from Springer.*

received enormous attention in various fields. Recently, hemicelluloses were used or modified to synthesize diverse hydrogels with excellent properties, and novel synthesis methods and biobased cross-linkers have been developed. Both hydrogel structures and synthesis methods affected the properties and applications of hemicellulose-based hydrogels. Up to now, synthesis methods and drug release properties of hemicelluloses-based hydrogels have not been discussed in detail. This chapter reviewed the recent studies in hemicelluloses-based hydrogels, focusing on the synthesis methods and properties as well as applications. Table 6.1 lists synthesis methods of hemicelluloses-based hydrogels.

6.2 Synthesis methods of hemicelluloses-based hydrogels

Hemicelluloses are mainly comprised of xylans and mannans that occur in wood and other plants with different contents and structures. The polyhydroxylated structure renders hemicelluloses open to chemical modification and to prepare hemicelluloses-based hydrogels easily by chemical, physical, and enzymatic cross-linking methods. In the networks of physically cross-linked hydrogels, the physical crossing points are formed through diversified forms, such as electrostatic interactions, hydrogen bonding, hydrophobic associations, and so on, whereas for the chemically cross-linked hydrogels, covalent bonds are formed through chemical reactions, which forms the three-dimensional networks with the presence of cross-linkers or by energy irradiation. Recently, enzymatic cross-linking also became another method to synthesize hemicellulose-based hydrogels, avoiding the use of toxic chemicals.

6.2.1 Physical cross-linking

Some physical methods, such as freezing or ultrasounding irradiation, are utilized to form the hydrogels where the use of cross-linkers and organic solvents can be avoided because they are toxic and can damage the loaded drugs [62]. These hydrogels could be sensitive, showing the change of the morphology or swelling ratio (volume), to the changes of environmental conditions, such as temperature, pH, or other stimuli. This property makes them prospect for application as an intelligent drug release system [63].

It is evident that mechanical properties of polysaccharides-based hydrogels are relatively weak. To improve mechanical strength of these gels, the structure of a semi- or full-interpenetrating polymer network was introduced to these gels where the hydrogen bond, microcrystallization, ionic interaction, or hydrophobic interaction exist between the polymers [64]. Gabrielii et al. first prepared hemicellulose-chitosan physical hydrogel

TABLE 6.1 Synthesis methods of hemicelluloses-based hydrogels.

Synthesis methods		Components/mechanism	References
Physical cross-linking	Hydrogen bond, microcrystallization, ionic interaction, or hydrophobic interaction exists between the polymers	Hemicellulose/chitosan	[29–31]
		Xylan-MA/PVA hydrogels	[32]
		Xylan/poly(acrylic acid)	[33]
		Xylan/poly(methacrylic acid)	[34]
		Phosphorylated poly(vinyl alcohol)/hemicellulose-*g*-poly(acrylic acid)	[35]
		Hemicellulose, polyvinyl alcohol, and chitin nanowhiskers by freeze-thaw cycle	[36]
Chemical cross-linking	Cross-linkers	*N-N'*-Methylenebisacrylamide	[37, 38]
		Glutaraldehyde	[39]
		Acrylamido end-capped poly(amidoamine) oligomers	[40]
		N,N'-Diallylaldardiamides	[41]
		Cellulose nanowhiskers	[42]
	Radical polymerization cross-linking	Redox initiation or photo initiation	[37, 43]
		Atom transfer radical polymerization	[44]
		Glow discharge electrolysis plasma	[45]
	"Click chemistry" cross-linking	Copper catalyzed azide-alkyne cycloaddition method	[46]
		Thiol-ene reaction	[47, 48]

Continued

TABLE 6.1 Synthesis methods of hemicelluloses-based hydrogels—cont'd

Synthesis methods		Components/mechanism	References
Enzymatic cross-linking		Horse radish peroxidase	[49, 50]
		Laccase	[51]
Hemicellulose-inorganic composite hydrogels		Fe_3O_4	[52–54]
		Carbon nanotube	[55, 56]
		TiO_2	[57]
		Montmorillonite	[58, 59]
		Ag	[60]

in acidic conditions using the hemicellulose isolated from aspen and chitosan [29], and both electrostatic interactions between amine groups of the chitosan and acidic groups of the hemicellulose and of the crystalline arrangement of two polysaccharides resulted in the cohesive forces of the physical hydrogels. The swelling test showed that the swelling ratio relied strongly on the amount of added chitosan. The addition of 15%–20% chitosan was considered to increase the water uptake, while the hydrogels with more than 20% chitosan content dissolved during the swelling test. In addition, the two different phases were also observed through atomic force microscopy and dynamic mechanical measurements in their works [19]. Recently, a xylan/chitosan composite hydrogel was synthesized by Bush and collaborators; the ratio of xylan to chitosan was 1:3, and the ammonium hydrogen phosphate solution was added to initiate gelation [30]. The prepared injectable and temperature-sensitive hydrogel is a gel state at physiological temperature but a liquid state at room temperature, and it can be applied in tissue engineering or regenerative medicine.

The polyelectrolytes complexes formed by strong electrostatic interaction can be used to fabricate hydrogels. A novel hydrogel has been obtained by blending the bagasse xylan phosphate, an anionic polyelectrolyte, and the chitosan as the cationic polyelectrolyte [31, 65]. Meanwhile, sodium tripolyphosphate was employed to be the ion cross-linker. The drug loading capacity of these gels for vitamin B1, a model drug, was enhanced, and the release rate in the simulation duodenum solution was lower with a higher content of sodium tripolyphosphate. pH 4.8 was the desirable drug delivery condition with sodium tripolyphosphate of 0.2 mol/L.

Some hydrophilic synthetic polymers have attracted more attention to fabricate hydrogels due to their superior advantage to natural polymers hydrogels, such as good mechanism properties, easy control of architecture and chemical structure, but most synthetic polymers are hazardous to the environment and nonbiodegradable. However, the natural hydrogels have predominant biocompatibility and biodegradability but weak strength. Therefore, the combination of synthetic and natural polymers has been developed to prepare desired composite hydrogels with prospect properties. The xylan derivative synthesized by esterification reaction using maleic anhydride (MA) was incorporated into polyvinyl alcohol (PVA) solution at a high temperature of 70°C to obtain xylan-MA/PVA hydrogels [32]. The hydrogels exhibited very high water-uptake ability: up to 30 times that of dry hydrogel mass. According to the results, the swelling degree and compressive strength obviously depended on the cross-link density and hydrophilicity that related to the ratio of incorporated MA to PVA. Noncytotoxicity of the xylan-MA/PVA gel was confirmed by the L929 cells culture test, suggesting that the prepared hydrogel could be used in the biomedicine field. Sun et al. synthesized some semi-IPN hydrogels from xylan and poly(methacrylic acid) or poly(acrylic acid) by the hydrogen bonds [33, 34]. Semi-IPN hydrogel was also produced by blending hemicellulose-g-poly(acrylic acid) with phosphorylated poly(vinyl alcohol) (P-PVA) that was uniformly scattered in the polymeric network, forming a number of hydrogen bonds. Therefore, the thermal property of the hydrogel was improved, and the compressive strength increased because of the spread of P-PVA chains [35].

A physical method, freeze-thaw cycle technique, was employed to prepare the hydrogels with good mechanical property, and the chemical cross-linkers are avoided. The stability of the formed hydrogels relies on the pH, temperature, freezing time, and cycle times of freeze-thaw [66–68]. The hemicellulose, chitin nanowhiskers, and PVA were mixed and subjected to freeze-thaw cycles [36]. The freeze-thaw cycles led to physical cross-linking through intermolecular hydrogen bonds and formed a stiff structure, which resulted in high thermal stability and mechanical strength. It was found that the compressive strength reached 10.5 MPa after 9 times cycle. However, the water uptake capacity of the prepared hydrogels reduced after 3 times of freeze and thaw cycle because a lamellar structure was formed.

6.2.2 Chemical cross-linking

6.2.2.1 Cross-linkers

The high mechanical strength and water-uptake capacity of hemicelluloses-based hydrogels seriously rely on a chemical structure. Some difunctional molecules have been utilized as cross-linkers to fabricate three-dimensional hydrophilic networks. The N-N'-methylenebisacrylamide (MBA) was a common cross-linker [41, 69, 70]. Peng et al. have prepared hydrogels through cross-linking xylan-rich hemicellulose (XH) and acrylic acid with MBA as the cross-linker [37]. The cross-link density of gel networks significantly increased with increases in AA/XH and MBA/XH ratios, whereas the swelling ratio decreased. These hydrogels displayed high equilibrium swelling ratio and had multiple sensitivity to pH, ions, and organic solvents. In addition, the XH/AA hydrogels were also developed to adsorb heavy metal ions from aqueous solutions, such as Cd^{2+}, Pd^{2+}, and Zn^{2+}, and exhibited highly efficient regeneration after some repeated adsorption/desorption cycles [71].

A kind of pH-responsive copolymers were prepared by grafting copolymerization of 4-vinyl pyridine and hemicellulose, and then the copolymers solution was blended with PVA to obtain pH- and thermal-dual sensitive semi-IPN hydrogels using glutaraldehyde as a cross-linker [39]. If the hydrogels were employed for application in biomedicines and food fields, the cross-linkers must be nontoxic or should be easily removable from the gel systems [17]. However, MBA and glutaraldehyde are known toxic regents. Therefore, it is an important research direction to develop some efficient biocompatible cross-linkers to synthesize hemicelluloses-based hydrogels.

Two acrylamido end-capped poly(amidoamine) oligomers (PAAs) have been synthesized as cross-linkers to covalently combine O-acetylated galactoglucomannan (AcGGM) and poly(methacrylic acid) networks through the free radical copolymerization and cross-linking [40]. The structures and synthesis of PAA oligomers are showed in Fig. 6.2. Renewable hemicellulose/PAA hydrogels have been synthesized using AcGGM, and it displayed higher adsorption amounts for many metal ions such as Cd^{2+}, Cu^{2+}, Ni^{2+}, Pb^{2+}, Co^{2+}, Zn^{2+}, and CrO_4^{2-}. The hydrogels exhibited better

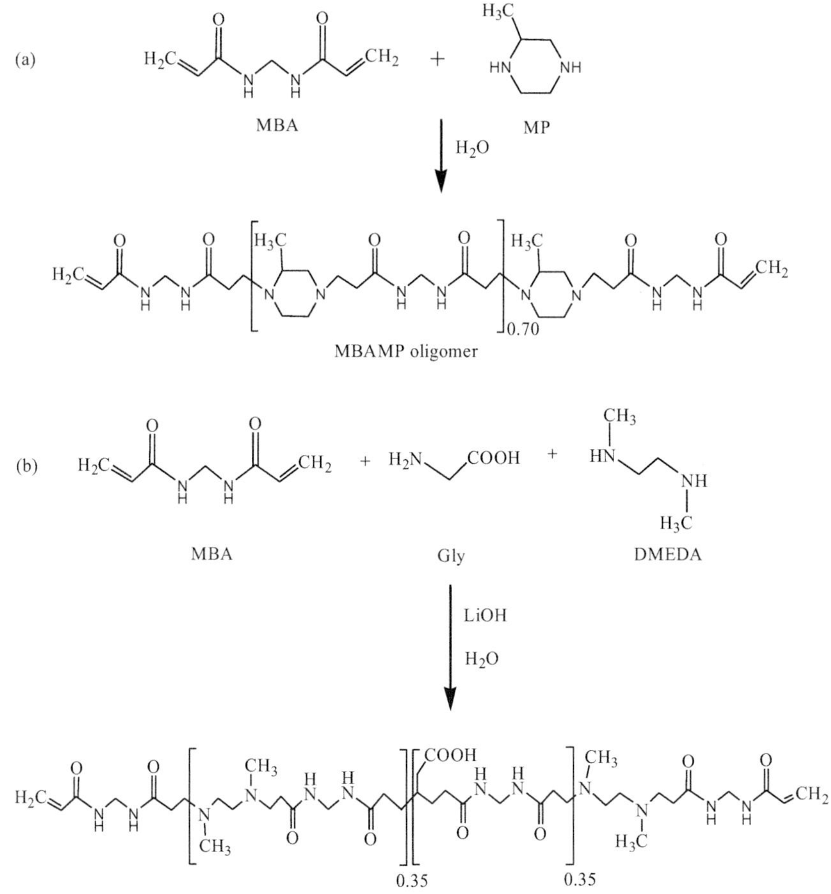

FIG. 6.2   Synthesis and structures of acrylamide-end-capped PAA oligomers. *Reproduced from Ferrari E, Ranucci E, Edlund U, Albertsson A-C. Design of renewable poly(amidoamine)/hemicellulose hydrogels for heavy metal adsorption. J Appl Polym Sci 2015;132:41695, Copyright (2015), with permission from Wiley.*

mechanical integrity than "homopolymeric" PAA hydrogels. All hydrogels were prepared by eco-friendly procedures.

A series of bio-based cross-linkers N,N'-diallylaldardiamides (DA) such as N,N'-diallylgalactardiamide (DAG), N,N'-diallylxylardiamide (DAX), N,N'-diallylarabinardiamide (DAA), and N,N'-diallyltartardiamide (DAT) were synthesized as novel cross-linkers, replacing the normal MBA. With the use of these biobased cross-linkers, some novel hemicelluloses-based hydrogels were prepared [41]. The swelling degree of these gels can reach 350%, and the addition of DA cross-linker can produce a more uniform pore structure, improving the water absorbency compared with pure xylan-derivative hydrogels. The influence of substituents in xylan derivatives such as 1-allyloxy-2-hydroxy-propyl (A) or hydroxypropyl groups on the swelling ratio of the prepared gels has been not found and needs to be explored further.

The freeze-casting technique, considered to be an easily implemented, promising, and versatile method, includes the formation of a porous structure by the freeze of a liquid solution/suspension and then sublimation of the used solvents under the condition of vacuum or negative pressure [72]. Many studies have been conducted on polysaccharides with the freeze-casting technique [73, 74]; however, hemicellulosic hydrogels have fallen behind. Köhnke et al. were pioneers to prepare nanoreinforced xylan-cellulose composite through blending xylan with cellulose nanocrystals (CNCs) [75], and the cross-linked xylan/CNCs hydrogel was prepared by using cellulose nanowhiskers as the cross-linker. The cross-linking took place between oxidized xylan-contained aldehyde group and CNCs in water during freeze-casting process, along with formation of the hemiacetal bonds [42].

6.2.2.2 Radical polymerization cross-linking

Radical polymerization has been used as the most common method to prepare hemicellulose-based hydrogels. There are two different preparation mechanisms: (1) The primary free radicals capture hydrogen from the polyhydroxyl groups of the polysaccharides to generate oxygen radicals and then to initiate the monomer polymerization [76–78]. The primary free radicals are generated from the decomposition of initiators, such as ammonium persulphate (APS), sodium metabisulfite, sodium peroxydisulfate, H_2O_2, or other initiating systems, the glow discharge electrolysis plasma (GDEP), and UV initiator [43, 45, 52]. (2) Hemicelluloses were modified with unsaturated groups, usually a vinyl group, which was employed to construct hydrogels after free radical polymerization using an initiating system [43, 79, 80].

In the polymerization, the monomer content can influence the cross-link density and then result in the changes of mechanical strength and swelling ratio of the hydrogels. In general, the swelling ratio of the hydrogel decreases as the ratio of monomers and hemicellulose increases. The hydrogels synthesized from hemicellulose (HC) and acrylamide (Am) with different Am/HC ratios were analyzed by SEM, and it was found that the produced pores became smaller in the higher Am/HC ratio hydrogels due to increased hydrogen bonding interactions and the enhanced homopolymerization reaction [81]. In addition, the obtained results suggested that the water molecules diffused into the hydrogel network with non-Fickian behavior, and the Schott second order dynamic equation was found to be suitable in describing the swelling kinetics.

For the second preparation mechanism, one prevalent approach to modify hemicelluloses was methacrylation through esterification reaction. Several examples of hemicellulose modification have been reported, for example, modifications with 2-[(1-imidazolyl)formyloxy]ethyl methacrylate (HEMA-Im) [79, 82], glycidyl methacrylate (GMA) [83], and MA [43]. DMF or DMSO was generally applied in the modification of galactoglucomannan as a solvent [84], and the temperature was set at 50°C to ensure significant modification yield. Using DMF can result in slightly higher conversion compared with DMSO while the DMSO was nontoxic. Albertsson et al. have explored a three-step route preparing AcGGM-based hydrogel [85], and it was found that the differences of the linked alkenyl species, the substitution degree of hemicellulose, and the cross-linking conditions had significant influences on the properties of gels using a redox initiation or photoinitiation. The three-step route is summarized in Fig. 6.3. This study provided an important method for adjusting the characters of the resulting gels through controlling all these factors.

Apart from some active vinyl monomers, acrylic acid (AA), acrylic amide, and hydroxyethylmethacrylate (HEMA), there are other specific vinyl monomers that are characterized with stimuli-response. The preparation of multiresponsive hydrogels with sensitivity to pH, light, and water/ethanol alternating solutions has been achieved through radicals copolymerizations of 4-[(4-acryloyloxyphenyl)azo]benzoic acid and xylan methacrylate [86]. The variation of hydrophobic/hydrophilic balance of the hydrogel would occur under UV irradiation because of the azobenzene transconformation. Itaconic acid and N-isopropylacrylamide (NIPAM) were used for preparing pH/thermal-response hemicellulose-containing hydrogels [87], and the pH/thermal sensitivity of the hydrogels could be modulated through altering the itaconic acid to NIPAM ratio. Dax and collaborators prepared new cationic hemicellulose-based hydrogels constructed using [2-(methacryloyloxy)ethyl]trimethylammonium chloride (MeDMA) as the monomers after the O-acetyl galactoglucomannan (AcGGM) was functionalized with GMA [84]. The cationic gels can be used to remove chromium and arsenic anions from highly contaminated wastewaters through electrostatic interaction. But the major drawback of the prepared hydrogels was low mechanical strength. Hence, the softwood

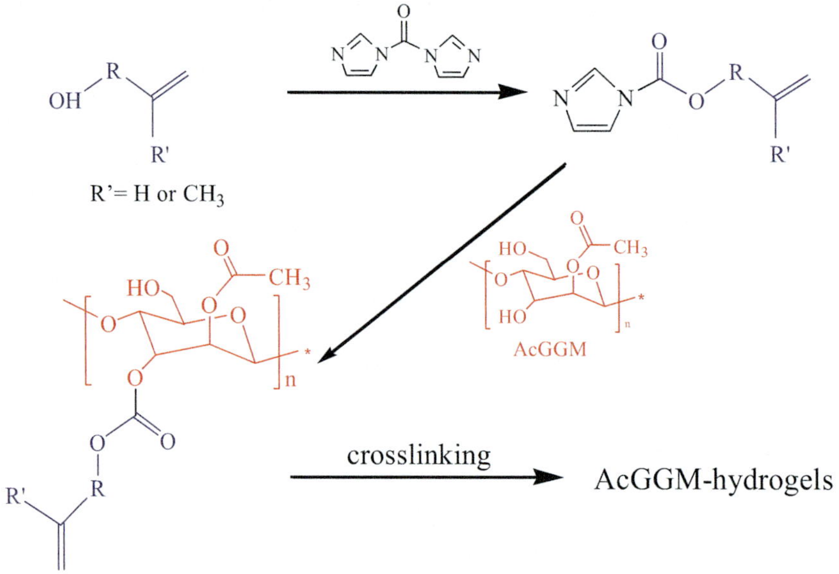

FIG. 6.3   Three-step route to synthesize alkenyl functionalized galactoglucomannan-based hydrogels. *Reproduced from Voepel J, Edlund U, Albertsson A-C. Alkenyl-functionalized precursors for renewable hydrogels design. J Polym Sci A Polym Chem 2009;47:3595–3606, Copyright (2009), with permission from Wiley.*

or hardwood nanofibrillated cellulose (NFC) was added as reinforcement material in the cationic hydrogels matrix [88] in which small amounts of NFC (5.3 wt%) resulted in a considerable improvement of the material properties (increased up to 8 times in the modulus).

An electrically conductive hemicellulose hydrogel was synthesized from conductive aniline tetramer (AT) and O-acetyl-galactoglucomannan (AcGGM), which was introduced into the hydrogel network through free radical copolymerization [89]. The swelling rate of the hydrogel can be adjusted from 228% to 548% through altering the content of added AT from 40% to 10% (w/w) while changing conductivities from 1.12×10^6 to 2.93×10^8 S/cm simultaneously. The robust pathway involved inorganic solvent, high temperature, and multiple step reactions. Afterward, the researchers improved these existing methods and designed a green one-pot method to obtain electrically conductive hemicellulosic hydrogel through cross-linking epichlorohydrin and AcGGM with the addition of aniline pentamer (AP) [90]. The findings proved that, with an increase in the content of added AP, the conductivity increased by triple magnitude and the thermal property of the hydrogels was improved. The swelling ratio could reach an ideal level through tuning the amount of cross-linker epichlorohydrin.

Atom transfer radical polymerization (ATRP), a synthesis method to realize living controllable radical polymerization [91], has been tried to apply for synthesizing hemicellulosic hydrogels [92, 93]. Zhou and Yang have prepared hemicellulose-based hydrogels successfully in the presences of NIPAM and ethylene glycol dimethacrylate (EDG) as the monomer and the cross-linker, respectively, using the ATRP technique under the UV light [44]. The produced hydrogels have exhibited obvious negative temperature responsive properties, apparently manifested as the swelling and deswelling behavior.

6.2.2.3 "Click chemistry" cross-linking

"Click chemistry", first raised by chemist Barry Sharpless [94], has been receiving much attention as a powerful bond-forming tool for combinatorial synthesis [95]. Huisgen 1,3-dipolar cycloaddition between terminal alkynes and azides with Cu(I) catalyst for 1,2,3-triazoles 5-membered heterocycles transformation is a representative click reaction, which was always carried out for the modification of polymers [96–102]. The modifications of polysaccharides using the azide-alkyne cycloaddition (CuAAC) catalyzed by copper have been widely explored [103–106]. However, there are limited reports about the modification of hemicelluloses using the CuAAC reaction. It still has very amplitude development space in the future. Enomoto-Rogers and Iwata have prepared novel xylan-based plastic materials, di-O-(6-azidohexanoyl)-xylan-$graft$-poly(L-lactide)s (XylC6N3-g-PLLAs), through grafting propargyl-terminated poly(L-lactide) onto di-O-(6-azidohexanoyl)-xylan (XylC6N3) by click reaction [107]. The introduction of poly(L-lactide) chains with desirable molecular weight has been found to effectively improve the thermal property of the copolymers. Subsequently, CuAAC was employed to synthesize a thermoresponsive hydrogel [46], and propargyl bifunctional PEG-PPG-PEG was reacted with the azide-functionalized xylan (DS values up to 0.28) (Fig. 6.4). The study showed that an increase in temperature (range from 7°C to 70°C) could lead to a decrease of swelling ratio and stiffness change, mainly depending on the length of the thermoresponsive PPG segment. According to the high selectivity and efficiency of click chemistry, we can effectively tune the structures through adjusting the DS of hemicellulose derivatives and then control their properties, such as swelling, stimulative responsibilities, or adsorb/release behavior.

The thiol-ene reaction [94, 108, 109], popularized by click chemistry concepts, has intrigued organic synthesis researchers because of its considerable merits, the mild reaction conditions without any metal catalysts, excellent selectivity and conversion, and the use of water solvent [110]. Some polysaccharides, for example, celluloses, hyaluronic acid, and dextran, have been tempted to be modified with ene or thiol-functionalities that were used for thiol-ene derivatization and cross-linking [111–114]. Utilizing the thiol-ene reaction for the functionalization of hemicellulose has been developed [110]. The thiol-functional xylans showed good

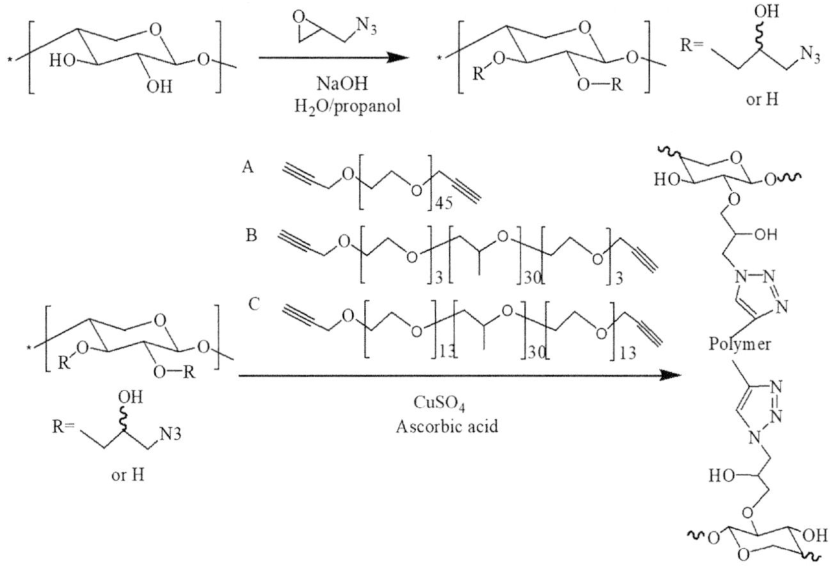

FIG. 6.4   Azide groups on xylan (top), cross-linking of azide-containing xylan with different polymers using CuAAC (bottom). PEG (A), PE6100 (B), PE6400 (C). *Reproduced from Pahimanolis N, Sorvari A, Luong ND, Seppälä J. Thermoresponsive xylan hydrogels via copper-catalyzed azide-alkyne cycloaddition. Carbohydr Polym 2014;102:637–644, Copyright (2014), with permission from Elsevier.*

adsorption performance on cellulosic surfaces, and this provided a way for enhancing the mechanical strengths of gels using nanocrystalline cellulose [115]. Moreover, the prepared mercaptopropyl xylan could be deprotected by undergoing simple hydrolysis. After that, the process of gelation would be achieved through thiol-thiol oxidative coupling reaction caused by hydrogen peroxide or atmospheric oxygen [116]. It has been discovered that the gelation was instantaneous, and the channel-networked hydrogel has been obtained after the xylans were contacted to the hydrogen peroxide [110]. Recently, Albertsson et al. explored the thiolation of AcGGM and gel formation via thiol-ene (AcGGM-S-G_t), thiol-Michael addition "click" reactions (AcGGM-S-G_m) with the difunctional N,N-methylenebis(acrylamide) (MBAA), and disulfide bond formation (AcGGM-S-G_s), and the obtained hydrogels as shown in Fig. 6.5 [47]. The porous hydrogels with three-dimensional network structure formed via thiol-ene click reaction with MBAA was observed, which led to swelling behavior in excess deionized water. A full interpenetrating hemicellulose hydrogel was also synthesized via thiol-ene click reaction between polyethylene glycol diacrylate and thiolated AcGGM [48], and the values of shear storage modulus of the prepared hydrogels were 35–40 times higher than the single network hydrogels.

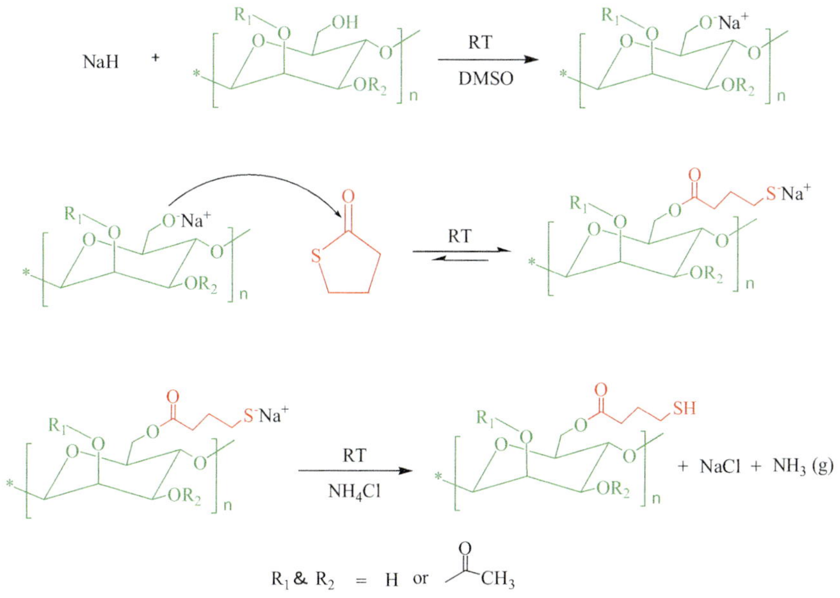

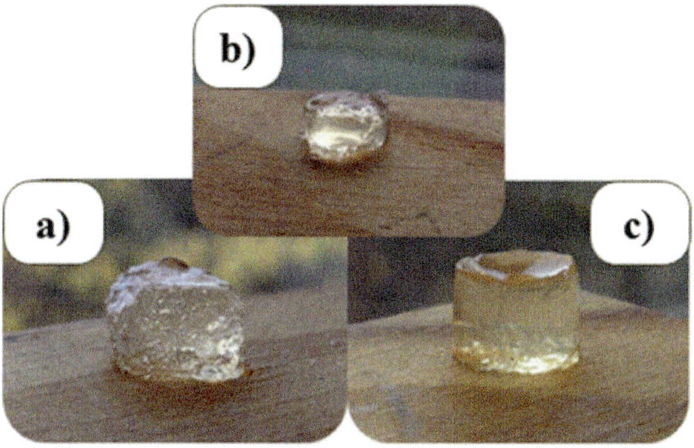

$$R_1 \& R_2 = H \text{ or } \overset{O}{\underset{}{\|}}\!\!-\!CH_3$$

FIG. 6.5 The pathway of one-pot thiolation of AcGGM in DMSO (top) and the obtained hydrogels images of (A) AcGGM-S-G$_m$, (B) AcGGM-S-G$_s$, and (C) AcGGM-S-G$_t$ (bottom). *Reproduced from Maleki L, Edlund U, Albertsson A-C. Thiolated hemicellulose as a versatile platform for one-pot click-type hydrogel synthesis. Biomacromolecules 2015:16:667–674, Copyright (2015), with permission from American Chemical Society.*

6.2.3 Enzymatic cross-linking

Enzymes have been used for the synthesis of hydrogels in situ with noninvasive behaviors and enable hydrogels suitable for controlled drug delivery and tissue engineering, overcoming traces of residual chemicals from chemically cross-linking methods and weak mechanical strength with physical cross-linking [117]. Oat spelt xylan was used for preparing hydrogels after selectively removing arabinose side chains by recombinant 1-1-arabinofuranosidase (AbfB), and the model bioactive agent horse radish peroxidase (HRP) loaded in the prepared hydrogels was studied for slow release [118]. HRP, a single-chain α-type hemoprotein, working as aromatic proton donors, is able to catalyze the coupling reaction of aniline derivatives or phenol induced under hydrogen peroxide [119, 120]. The precursor tyramine side groups-functionalized xylan was cross-linked in situ employing HRP and H_2O_2 accordingly to form an injectable hydrogel (Fig. 6.6) [49]. The hydrogels had sufficient mechanical performance because of forming a 3D network correlated with the rapid gelation, and they were reported to be innocuous, which were suitable for the cell immobilization. The tunable hydrogels have been synthesized from tyramine-functionalized

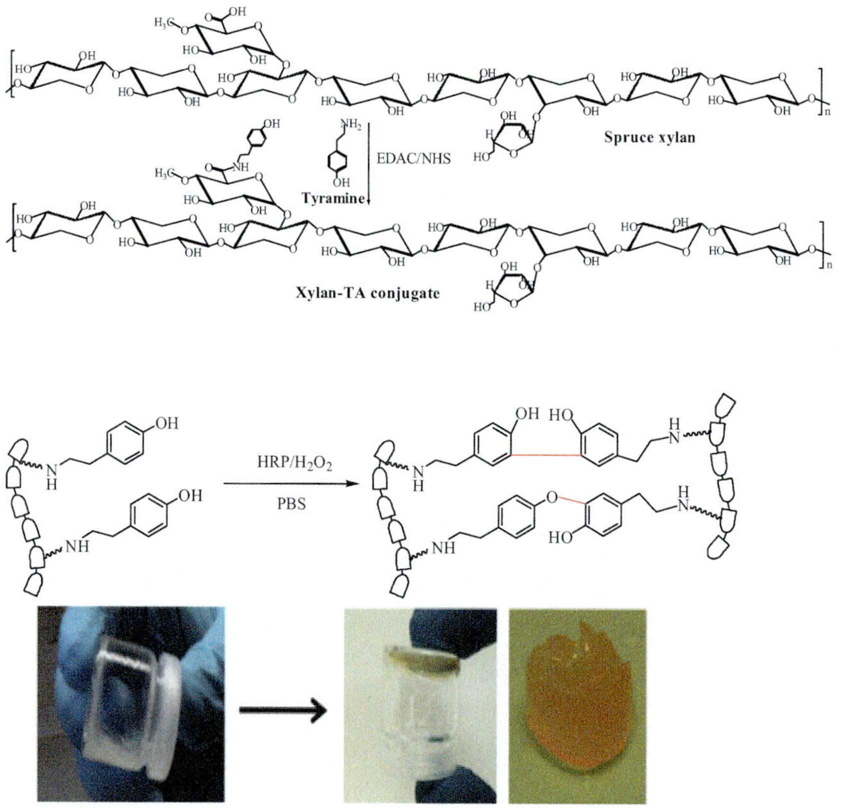

FIG. 6.6   Chemical reaction of conjugate formation from spruce xylan and tyramine (top); enzymatic cross-linking of xylan-TA conjugates and illustration of gels formation (bottom). *Reproduced from Kuzmenko V, Hägg D, Toriz G, Gatenholm P. In situ forming spruce xylan-based hydrogel for cell immobilization. Carbohydr Polym 2014;102:862–868, Copyright (2014), with permission from Elsevier.*

O-acetyl-galactoglucomannans, and the hydrogels were also formed via enzymatic cross-linking with HRP and peroxide additions [50]. Berlanga-Reyes et al. have prepared maize bran arabinoxylan (MBAX) hydrogels with laccase-inducing gelation [51], and the enzymatic cross-linking made the synthesis of MBAX hydrogel with β-lactoglobulin or insulin, which did not modify the rheological characters of the hydrogel.

6.3 Hemicelluloses-inorganic composite hydrogels

The organic-inorganic composite materials were studied with excellent mechanical strength and high thermal stability, which provided a direction to build hydrogels through introducing inorganic nanoparticles into degradable polysaccharide matrix. Some research groups have prepared various xylan-based nanocomposite hydrogels for applications in chemical and environmental engineering. Carbon nanotubes (CNT), with unique electrons, cavity structure, and adsorption property [121], have been combined with hemicellulose to prepare hydrogel as an adsorbent for water treatment [55]. The adsorption percentage for a model hazardous material methylene blue by this adsorbent was more than 98% with a concentration of $6\,g/L$ adsorbent, which attributed to the porous structure tunable by changing the CNT content and monomer ratio. Particularly, xylan can be modified with oxidized multiwalled carbon nanotubes (MWCNTs) to obtain the MWCNTs-xylan composites that participated in forming a novel superadsorbent during the polymerization of methacrylic acid with MBA as the cross-linker [56]. The synthesized composite hydrogels showed higher removal rate and adsorption capacity for methylene blue related to the superadsorbent dosage, ion strength, contact time, and pH value.

A magnetic hemicellulose-based hydrogel with covalently chemical cross-linked network has been prepared using H_2O_2-Vc redox initiator system to induce acrylated hemicellulose and functionalized Fe_3O_4 particles [52], and spherical Fe_3O_4 nanoparticles were distributed evenly in the hemicellulose matrices (Fig. 6.7). The magnetic hydrogels can efficiently adsorb the lysozyme, and both of the Freundlich and Temkin isotherm models could describe the adsorption behavior. Studies indicated that the Fe_3O_4 nanoparticles played a significant role in the physical and chemical structures, water uptake, and thermal and paramagnetic properties of the composite hydrogels [33, 53, 122]. Hemicelluloses-based magnetic hydrogels have been studied for application in these areas, such as controllable drug release or delivery, magnetic bioseparation, and H_2O_2 detection [53, 54]. Recently, photocatalyst titanium dioxide (TiO_2) was embedded firmly in the hemicellulose-based hydrogel networks [57], creatively endowing gels with great photocatalytic performance, and the study found that the TiO_2 content and pH value of solution influenced the degradation ratio of methylene blue. Zhang and collaborators produced a composite

wastewater streams, containing O-acetyl-galactoglucomannan (80%), arabinogalactan (15%), and arabino-4-O-methyl-glucuronoxylan (< 5%), was alkenyl-functionalized and then utilized to synthesize covalently cross-linked hydrogel, and the synthesized hydrogels can be used in the fields of biomedicine and agriculture due to its ability of delivering loaded molecules. The release of loaded BSA from the hydrogels exhibited Fickian diffusion behavior, and the hydrogels that incorporated growth-retardant agents were also developed for the coating of seeds to achieve tempo-rary inhibition of germination [38]. Sun and coworkers investigated the biodegradation of hemicellulose hydrogel and the controlled releases of theophylline and acetylsalicylic acid [125]; the hemicellulose extracted from wheat straw were mainly xylan, and the hydrogels synthesized from acrylic acid and wheat straw xylan by radical polymerization were pH sensitive. Fig. 6.8 shows that the prepared sensitive hydrogels can be

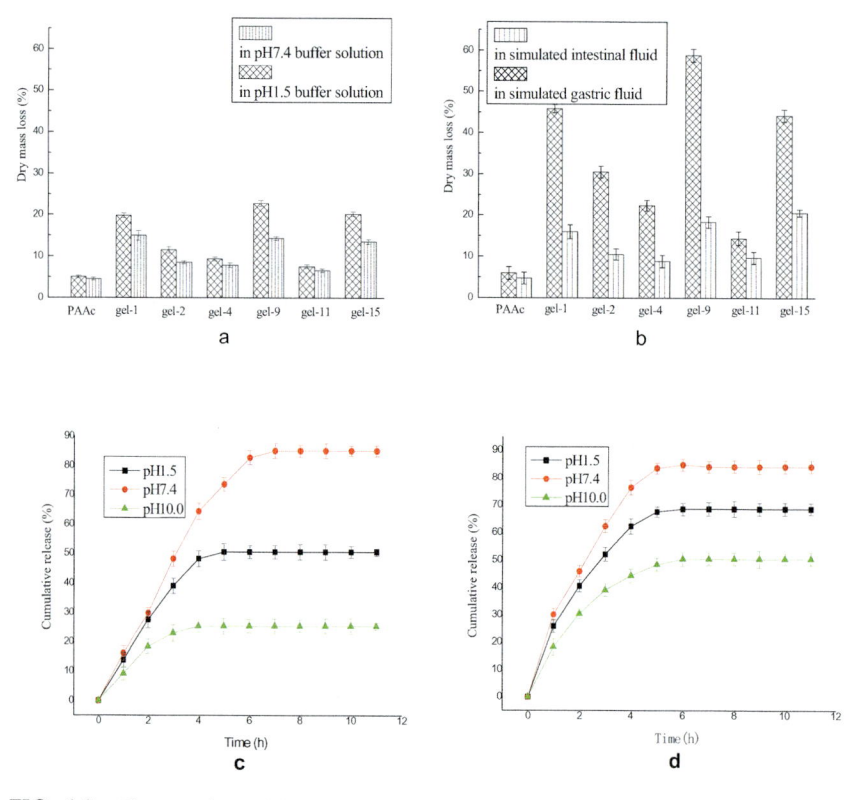

FIG. 6.8   The mass loss of the dry hydrogel samples after 96 h degradation: (A) in pH 1.5 and 7.4 buffer solutions; (B) in the simulated intestinal fluid and gastric fluid, and In vitro cu-mulative drug release from the hydrogels in different pH buffer solutions at 37°C; (C) acetyl-salicylic acid; and (D) theophylline. *Reproduced from Sun X-F, Wang H, Jing Z, Mohanathas R. Hemicellulose-based pH-sensitive and biodegradable hydrogel for controlled drug delivery. Carbohydr Polym 2013;92:1357–1366, Copyright (2013), with permission from Elsevier.*

significantly degraded in the simulated intestinal fluid, and degradation was enhanced with an increase of hemicellulose content in the hydrogels, indicating that hemicellulose accelerated the degradation of the prepared hydrogels. Fig. 6.8C and D also shows the cumulative releases of theophylline and acetylsalicylic acid with the prepared hydrogel; the acetylsalicylic acid can be uniformly released with a duration of 6h, and the zero order release kinetic could match the drug release dynamics, and initial burst release did not appear. The significant study indicated that hemicellulose hydrogels could be applied for controllable releases of drugs and bioactive molecules or other agents [125].

Modifications of hemicelluloses can improve their reactivity and drug delivery properties of the prepared hydrogels. For example, GMA-modified xylan was used to synthesize temperature/pH dual-responsive hydrogel, and the acetylsalicylic acid encapsulation ratio was up to 95.21% on the glycidyl methacrylate-modified xylan (GMAX)-based hydrogel [126]. The drug delivery rate of GMAX-based hydrogel for acetylsalicylic acid was 84.2% in the intestinal fluid, higher than that of xylan-based hydrogels (77.5%). Most importantly, the cumulative delivery rate of acetylsalicylic acid showed an increasing trend, and acetylsalicylic acid was continuously released up to 8h. In addition, the study of another temperature/pH dual-sensitive hydrogels prepared from MA-modified xylan showed that the hydrogels could release more acetylsalicylic acid cumulatively compared with theophylline, and only 24.26% of acetylsalicylic acids were released in gastric juice, but 90.5% of acetylsalicylic acids were released in simulated intestinal juice. Furthermore, the mechanical strength and drug release rate of the hydrogel can be adjusted by changing the substitution degree of modified xylan [127]. Xylan-β-cyclodextrin chemically cross-linked hydrogel was synthesized in alkaline medium with ethylene glycol diglycidyl ether as the cross-linking agent, and the in vitro release of 5-fluorouracil and curcumin was studied [128]. The hydrogel had the highest 5-fluorouracil loading (98%) and less curcumin loading (26%) because β-cyclodextrin and xylan have hydrophilic surface, which provides many binding sites for 5-fluorouracil, while only one aromatic ring of curcumin or one 5-fluorouracil molecule can be accommodated by the hydrophobic cavity of β-cyclodextrin. The high cumulative releases of 5-fluorouracil (56%) and curcumin (37%) was achieved in PBS buffer after 24h. Furthermore, the prepared hydrogels also presented good results for cell encapsulation and tumor treatment [128]. In addition, Chang et al. studied the effect of different pore-producing agents on the performances of hemicellulose hydrogels, such as polyethylene glycol 2000, polyvinylpyrrolidone K30, carbamide, $CaCO_3$, $NaHCO_3$, and NaCl [129]. The results showed that the release rate of 5-fluorouracil was significantly increased after $NaHCO_3$ was used as a pore-producing agent, and the drug delivery ratio raised to 71.05% in the simulated intestinal fluid in 4h.

To study the vitamin B12 delivery of hemicellulose hydrogels, xylan methacrylate-based multiresponsive hydrogels containing vitamin B12 were prepared and set under UV irradiation for the cumulative release study, and the highest release ratios were acquired, which were 78.2% and 89.3% in pH 2.2 and 7.4 solutions, respectively [86]. Because xylan methacrylate-based hydrogel had better cumulative release property with UV than that without UV, the modified xylan-based hydrogels can be applied in the field of drug release under the control of UV. Carboxymethyl cellulose-xylan homopolymerized and copolymerized hydrogels were synthesized in alkaline medium, using a cross-linking agent, ethylene glycol diglycidyl ether, and its drug delivery property was studied [130]. The synthesized hydrogels had a relatively high vitamin B12 loading of 36.59% and cumulative releases of 80%–88% in artificial intestinal fluid, 93%–98% in phosphate-buffered saline, and 19%–28% in artificial gastric fluid. The carboxymethyl cellulose-xylan copolymerized hydrogels had a relatively high release rate and long delivery duration in artificial intestinal fluid and phosphate-buffered saline, while it had a weak ability to release vitamin B12 in the artificial gastric fluid. The maximum delivery ratios of all carboxymethyl cellulose-xylan hydrogels were 93%–99% for vitamin B12 under desirable conditions. In all, the carboxymethyl cellulose-xylan hydrogel can deliver more than 90% of vitamin B12 within 10 h.

Hemicelluloses-based magnetic hydrogels have been prepared for drug or enzyme encapsulation and release [52, 53, 131]. Immobilization of lysozyme on semi-IPN magnetic hydrogel prepared from xylan and poly(acrylic acid) was studied, and the results showed that the adsorption amount of lysozyme was affected by the initial lysozyme concentration. The immobilization amount of the magnetic hydrogel for lysozyme was 180 mg/g, which was higher than that of the nonmagnetic hydrogel (165 mg/g) [131]. However, chemically cross-linked hemicellulose-g-poly(acrylic acid) magnetic hydrogel prepared from acryloyl hemicellulose and functional Fe_3O_4 particles using a green redox initiator system (H_2O_2-Vc) had higher lysozyme adsorption amount (220 mg/g) [52], and this may be due to the formed dense and uniform pore structure, and Fe_3O_4 particles that chemically linked with polymers were also dispersed uniformly in the hydrogel matrix in this method (Fig. 6.9). Hemicellulose hydrogels with magnetic sensitivity, prepared from O-acetyl-galactoglucomannan and Fe_3O_4 nanoparticles, also showed high adsorption capacity of BSA and controllable delivery ability, and the magnetic hydrogel (M-15) had high adsorption capacity for BSA (146.5 mg/g), higher than the amount (100.2 mg/g) of the hydrogel without Fe_3O_4 nanoparticles. Therefore, the addition of Fe_3O_4 particles in the hydrogels is very significant in improving adsorption capacity of the prepared hydrogels for drugs or enzymes; 74% of BSA was released from the magnetic hydrogel in 5 days, indicating that the hemicelluloses-based magnetic hydrogel could be applied in

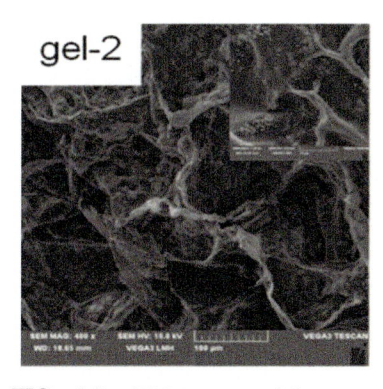
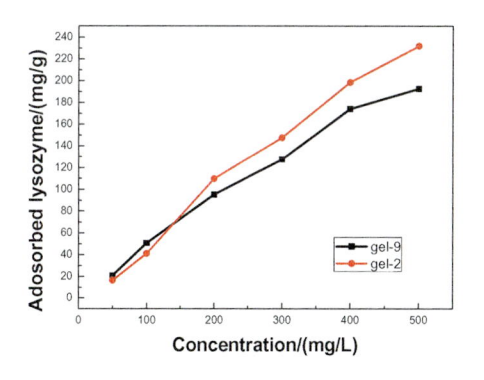

FIG. 6.9 SEM image and lysozyme adsorption data on magnetic hemicellulose hydrogel and nonmagnetic hydrogel. *Reproduced from Li Y-J, Sun X-F, Ye Q, Liu B-C, Wu Y-G. Preparation and properties of a novel hemicellulose-based magnetic hydrogel. Acta Phys - Chim Sin 2014;30:111–120, Copyright (2014), with permission from publisher: Editorial Office of Acta Physico-Chimica Sinica.*

the biomedicine field because of the excellent delivery property and high loading capacity for drugs or enzymes [53].

6.5 Tissue engineering

Polysaccharide dressings, such as hemicellulose dressing (Veloderm), calcium alginate dressing (Algisite M), and hyaluronic acid ester dressing (Jaloskin), have attracted increasing attention as temporary skin materials to heal the damage of superficial epidermal layers in tissue engineering. Hemicellulose dressing has been used to treat wounds, burns, ulcers, abrasions, sores, and autograft donor areas [132]. The performances of Veloderm were compared with Jaloskin and Algisite M on 23 adult burn patients (Fig. 6.10). After dressing with Veloderm, within 10–13 days, a high proportion of the split-thickness skin graft donor site area (47.6%) was healed, which was better than the Algisite M (26.3%) and Jaloskin (10%). In addition, Veloderm not only reduced the exudate near the wound, it also decreased the incidence of perilesional erythema during the whole study. Veloderm gave better aesthetic outcome after healing ($P = .0016$), and few medicines were renewed in the beginning week. Veloderm has been considered a better wound dressing than Algisite M and Jaloskin because of its advantages such as easy use ($P < .001$), acceptability ($P < .001$), and efficacy ($P < .00001$). Throughout all treatments, the use of Veloderm as a wound dressing produced little pain, and scars and local infections did not appear in the split-thickness skin graft donor site area. Therefore,

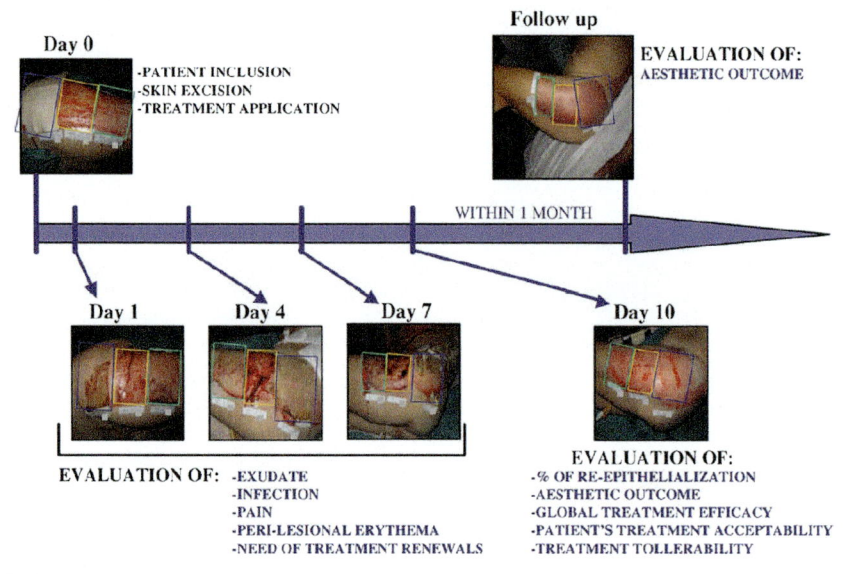

FIG. 6.10   Protocol summary. The *squared-green-areas* are dressed with Veloderm; the *squared-blue areas* are dressed with Algisite M; the *squared-yellow areas* are dressed with Jaloskin. *From Melandri D, Angelis AD, Orioli R, Ponzielli G, Lualdi P, Giarratana N, Reiner V. Use of a new hemicellulose dressing (Veloderm1) for the treatment of split-thickness skin graft donor sites: a within-patient controlled study. Burns 2006;32:964–972, Copyright (2006), with permission from Elsevier.*

the hemicellulose dressing is an anticipated dressing for skin graft donor sites because of its safety and efficacy. A study also compared the effectiveness of rayon and hemicellulose dressings to heal the skin graft donor site with 28 patients, all of whom completed re-epithelialization within 14–21 days [133]. Hemicellulose dressings exhibited very similar performances to rayon dressings in some respects such as pain, exudate, pruritus, hyperemia, and final appearance after treatment. The same results were also achieved when evaluating the therapeutic parameters of hemicellulose dressing and rayon dressing.

Xyloglucan and xylan have been fabricated into scaffolds for regenerating damaged tissues because of their bioactivity and special gelling properties [134, 135]. Xyloglucan was found to increase corneal wound healing, and 1% xyloglucan from tamarind seed can promote cell adhesion to laminin and spheroid formation, because the galactose groups on the backbone can bind with asialoglycoprotein receptors on hepatocytes [135]. Xyloglucan can form a thermally sensitive hydrogel after removing 35%–50% of the galactose groups, and the partial removal of galactose moieties reduces steric hindrance, resulting in thermal gelation because the polymer backbones of xyloglucan may associate or interact via hydrophobic interactions, so this gel has the sol-gel behaviors of becoming gel when heating and returning to sol states after cooling [136]. Biological hydrogel scaffolds have been prepared based on functionalization of xyloglucan for neural tissue engineering [137]. The results showed that the xyloglucan hydrogel exhibited the same mechanical strength as that of natural spinal cords, which provided greater support to the survival of in vitro neurons, differentiation of primary cortical neurons, and the neurite extension under 3D and 2D culture conditions.

Furthermore, functionalization of xyloglucan provided ways to control and optimize the cell number, diameter, migration, neurite density, as well as growth direction. Tissue engineering scaffolds for cardiovascular system must be noncytotoxic, biodegradable, biocompatible, highly porous, and mechanically stable for the appropriate functions. Venugopal et al. selected the xylan of beech wood to function infarcted myocardium and prepared nanofibrous scaffolds that cross-linked with glutaraldehyde vapor for cardiac tissue engineering [134]. The results showed that the mechanical strength and Young's modulus of the xylan/PVA nanofibers (427 nm) that cross-linked with glutaraldehyde vapor for 24 h were 2.43 and 3.74 MPa, respectively, which were desirable to cardiomyocyte cells culture, enhancing the proliferation of cardiomyocytes by 11%. In addition, the xylan-based nanofiber scaffold could directly deliver the nanofibers into the heart muscle, eliminating the requirement for open heart surgery.

6.6 Relationship between the structure and property

The performances of hemicelluloses-derived hydrogels are influenced by the structural and physiochemical properties of hemicelluloses [138]. Table 6.2 lists the relationship between hemicellulose structure and hydrogel property. Hydrogels based on hemicellulose containing acetyl groups are stiffer and have a low water absorption capacity, but acetylated xylan has a higher drug release rate against doxorubicin, which is twice that of hemicellulose hydrogels without acetyl groups. The nanofibrillated cellulose (NFC) hydrogel was reinforced by various hemicellulosic polysaccharides including xylan, xyloglucan (XG), and galactoglucomannan (GGM) [139]. It was found that the type and amount of incorporated hemicelluloses can influence the growth of cells through changing the mechanical properties and pore structure of the composite hydrogel scaffolds. The NFC hydrogel containing XG exhibited the highest mechanical strength, and XG can promote cell growth and show excellent adsorption ability on NFC. In addition, preparations of nanoreinforced hydrogels have also been achieved via absorbing the methacrylate-modified hemicellulose onto the cellulose nanowhiskers before in situ radical polymerization [140]. The prepared hydrogel exhibited increased viscoelasticity, enhanced tenacity

TABLE 6.2   Relationship between hemicellulose structure and hydrogel property.

Hemicellulose structure	Hydrogel property	Reference
Acetyl groups	Reducing equilibrium swelling ratio but improving drug delivery rate	[129]
Xyloglucan	The highest reinforcement effect and the highest adsorption capacity on the NFC	[130]
Methacrylate modified hemicellulose	Enhancing toughness and increasing viscoelasticity and recovery behavior	[131]
Carboxymethyl xylan	pH sensitivity	[76]
Molecular chain extension of hemicelluloses	Mechanical performance was enhanced	[132]
Glycidyl methacrylate-modified xylan	A high drug encapsulation efficiency, low drug release rate, and high cell viability	[126]
Maleic anhydride-modified xylan	Biocompatibility with NIH3T3 cells, promoting cell proliferation	[127]

and recoverability, and was considered a substitute of articular cartilage in load-bearing biomedical fields.

Modifications of hemicellulose can impart new properties or improve some properties of its derived hydrogel, for example, carboxymethylation of xylan gave pH sensitivity of xylan hydrogel (Fig. 6.11) [76]. The extension of hemicellulosic polymer chains could enhance the mechanical strength of hemicellulose-derived hydrogel [141]. GMAX-derived hydrogel had relatively low drug delivery ratio and high drug loading efficiency, and NIH3T3 cells kept high cell viability in GMAX-derived hydrogel [126]. Maleic anhydride-modified xylan (MAHX)-derived hydrogel had desirable biocompatibility with NIH3T3 cells, promoting cell proliferation, and the substitution degree of MAHX can determine the drug delivery, mechanical strength, and pore structure of the hydrogel [127].

Besides hemicellulose, the structure and content of other polymers in hydrogels, such as lignin and cellulose, also affected the performances of the hemicellulose hydrogels. Previous studies have shown that lignin can affect the performances of hemicellulose hydrogels [142, 143]. For example, lignosulfonates content in hydrogel affected adsorption capacity, mechanical strength, and chemical and thermal properties, and the maximum adsorption capacity of hemicellulose-lignin composite hydrogel toward methylene blue was 2691 mg/g [143]. The addition of CNC into xylan hydrogel can improve the mechanical property [144]. Lindblad and his collaborator first investigated the rheological characterization of hemicellulosic hydrogels [145]. The results showed that hydrogels presented a stronger elastic response than viscous response, indicating that solid-like

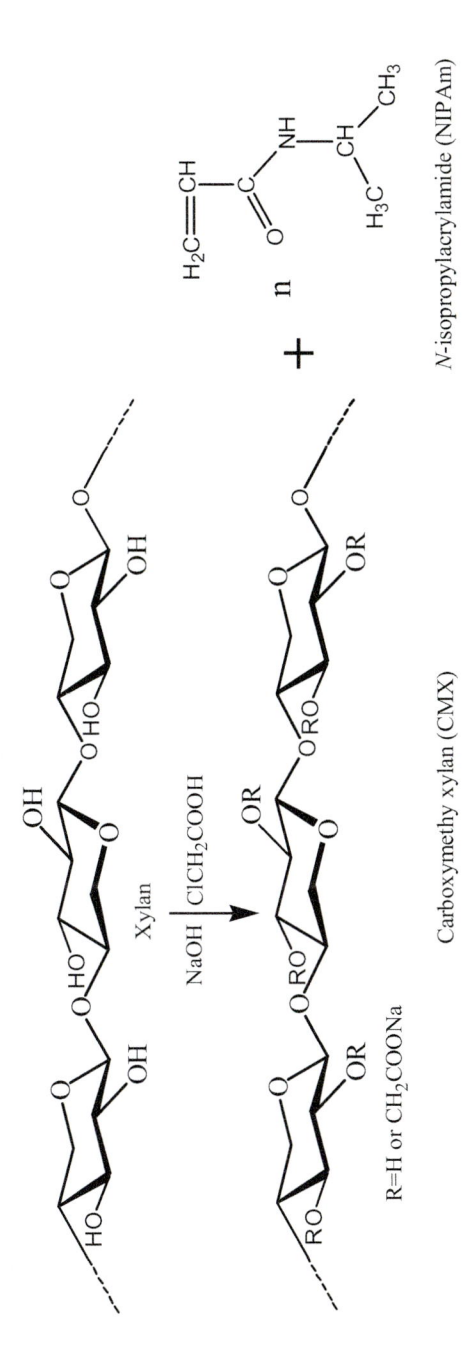

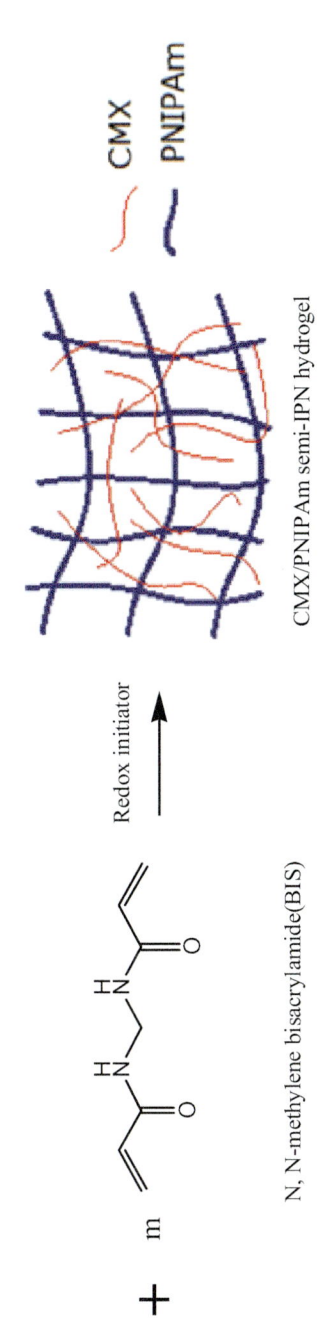

FIG. 6.11 Synthetic scheme of pH- and temperature-sensitive xylan hydrogel. *Reproduced from Sun X-F, Zeng QH, Wang HH, Hao YW. Preparation and swelling behavior of pH/temperature responsive semi-IPN hydrogel based on carboxymethyl xylan and poly(N-isopropyl acrylamide). Cellulose 2019;26:1909–1922, Copyright (2019), with permission from Springer.*

behavior was predominant in the hemicellulosic hydrogel system, and the properties of the hemicellulosic hydrogels were also affected by the property of synthetic comonomer. The incorporation of synthetic polymers like polyacrylamide and poly(acrylic acid) resulted in higher adsorption amount for dye and heavy metal ions [78, 146, 147].

Liu et al. prepared carboxymethyl xylan-g-poly(acrylic acid) composite hydrogel with high strength and shape memory property [148]. This study presented that the composite hydrogels that incorporated with hydroxylate MWCNTs and metal coordination had excellent mechanical property and rapid recovery property, and the highest breaking elongation (1032%) and compressive strength (10.4 MPa) of the hydrogels (1032%) had been detected in this study. Even after 30 compression cycles, the hydrogel can almost return to its original structure once removing the external force. The addition of acid-treated CNTs in the hydrogels not only changed mechanical strength, physical-chemical structures, and swelling property but also gave some new features, such as photothermal conversion and electrical conductivity [149]. The incorporation of Fe_3O_4 particles in xylan hydrogel not only demonstrated excellent mechanical and magnetic properties but also exhibited desirable H_2O_2 detection sensitivity and catalytic action [54].

6.7 Conclusion and further outlook

Because of the scarcity of fossil resources and deterioration of ecological environment problems, the transformation of plant sources becomes a key point of research direction. Hemicelluloses from plants have attracted much attention because of its abundant storage in nature, and the hemicelluloses-based hydrogels have been extensively studied recently. The synthesis methods of hemicelluloses-based hydrogels can be divided into physical cross-linking, chemical cross-linking, enzymatic cross-linking, and others. The mechanical property of the hemicellulose hydrogel was significantly enhanced through blending with PVA, forming a semi- or full-interpenetrate network structure with chitosan or adopting a physical method, freeze-thaw cycle technique. For chemical cross-linking, biobased cross-linkers have been developed to fabricate green and biodegradable hydrogels. The hydrogels with stimulative responsibility, such as temperature, pH, or light sensitivity and special performances, superabsorbent, or others, have been synthesized via radical polymerization or click chemistry methods. Enzymatic cross-linking could prepare the hemicellulose hydrogels in situ. Additionally, many inorganic nanoparticles have been introduced into hydrogels network matrices for preparing the hemicellulose-inorganic composite hydrogels. The developments of green methods and biobased cross-linkers made hemicelluloses-based hydrogels applicable in biomedical and other fields.

Hemicelluloses-based hydrogels have perfectly combined the advantages of both hemicelluloses and hydrogels, including hydrophilicity, biocompatibility, biodegradability, swelling property, excellent mechanical property, and other performances, which determined the wide application prospects in biomedicine, drug delivery, water treatment, and other fields. But on the basis of previous studies, some suggestions and research orientations should be put forward. The theoretical study would be strengthened on the interactions between hemicelluloses and other components and the relationship between the gel structure and their properties. These are vital to design multifunctional and smart hemicelluloses-based hydrogels to meet the application requirements of different fields. Therefore, how to fabricate and synthesize novel hemicelluloses-based hydrogels and expand application fields will be future research directions.

Acknowledgments

The authors are grateful to the financial support by the Fundamental Research Funds for the Central Universities (No. 310201911cx012) and the Sustainable Development Science and Technology Project of Shenzhen (2021N030).

References

[1] Wichterle O, Lim D. Hydrophilic gels for biological use. Nature 1960;185:117–8.

[2] Gao C, Ren J, Zhao C, Kong W, Dai Q, Chen Q, Liu C, Sun R. Xylan-based temperature/pH sensitive hydrogels for drug controlled release. Carbohydr Polym 2016;151:189–97.

[3] Kong BJ, Kim A, Park SN. Properties and in vitro drug release of hyaluronic acid-hydroxyethyl cellulose hydrogels for transdermal delivery of isoliquiritigenin. Carbohydr Polym 2016;147:473–81.

[4] Van Vlierberghe S, Dubruel P, Schacht E. Biopolymer-based hydrogels as scaffolds for tissue engineering applications: a review. Biomacromolecules 2011;12:1387–408.

[5] Buenger D, Topuz F, Groll J. Hydrogels in sensing applications. Prog Polym Sci 2012;37:1678–719.

[6] Caló E, Khutoryanskiy VV. Biomedical applications of hydrogels: a review of patents and commercial products. Eur Polym J 2015;65:252–67.

[7] Cong H-P, Qiu J-H, Yu S-H. Thermoresponsive poly(N-isopropylacrylamide)/graphene/Au nanocomposite hydrogel for water treatment by a laser-assisted approach. Small 2015;11:1165–70.

[8] Soto D, Urdaneta J, Pernia K, León O, Muñoz-Bonilla A, Fernández-García M. Itaconic acid grafted starch hydrogels as metal remover: capacity, selectivity and adsorption kinetics. J Polym Environ 2016;24:343–55.

[9] Hoffman AS. Hydrogels for biomedical applications. Adv Drug Deliv Rev 2002;54:3–12.

[10] Hoffman AS. Conventional and environmentally-sensitive hydrogels for medical and industrial uses: a review paper. In: DeRossi D, Kajiwara K, Osada Y, Yamauchi A, editors. Polymer gels. Boston, MA: Springer; 1991. p. 289–97.

[11] Rassu G, Salis A, Porcu EP, Giunchedi P, Roldo M, Gavini E. Composite chitosan/alginate hydrogel for controlled release of deferoxamine: a system to potentially treat iron dysregulation diseases. Carbohydr Polym 2016;136:1338–47.

[12] Baei P, Jalili-Firoozinezhad S, Rajabi-Zeleti S, Tafazzoli-Shadpour M, Baharvand H, Aghdami N. Electrically conductive gold nanoparticle-chitosan thermosensitive hydrogels for cardiac tissue engineering. Mater Sci Eng, C 2016;63:131–41.

[13] Elviri L, Asadzadeh M, Cucinelli R, Bianchera A, Bettini R. Macroporous chitosan hydrogels: effects of sulfur on the loading and release behaviour of amino acid-based compounds. Carbohydr Polym 2015;132:50–8.

[14] Li C, Jia J, Yi G, Yun L, Ping Z. Preparation and characterization of IPN hydrogels composed of chitosan and gelatin cross-linked by genipin. Carbohydr Polym 2014;99:31–8.

[15] Huerta-Angeles G, Němcová M, Příkopová E, Šmejkalová D, Pravda M, Kučera L, Velebný V. Reductive alkylation of hyaluronic acid for the synthesis of biocompatible hydrogels by click chemistry. Carbohydr Polym 2012;90:1704–11.

[16] Wang J, Hong S, Li J, Dong D, Zhang Y, Yao F. Ionic starch-based hydrogels for the prevention of nonspecific protein adsorption. Carbohydr Polym 2015;117:384–91.

[17] Chang C, Zhang L. Cellulose-based hydrogels: present status and application prospects. Carbohydr Polym 2011;84:40–53.

[18] Peng N, Wang Y, Ye Q, Liang L, An Y, Li Q, Chang C. Biocompatible cellulose-based superabsorbent hydrogels with antimicrobial activity. Carbohydr Polym 2016;137:59–64.

[19] Gabrielii I, Gatenholm P. Preparation and properties of hydrogels based on hemicellulose. J Appl Polym Sci 1998;69:1661–7.

[20] Ismail H, Irani M, Ahmad Z. Starch-based hydrogels: present status and applications. Int J Polym Mater Polym Biomater 2013;62:411–20.

[21] Schulze E. Zur Kentniss der chemischen Zusammensetzung der pflanzlichen Zellmembranen. Ber Dtsch Chem Ges 1891;24:2277–87.

[22] Fang JM, Sun RC, Tomkinson J, Fowler P. Acetylation of wheat straw hemicellulose B in a new non-aqueous swelling system. Carbohydr Polym 2000;41:379–87.

[23] Tokoh C, Takabe K, Sugiyama J, Fujita M. CP/MAS 13C NMR and electron diffraction study of bacterial cellulose structure affected by cell wall polysaccharides. Cellulose 2002;9:351–60.

[24] Puls J, Schuseil J. In: Coughlan MP, Hazlewood GP, editors. Hemicellulose and hemicellulases. London, Chapel Hill: Portland Press; 1993. p. 1.

[25] Cai ZS, Paszner L. Salt catalyzed wood bonding with hemicellulose. Holzforschung 1988;42:11–20.

[26] Sun XF, Sun RC, Fowler P, Baird MS. Extraction and characterization of original lignin and hemicelluloses from wheat straw. J Agric Food Chem 2005;53:860–70.

[27] Sun XF, Fowler P, Zhang GC, Rajaratnam M. Extraction and characterization of hemicelluloses from maize stem. Phytochem Anal 2010;21:406–15.

[28] Sun XF, Jing ZX, Fowler P, Wu YG, Rajaratnam M. Structural characterization and isolation of lignin and hemicelluloses from barley straw. Ind Crop Prod 2011;33:588–98.

[29] Gabrielii I, Gatenholm P, Glasser WG, Jain RK, Kenne L. Separation, characterization and hydrogel-formation of hemicellulose from aspen wood. Carbohydr Polym 2000;43:367–74.

[30] Bush JR, Liang H, Dickinson M, Botchwey EA. Xylan hemicellulose improves chitosan hydrogel for bone tissue regeneration. Polym Adv Technol 2016;27:1050–5.

[31] Li HP, Hu Y, Yang G, Yang Y, Zhang Y. Preparation of bagasse xylan phosphate-chitosan hydrogel and drug release effect. Chem Res Appl 2013;25:399–406 [in Chinese].

[32] Tanodekaew S, Channasanon S, Uppanan P. Xylan/polyvinyl alcohol blend and its performance as hydrogel. J Appl Polym Sci 2006;100:1914–8.

[33] Sun X-F, Jing Z, Wang H, Liu Y. Physical–chemical properties of xylan/PAAc magnetic semi-interpenetrating network hydrogel. Polym Compos 2015;36:2317–25.

[34] Sun X-F, Feng Y, Shi X, Wang Y. Preparation and property of xylan/poly(methacrylic acid) semi-interpenetrating network hydrogel. Int J Polym Sci 2016;, 8241078.

[35] Peng F, Guan Y, Zhang B, Bian J, Ren J-L, Yao C-L, Sun R-C. Synthesis and properties of hemicelluloses-based semi-IPN hydrogels. Int J Biol Macromol 2014;65:564–72.

[36] Guan Y, Bian J, Peng F, Zhang X-M, Sun R-C. High strength of hemicelluloses based hydrogels by freeze/thaw technique. Carbohydr Polym 2014;101:272–80.

[37] Peng X-W, Ren J-L, Zhong L-X, Peng F, Sun R-C. Xylan-rich hemicelluloses-graft-acrylic acid ionic hydrogels with rapid responses to pH, salt, and organic solvents. J Agric Food Chem 2011;59:8208–15.

[38] Albertsson AC, Voepel J, Edlund U, Dahlman O, Lindblad MS. Design of renewable hydrogel release systems from fiberboard mill wastewater. Biomacromolecules 2010;11:1406–11.

[39] Ge MC, Zhou XS. The synthesis and property of hemicelluloses/PVA semi-IPN hydrogel. Pap Sci Technol 2015;34:28–32 [in Chinese].

[40] Ferrari E, Ranucci E, Edlund U, Albertsson A-C. Design of renewable poly(amidoamine)/hemicellulose hydrogels for heavy metal adsorption. J Appl Polym Sci 2015;132:41695.

[41] Pohjanlehto H, Setälä H, Kammiovirta K, Harlin A. The use of N,N'-diallylaldardiamides as cross-linkers in xylan derivatives-based hydrogels. Carbohydr Res 2011;346:2736–45.

[42] Köhnke T, Elder T, Theliander H, Ragauskas AJ. Ice templated and cross-linked xylan/ nanocrystalline cellulose hydrogels. Carbohydr Polym 2014;100:24–30.

[43] Yang JY, Zhou XS, Fang J. Synthesis and characterization of temperature sensitive hemicellulose-based hydrogels. Carbohydr Polym 2011;86:1113–7.

[44] Yang J, Zhou X. Properties of hemicellulose-based hydrogels synthesized via ATRP. Polym Mater Sci Eng 2014;30:21–5 [in Chinese].

[45] Zhang W, Zhu S, Bai Y, Xi N, Wang S, Bian Y, Li X, Zhang Y. Glow discharge electrolysis plasma initiated preparation of temperature/pH dual sensitivity reed hemicellulose-based hydrogels. Carbohydr Polym 2015;122:11–7.

[46] Pahimanolis N, Sorvari A, Luong ND, Seppälä J. Thermoresponsive xylan hydrogels via copper-catalyzed azide-alkyne cycloaddition. Carbohydr Polym 2014;102:637–44.

[47] Maleki L, Edlund U, Albertsson A-C. Thiolated hemicellulose as a versatile platform for one-pot click-type hydrogel synthesis. Biomacromolecules 2015;16:667–74.

[48] Maleki L, Edlund U, Albertsson A-C. Synthesis of full interpenetrating hemicellulose hydrogel networks. Carbohydr Polym 2017;170:254–63.

[49] Kuzmenko V, Hägg D, Toriz G, Gatenholm P. In situ forming spruce xylan-based hydrogel for cell immobilization. Carbohydr Polym 2014;102:862–8.

[50] Markstedt K, Xu W, Liu J, Xu C, Gatenholm P. Synthesis of tunable hydrogels based on O-acetyl-galactoglucomannans from spruce. Carbohydr Polym 2017;157:1349–57.

[51] Berlanga-Reyes CM, Carvajal-Millán E, Lizardi-Mendoza J, Rascón-Chu A, Marquez-Escalante JA, Martínez-López AL. Maize arabinoxylan gels as protein delivery matrices. Molecules 2009;14:475–1482.

[52] Li Y-J, Sun X-F, Ye Q, Liu B-C, Wu Y-G. Preparation and properties of a novel hemicellulose-based magnetic hydrogel. Acta Phys -Chim Sin 2014;30:111–20.

[53] Zhao W, Odelius K, Edlund U, Zhao C, Albertsson A-C. In situ synthesis of magnetic field-responsive hemicellulose hydrogels for drug delivery. Biomacromolecules 2015;16:2522–8.

[54] Dai QQ, Ren JL, Peng F, Chen XF, Gao CD, Sun RC. Synthesis of acylated xylan-based magnetic Fe_3O_4 hydrogels and their application for H_2O_2 detection. Materials 2016;9:690. https://doi.org/10.3390/ma9080690.

[55] Sun X-F, Ye Q, Jing Z, Li Y. Preparation of hemicellulose-g-poly(methacrylic acid)/carbon nanotube composite hydrogel and adsorption properties. Polym Compos 2014;35:45–52.

[56] Jing Z, Zhang G, Sun X-F, Shi X, Sun W. Preparation and adsorption properties of a novel superabsorbent based on multiwalled carbon nanotubes–xylan composite and poly(methacrylic acid) for methylene blue from aqueous solution. Polym Compos 2014;35:1516–28.

[57] Sun X-F, Li C, Xia X-Y, Zhou R, Wang Y-X, Feng Y. Photocatalytic degradation property of hemicellulose/TiO$_2$ composite gel. Huagong Xuebao/CIESC J 2016;67:2070–7.

[58] Zhang S, Guan Y, Fu GQ, Chen BY, Peng F, Yao CL, Sun RC. Organic/inorganic superabsorbent hydrogels based on xylan and montmorillonite. J Nanomater 2014;3669–76.

[59] Qi X, Guan Y, Chen G, Zhang B, Ren J, Peng F, Sun R. A non-covalent strategy for montmorillonite/xylose self-healing hydrogels. RSC Adv 2015;5:41006–12.

[60] Guan Y, Chen J, Qi X, Chen G, Peng F, Sun R. Fabrication of biopolymer hydrogel containing Ag nanoparticles for antibacterial property. Ind Eng Chem Res 2015;54:7393–400.

[61] Kong W, Dai Q, Gao C, Ren J, Liu C, Sun R. Hemicellulose-based hydrogels and their potential application. In: Thakur V, Thakur M, editors. Polymer gels. Gels horizons: from science to smart materials. Singapore: Springer; 2018. p. 87–127.

[62] Yan S, Yin J, Tang L, Chen X. Novel physically crosslinked hydrogels of carboxymethyl chitosan and cellulose ethers: structure and controlled drug release behavior. J Appl Polym Sci 2011;119:2350–8.

[63] Overstreet DJ, Dutta D, Stabenfeldt SE, Vernon BL. Injectable hydrogels. J Polym Sci Polym Phys 2012;50:881–903.

[64] Karaaslan MA, Tshabalala MA, Buschle-Diller G. Semi-interpenetrating polymer network hydrogels based on aspen hemicellulose and chitosan: effect of crosslinking sequence on hydrogel properties. J Appl Polym Sci 2012;124:1168–77.

[65] Li H, Li D, Lu Y. Synthesis and characterization of bagasse xylan phosphate. Chem Res Appl 2011;23:1353–8 [in Chinese].

[66] Hennink WE, van Nostrum CF. Novel crosslinking methods to design hydrogels. Adv Drug Deliv Rev 2012;64S:223–36.

[67] Zhang H, Zhang F, Wu J. Physically crosslinked hydrogels from polysaccharides prepared by freeze–thaw technique. React Funct Polym 2013;73:923–8.

[68] Zhao Y, Shen W, Chen Z, Wu T. Freeze-thaw induced gelation of alginates. Carbohydr Polym 2016;148:45–51.

[69] Fekete T, Borsa J, Takács E, Wojnárovits L. Synthesis of cellulose-based superabsorbent hydrogels by high-energy irradiation in the presence of crosslinking agent. Radiat Phys Chem 2016;118:114–9.

[70] Zhou Y, Fu S, Zhang L, Zhan H. Superabsorbent nanocomposite hydrogels made of carboxylated cellulose nanofibrils and CMC-g-p(AA-co-AM). Carbohydr Polym 2013;97:429–35.

[71] Peng X-W, Zhong L-X, Ren J-L, Sun R-C. Highly effective adsorption of heavy metal ions from aqueous solutions by macroporous xylan-rich hemicelluloses-based hydrogel. J Agric Food Chem 2012;60:3909–16.

[72] Deville S. Freeze-casting of porous ceramics: a review of current achievements and issues. Adv Eng Mater 2008;10:155–69.

[73] Madihally SV, Matthew HWT. Porous chitosan scaffolds for tissue engineering. Biomaterials 1999;20:1133–42.

[74] Zmora S, Glicklis R, Cohen S. Tailoring the pore architecture in 3-D alginate scaffolds by controlling the freezing regime during fabrication. Biomaterials 2002;23:4087–94.

[75] Köhnke T, Lin A, Elder T, Theliander H, Ragauskas AJ. Nanoreinforced xylan-cellulose composite foams by freeze-casting. Green Chem 2012;14:1864–9.

[76] Sun X-F, Zeng QH, Wang HH, Hao YW. Preparation and swelling behavior of pH/temperature responsive semi-IPN hydrogel based on carboxymethyl xylan and poly(N-isopropyl acrylamide). Cellulose 2019;26:1909–22.

[77] Zhang J, Xiao H, Li N, Ping Q, Zhang Y. Synthesis and characterization of superabsorbent hydrogels based on hemicellulose. J Appl Polym Sci 2015;132:42441.

[78] Sun X-F, Gan Z, Jing Z, Wang H, Wang D, Jin Y. Adsorption of methylene blue on hemicellulose-based stimuli-responsive porous hydrogel. J Appl Polym Sci 2015;132:41606.

[79] Lindblad MS, Ranucci E, Albertsson A-C. Biodegradable polymers from renewable sources. new hemicellulose-based hydrogels. Macromol Rapid Commun 2001;22:962–7.

[80] Ren J-L, Peng X-W, Sun R-C, Wu H. Progress in functional materials-hydrogel based on hemicellulose. Trans China Pulp Pap 2011;26:49–53 [in Chinese].

[81] Sun X-F, Jing Z, Wang G. Preparation and swelling behaviors of porous hemicellulose-g-polyacrylamide hydrogels. J Appl Polym Sci 2013;128:1861–70.

[82] Lindblad MS, Albertsson A-C, Ranucci E. New hemicellulose-based hydrogels. In: Hemicelluloses: science and technology. ACS symposium series 2004, vol. 864. American Chemical Society; 2004. p. 347–59.

[83] Peng X, Ren J, Zhong L, Sun R, Shi W, Hu B. Glycidyl methacrylate derivatized xylan-rich hemicelluloses: synthesis and characterizations. Cellulose 2012;19:1361–72.

[84] Dax D, Chávez MS, Xu C, Willför S, Mendonça RT, Sánchez J. Cationic hemicellulose-based hydrogels for arsenic and chromium removal from aqueous solutions. Carbohydr Polym 2014;111:797–805.

[85] Voepel J, Edlund U, Albertsson A-C. Alkenyl-functionalized precursors for renewable hydrogels design. J Polym Sci A Polym Chem 2009;47:3595–606.

[86] Cao X, Peng X, Zhong L, Sun R. Multiresponsive hydrogels based on xylan-type hemicelluloses and photoisomerized azobenzene copolymer as drug delivery carrier. J Agric Food Chem 2014;62:10000–7.

[87] Liu S, Chen F, Song X, Wu H. Preparation and characterization of temperature- and pH-sensitive hemicellulose-containing hydrogels. Int J Polym Anal Charact 2017;22:187–201.

[88] Dax D, Bastidas MSC, Honorato C, Liu J, Spoljaric S, Seppälä J, Mendonça RT, Xu C, Willför S, Sánchez J. Tailor-made hemicellulose-based hydrogels reinforced with nanofibrillated cellulose for the removal of chromium ions from aqueous solutions. Nord Pulp Pap Res J 2015;30:369–72.

[89] Zhao W, Glavas L, Odelius K, Edlund U, Albertsson A-C. A robust pathway to electrically conductive hemicellulose hydrogels with high and controllable swelling behavior. Polymer 2014;55:2967–76.

[90] Zhao W, Glavas L, Odelius K, Edlund U, Albertsson A-C. Facile and green approach towards electrically conductive hemicellulose hydrogels with tunable conductivity and swelling behavior. Chem Mater 2014;26:4265–73.

[91] Matyjaszewski K, Xia J. Atom transfer radical polymerization. Chem Rev 2001;101:2921–90.

[92] Vivek AV, Dhamodharan R. Amphiphilic polystyrene-graft-poly(N,N-dimethylamino-2-ethyl methacrylate) hydrogels synthesized via room temperature ATRP: studies on swelling behaviour and dye sorption. React Funct Polym 2008;68:967–73.

[93] Yoon JA, Kowalewski T, Matyjaszewski K. Comparison of thermoresponsive deswelling kinetics of poly(oligo(ethylene oxide) methacrylate)-based thermoresponsive hydrogels prepared by "graft-from" ATRP. Macromolecules 2011;44:2261–8.

[94] Kolb HC, Finn MG, Sharpless KB. Click chemistry: diverse chemical function from a few good reactions. Angew Chem Int Ed 2001;40:2004–21.

[95] Mamidyala SK, Finn MG. In situ click chemistry: probing the binding landscapes of biological molecules. Chem Soc Rev 2010;39:1252–61.

[96] Binder WH, Sachsenhofer R. 'Click' chemistry in polymer and materials science. Macromol Rapid Commun 2007;38:15–54.

[97] Gerstel P, Klumpp S, Hennrich F, Altintas O, Eaton TR, Mayor M, Barner-Kowollik C, Kappes MM. Selective dispersion of single-walled carbon nanotubes via easily accessible conjugated click polymers. Polym Chem 2012;3:1966–70.

[98] Lutz J-F. 1,3-Dipolar cycloadditions of azides and alkynes: a universal ligation tool in polymer and materials science. Angew Chem Int Ed 2007;46:1018–25.

[99] Nielsen TT, Wintgens V, Amiel C, Wimmer R, Larsen KL. Facile synthesis of β-cyclodextrin-dextran polymers by "click" chemistry. Biomacromolecules 2010;11:1710–5.

[100] Oshima K, Fujimoto T, Minami E, Mitsukami Y. Model polyelectrolyte gels synthesized by end-linking of tetra-arm polymers with click chemistry: synthesis and mechanical properties. Macromolecules 2014;47:7573–80.

[101] Park JS, Kim YH, Song M, Kim C-H, Karim MA, Lee JW, Gal Y-S, Kumar P, Kang S-W, Jin S-H. Synthesis and photovoltaic properties of side-chain liquid-crystal click polymers for dye-sensitized solar-cells application. Macromol Chem Phys 2010;211:2464–73.

[102] Rostovtsev VV, Green LG, Fokin VV, Sharpless KB. A stepwise huisgen cycloaddition process: copper(I)-catalyzed regioselective "ligation" of azides and terminal alkynes. Angew Chem Int Ed 2002;41:2596–9.

[103] Koschella A, Hartlieb M, Heinze T. A "click-chemistry" approach to cellulose-based hydrogels. Carbohydr Polym 2011;86:154–61.

[104] Meng X, Edgar KJ. "Click" reactions in polysaccharide modification. Prog Polym Sci 2016;53:52–85.

[105] Tirino P, Laurino R, Maglio G, Malinconico M, d'Ayala GG, Laurienzo P. Synthesis of chitosan–PEO hydrogels via mesylation and regioselective Cu(I)-catalyzed cycloaddition. Carbohydr Polym 2014;112:736–45.

[106] Zhang J, Xu X-D, Wu D-Q, Zhang X-Z, Zhuo R-X. Synthesis of thermosensitive P(NIPAAm-co-HEMA)/cellulose hydrogels via "click" chemistry. Carbohydr Polym 2009;77:583–9.

[107] Enomoto-Rogers Y, Iwata T. Synthesis of xylan-graft-poly(l-lactide) copolymers via click chemistry and their thermal properties. Carbohydr Polym 2012;87:1933–40.

[108] Hoyle CE, Bowman CN. Thiol–ene click chemistry. Angew Chem Int Ed 2010;49:1540–73.

[109] Xu Y. Thiol-ene click chemistry. Prog Chem 2012;24:385–94.

[110] Pahimanolis N, Kilpeläinen P, Master E, Ilvesniemi H, Seppälä J. Novel thiol- amine- and amino acid functional xylan derivatives synthesized by thiol–ene reaction. Carbohydr Polym 2015;131:392–8.

[111] Hachet E, Sereni N, Pignot-Paintrand I, Ravaine V, Szarpak-Jankowska A, Auzély-Velty R. Thiol-ene clickable hyaluronans: from macro-to nanogels. J Colloid Interface Sci 2014;419:52–5.

[112] Li M, Tang Z, Wang C, Zhang Y, Cui H, Chen X. Efficient side-chain modification of dextran via base-catalyzed epoxide ring-opening and thiol-ene click chemistry in aqueous media. Chin J Polym Sci 2014;32:969–74.

[113] Rosilo H, Kontturi E, Seitsonen J, Kolehmainen E, Ikkala O. Transition to reinforced state by percolating domains of intercalated brush-modified cellulose nanocrystals and poly(butadiene) in cross-linked composites based on thiol–ene click chemistry. Biomacromolecules 2013;14:1547–54.

[114] Tingaut P, Hauert R, Zimmermann T. Highly efficient and straightforward functionalization of cellulose films with thiol-ene click chemistry. J Mater Chem 2011;21:16066–76.

[115] Wallenius J, Pahimanolis N, Zoppe J, Kilpeläinen P, Master E, Ilvesniemi H, Seppälä J, Eerikäinen T, Ojamo H. Continuous propionic acid production with Propionibacterium acidipropionici immobilized in a novel xylan hydrogel matrix. Bioresour Technol 2015;197:1–6.

[116] Shu XZ, Liu Y, Luo Y, Roberts MC, Prestwich GD. Disulfide cross-linked hyaluronan hydrogels. Biomacromolecules 2002;3:1304–11.

[117] Lee F, Chung JE, Kurisawa M. An injectable enzymatically crosslinked hyaluronic acid-tyramine hydrogel system with independent tuning of mechanical strength and gelation rate. Soft Matter 2008;4:880–7.

[118] Chimphango AFA, van Zyl WH, Görgens JF. In situ enzymatic aided formation of xylan hydrogels and encapsulation of horse radish peroxidase for slow release. Carbohydr Polym 2012;88:1109–17.

[119] Kobayashi S, Uyama H, Kimura S. Enzymatic polymerization. Chem Rev 2001;101:3793–818.

[120] Sakai S, Hirose K, Taguchi K, Ogushi Y, Kawakami K. An injectable, in situ enzymatically gellable, gelatin derivative for drug delivery and tissue engineering. Biomaterials 2009;30:3371–7.

[121] Hu L, Hecht DS, Grüner G. Carbon nanotube thin films: fabrication, properties, and applications. Chem Rev 2010;110:5790–844.

[122] Sun X-F, Liu BC, Jing ZX, Wang HH. Preparation and adsorption property of xylan/poly(acrylic acid) magnetic nanocomposite hydrogel adsorbent. Carbohydr Polym 2015;118:16–23.

[123] Sun RC, Sun XF, Tomkinson J. Hemicelluloses and their derivatives. ACS Symp Ser 2004;864:2–22.

[124] Edlund U, Albertsson AC. A microspheric system: hemicellulose-based hydrogels. J Bioact Compat Polym 2008;23:171–86.

[125] Sun X-F, Wang H, Jing Z, Mohanathas R. Hemicellulose-based pH-sensitive and biodegradable hydrogel for controlled drug delivery. Carbohydr Polym 2013;92:1357–66.

[126] Gao C, Ren J, Kong W, Sun R, Chen Q. Comparative study on temperature/pH sensitive xylan-based hydrogels: their properties and drug controlled release. RSC Adv 2015;5:90671–81.

[127] Kong W-Q, Gao C-D, Hu S-F, Ren J-L, Zhao L-H, Sun R-C. Xylan-modified-based hydrogels with temperature/pH dual sensitivity and controllable drug delivery behavior. Materials 2017;10:304. https://doi.org/10.3390/ma10030304.

[128] Gami P, Kundu D, Seera SDK, Banerjee T. Chemically crosslinked xylan–β-Cyclodextrin hydrogel for the in vitro delivery of curcumin and 5-fluorouracil. Int J Biol Macromol 2020;158:18–31.

[129] Chang M, Liu X, Meng L, Wang X, Ren J. Xylan-based hydrogels as a potential carrier for drug delivery: effect of pore-forming agents. Pharmaceutics 2018;10:261. https://doi.org/10.3390/pharmaceutics10040261.

[130] Kundu D, Banerjee T. Carboxymethyl cellulose–xylan hydrogel: synthesis, characterization, and in vitro release of vitamin B12. ACS Omega 2019;4:4793–803.

[131] Ma J, Sun XF, Yao XY, Zeng QH. Hemicellulose-based magnetic hydrogel for enzyme drug immobilisation. J Invest Med 2017;65:A2.

[132] Melandri D, Angelis AD, Orioli R, Ponzielli G, Lualdi P, Giarratana N, Reiner V. Use of a new hemicellulose dressing (Veloderm1) for the treatment of split-thickness skin graft donor sites: a within-patient controlled study. Burns 2006;32:964–72.

[133] Ferreira LM, Blanes L, Gragnani A, Veiga DF, Veiga FP, Nery GB, Rocha GHHR, Gomes HC, Rocha MG, Okamoto R. Hemicellulose dressing versus rayon dressing in the re-epithelialization of split-thickness skin graft donor sites: a multicenter study. J Tissue Viability 2009;18:88–94.

[134] Venugopal J, Rajeswari R, Shayanti M, Sridhar R, Sundarrajan S, Balamurugan R, Ramakrishna S. Xylan polysaccharides fabricated into nanofibrous substrate for myocardial infarction. Mater Sci Eng C 2013;33:1325–31.

[135] Burgalassi S, Raimondi L, Pirisino R, Saettone MF. Effect of xyfoglucan (tamarind seed polysaccharide) on conjunctival cell adhesion to laminin and on corneal epithelium wound healing. Eur J Ophthalmol 2000;10:71–6.

[136] Shirakawa M, Yamotoya K, Nishinari K. Tailoring of xyloglucan properties using an enzyme. Food Hydrocoll 1998;12:25–8.

[137] Nisbet DR, Moses D, Forsythe JS, Finkelestain DI, Horne MK. Enhancing neurite outgrowth from primary neurones and neural stem cells using thermoresponsive hydrogel scaffolds for the repair of spinal cord injury. J Biomed Mater Res 2009;89A:24–35.

[138] Silva TCF, Habibi Y, Colodette JL, Lucia LA. The influence of the chemical and structural features of xylan on the physical properties of its derived hydrogels. Soft Matter 2010;7:1090–9.

[139] Liu J, Chinga-Carrasco G, Cheng F, Xu W, Willfor S, Syverud K, Xu C. Hemicellulose-reinforced nanocellulose hydrogels for wound healing application. Cellulose 2016;23:3129–43.

[140] Karaaslan MA, Tshabalala MA, Yelle DJ, Buschle-Diller G. Nanoreinforced biocompatible hydrogels from wood hemicelluloses and cellulose whiskers. Carbohydr Polym 2011;86:192–201.

[141] Qi X-M, Chen G-G, Gong X-D, Fu G-Q, Niu Y-S, Bian J, Peng F, Sun R-C. Enhanced mechanical performance of biocompatible hemicelluloses based hydrogel via chain extension. Sci Rep 2016;6:33603. https://doi.org/10.1038/srep33603.

[142] Al-Rudainy B, Galbe M, Hernandez MA, Jannasch P, Wallberg O. Impact of lignin content on the properties of hemicellulose hydrogels. Polymers 2019;11:35. https://doi.org/10.3390/polym11010035.

[143] Song X, Chen F, Liu S. A lignin-containing hemicellulose-based hydrogel and its adsorption behavior. BioResources 2016;11:6378–92.

[144] Ren J, Dai Q, Zhong H, Liu X, Meng L, Wang X, Xin F. Quaternized xylan/cellulose nanocrystal reinforced magnetic hydrogels with high strength. Cellulose 2018;25:4537–49.

[145] Lindblad MS, Albertsson A-C, Ranucci E, Laus M, Giani E. Biodegradable polymers from renewable sources: rheological characterization of hemicellulose-based hydrogels. Biomacromolecules 2005;6:684–90.

[146] Zhong L, Peng X, Song L, Yang D, Cao X, Sun R. Adsorption of Cu2+ and Ni2+ from aqueous solution by arabinoxylan hydrogel: equilibrium, kinetic, competitive adsorption. Sep Sci Technol 2013;48:2659–69.

[147] Lian Y, Zhang J, Li N, Ping Q. Preparation of hemicellulose-based hydrogel and its application as an adsorbent towards heavy metal ions. BioResources 2018;13:3208–18.

[148] Liu X, Chang M, He B, Meng L, Wang X, Sun R, Ren J, Kong F. A one-pot strategy for preparation of high-strength carboxymethyl xylan-g-poly(acrylic acid) hydrogels with shape memory property. J Colloid Interface Sci 2019;538:507–18.

[149] Liu X, Song T, Chang M, Meng L, Wang X, Sun R, Ren J. Carbon nanotubes reinforced maleic anhydride-modified xylan-g-poly(N-isofigpropylacrylamide) hydrogel with multifunctional properties. Materials 2018;11:354. https://doi.org/10.3390/ma11030354.

Locust bean gum-derived hydrogels

Vipul D. Prajapati[a], Pankaj M. Maheriya[b], and Salona D. Roy[a]

[a]Department of Pharmaceutics, SSR College of Pharmacy, Saily, Silvassa, Union Territory of Dadra Nagar Haveli and Daman Diu, India, [b]Department of Formulation & Development, Ajanta Research Centre, Mumbai, India

7.1 Introduction

Hydrogels are hydrophilic, three-dimensional (3D), polymeric, macromolecular-swelled networks. They are proficient to retain a large volume of water depending on the polymer's type of inherent physicochemical characteristics [1]. The hydrophilic groups (such as $-OH$, $-CONH$, $-CONH_2$, and $-SO_3H$) present in the polymers enable the absorption of a large volume of water, while their cross-linked grid structure delays their dissolution due to either covalent bonding, hydrogen bonding, and/or Van der Waals interactions along with physical entanglements, known as crystallites [2, 3]. Hydrogels can be derived both from natural polymers (natural or biohydrogels) and synthetic polymers (synthetic hydrogels).

Naturally derived hydrogels are advantageous due to their biocompatibility, biodegradability, nontoxic, economic source, and flexible properties for diversified use compared with synthetic polymer-based hydrogels. Diversities of natural biodegradable polysaccharides such as alginates, agar, chitosan, dextran, gellan gum, guar gum, hyaluronic acid, karaya gum, locust bean gum, pectin, psyllium, sterculia gum, tamarind seed gum, tragacanth, xanthan gum, etc., and proteins such as silk fibroin, fibroin from spider webs, fibrin from blood clots, gelatin, collagen from skin, keratin from wool/hair, bone, tendons, elastin from elastic tissues, and resilient from insect tendons, etc. have been reported for their versatile use in the preparation of hydrogels-derived formulations for various applications. Among these naturally originated polysaccharides or proteins, the hydrogels made from the natural gums have been considered more useful in terms of biodegradability, biocompatibility, material cost, ease of production, and wide array of applications in different fields [4–7].

Gums originated from varied natural sources such as plants, animals, microbials, and marine forms have been utilized for the formulation of different types of hydrogels for suitable applications in various fields. Many field reports, review, and research articles on naturally derived gums-based hydrogels including their commercial applications in areas like food, pharmaceuticals, biomedicals, cosmetics, etc. are available. To get the desired hydrogel-derived drug delivery systems of molecules, the inherent properties of these naturally derived gums have been modified either physically or chemically using suitable cross-linkers with or without the addition of other compatible polymers for improvement of their mechanical gel strength and delaying release pattern of entrapped molecules for the need of its desired scientific requirements.

Among them, locust (carob) bean gum (LBG), a plant originated nonionic seed (kernel) gum, has been utilized as a therapeutic agent or carrier in hydrogel-derived drug delivery systems for the last decade. It has been commonly used as a stabilizer and thickener in dairy products and also replaced the fat in many milk products due to its property to form viscous suspensions at a low proportion and maintain the stability of suspensions/emulsions [8–10].

Based on thorough reference of reported literature on LBG for various purposes, this chapter is prepared to describe LBG's profile in detail following its hydrogel-derived formulations for versatile applications in several fields either in its native form or in combination with many compatible polymers [11] to improve the functionality of the end product to make it attentive for extension of its research work in various fields.

7.1.1 Historical perspective of locust bean gum and its derived hydrogel formulations

LBG is known by many names in different countries for years. The most common names are Carob and Locust bean, while other regional names include Johannis brotbaum (Germany), Alfarrobeira (Portugal), Garrofer, and Garrover (Catalonia). It earlier originated in the Middle East where it grew in dry areas with poor soil quality and lesser in quantity; the ancient Greeks cultivated the tree from its native lands to the Mediterranean basin from where Arabs took this tree to cultivate into Spain and Portugal along with the North Africa coast. It was then introduced in the U.S. and patented by the Patent Office in 1854 [12,13].

LBG has been utilized in food since 1854 and in pharmaceutical formulations due to its interaction with water via hydrogen bonding; its combination with various compatible polymers for desired functions has been used in various fields since 1990. After 1991 to date, its use in various fields has been increased due to its flexible properties. The historical growth of LBG as well as its derived hydrogel formulations for various purposes in different fields [13–33] is shown in Fig. 7.1.

7.2 Sources, structure, and properties of LBG with special emphasis on hydrogel formation

7.2.1 Sources of locust bean gum

LBG (Chemical Abstract Serial Number 9000-40-2), a plant-based non-ionic neutral galactomannan gum, is obtained from the seed's endosperm of *Ceratonia siliqua* L. of Leguminosae/Fabaceae family [34]. The parts of the carob tree, foliage, flower, fruit, wood, bark, and roots have been utilized for its pharmacological and nonpharmacological characteristics since ancient times [13]. It is a leguminous tree (an endemic tree in Algeria) indigenous to Spain having chromosome number of $2n = 24$ [35]. Reported common traditional names of LBG are *Kharoub* or *Karruba* in Arabic, *Algarrobo* or *Garrofero* in Spanish, *Alfarrobeira* in Portuguese, *Carrubo* in Italian, *Caroubier* in French, carob (in English), *Karubenbaum* in German, *Keration* or *Charaoupi* in Greek, *Keciboynuzu, Harnup (Charnup)* in Turkish [36], as well as *Taslighoua, Tikharroubt, Tikida* and *St. Johńs Bread* [12,13]. It is the widely used industrial crop for gelling functionality. The most prominent role of LBG is acting as a gelling agent in plant culturing or tissue engineering as it provides support to inhibit contact between the medium and the plant material.

7.2.1.1 Cultivation of locust bean gum

Ceratonia siliqua L. (Leguminosae/Fabaceae) has been considered as a Mediterranean spontaneous or cultivated tree growing to a height of 12 to 15m with a productive life span of more than 100 years. It is an evergreen tree cultivated for more than 4000 years [37] or naturally grown in the Mediterranean area such as the Maghreb countries in North-Africa including Tunisia, Algeria, and Morocco [12]. The worldwide production of carob bean pods was estimated to be approximately 300,000 to 350,000 tons/year, out of which 9000 to 10,000 tons are consumed in the food industry. The principal locust bean producing and exporting countries are Spain, Italy, Portugal, Morocco, Greece, Cyprus, Turkey, Algeria, and Tunisia [14,35,38,39]. Depending on the cultivar, region, and farming practices, the reported annual production of carob pods is 374,800 to 441,000 tons on 200,000ha with very variable yields [12]. Carob kernels are very important for the LBG industry. The United States and Cyprus have established the two gene banks of LBG. The wild carob genotype

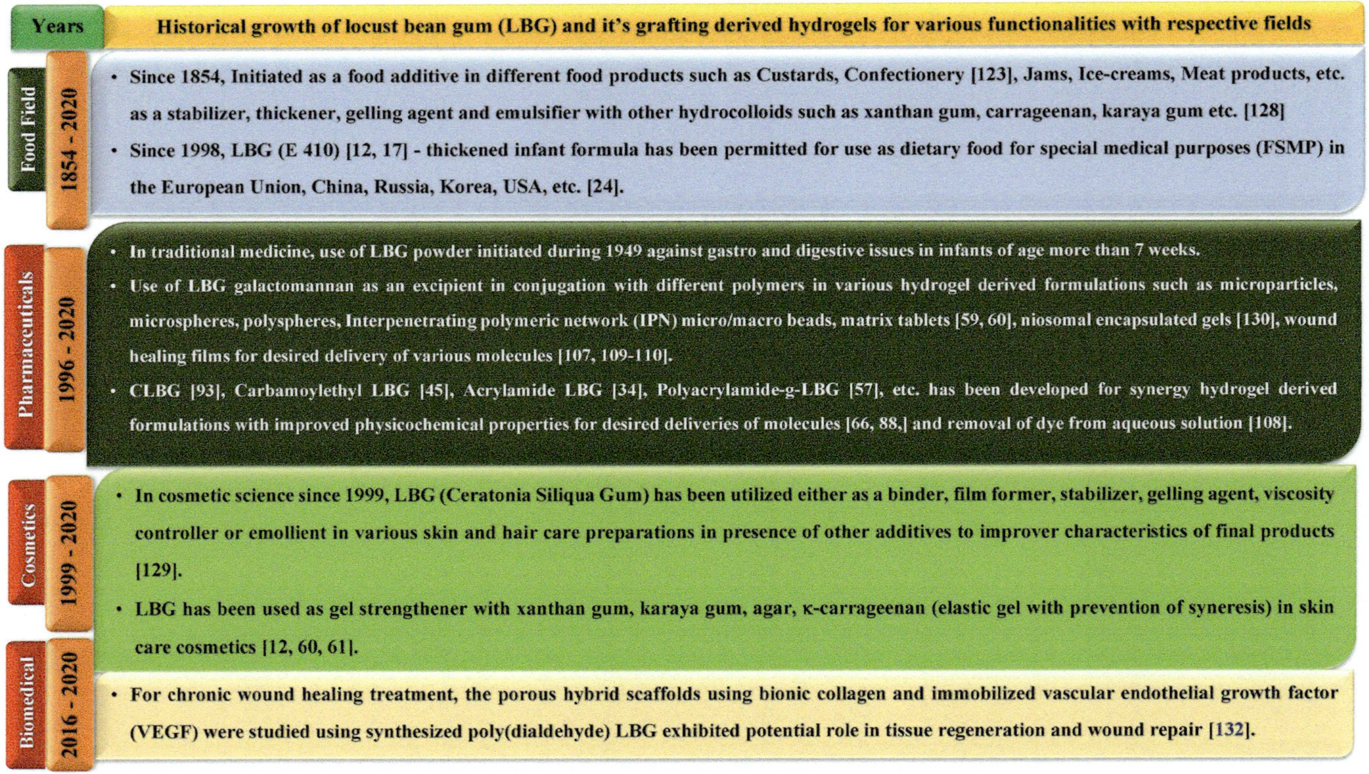

Years	Historical growth of locust bean gum (LBG) and it's grafting derived hydrogels for various functionalities with respective fields
Food Field 1854 – 2020	• Since 1854, Initiated as a food additive in different food products such as Custards, Confectionery [123], Jams, Ice-creams, Meat products, etc. as a stabilizer, thickener, gelling agent and emulsifier with other hydrocolloids such as xanthan gum, carrageenan, karaya gum etc. [128] • Since 1998, LBG (E 410) [12, 17] - thickened infant formula has been permitted for use as dietary food for special medical purposes (FSMP) in the European Union, China, Russia, Korea, USA, etc. [24].
Pharmaceuticals 1996 – 2020	• In traditional medicine, use of LBG powder initiated during 1949 against gastro and digestive issues in infants of age more than 7 weeks. • Use of LBG galactomannan as an excipient in conjugation with different polymers in various hydrogel derived formulations such as microparticles, microspheres, polyspheres, Interpenetrating polymeric network (IPN) micro/macro beads, matrix tablets [59, 60], niosomal encapsulated gels [130], wound healing films for desired delivery of various molecules [107, 109-110]. • CLBG [93], Carbamoylethyl LBG [45], Acrylamide LBG [34], Polyacrylamide-g-LBG [57], etc. has been developed for synergy hydrogel derived formulations with improved physicochemical properties for desired deliveries of molecules [66, 88,] and removal of dye from aqueous solution [108].
Cosmetics 1999 – 2020	• In cosmetic science since 1999, LBG (Ceratonia Siliqua Gum) has been utilized either as a binder, film former, stabilizer, gelling agent, viscosity controller or emollient in various skin and hair care preparations in presence of other additives to improver characteristics of final products [129]. • LBG has been used as gel strengthener with xanthan gum, karaya gum, agar, κ-carrageenan (elastic gel with prevention of syneresis) in skin care cosmetics [12, 60, 61].
Biomedical 2016 – 2020	• For chronic wound healing treatment, the porous hybrid scaffolds using bionic collagen and immobilized vascular endothelial growth factor (VEGF) were studied using synthesized poly(dialdehyde) LBG exhibited potential role in tissue regeneration and wound repair [132].

FIG. 7.1 A flowchart of the historical perspective of LBG and its derived hydrogel formulations with respect to various fields.

is mainly found in Arabia, Egypt, Jordan, Lebanon, Syria, Tunisia, and Turkey, although its localization also extends to different regions of North Africa, South America, and Asia. Three types of LBG are grown in Turkey, i.e., wild, fleshy and Sammie, which differ in their physical properties.

LBG is a fruit pod of the carob tree that can be classified into two parts: the kibble (locust bean) and the seeds (locust kernel gum) [36,40]. Approximately, 80% to 90% of the carob pod is the kibble and 10% to 20% of carob pod is seeds [40]. The seed-to-kibble ratio is increased from cultivated type to wild type [40]. The kibble part of the wild type is smaller than the cultivated type. The carob seed in the fruit pod has three main layers, namely husk, endosperm, and germ. This is available in white to cream powder form after mechanical treatment, i.e., milling of carob seed endosperm.

The sequential stagewise development of LBG in nature is shown in Fig. 7.2 with its powder form that can be processed from the seeds of the carob tree.

Depending on the area and environmental condition of cultivation of the locust tree, the locust seed contains 30% to 33% husk (seed coat), 23% to 25% germ, and 42% to 46% endosperm, and molecular weight ranges from 5×10^4 to 3×10^6 Da [41,42]. The composition of low-quality crude LBG (cLBG) and high-quality refined LBG (rLBG) exhibited the mannose-to-galactose (M/G) ratio in the range from 3.1 to 3.9 [10]. The cCBG contains significant levels of arabinose, fat, protein, and ash, more so than

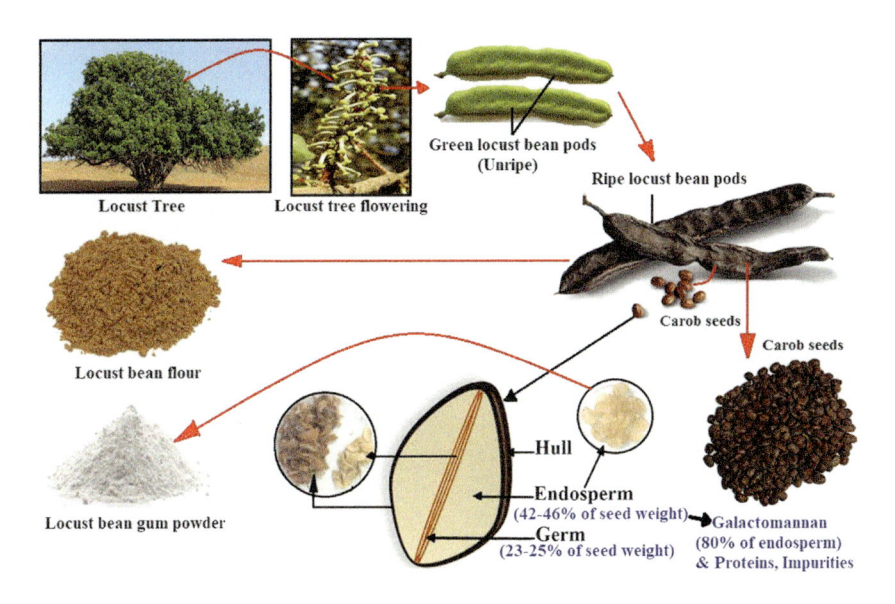

FIG. 7.2 An image showing the development stages of locust bean from the flowering to the final powder.

those of rCBG, by which functional and gelling properties were affected and quality of gum was compromised. Due to nongalactomannan content, thermal stability of gum fraction of the crude and refined sample was different [10,15,43]. Through various sequential stepwise processing from the mature carob pods, the powdered form of LBG can be obtained.

7.2.1.2 Processing

Many authors have reported isolation, extraction, and purification methodology of LBG powder from its sources that can be utilized at various scales of production [38,43–45]. The fruit carob pod has been used as feed for both human and livestock. The mature pod is 10 to 25 cm in length and is made up of about 90% pulp and 10% seeds [11]. The harvested carob pod is kibbled to separate its two main constituents, the carob seed/ kernel and the pulp. LBG powder is mainly composed of galactomannan that, when purified, constitutes the food additive (coded E410 in the European Union) used frequently in food, pharmaceutical, cosmetic, paper, petroleum, paint, and textile industries as a viscosifier, thickening, gelling, binding, and stabilizing agent in products such as juices, dietetic beverages, desserts, and baby and pet foods [12,13,34,46,47], while the pulp of the carob pod is used as an animal food, human food, and in the manufacturing of sugars and alcohols at an industrial scale. The extremely hard carob seed comprises of about 10% to 20% of the carob fruit pod, and carob endosperm contains 30% to 40% by weight of galactomannan with mannose and galactose sugar units. LBG powder is mostly extracted from the endosperm seeds, which is responsible for energy reservation and hydration. The endosperm has special properties like high molecular mass, water solubility, and nonionic neutral characteristics that direct their potential use as films/coating, a gelling agent, a part of a mixed matrix system with retention of a large quantity of water-known as hydrogel, an emulsion stabilizer, and a thickener.

The carob seeds are processed sequentially to obtain the endosperm, i.e., the outer layers such as the husk and germ layers. Due to the hardness of the carob seed coat, their endosperms are quite difficult to separate from the seeds by normal process. Hence, using various steps of an isolation process, the carob seeds kernels are peeled (dehusked) leaving behind the endosperm and germ layer (embryos) [43–45,48]. The peeling process involves two major methods: acid peeling or thermal peeling. The proper treatment can be achieved by washing and brushing the endosperm separated at the end of the acid peeling process. The acid peeling involves the treatment of kernels/seed coat with dilute sulfuric acid at a specific temperature, i.e., carbonized to obtain the endosperm or roasting the kernels to break the layer of seeds. Roasting can be carried out between 150°C to 200°C for 30, 60, and 90 min in a hot air oven. The roasted kernels are then further processed. The obtained crude material is in the form of a dry powder/flour. The dry powder is then further processed to obtain the clarified gum using the precipitation reactions (Fig. 7.3). Here, the gum is first dissolved into a suitable solvent (water) under the application of heat and then made to precipitate using another solvent (ethanol or isopropanol) and then filtered, evaporated, and dried.

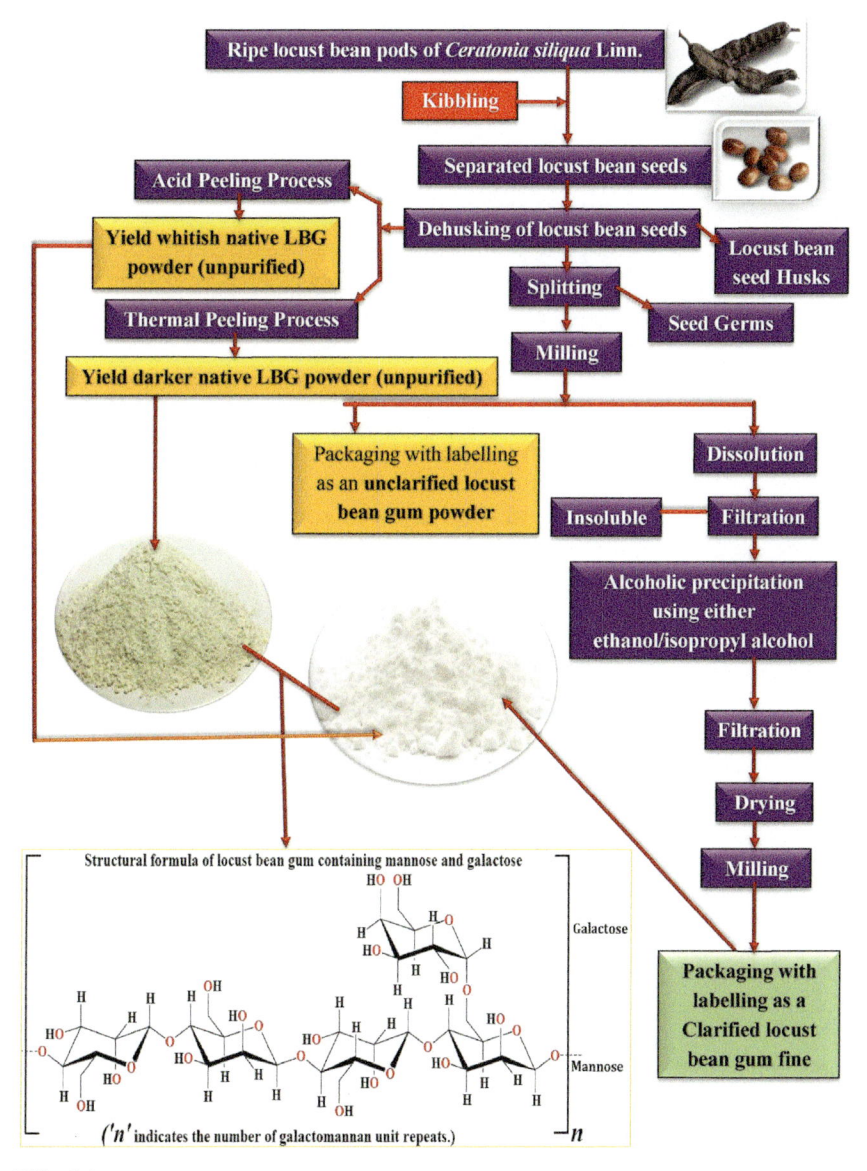

FIG. 7.3 The outlook sequential steps of extraction and processing of the ripe locust bean pods with unit operations to get powdered locust bean gum.

The thermal peeling process involves the roasting of kernels at very high temperature in a rotating furnace to separate the seed coat from the endosperm. The extract obtained by this process is darker than the extract obtained by the acid peeling process because sulfuric acid isn't involved. The peeled material is then dried followed by hull cracking resulting in kernels that are easily cracked and crushed. The endosperm is milled and sieved to get the fine powder of LBG. The next process involves clarification in which various steps are involved from precipitation to clarified LBG powder. Hence it is followed by precipitation, filtration, drying, milling, and packaging. [46]. The whitest colored and highest gel strength is obtained from Portuguese LBG with a gradual deterioration in properties. Acid peeling process yields white to off-white LBG powder from the carob seeds, while that of a darker color is yielded through the thermal peeling process [38,43,47,49]. The stepwise extraction and complete processing that can be carried out for isolation and purification of LBG powder in the laboratory as well as in an industrial scale with needful conditions are summarized in Fig. 7.3.

7.2.1.3 Phytochemical constituents

The seeds of a locust bean tree are approximately 10 mm in size [50] composing the major portion of carbohydrates; polyphenolic compounds such as tannins, fibers, and minerals; and a lesser number of proteins and lipids. The presence of tannins, especially hydrolyzable tannins and glycosides due to polyphenolic compounds, have also been reported in many articles and literature reviews. Added derivatives of polyphenolic compounds have also been found such as kaempferol, tannic acid, catechin hydrate, and polydation in varied percentages. The immature LBG contains a higher amount of pyrogallol, catechin, tannic acid, chlorogenic acid, epicatechin, gallic acid, epicatechin gallate, epigallocatechin, epigallocatechin allotted, myrectin, and quercetin [51,52]. It also contains cellulose and hemicellulose in varied quantities. Carob trees grown in different environments produce variations in constituents as found through analytical methods [43]. Some important compositional elements of green and mature dried carob pods are summarized in Fig. 7.4, while that of carob flour, seeds, germ flour, and leaves are in Fig. 7.5.

7.2.1.4 Purity of locust bean gum

The fine LBG powder obtained after clarification has been analyzed for its purity through purity parameters such as loss on drying (LOD), and contents of total ash, acid insoluble matter, protein, starch, ethanol and isopropanol, lead, and microbiological criteria as mentioned in an official pharmacopeia:

- Not more than 14% LOD at 105°C for 5 h.
- Total ash should not be more than 1.2% at 800°C for 3–4 h.

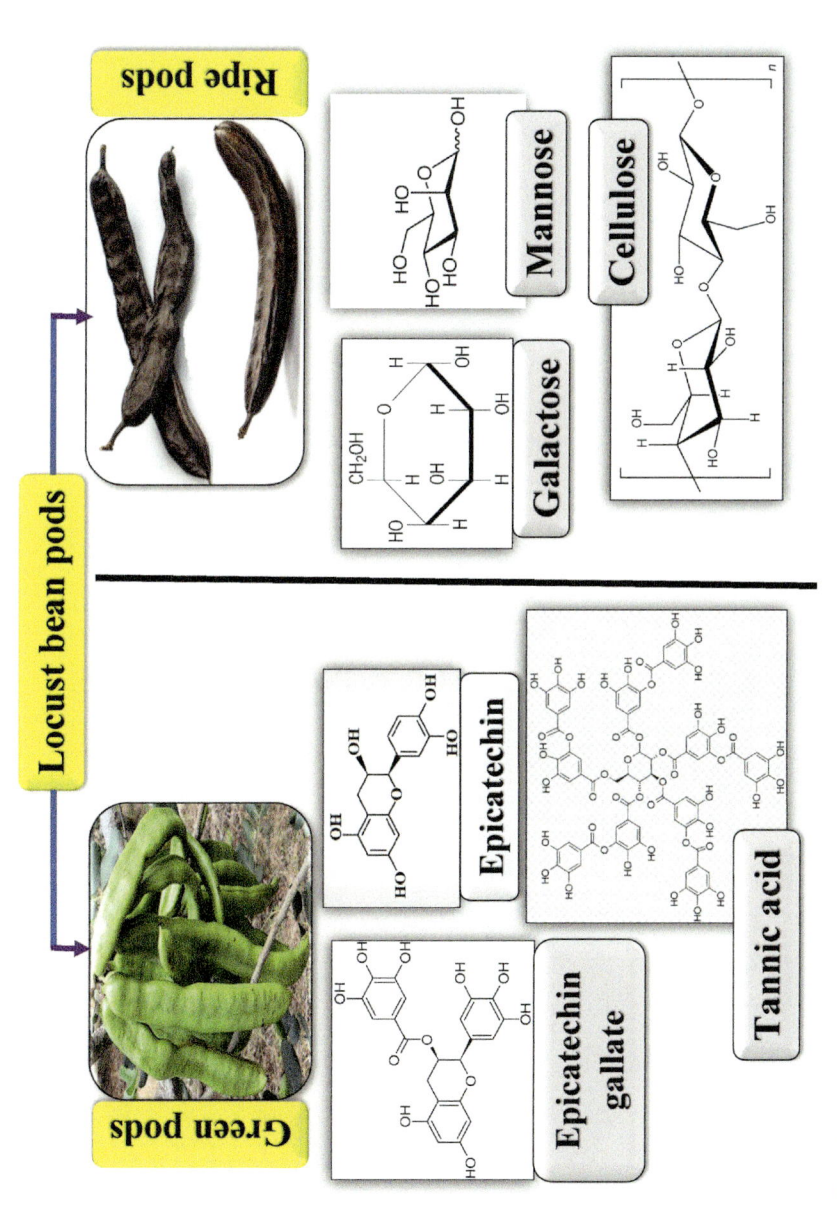

FIG. 7.4 An image showing a few compositional elements of green and dried carob pods [43,51–53].

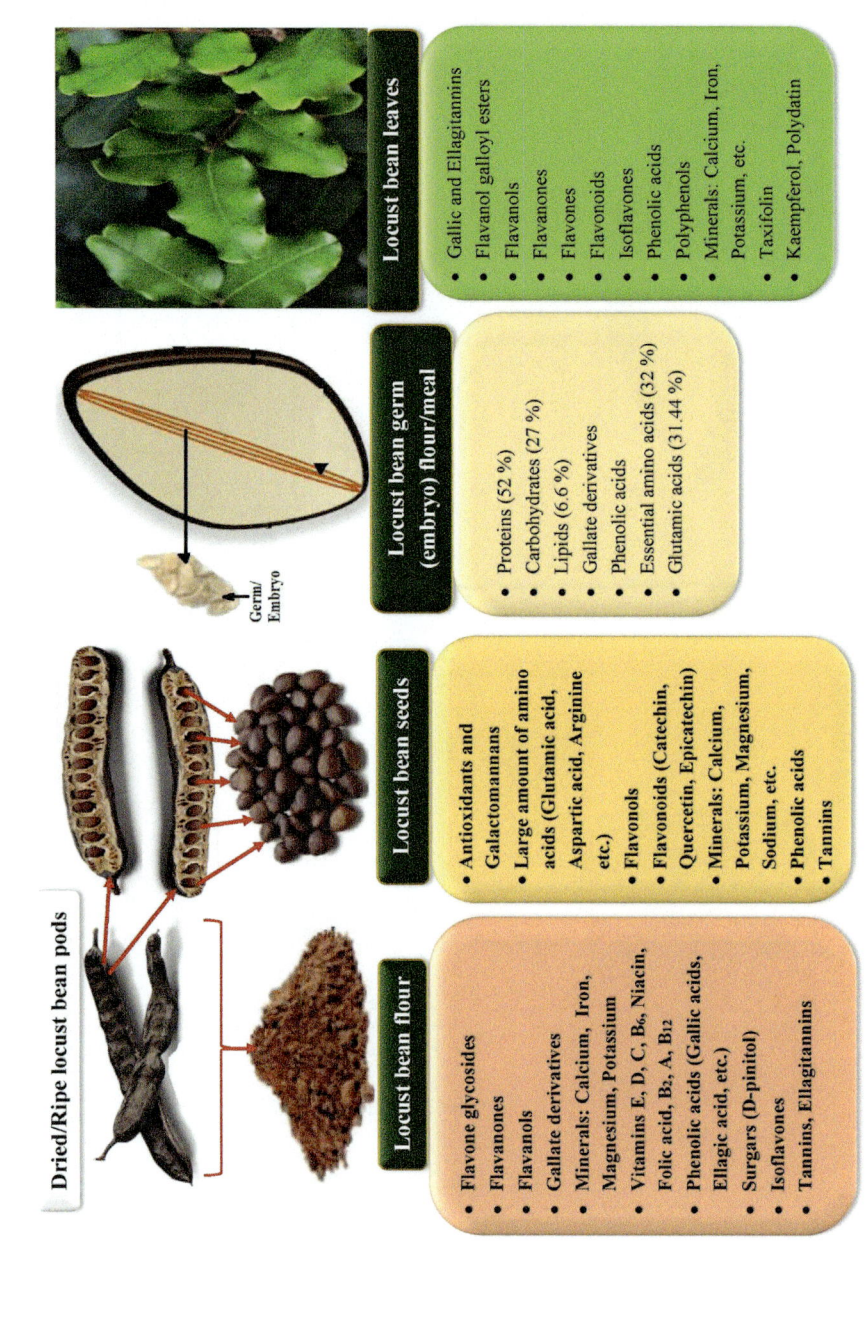

FIG. 7.5 An illustration showing a few compositional elements of carob flour, seeds, germ flour, and leaves [50–53].

- Acid insolubility should not be not more than 40%.
- Protein content should not be more than 7.0% by Kjeldahl method.
- Starch should not be present.
- Ethanol and isopropanol content should not be more than 1%.
- Lead content should not be more than 2 mg/kg.
- Total plate count should not be more than 5000 CFU/g.

Commercial grade of LBG contains moisture (5%–12%), acid-soluble ash (1.7%–5%), ash (0.4%–1.0%), and mixed proteins (3%-7%), while clarified LBG contains moisture (3%–10%), acid-soluble matter (0.1%–3%), ash (0.1%–1%), and mixed proteins (0.1%–0.7%). The possible impurities identified in processing parts of LBG are as in husk (acid-insoluble-matter), germ layer (protein), extracting solvent (< 1% either alone or in combination), or any microbiological contaminations and metallic impurities (lead, 0.040 mg/kg; aluminum, 0.24 mg/kg; arsenic, 1.00 mg/kg; cadmium and mercury, 0.005 mg/kg) [40,46–48,50].

7.2.2 Structure and properties of locust bean gum and its derived hydrogel

LBG is a branched heteroglycan consisting of a (1,4)-linked β-D-mannopyranose skeleton having axial points from the 6-positions linked to α-D-galactose (1,6-linked to α-D-galactopyranose) consisting of galactose and mannose units (Fig. 7.3), combined through glycosidic linkage in a ratio of 1:4, chemically known as a galactomannan [14–16,37–39, 41–46,48,49,54,55]. The mannose elements from a linear chain linked to the branched galactopyranosyl residues at varying distances of a parent chain are a function of the plant origin [56]. The mannose units are randomly dispersed throughout its backbone in multiple units in a row that can allow for self-association, while the galactose units prevent strong chain interactions [57]. M/G ratio differs due to varying origins of LBG and growth conditions of the carob tree during production. The physicochemical characteristics of LBG are strongly influenced by D-galactose contents and its distribution on the main chain. Longer galactose side chains produce stronger synergistic interaction with many compatible polymers [58] like xanthan gum (XG), karaya gum (KG), κ-carrageenan (kC), etc. with improved functionality of the yield. It has a nonstatistically random distribution of D-galactose. It has the lowest galactose content of about 20% [59]. LBG is a straight backbone chain of D-mannopyranosyl residues bonded through β-(1 → 4) linkages with side branching units of D-galactopyranosyl residues linked by α-(1 → 6) linkages [43,60,61]. The distribution of galactopyranosyl (G) residues on mannopyranosyl (M) backbone can be random, regular, or blockwise in a ratio 7:2 (M/G) [15,17,20,43,62,63]. To modify LBG for desired hydrogel composite formulation, the hydroxy (-OH) group present in its mannose and galactose units can be replaced with a variety of functional groups [61,63]. Due to its insolubility in cold water and formation of highly viscous solutions in hot or lukewarm water, it has been chemically modified by carboxymethylation [60,61,63], sulfation [64,65], and carboxylation [24,63,66]. Carbamoylethylation involves addition of an amide group ($-CH_2-CH_2-CONH_2$) at the 6th position of galactose/glucose/mannose units present in gums by replacing their $-OH$ moieties [5,10,17,61]. It significantly decreases the viscosity of polymer, enhances its solubility, and has a positive influence on oxygen-neutralizing capacity and adhesive strength of polymer [63,67].

LBG in water exists as a random coil [68]. Due to presence of numerous -OH groups, LBG exhibits a significant capacity to form harmonious interaction with other polysaccharides revealing an enhancement of flexibility in the production of a gelling structure for important biopharmaceutical applications [13,41,48]. The molecular size, M/G ratio, and galactose distribution in the mannose backbone chain influences the solubility and also controls the rheological properties of LBG [43]. LBG has high molecular weight, approximately 2000–3000 kDa. The properties of LBG depend upon its interaction in an aqueous medium.

7.2.2.1 Physicochemical properties of locust bean gum

LBG, the high molecular weight branched polysaccharide, occurs as a white to yellow-white powder, odorless and tasteless, but it acquires a leguminous taste when boiled in water [69]. It is reported as a biocompatible, bioabsorbable, biodegradable, nonteratogenic, nonmutagenic, mucoadhesive, and nonionic organic galactomannan whose degradation products are excreted readily [34,66,70]. It is classified by the Food and Drug Administration as a Generally Recognized as Safe (GRAS) material [17,43,62,63,66].

Solubility

The mannose chains are relatively hydrophobic, and the galactose units are more hydrophilic. LBG has a M/G ratio of approximately 4:1 representing limited water solubility and propensity to form aggregates in cold water. In general, a gum with higher percentage of galactose has good cold water dispersibility and higher viscosity but poor gelling properties [12]. Its solubility can be increased by increasing the temperature, depending on its strength and molecular weight. A report showed 70% to 85% solubilization of LBG upon 30 min stirring at 80°C [44]. The difference of stabilization as a function of temperature has been due to high molecular weight galactomannan with low galactose substitution [12]. It is partially soluble in cold water, hence heating is required to reach its maximum solubility in water, but very high temperature may degrade its polymeric structures resulting in depolymerization. Hence, a suitable temperature range is required to obtain either its high aqueous solubility or gel characteristic. For complete solubilization of LBG in water, it requires heating above 85°C for 10 min. It can dissolve in water at a temperature range of 80°C to 85°C $\pm$ 0.5°C to form a viscous solution with a pH range of 5.4 to 7.0, and the solution can further form gel by adding the small amount of either sodium borate or sodium tetraborate at pH 7.5 or higher [71,72]. The maximum solubility achieved by LBG is about 90% due to the internal factors such as particle size, particle number, impurity, etc. [43]. LBG has the capacity to form very viscous solutions at relatively low concentrations. Due to its nonionic nature, its aqueous solubility is unaffected by pH, salts, adsorption on solid surface, or ionic strength of the liquid medium [48,73]. The molecular size and structure of LBG decides the viscosity and solubility property [48]. The pH requirement is 4 to 7 and shows good acid stability. Its viscosity and solubility are little affected by pH changes within a range of 3 to 11. To improve the solubility of LBG, it has been synthesized as a sulfate, carboxylate, and aminate derivatives for utilization in desired drug delivery by polyelectrolyte complexation with other polymers [13,74]. This gum is also soluble in a LiCl-DMSO solution. It is insoluble in most organic solvents including ethanol.

Gel formation

The gelation mechanism mainly depends on the gelling agents, nature, and synergistic effects of different constituents. Under normal conditions, LBG does not form a gel [43,75]. The C-6 atoms of the monomer chain molecules potentially react with acids or base [76,77]. LBG is flexible to modify its structure for desired viscoelasticity and gel strength in the final hydrogel-derived formulation using cross-linkers such as carboxylic group of citric acid in the presence of HCl and UV-irradiation [78] and amide group of acrylamides in the case of acrylamide-grafted LBG [77]. Some studies have been reported on irradiation-induced acrylamide/citric acid LBG-derived hydrogel formulations for desired drug delivery due to a change of swelling behavior and diffusion path for release [18,77–81]. A metal ion Ca^{2+} from $CaCl_2$ has been utilized as a cross-linker for modified release interpenetrating polymeric network (IPN) microbeads of capecitabin using LBG and sodium alginate (NaAlg) [80], and gastroretentive LBG-derived IPN hydrogel beads with NaAlg [82]. Fig. 7.6 shows a schematic diagram of cross-linking of LBG for hydrogel-derived formulations as a drug delivery carrier.

LBG forms a weak gel by freeze-thaw treatment [73,83] but also forms a proper gel with the addition of a large amount of sucrose and lesser amount of water. The gel strength can be determined by the moisture content present in LBG along with the proportion of sugar. Increasing the quantity of water leads to breakage of polymeric long chains by the hydrolytic action of water hence the decreased gel strength from decreasing

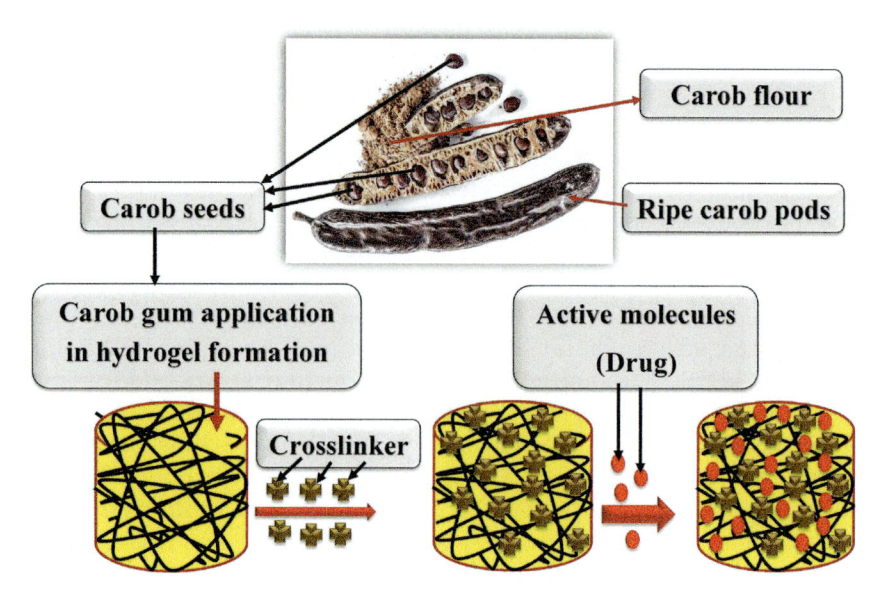

FIG. 7.6   A schematic diagram showing cross-linking of locust bean gum with cross-linker as a carrier in hydrogel derived formulation for drug deliveries.

binding strength. Maximum gel strength can be obtained by adding 45% (by weight) fructose, 50% (by weight) sucrose or sorbitol, and 55% (by weight) glucose but increased in the same order: fructose < sucrose ≈ sorbitol < glucose [43,73,75].

LBG, due to numerous hydroxyl groups, exhibits a significant role in synergistic gel formation with a number of polymers such as guar gum, tara gum, okra gum, κC, KG, XG, etc. to increase gel strength [22,43]. Hence, it forms a viscous shear-thinning system, but in combination with κC [84] and XG, it produces the elastic nature with no syneresis [20,21] due to synergy between LBG and XG in the same weight ratio formed a stronger elastic thermoreversible hydrogel [84,85]. X-ray diffraction studies exhibited a random aggregation between LBG and κC indicating a small degree of intermolecular binding resulting in an increase in the gel strength indexed by dynamic rigidity modulus and compressive Young's modulus. This increase in gel strength increases with the increase in concentration of LBG and then decreases after a peak point in the mixed gel known as the synergistic effect [10,43]. Unsubstituted block of LBG interacted with κC helix exhibited increased in gel strength, elasticity, and reduced tendency to syneresis [84].

Viscosity

The gelling behavior of LBG in hot water is due to its hydration to produce a viscous system that has drawn the attention of many researchers to utilize it in a drug delivery system more efficiently. Certain factors such as particle size, polymer concentration, molecular weight distribution, shear rates, solubilization methods, and impurities decide its thickening capacity. Viscosity of LBG increases upon increasing its concentration. Its intrinsic viscosity is related to its molecular weight through a power-law equation known as the Mark-Houwink-Sakurada equation with 0.77 as a power-law exponent α when water is used as a solvent. LBG is the stiffer one due to more unsubstituted mannan regions exhibiting a higher propensity to form gels as a result of synergism due to formation of "junction zones" [86,87]. Based on molecular mass, it possesses low viscosity in comparison to the other galactomannans [22,86–88]. Its viscosity is stable in the pH range of 3.5 to 9.0 and is not affected by Ca^{2+} and Mg^{2+} ions. But the acid or oxidizer will make the LBG salt out and reduce the viscosity.

Hydration rate

Hydration rate depends on different grades based on particle size and content of LBG powders. It requires 30 min heating at 80°C for its complete hydration, whereas to obtain maximum viscosity, 2 h heating is required [43]. The smaller the particle size of gum, the more easily it is hydrated. Commercial grade LBG is available as a fine powder for quick hydration. For the preparation of a good quality hydrogel of LBG, its particle size with respect to grade is required as it depends on the hydration rate.

Rheology

LBG in an aqueous phase exhibits a non-Newtonian flow, i.e., shear-thinning or pseudoplastic steady flow behavior at high shear rates, while at low shear rates it exhibits a Newtonian flow [43]. This is due to the fact that new polymeric chains start to form after the breakage of older ones upon low shear force, so the equilibrium between them is maintained hence the viscosity of LBG remains constant. In the case of high shearing forces, the equilibrium is disturbed, the disruption of polymeric chains predominates over their formation, and molecules are set in the direction of flow, which leads to a decrease in its viscosity and thus exhibits a non-Newtonian flow. Lower concentration of LBG aqueous solution acts as a macromolecule polymer. It shows liquid behavior at a low frequency yet solid behavior at a high frequency [89–91]. The higher amounts of arabinose in LBG indicate the impurity as a crude material, and it can be detected easily through rheological analysis [15,42].

7.2.2.2 Pharmacological properties

Antioxidant

LBG blocks myeloperoxidase activity and thereby decreases hypochlorous acid formation due to its engulfing effect on reactive oxygen species, and free radicals found the potential of LBG to inhibit the phosphorylation of p47phox-Ser-328 [51]. It also inhibits the lipid peroxidation and hence reduces the harmful effects of its generated products.

Antidiarrheal

LBG possess the activity to inhibit *Escherichia coli* in the small intestine, which probed a problem of imbalance between the absorption and secretion process. Hence, LBG proved to be beneficial for gut microflora and microfauna. Conversely, immature extract of LBG can cause a slowdown in intestinal secretion because it is rich in tannin content, which provides the astringent property and therefore inhibits GIT hypersecretion as well as diarrhea-like conditions [51].

Anti-ulcer

Peptic ulcer is the main consequence of increase in *Helicobacter pylori* in the stomach environment, which causes the GI hypersecretion. LBG aqueous extract inhibits the cytokines factors such as TNF-α and IL-1β. Also, LBG water extracts also possess the property to treat gastric mucosa lesions [51].

7.3 Formulation development and evaluations of locust bean gum-derived hydrogels

Hydrogel fabricated by LBG is a hydrophilic polymer network made by physical cross-linking or chemical cross-linking gelation mechanism of its polymeric chain. The physical mechanism includes strong and weak bond formation, whereas chemical mechanism includes condensation, addition, and cross-linking reactions. By suitable formulation method of hydrogel, LBG can be used for encapsulation of various molecules for desired drug delivery systems. LBG-based hydrogel beads were formulated with the addition of carboxymethyl in LBG through a cross-linking reaction mechanism as reported by Maiti et al. [69,76,92].

7.3.1 Method of preparation of LBG-derived hydrogels

In general, hydrogels of any polymeric materials can be prepared or synthesized through several methods with a principle of cross-linking of polymeric chains [93]. Plant-originated gums and mucilages have been widely used as a carrier for delivering various molecules at a definite rate from hydrogels due to their economic abundant source, nontoxic, biocompatible, biodegradable, and its vulnerability to combine with other polymeric materials [4,5]. Cross-linking of polymeric chains is the fundamental principle behind hydrogel preparation. This should be possible by either chemical modification, using an external cross-linker, or by exposure to high energy radiation. The chemical cross-linking [67,93–95], physical cross-linking [67,93–95], radiation cross-linking [67,93–96], and polymerization grafting [49,67,72,73,93,94,96] have been utilized for the preparation of LBG-derived hydrogels. A decent variety of cross-linking strategies including amide cross-linking, click chemistry, enzyme-mediated cross-linking, photoinduced cross-linking, Schiff-base reactions, thiol-disulfide exchange, etc. have been utilized for the synthesis of hydrogels.

In the preparation of less-dense LBG-derived hydrogel occupying less volume of water due to its branch heterogeneous gummy nature, a suitable method can be used with or without blending other polymeric materials in suitable proportion for desired functionality. A few reported methods for the preparation of LBG-derived hydrogels for various purposes are as follows.

7.3.1.1 Physical cross-linking methods of locust bean gum-derived hydrogels

Freeze-thawing method

A study showed that LBG forms lyotropic thermotropic liquid crystals at water content ranging from 0.5 to 2.0 g/g (gram of water/gram of dry sample) [83]. The liquid crystalline state of the LBG-water system is similar to that of aqueous systems of polyelectrolyte polysaccharides such as XG [97–99], gellan gum [100], and cellulose derivatives [97,99–101]. The liquid crystalline state is formed when 4 to 20 water molecules in one repeating unit are bound by the polysaccharide molecules, suggesting that LBG forms a tight junction in aqueous media, but no distinct hydrogel is formed from its aqueous solution. Gel-forming properties are closely related to the molecular mobility of polymer chains associated with bound water molecules. The molecular chain of LBG is too mobile in an excess amount of water to stabilize junction zones via freeze-thawing to create its hydrogel. Using rheological and calorimetric methods, the freezing-thawing gelation of the LBG-water system was invented [83]. An appropriate amount of LBG contained in a 20-mL glass container with approximately 10 g of deionized water was heated at 105°C for 30 min. The heated LBG aqueous solution was cooled at about 25°C, and then it was frozen in a freezer (about − 15°C) for approximately 18 h and then thawed slowly at about 25°C for at least 6 h, known as a single freezing-thawing cycle. Gelation using various concentrations of LBG and various freezing-thawing cycles was performed to increase the strength of the LBG hydrogel. The strength was prominent during the first three cycles and dependent on the cooling rate for freezing, suggesting that the size of ice crystals formed in the LBG-water system is strongly related to hydrogen bonds between –OH groups of the LBG molecules [83].

Ionic interaction method

Hydrogel preparation by ionic interaction method does not require the presence of ions in the polymeric chain under conditions such as pH and temperature. LBG is a nonionic organic galactomannan solubilized in water at temperature above 80°C and it produces low viscose, moderate strength hydrogel that can't be ionically cross-linked using polyvalent cations. But with the addition of anionic polymers such as guar gum, agar, sodium alginate, κ-carrageenan, gellan gum, hyaluronic acid, etc., LBG produces an IPN-based hydrogel formulation that can be cross-linked using various inorganic cations such as $CaCl_2$, and $AlCl_3$ for various drug delivery purposes. With various natural polymers, LBG or its modified form have been used for hydrogels-derived IPN micro/macrobeads, microparticles/nanocomposites/matrix tablets, polyspheres for desired delivery of drugs, and probiotics, while synergism formed hydrogels-derived films for edible packaging, wound dressing application, and hard capsules formation (Table 7.1).

Hydrogen bonding method

The polar groups of the polymer strongly bind the water molecules during its interaction by forming hydrogen (H–) bonds, a strong intermolecular force, causing hydrophobic effects [113] to design physically cross-linked hydrogels that exhibit self-healing abilities. Self-healing hydrogels can automatically recover their structure when the hydrogels are damaged. Through H-bonding, elastic mechanical properties and water-holding capacity of hydrogel increases. Physical self-healing polymeric hydrogels can be prepared by H-bonding having low mechanical properties and shape stability but enhanced with the addition of dynamic covalent "borate ester bonds" [114]. Due to fewer galactose units, LBG has limited solubility in cold water, and unsubstituted mannose units are prone to undergo aggregation [91]. This hydrophobic mannose zone permits the formation of strong H-bonds, unstable at higher temperature, which reduces the hydration of the LBG. Some factors such as proportion of polymers, presence and types of other polymers with parent polymer, types of solvent, and temperature affect the strength of H-bonding in hydrogel formation. Hydrogel-based film properties of LBG with κ-carrageenan was improved due to H-bond interactions between κC and LBG observed via Fourier Transform Infrared (FTIR) spectroscopy [23].

Thermoreversible hydrogel method

Thermally reversible gels of interest for tissue engineering and drug delivery purposes were reported using LBG with XG in suitable proportion for desired loading of silicon dioxide (SiO_2) [115]. SiO_2 nanoparticles loaded 1% solutions of XG, LBG, and XG/LBG (1:1) mixed gels (LX) were rheologically characterized for nanoparticle concentration and temperature. With 10% SiO_2 nanoparticles, XG formed larger domains of associated polymer, resulting in enhanced viscosity and viscoelastic moduli, while LBG exhibited transient viscosity and a gel-sol transition due to particle bridging and aggregation, but in the case of LX, 10% SiO_2 nanoparticles showed an increase in elasticity. Under heat treatment in a

TABLE 7.1 The summary of the few reported studies of LBG in combination with other natural polymers and modified grafted LBG for different applications.

Sr. no.	Primary polymer	Secondary polymer	Utilized method of preparation of hydrogel formulation	Purpose with significant outcome
1.	LBG	Agar	Solvent casting method for hydrogel-derived film formulation	Incorporation of LBG into agar film exhibited higher water vapor permeability, low solubility in water and in phosphate buffer solutions, low tensile strength, and appropriate thickness for wound dressing applications with higher antimicrobial and cell viability [25]
2.	LBG	Chitosan	Simple dispersion of polymeric blends containing aceclofenac with pH 5.4 adjustment following cross-linking using glutaraldehyde and centrifugation at 6000 RPM for 30 min [102]	Aceclofenac loaded IPN-nanocomposites based on chitosan and LBG using glutaraldehyde cross-linker was studied for oral sustained release [102]. The proportion of LBG exhibited its effect on drug release rate based on its swelling behavior by reducing the burst release at stomach pH
3.	LBG	κC	The temperature changed sol-gel transmission using a cross-linker citric acid [27] or potassium citrate [28]	• Smart wound dressing based on κC, LBG, and cranberry extract as a pH-responsive hydrogel film was developed with needful characterizations. This anthocyanin-rich extract containing hydrogel film exhibited a better visual system for monitoring bacterial wound infections [27] • The blend of LBG and κC in the ratio of 1:3 and K + in 0.2%w/w exhibited good proportion for hard capsules to overcome the brittle defects of κC. LBG significantly influenced the physicochemical properties of the resultant hard capsules in presence of κC, showing good mechanical properties and storage stability [28]

Continued

TABLE 7.1 The summary of the few reported studies of LBG in combination with other natural polymers and modified grafted LBG for different applications—cont'd

Sr. no.	Primary polymer	Secondary polymer	Utilized method of preparation of hydrogel formulation	Purpose with significant outcome
4.	LBG	NaAlg	[a]Using a cross-linker either $CaCl_2$ [103,104] or $AlCl_3$ [82]	• IPN based microbeads for oral controlled delivery of capecitabine (CAP) in the treatment of colonic cancer [104]. Proportion of LBG in hydrogel-based drug-loaded IPN microbeads exhibited its effect on the drug release rate based on its swelling due to mannose content and strength of a cross-linker against pH of the media • Hydrogel-derived buoyant IPN microbeads of LBG and NaAlg-containing CAP was studied for oral sustained delivery, exhibited good buoyancy in gastric pH, better mucoadhesion in intestinal pH, improved systemic circulation, bioavailability, and extended half-life of entrapped CAP [82,105] • IPN hydrogel-based mucoadhesive macromolecules of aceclofenac, for oral sustained delivery, affected by pH of the media on its swelling, diffusion path length, and release rate depending on its content with respect to NaAlg and the strength of $CaCl_2$ [103]
5.	CLBG	NaAlg	[a]Using a counter-ion "$AlCl_3$"	• Oral-controlled delivery of glipizide from hydrogel-derived IPN beads using CLBG with NaAlg and aqueous $AlCl_3$ as gelation medium was studied [106]. pH-dependent swelling behavior of hydrogel-derived IPN beads at stomach pH was due to unionized form of the carboxyl groups, and hence low swelling at acidic pH led to lower drug release. At intestinal pH, ionization of the carboxyl groups and generation of an electrostatic repulsive force inside the beads led to higher swelling propensity of the beads. This is also due to swelling involving an exchange of aluminum ions with monovalent cations [107] and sequestering effect of phosphate ions on Al^{3+} resulting in high water-holding capacity and higher drug release rate in alkaline media [108,109]

6.	CLBG	KG	[a]Using a counter-ion "AlCl$_3$"	Oral-sustained release carvedilol phosphate-loaded IPN hydrogel microparticles of KG and CLBG in different ratios exhibited higher swelling and mucoadhesion in simulated intestinal fluid due to COO– groups of CLBG [110]
7.	LBG	Hyaluronic acid (HA)	Temperature- and pH-controlled blending of LBG and HA in different ratios	Mixture of LBG:HA as synergism hydrogels exhibited good viscoelasticity and the best synergism at 50%w/w strength with formation of physical gel [111] that can be utilized for economic hydrogels formulation in nutraceutical foods, support for tissue engineering, and cosmetic products
8.	LBG	Tragacanth gum	Blending of gums at different ratios in controlled conditions following drying to produce edible film	A distinct synergism hydrogel-derived film was identified at all ratios of both gums with the existence of noncovalent intermolecular interactions between them, proved by FTIR [112]. The blended film exhibited improvement in transparency, water vapor barrier, and mechanical properties suggesting its use as a new degradable food packaging material
9.	LBG	Gellan gum (Gg)	Chemical and physical cross-linking by pH-sensitive borate-ester bond in LBG network and hydrogen-bond-associated double-helix structure of Gg [90]	Temperature- and pH-sensitive double network hydrogel for desired drug delivery systems due to improvement of mechanical strength and viscoelasticity
10.	Polyacrylamide-g-LBG (PAAm-g-LBG)	NaAlg	[a]Using CaCl$_2$ and glutaraldehyde as cross-linkers of NaAlg in the presence of PAAm-g-LBG containing ketoprofen	With minimization of gastric side effects and targeting to small intestine of ketoprofen, pH-sensitive hydrogel-derived IPN-polyspheres was studied [18]. They showed reversible swelling-shrinking behavior with the inner change of surrounding pH between 1.2 and 7.4 due to carboxylic groups of PAAm-g-LBG. In alkaline medium, the carboxyl groups of IPN polyspheres undergoes ionization thereby increasing osmotic pressure inside the matrix of IPN causing increased swelling and exhibited control (about 10% in 1.2 pH buffer and about 88% in 7.4 pH buffer) from dual cross-linked IPN polyspheres [18]

[a] Ionotropic gelation method was used.

temperature range from 25°C to 85°C under conditions of constant strain and frequency, the solutions sustained a nearly constant measured complex modulus with 10% loading indicating the particle-mediated network structure counteracts the effect of temperature on the material properties. This study showed the use of LBG with XG-type biopolymers for the development of biopolymeric hydrogel systems in biomedical and food processing applications where property prediction and control are critical [115].

7.3.1.2 Chemical cross-linking methods

Grafting method

Grafting is a way to add desired properties in a polymer without significant loss of initial characteristics of the polymer [116]. LBG contains a number of –OH groups in its structure based on its proportion. The extent of degree of substitution/modifications also depends upon stearic hindrance caused by the –OH group present in it.

LBG is grafted with methacrylic acid [117] to improve and/or enhance the physical and chemical properties of LBG for a drug delivery system as hydrogel beads. Grafting ensures the method for tailoring material characteristics for utilization as a macro molecular chain in which free radicals initiate the chain propagation step and hence forms the grafted chains [16,72]. The acrylamide-grafted LBG was synthesized through microwave irradiation with the help of ceric ammonium nitrate as a redox initiator and was found to be biocompatible and biodegradable, which successfully mediated the controlled release of matrix tablet of Buflomedil hydrochloride [16,72].

Cross-linking by covalent bond

Dynamic covalent borate ester bonds can be used to prepare self-healing polymeric hydrogels [114]. LBG's structural unit consists of four 1,4-linked β-D-mannopyranosyl as the main chain and one 1,6-linked α-D-galactopyranosyl as the side chain (Fig. 7.3). Since LBG contains a large amount of 1,3-diol structure, it can be complexed with borax in aqueous solution to form borate ester bonds, imparting excellent self-healing properties to the hydrogel [94].

Cross-linking by enzymatic reaction

The galactose oxidase (GO)-catalyzed oxidation of galactose-containing high molecular weight galactomannans produced thermally stable gels having potential applications in the food and biomedical industries requiring thermal stability [118]. The GO-catalyzed oxidation-producing hydrogel of LBG is due to the formation of hemiacetal bonds between the hydroxyl groups and the new carbonyl groups of polymer chains. After enzymatic reaction using oxidation, the hydrogel strength of galactomannan depends on their molecular weight. LBG produced stronger hydrogel after oxidase-catalyzed oxidation [118]. The hydrogel properties of LBG can be altered with its concentration and degree of oxidation. To enhance the GO enzymatic action, horseradish peroxidase (HRP) and catalase can be incorporated in LBG-derived hydrogel formulation. The amount of addition of GO depends on the approximate amount of terminal galactose present in galactomannan. The reaction dosage of enzymes and reaction conditions govern the hydrogel development of galactomannans. A study showed that 21 U of GO, 400 U of HRP, and 46 kU of catalase were used in the oxidation of 1 g of guar gum containing ca. 400 mg of galactose (ca. 40% of total sugars) [118]. The degrees of oxidation for LBG were 10% to 16% calculated from the ratio of oxidized galactose units and total carbohydrates. The oxidized LBG formed stable gels at low concentrations (0.2%–0.4% w/v) throughout 20°C to 90°C.

Cross-linking by high energy radiation

Radiation processing of LBG exhibited in reduction of molecular weight due to its depolymerization and thus affected its viscosity, gelation, solubility, and swelling in a dose-dependent manner. Irradiation of the LBG leads to depolymerization making its improved prebiotic potential and hence makes it more useful and amenable for the probiotics [96]. LBG's functionality as a source of dietary fiber in enteral feed without compromising the rheological properties of the feed has been improved using gamma irradiation. Due to hydrogel formation of LBG under exposure to gamma radiation processing using ^{60}Co gamma irradiation having a dose rate of 1.9 kGy/h, 5 to 50 kGy/h at 28°C ± 2°C, it improved the survivability of the probiotic organism during its transit in gastrointestinal conditions [96].

A process has been reported to modify natural polysaccharides in solid-state by high energy radiation [119] to obtain hydrogel [24]. In the presence of a suitable mediating gas (alkyne or acetylene), their structure in solid-state can be controlled/modified using ionizing radiation. The polysaccharides, when irradiated in the presence of acetylene gas, undergo cross-linking leading to formation of macromolecules with increased molecular weight and functionalities [24]. Highly branched polysaccharides can produce hydrogels with high energy radiation of doses up to 50 kGy, but with straight chain polysaccharides, it produces hydrogels at doses of 1 to 3 kGy.

A carboxylated LBG (CLBG) was synthesized using TEMPO (2,2,6,6-tetramethylpiperidin-1-yl)oxyl)-mediated oxidation method [24]. In the presence of acetylene gas or in the pastelike state, synthesized CLBGs' hydrogel was prepared by irradiation with gamma rays utilizing a ^{60}Co gamma-ray source in a Gamma cell 220 type ^{60}Co-gamma irradiator at room temperature, in air at the dose rates of 30 Gy/h and 300 Gy/h up to 10 kGy. CLBG hydrogels exhibited the highest swelling capacity (~ 34,000%) in the case of CLBG hydrogels prepared in the presence of acetylene gas but lowest swelling capacity (4700%) in the pastelike state. A decrease in degree of gelation was observed when the irradiation dose was increased from 5 to 10 kGy for all carboxylation degrees in CLBG. The irradiation dose of 5 kGy and a carboxylation degree of 26% were identified as the optimal conditions for hydrogels of CLBGs [24].

7.3.2 Evaluation tests of LBG-derived hydrogel formulations

7.3.2.1 Important evaluation parameters

Various major evaluation parameters for determination of LBG-derived hydrogel formulations[18–20,25,28,68,80,82,84,102–106,120–123] are summarized in Figs. 7.7, 7.8, and 7.9 that can be used after general preformulation characterization of the raw materials.

7.3.2.2 Controlled release mechanism of LBG-derived hydrogels

Drug release pattern from LBG is predetermined when some criteria are justified. The disposition of drug in the body should follow first order kinetics; the release of drug from polymer complex is the rate-limiting step that also limits its absorption, and the released drug from the complex should be completely absorbed and bioavailable through the four-model theory, i.e., slow zero order release [124], slow first order release, initial loading dose rapid release through slow zero order release, and initial loading dose rapid release through slow first order release.

The system that governs the rate of release of controlled drug release is the stimuli-based drug delivery system. Here in this system, drug release is modified by various physical, chemical, or biological stimuli [2]. These systems are also called a smart drug delivery system or environment-sensitive drug delivery system as they are capable of releasing the drug when stimulated by external factors/stimulus (Fig. 7.10) [2,125].

Physical stimulus

Osmotic pressure

LBG-XC (XLBG) system follows typical zero order kinetics on the basis of osmosis, which is the movement of solvent from a higher concentration to lower concentration through a semipermeable membrane [19,20]. The entry of water from the body fluids leads to swelling of the DDS and generates an orifice through which the drug molecule is released.

Hydration pressure

This is different from osmotic pressure, which is a hydrodynamic pressure-generating system. Here the compartment-based system of LBG is generated having rigid housing in which one compartment contains the drug and other compartment contains water-swelling hydrocolloids such as hydroxypropyl methylcellulose (HPMC).

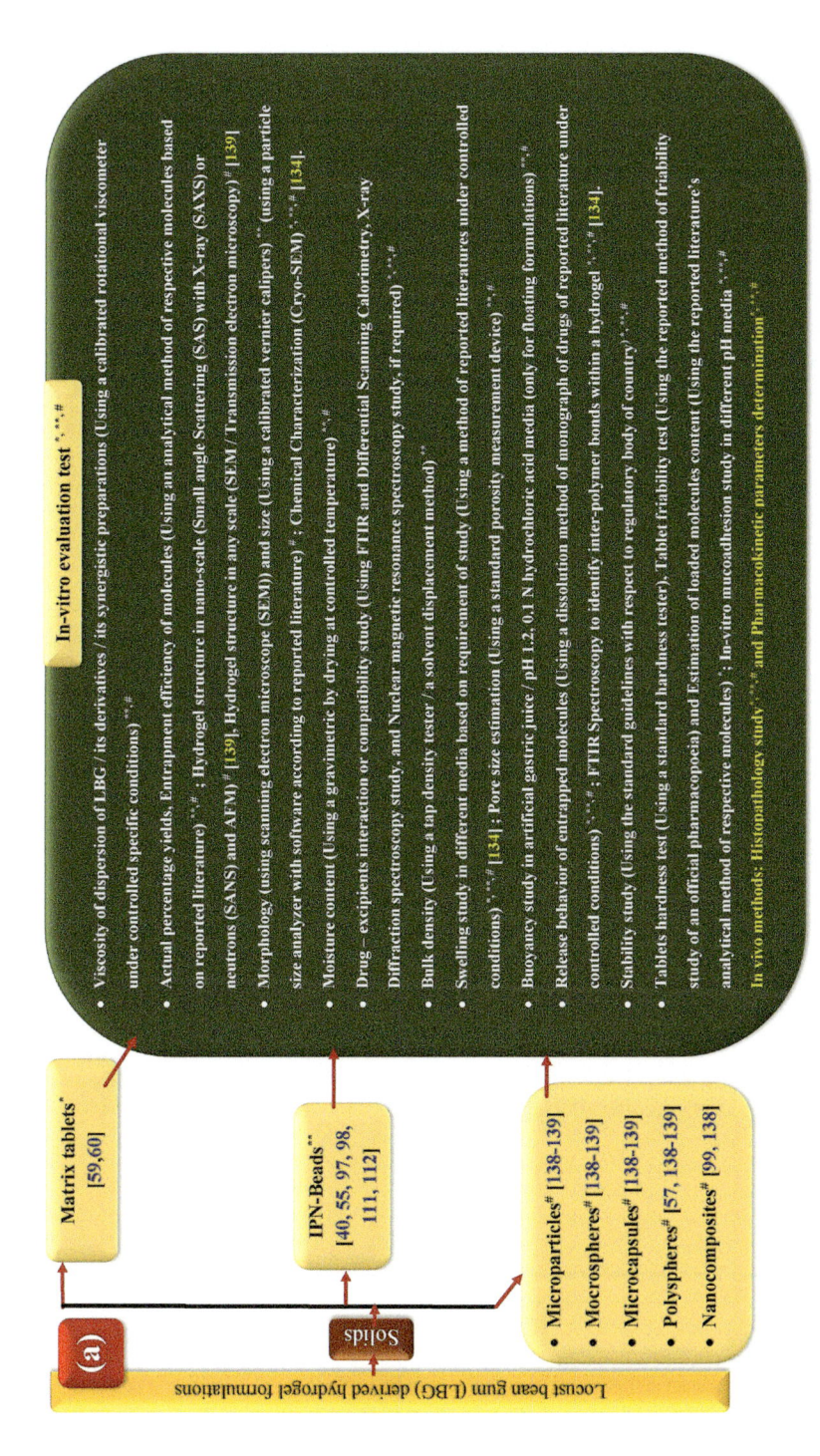

FIG. 7.7 A flowchart showing the list of major evaluation tests of LBG-derived hydrogels solid formulation: Matrix tablets, IPN beads, and particulates (a).

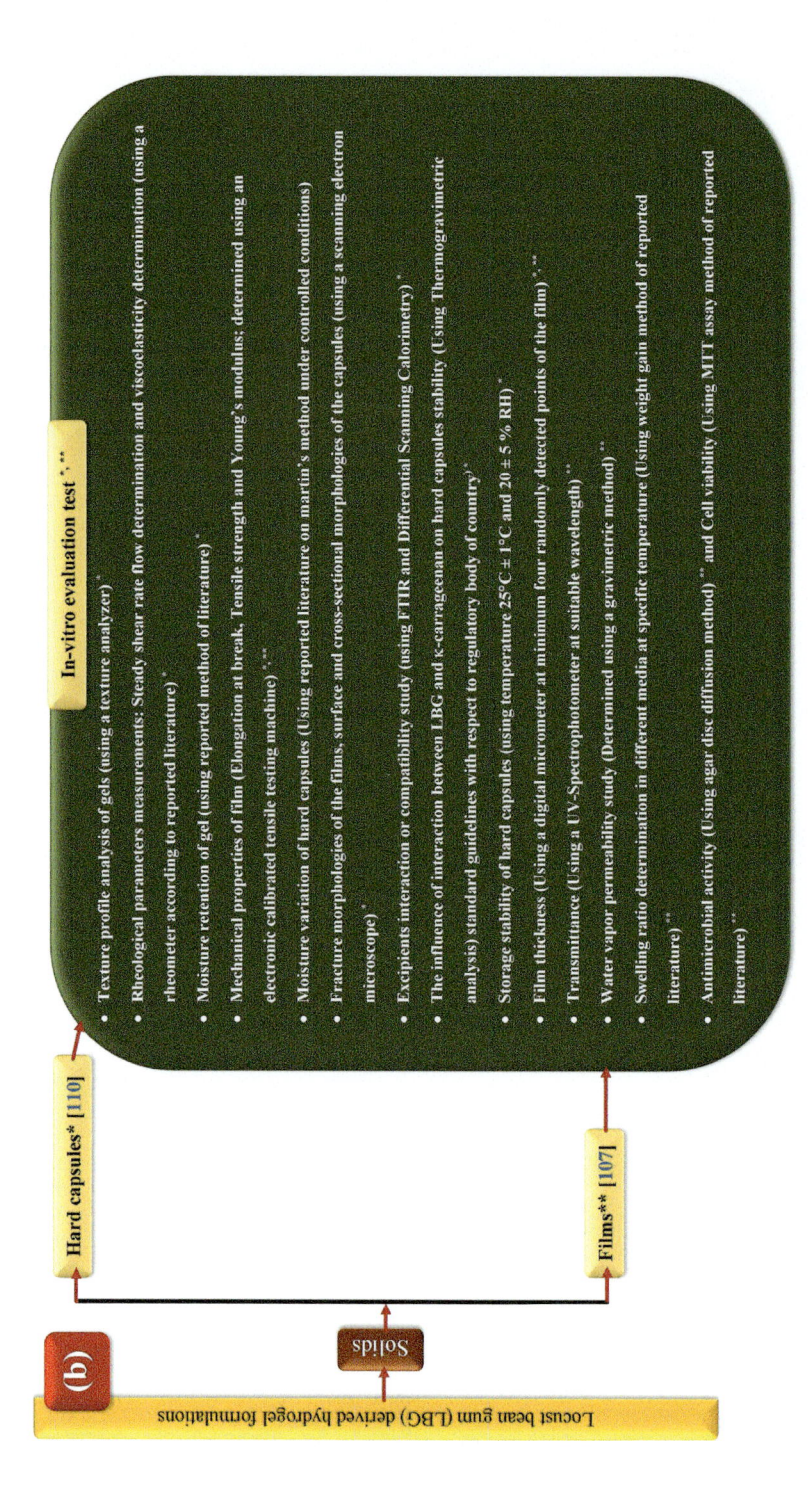

FIG. 7.8 A flowchart showing the list of major evaluation tests of LBG-derived hydrogels solid formulations: hard capsules and films (b).

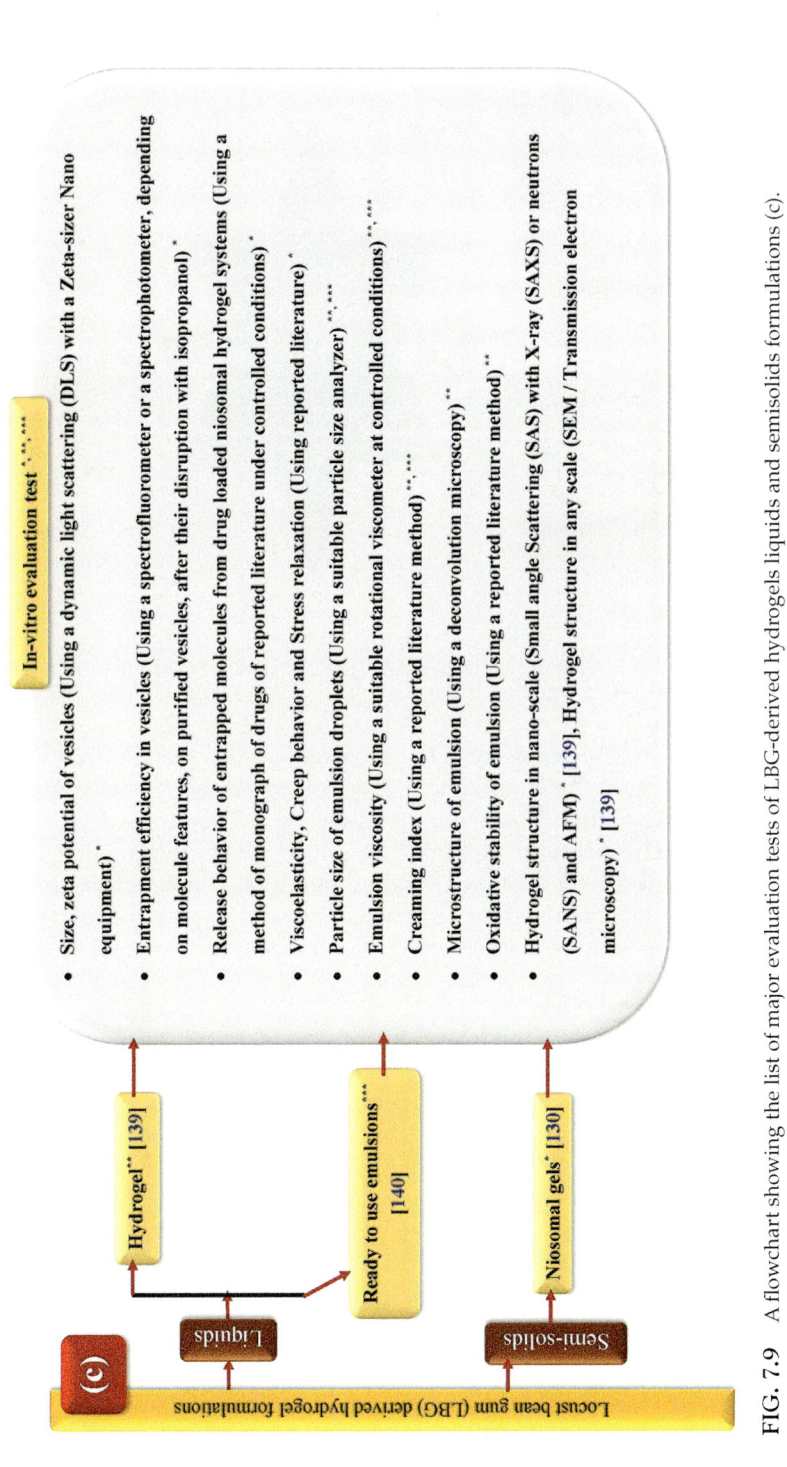

FIG. 7.9   A flowchart showing the list of major evaluation tests of LBG-derived hydrogels liquids and semisolids formulations (c).

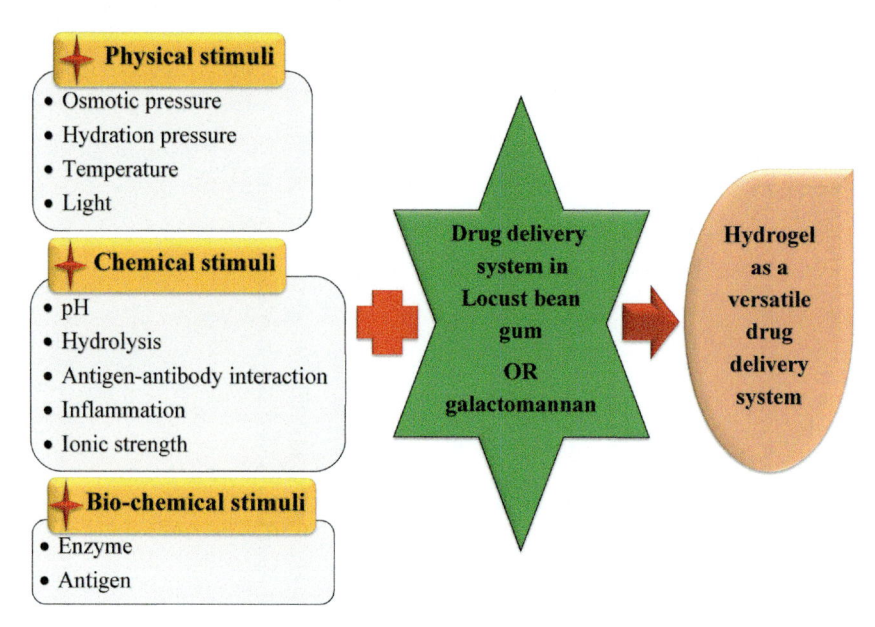

FIG. 7.10   Different types of stimulus that cause the release of a drug from extensive polymeric chains of locust bean gum.

The water-swelling capacity of hydrocolloids is such that they absorb water molecules from the environment due to the presence of heterogeneous groups of polysaccharides resulting in swelling, pushing the drug toward the orifice and is released through that orifice. XLBG formulation with a drug gum ratio of 1:2 exhibited better dissolution characteristics of drug molecules, and it continued for 8h [19,20]. The swelling starts due to hydration pressure as soon as matrices of XLBG came into contact with the liquid.

Thermal responsive
The thermal-responsive polymers can be of two types, either polymers that interact with water with no polymer-polymer interaction or polymers that interact with both water as well as show polymer-polymer interaction. The polymers acting by thermal stimuli are defined by lower critical solution temperature (LCST) property. LCST indicates the positive enthalpy whenever a polymer swells in water but exerts an opposite effect on the system, and this function governs the polymer property of swelling, i.e., temperature above LCST-polymer shrinks whereas temperature below LCST-polymer swells. It can affect the release pattern of a controlled release drug delivery system [126].

Light responsive
The polymeric structures are altered in the presence of light (photo radiation) leading to a change in physical or chemical properties. The photochrome group in the gel absorbs the light and causes the released mechanism [126].

Chemical stimuli

pH-induced drug release

The pH stimuli enhance the solubility, degradation, and swelling of polymeric complexes, i.e., LBG hydrogels. Solubility enhancement by pH is especially made for acid-sensitive drugs or drugs that irritate gastric mucosa and hence are meant for delayed released drug by the use of intestinal fluid-soluble polymers. In the case of degradation of bioerodible polymers, the influence of pH is utilized for drug release based on the targeted site of drug dissolution. Swelling of LBG is influenced at neutral pH [2].

Hydrolysis-induced drug release

In this system, a drug that is packed or trapped in polymeric chains of LBG are released from the polymeric matrix once it is hydrolyzed and hence drug delivery can be controlled by this mechanism for longer desired periods of time.

Enzyme as stimuli

The drug that is entrapped in the reservoir of many polymers is made to release through enzymatic hydrolysis into the body cavities.

7.4 Applications of LBG-derived hydrogel formulation

LBG, a natural GRAS-approved hydrocolloidal, is widely used in the food and pharmaceutical industries [10,13–15,45,93]. In pharmaceuticals, it has a wide range of application, especially in viscous liquid and gel formulations, and also performs varied functions such as binder, viscosity enhancer, stabilizer, matrix former, drug release modifier, disintegrator, emulsifier, suspending agent, gelling agent [127], and bio/mucoadhesive [15,102]. It is also used in the textile industry due to its film-forming property that makes it ideal as a sizing and finishing agent. It also plays a significant role as a prebiotic due to the presence of oligosaccharides, i.e., mannose and galactose [10,86].

The use of LBG with various polymers such as IPN-based hydrogel formulations are the most recent advancement in the drug delivery system for the modified release of loaded molecules with the function of predetermined time [82,102,103,127]. IPN is a network of at least two polymers that are not covalently bonded but overlap each other, and drug deliveries have been reported for LBG-derived hydrogel formulations [82,102,103,117]. The frequent approach of drug delivery is the utilization of a combination of LBG with other compatible polysaccharides such as hydrogel formulation for better mechanical strength and enhancing the drug-releasing performance [13]. LBG, its possible interactions with other polymeric materials, and grafted LBG's derived hydrogel formulations for various applications in different fields are summarized in Fig. 7.11 and Table 7.2.

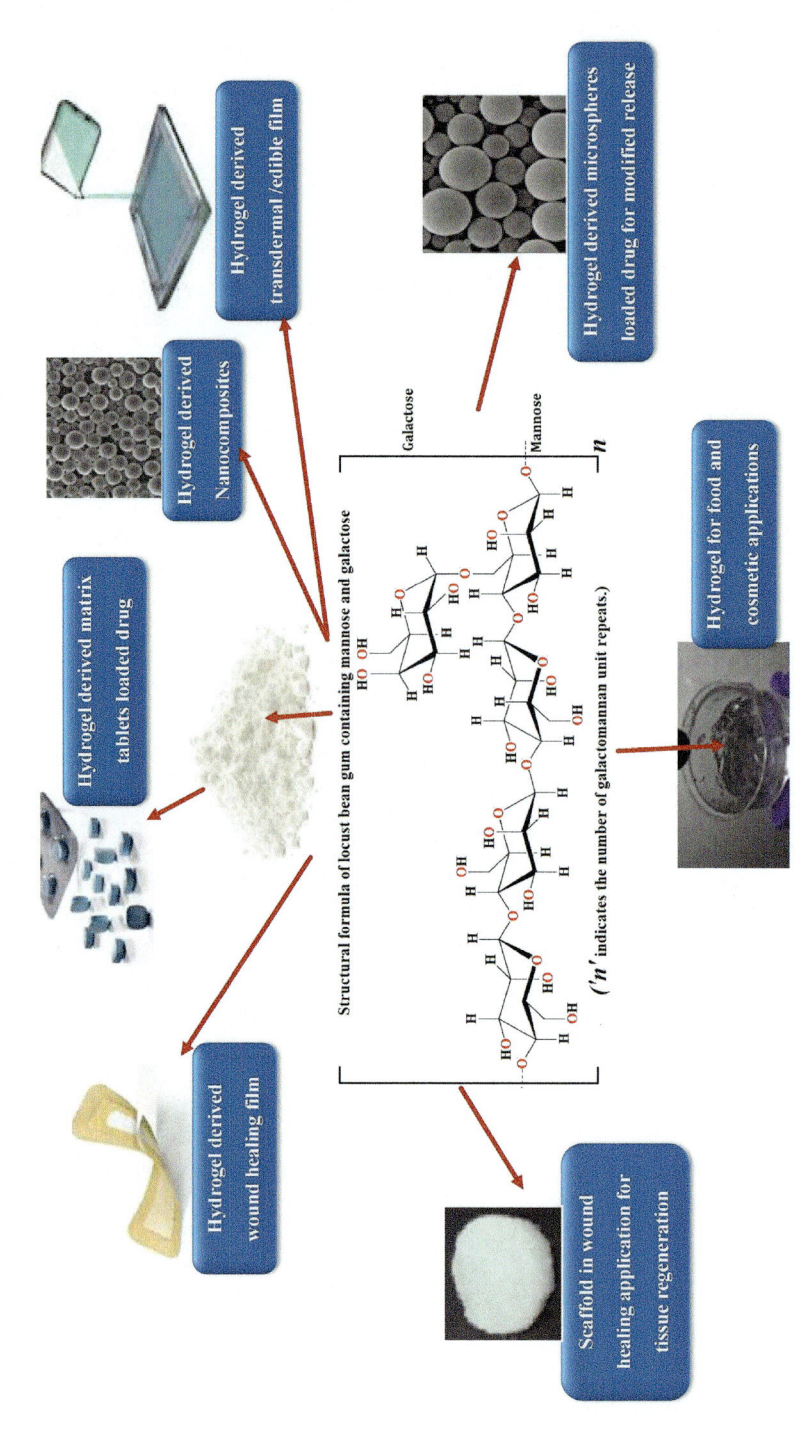

FIG. 7.11 An illustration showing applications of locust bean gum and its derived hydrogel formulations.

TABLE 7.2 The summary of working patents on locust bean gum as a material for various application in its native and in combination form with other polymers.

Patent number	Title, filing date and inventor(s)	Assignee	Remarkable outcomes
US3855149	Method of increasing cold water solubility of locust bean gum, 13/11/1972, Bielskis E	Patterson C Co, U.S.	Improving cold water solubility of LBG; suggested to be used in cold products [128]
US4038206	Hydroxyalkyl locust bean/ xanthomonas hydrophilic colloid blends, 01/15/1976, Karl CL	General Mills Chemicals, Inc. (Minneapolis, MN)	The thickening property of a blend useful in drilling oil wells and in oil well fracturing fluids [129]
US4136178A	Locust bean gum therapeutic compositions; 01/31/1977, Lin Song-ling, Pramoda MK. (Rouses Point, NY)	American Home Products Corp. (New York, NY)	Exhibited role of LBG in the manufacturing of ophthalmic preparation with remarkable viscoelasticity [130]
US4162925	Phosphated locust bean gums; 05/10/1978, Tiefenthaler, Karl HO, Nittnerich WK	Meyhall Chemical AG (Kreuzlingen, Ch)	High viscous blend of phosphated LBG and XG in fluid drilling planting operations as a suspending media [131]
US4219582	Xanthan gum and locust bean gum in confectionery use; 03/29/1979, Cheng H. (San Diego, CA)	Merck & Co., Inc. (Rahway, NJ)	Suitable in the manufacturing of high solids starch jelly confectionery product due to synergism hydrogel of LBG with XG [29]
US4829056	Buccal tablet comprising etorphine or a salt thereof; 04/10/1987, Sugden K. (Beverley, GB3)	Reckitt & Colman Products Limited (London, GB)	Improved bioavailability of buccal tablet due to synergy of LBG with XG in hydrogel-based matrix tablets [132]
US5169639	Controlled release verapamil tablets; 07/25/1991, Baichwal AR (Wappingers Falls, NY), Staniforth JN. (Bath, GB2)	Edward Mendell Co., Inc. (Patterson, NY)	Blend of XG and LBG in all proportion exhibited its role in oral controlled release verapamil hydrogel matrix tablets due to pH-dependent swelling and diffusion path length [133]

Continued

TABLE 7.2 The summary of working patents on locust bean gum as a material for various application in its native and in combination form with other polymers—cont'd

Patent number	Title, filing date and inventor(s)	Assignee	Remarkable outcomes
US7037653	Molecular methods for detecting guar gum additions to locust bean gum; 03/02/2001, Benedi BVJ, Domenech SA, Alberti SS (Palma de Malloraca, ES), Hernandez VML, Rossello PJA (Valencia, ES)	Consejo Superior de Investigaciones Cientificas (Madrid, ES)	Suitable method for extracting, amplifying, and detecting DNA using a mixture of guar gum and LBG or alone [134]
US7179782	Detergent compositions; 01/16/2004, Gibbs, CD, Parry AJ, Rogers SH (Bebington, GB)	Unilever Home & Personal Care USA, Division of Conopco, Inc. (Greenwich, CT, U.S.)	Improved antiredeposition property of detergent using LBG [135]
US20080299267	Packaged concentrate for preparing a bouillon, soup, sauce, gravy, or for use as a seasoning; the concentrate comprising xanthan and locust bean gum; 08/04/2008, Achterkamp G, Ackermann DKK, Kohlus R, Kuhn M (Heilbronn, DE), Inoue C (Vlaardingen, NL).	Conopco, Inc., d/b/a UNILEVER (Englewood Cliffs, NJ, U.S.)	Gelling property imparted by XG and LBG for preparing various household products [30]
US20110256087	Cosmetic composition containing a locust bean gum hydrolysate; 12/23/2009, Fabre B (Belberaud, FR), Fiorini-puybaret C (L'Union, FR)	Pierre Fabre Dermo-Cosmetique (Boulogne-billancourt, FR)	Exhibited compatible role in the manufacturing of hair cosmetics containing LBG hydrolysate [31]

7.4.1 Locust bean gum and its hydrogel-derived formulations for oral drug delivery

Oral delivery of LBG as well as its hydrogel-derived formulations is the most effective biopharmaceutical formulations. Due to the presence of β-mannanase in the human colonic region, oral delivery ensures ease and effective biodegradation of LBG macromolecules [13]. Due to pH-dependent swellability of LBG, it has been utilized in matrix tablet formulation for oral modified release of various drugs [13].

To improve LBG's functionality in desired oral drug delivery, it was chemically modified by carboxymethylation [61,136], which altered its physicochemical properties such as primary structures, hydrophilicity, polyelectrolytic nature, solution rheology, and gel-forming behavior. Numerous hydroxyl groups present in the structure of LBG can be substituted by carboxymethyl groups [60]. LBG either alone or in combination with other polysaccharides have been used as matrix materials to study the release behavior of various drugs depending on their rheological or gel strength characteristic [13]. LBG, in contact with water, produced a strong elastic gel that swelled less due to lower penetration of water resulting in slower drug release, while carboxymethylated locust bean gum (CMLBG) formed a viscous polymer solution through which higher influx of water resulted in rapid swelling of the matrix and faster drug release [60].

CMLBG was synthesized, characterized, and utilized as a possible carrier system using trivalent Al^{3+} cross-linked hydrogel beads for the oral controlled delivery of glipizide [68]. CMLBG became soluble in distilled water at room temperature and formed a clear solution that could be attributed to the hydrophilic nature of carboxylate functional groups of CMLBG. Glipizide release from the Al^{3+} cross-linked hydrogel beads of CMLBG was controlled by a combination of diffusion as well as polymer relaxation phenomena. The Al^{3+} cross-linked hydrogel beads of CMLBG-loaded glipizide exhibited in vitro release up to 10 h in alkaline dissolution media due to high swelling ability [68].

7.4.2 Buccal drug delivery

Buccal delivery is largely used for various drugs' formulation as it avoids first pass metabolism thus avoiding the degradation of the drug before reaching systemic circulation and ensures improving bioavailability of poor soluble drugs in the intestine [13,69]. LBG has buco/mucoadhesive property [69] and hence its hydrogel-derived formulations have an affinity to control the release rate of entrapped molecules [85,125]. In the case of metoprolol, a tablet containing a mixture of LBG and Xanthan gum in the ratio 2:1 with 1% sodium lauryl sulfate exhibited drug release within 45 min and good permeation across the buccal mucosa [19,20]. A buccal tablet of propranolol hydrochloride with a mixture of LBG and chitosan in 2:3 ratio exhibited good bioavailability [137].

7.4.3 Nasal drug delivery

LBG microparticles have been utilized for pulmonary delivery of first-line antitubercular drugs rifabutin and isoniazid having proper aerodynamic property [138]. These microparticles showed the highest affinity for macrophages as revealed in flow cytometry assay with no toxicity as a more popular alternative drug system for tuberculosis therapy.

7.4.4 Ocular drug delivery

Gentamicin encapsulated in microparticles of LBG with i-carrageenan is further incorporated in a polyvinyl alcohol gel for topical ocular use [139]. This study exhibited prevention of burst release of the drug with delay release by incorporation of 10% LBG with i-carrageenan. The stability of this combination is greatly affected by molecular weight and degree of substitution of LBG.

7.4.5 Transdermal drug delivery

A new niosomal vesicle-loaded hydrogel system using a blend of LBG and XG in 1:1 ratio was used for topical application [32]. This system showed a slow release of the loaded molecules from niosomal hydrogels up to 50 h with a protective effect on vesicle integrity.

7.4.6 Other applications of the hydrogel of locust bean gum and its derivatives

In the literature, Akkaya et al. [25] demonstrated the antibacterial property of agar-LBG and agar-salep film as a wound dressing system against the Gram-positive, Gram-negative, and fungi agar disc diffusion method. The agar alone does not possess any antibacterial activity but with 25% LBG antibacterial activity was increased but less than agar-salep films.

LBG also plays a vital role in a colon drug delivery system formulated along with chitosan in the ratio 2:3, respectively. They both proved to be effective in prevention of drug release in the stomach and hence the drug was released in the colon [14]. LBG also acts as a hypolipidemic agent by decreasing low density lipoprotein (LDL) cholesterol, an antidiabetic agent, by causing a fullness sensation upon ingestion.

The stable novel low-cost sorbent LBG-cl-Poly(DMAAm) hydrogel, prepared via free radical in situ polymerization of N, N-dimethyl acrylamide by employing N, N'-methylene bis(acrylamide) as cross-linkers, can be used as an alternative and promising adsorbent in the treatment of effluents containing the water-soluble cationic dye Brilliant green (BG) [26]. The adsorption efficiency of the LBG-cl-Poly(DMAAm) hydrogel adsorbent was determined using parameters such as chemical structural of adsorbent and dye molecule, swelling behavior of adsorbent, and solubility parameter of the dye. The leading mechanism of BG dye adsorption tends to be simply strong electrostatic interactions between (− ve)-charged (–COO⁻) groups on the LBG-cl-Poly(DMAAm) hydrogel and (+ ve)-charged (N +) groups on the cationic BG [26]. The LBG-cl-Poly(DMAAm) hydrogel showed high swelling and high adsorption efficiency for BG dye. The adsorption behavior of this hydrogel matched very well with the model's "pseudo-second order model and Langmuir adsorption isotherm." Hence the LBG-cl-Poly(DMAAm) hydrogel can be used as a promising functional regenerable adsorbent with high capacity to remove cationic dye from a liquid media.

7.4.7 Commercial application of LBG-derived hydrogel formulations

The appealing characteristics like gelling properties and synergistic interaction with other polysaccharides made it possible in the field of drug delivery system for efficient drug delivery with less or no adverse effects [65]. LBG has been used synergistically with xanthan gum or carrageenan gum in many food and non-food industries such as paper industry, textile industry, pharmaceutical industry, cosmetic industry, and food industry as edible films, jellies, beads, matrix hydrogel films, and patches for either therapeutic or nontherapeutic purposes. Commercially, five different grades of brand PALGUM based on viscosity and particle size LBG gum powder developed by Carob, S.A., Mallorca, Spain, is available for various applications. Commercial LBG-derived hydrogel formulations is not available from any industries, even though numerous research applications of the same have been reported (Table 7.1).

7.5 LBG-derived hydrogels in tissue engineering

Tissue engineering is the biomedical engineering discipline that involves a combination of cells or cell lines, engineering techniques, or material methods along with the biophysicochemical requirements to replace damaged tissues or modify them for treatment purposes. It is designed and fabricated in such a way as a therapeutic agent [63]. The hydrophilic nature of engineered LBG-based hydrogel due to numerous –OH groups serves a function to attach at different cellular sites and provides specificity to the molecule to attach at target sites [71]. Tissue scaffolds are a 3D structure having vivid polymeric networks including large porosity within it. It is incorporated as scaffolds into seeding cells (as in cell line culture) for tissue damage repair, modification, or rejuvenation process. These scaffolds can be of a natural or synthetic type and are utilized widely based on the requirement of procedure. Tissue scaffolds again can be of two types, permanent or temporary scaffolds based on their retention into the body. The permanent scaffolds are those that are retained in the body throughout the process of tissue damage repair, while temporary scaffolds are those that are degraded after a certain course of time in the body itself [98,117].

7.5.1 Objectives and formulation method of hydrogels of locust bean gum in tissue engineering

To repair and/or regenerate defective tissue using a tissue bionic in wound healing dressings and a suitable growth factor incorporated tissue engineering using LBG-derived hydrogel construction as the main objective to stimulate cellularization, vascularization, vasculogenesis, and angiogenesis [33].

Perestrelo et al. [140] worked to evaluate the potential of pluripotent embronic stem cells (ESCs) to differentiate into different types of cells and/or tissues in which they utilized LBG as a coating for ESC culture, and the cells were able to maintain their viability and supported the mouse ESC differentiation capacity. LBG solution was prepared in sterile milliQ water, and simultaneously gelatin solution was also prepared; both were processed, mixed, and poured on TCPS 6 well plate and incubated for the preparation of growth area for ESC.

7.5.2 Research approaches of locust bean gum-derived hydrogel in tissue engineering

To promote early in vivo wound repair and regenerate tissue formation in wound healing applications on open excision wound model in Wistar albino rats for stabilizing collagen and immobilizing vascular endothelial growth factor (VEGF), bionic collagen-poly(dialdehyde) LBG (PDALBG) hybrid scaffolds were prepared using synthesized PDALBG [33]. These hybrid porous scaffolds exhibited improved collagen stability, biostability, and immobilization of VEGF due to incorporation of dialdehyde functionalities in LBG. The proportion of PDALB in collagen significantly improved the thermal, 3D-porous topography, swelling, and biodegradation abilities in the hybrid scaffolds. The collagen deposition, wound closure, re-epithelialization, and blood vessel formation were identified by in vivo wound healing study using the collagen-PDALB-VEGF hybrid porous scaffolds [33].

7.6 Patents of LBG-derived hydrogel formulations

Various works on LBG-derived hydrogels have been carried and patented by researchers throughout the world in building up new platforms due to its flexible inherent properties to combine with various polymers in suitable ratios for achieving functionality in food, pharmaceuticals, biomedicals, and cosmetics. Table 7.2 shows the summary of a few reported working patents of the U.S. on LBG as a nonionic, biodegradable, galactomannan-derived hydrogel preparation in various forms in its native form as well as its combination with other polymers.

7.7 Conclusion

Due to the evergreen cultivation of carob trees in various regions of the world, and the economic production of LBG from its seed coat and fundamental properties, the use of LBG has immensely increased in various fields. Based on reported literature on LBG and its derived hydrogels' formulation for various purposes in society, it can be concluded that the use of LBG-derived hydrogels has been increased gradually in food, pharmaceuticals, biomedical, cosmetics, and other industries. For the development of desired hydrogel-derived drug delivery using LBG in combination with other compatible polymers, it is required to digest the fundamental properties of LBG through this chapter, and it will be helpful in quality innovation work using clarified LBG. LBG-derived hydrogel formulations have been utilized as a carrier-based delivery system for various molecules for modified release purposes due to its grafting or synergy effect with a number of polymers. Moreover, it is framed to provide an idea in building up novel platforms for desired design and delivery of various classes of molecules, nutraceuticals, and probiotics in pharmaceutical, food, biomedical, and cosmetic industries. In the coming future, LBG-derived hydrogel formulations for suitable purposes in society will be commercialized with consideration of its fundamental flexible physicochemical properties, biocompatibility, biodegradability, nonmutagenic, nontoxic, economic processing of production of LBG, excellent swelling, and gelling ability.

References

[1] Pal P, Pandey JP, Sen G. Sesbania gum based hydrogel as platform for sustained drug delivery: an in vitro study of 5-FU release. Int J Biol Macromol 2018;113:1116–24.
[2] Abdollahiyan P, Baradaran B, De La Guardia M, Oroojalian F, Mokhtarzadeh A. Cutting-edge progress and challenges in stimuli responsive hydrogel microenvironment for success in tissue engineering today. J Control Release 2020;328:514–31.
[3] Buwalda SJ, Boere KWM, Dijkstra PJ, Feijen J, Vermonden T, Hennink WE. Hydrogels in a historical perspective: from simple network to smart materials. J Control Release 2014;190:254–73.
[4] Rana V, Rai P, Tiwary AK, Singh RS, Kennedy JF, Knill CJ. Modified gums: approaches and applications in drug delivery. Carbohydr Polym 2011;83:1031–47.
[5] Ahmad S, Ahmad M, Manzoor K, Purwar R, Ikram S. A review on latest innovations in natural gums based hydrogels: preparations & applications. Int J Biol Macromol 2019;136:870–90.

[6] Calo E, Khutoryanskiy VV. Biomedical applications of hydrogels: a review of patents and commercial products. Eur Polym J 2015;65:252–67.

[7] Dea IC, Morrison A. Chemistry and interactions of seed galactomannans. Adv Carbohydr Chem Biochem 1975;31:241–312.

[8] Dakia PA, Blecker C, Robert C, Wathelet B, Paquot M. Composition and physicochemical properties of locust bean gum extracted from whole seeds by acid or water dehulling pre-treatment. Food Hydrocoll 2008;22(5):807–18.

[9] El Bouzdoudi B, Saïdi R, Embarch K, El Mzibri M, Nejjar El Ansari Z, El Kbiach ML, Badoc A, Patrick M, Lamarti A. Mineral composition of mature carob (Ceratonia siliqua L.) pod: study. Int Food Sci Nutr Eng 2017;7(4):91–103.

[10] Sharma P, Sharma S, Ramakrishna G, Srivastava H, Gaikwad K. A comprehensive review on leguminous galactomannans: structural analysis, functional properties, biosynthesis process and industrial applications. Crit Rev Food Sci Nutr 2020;1–24.

[11] Karababaa E, Coskuner Y. Physical properties of carob bean (Ceratonia siliqua L.): an industrial gum yielding crop. Ind Crop Prod 2013;42:440–6.

[12] Boublenza I, AEl H, Ghezlaoui S, Mahdad M, Vasai F, Chemat F. Algerian carob (Ceratonia siliqua L.) populations. Morphological and chemical variability of their fruits and seeds. Sci Hortic 2019;256:108537.

[13] Dionisio M, Grenha A. Locust bean gum: exploring its potential for biopharmaceutical applications. J Pharm Bioallied Sci 2012;4(3):175–85.

[14] Prajapati VD, Jani GK, Moradiya NG, Randeria NP, Nagar BJ. Locust bean gum: a versatile biopolymer. Carbohydr Polym 2013;94:814–21.

[15] Barak S, Mudgil D. Locust bean gum: processing, properties and food applications—a review. Int J Biol Macromol 2014;66:74–80.

[16] Giri TK, Pure S, Tripathi DK. Synthesis of graft copolymers of acrylamide for locust bean gum using microwave energy: swelling behavior, flocculation characteristics and acute toxicity study. Polimeros 2015;25(2):168–74.

[17] Singh RS, Kaur N, Rana V, Singla RK, Kang N, Kaur G, Kaur H, Kennedy JF. Carbamoylethyl locust bean gum: synthesis, characterization and evaluation of its film forming potential. Int J Biol Macromol 2020;149:348–58.

[18] Rashmi B, Sushil YR, Krishna M, Biswanath S, Srinivas M, Kakarla RR, Kusal KD, Mallanagouda SB, Raghavendra VK. Novel pH-sensitive interpenetrated network polyspheres of polyacrylamide-g-locust bean gum and sodium alginate for intestinal targeting of ketoprofen: in vitro and in vivo evaluation. Colloids Surf B: Biointerfaces 2019;362–70.

[19] Venkataraju MP, Gowda DV, Rajesh KS. Xanthan and locust bean gum (from Ceratonia siliqua) matrix tablets for oral controlled delivery of metoprolol tartrate. Curr Drug Ther 2008;3(1):70–7.

[20] Venkataraju MP, Gowda DV, Rajesh KS, Shiva KH. Xanthan and locust bean gum (from Ceratonia siliqua) matrix tablets for oral controlled delivery of propranolol hydrochloride. Asian J Pharm Sci 2007;2(6):239–48.

[21] Dunstan DE, Cheng Y, Liao ML, Salvatore R, Boger DV, Prica M. Structure and rheology of the κ-carrageenan/locust bean gum gels. Food Hydrocoll 2001;15(4-6):475–84.

[22] Copetti G, Lapasin R, Grassi M, Pricl S. Synergistic gelation of xanthan gum with locust bean gum: a rheological investigation. Glycoconj J 1997;14:951–61.

[23] Martins JT, Cerqueira MA, Bourbon AI, Pinheiro AC, Souza BWS, Vicente AA. Synergistic effects between κ-carrageenan and locust bean gum on physicochemical properties of edible films made thereof. Food Hydrocoll 2012;29:280–9.

[24] Hayrabolulu H, Sen M, Celik G, Kavaklı PA. Synthesis of carboxylated locust bean gum hydrogels by ionizing radiation. Radiat Phys Chem 2014;94:240–4.

[25] Akkaya NE, Ergun C, Saygun A, Yesilcubuk N, Akel-Sadoglu N, Kavakli IH, Turkmen HS, Giz HC. New biocompatible antibacterial wound dressing candidates; agar-locust bean gum and agar salep films. Int J Biol Macromol 2020;430–8.

[26] Pandey S, Do JY, Kim J, Kang M. Fast and highly efficient removal of dye from aqueous solution using natural locust bean gum-based hydrogels as adsorbent. Int J Biol Macromol 2020;143:60–75.

[27] Karine MZ, Maryane MM, Morgana SM, Julia MH, Fernando DPM, Marina GM, Ana LZ, Luiz AK. Smart wound dressing based on κ-Carrageenan/locust bean gum/cranberry extract for monitoring bacterial infections. Carbohydr Polym 2019;362–70.

[28] He H, Ye J, Zhang X, Huang Y, Li X, Xiao M. κ-Carrageenan/locust bean gum as hard capsule gelling agents. Carbohydr Polym 2017;175:417–24.

[29] Hsiung C. Xanthan gum and locust bean gum in confectionery use. US4219582; 1979.

[30] Achterkamp G, Ackermann DKK, Inoue C, Kohlus R, Kuhn M. Packaged concentrate for preparing a bouillon, soup, sauce, gravy or for use as a seasoning, the concentrate comprising xanthan and locust bean gum. US20080299267; 2008.

[31] Fabre B, Christel FP. Cosmetic composition containing a locust bean gum hydrolysate. US20110256087; 2009.

[32] Carafa M, Marianecci C, Di Marzio L, Rinaldi F, Meo C, Matricardi P, Alhaique F, Coviello T. A new vesicle-loaded hydrogel system suitable for topical applications: preparation and characterization. J Pharm Pharm Sci 2011;14(3):336–46.

[33] Murali R, Thanikaivelan P. Bionic, porous, functionalized hybrid scaffolds with vascular endothelial growth factor promote rapid wound healing in Wistar albino rats. RSC Adv 2016;6:19252–64.

[34] Yatmaz E, Turhan I. Carob as a carbon source for fermentation technology. Biocatal Agric Biotechnol 2018;16:200–8.

[35] Catarino F. The carob tree: an exemplary plant. Naturopathy 1993;73:14–5.

[36] Barracosa P, Lima MB, Cravador A. Analysis of genetic diversity in Portuguese *Ceratonia siliqua* L. Cultivars using RAPD and AFLP markers. Sci Hortic 2008;189–99.

[37] Albanell E, Caja G, Plaixats J. Characterization of carob fruits (*Ceratonia siliqua* L.), cultivated in Spain for agroindustrial use. Int Tree Crops J 1996;9(1):1–9.

[38] Vardar Y, Secmen O, Ozturk M. Some distributional problems and biological characteristics of ceratonia in Turkey. Port Acta Biol 1980;16:75–86.

[39] Yatmaz E, Turhan I. Carob as a carbon source for fermentation technology. Biocatal Agric Biotechnol 2018;16:200–8.

[40] Sebastien G, Christophe B, Mario A, Pascal L, Michel P, Aurore R. Impact of purification and fractionation process on the chemical structure and physical properties of locust bean gum. Carbohydr Polym 2014;108:159–68.

[41] Kok MS, Hill SE, Mitchell JR. Viscosity of galactomannans during high temperature processing: influence of degradation and solubilisation. Food Hydrocoll 1999;13(6):535–42.

[42] Kok MS. A comparative study on the compositions of crude and refined locust bean gum: in relation to rheological properties. Carbohydr Polym 2007;70:68–76.

[43] Dakia P, Blecker C, Robert C, Whatelet B, Paquot M. Composition and physicochemical properties of locust bean gum extracted from whole seeds by acid or water dehulling pre-treatment. Food Hydrocoll 2008;22:807–18.

[44] Richarsdon P, Willmer J, Foster T. Dilute properties of guar and locust bean gum in sucrose solutions. Food Hydrocoll 1998;12:339–48.

[45] Verma A, Tiwari A, Panda PK, Sharaf S, Jain A, Jain SK. Locust bean gum in drug delivery application. Chapter 8, In: Natural polysaccharides in drug delivery and biomedical applications; 2019. p. 203–22.

[46] Ayaz FA, Torun H, Glew RH, Bak ZD, Chuang LT, Presley JM, Andrews R. Nutrient content of carob pod (*Ceratonia silique* L.) flour prepared commercially and domestically. Plant Foods Hum Nutr 2009;64:286–92.

[47] Benkovic M, Belscak-Cvitanovik A, Bauman I, Komes D, Srecec S. Flow properties and chemical composition of carob (*Ceratonia siliqua* L.) flours as related to particle size and seed presence. Food Res Int 2017;100:211–8.

[48] Srivastava M, Kapoor V. Seed galactomannans: an overview. Chem Biodivers 2005;2:295–317.

[49] Kıvrak NE, Askın B, Kucukone E. Comparison of some physicochemical properties of locust bean seeds gum extracted by acid and water pre-treatments. Food Nutr Sci 2015;6:278–86.

[50] Rtibi K, Selmi S, Grami D, Amri M, Eto B, El-benna J, Sebai H, Marzouki L. Chemical constituents and pharmacological actions of carob pods and leaves (*Ceratoia siliqua* L.) on the gastrointestinal tract: a review. Biomed Pharmacother 2017;93:522–8.

[51] Stavrou IJ, Christou A, Kapnissi-Christodoulou CP. Polyphenols in carobs: a review on their composition, antioxidant capacity and cytotoxic effects, and health impact. Food Chem 2018;269:355–74.

[52] Feng B, Peng J, Zhang W, Ning X, Guo Y, Zhang W. Use of locust bean gum in flotation separation of chalcopyrite and talc. Miner Eng 2018;122:79–83.

[53] Lakkab I, HEL H, Lachkar N, BEL B, Lachkar M, Ciobica A. Phytochemistry, bioactivity: suggestion of *Ceratonia siliqua* L. as neurodegenerative disease therapy. J Complement Integr Med 2018;15(4), 20180013.

[54] Mirhosseini H, Amid BT. A review study on chemical composition and molecular structure of newly plant gum exudates and seed gums. Food Res Int 2012;46(1):387–98.

[55] Sharma BR, Dhuldhoya NC, Merchant SN. Glimpses of galactomannans. Science Tech Entrepreneur 2008;3:1–10.

[56] Mao CF. Self- and cross-associations in two-component mixed polymer gels. J Polym Sci B Polym Phys 2008;46:80–91.

[57] Richarsdon PH, Willmer J, Foster TJ. Dilute solution properties of guar and locust bean gum in sucrose solutions. Food Hydrocoll 1998;12(3):339–48.

[58] Prajapati VD, Jani GK, Moradiya NG, Randeria NP, Nagar BJ, Naikwadi NN, Variya BC. Galactomannan: a versatile biodegradable seed polysaccharide. Int J Biol Macromol 2013;60:83–92.

[59] Oliveira F, Monteiro SR, Barros-Timmons A, Lopes-da-Silva JA. Weak-gel formation in dispersions of silica particles in a matrix of a non-ionic polysaccharide: structure and rheological characterization. Carbohydr Polym 2010;82:1219–27.

[60] Chakravorty A, Barman G, Mukherjee S, Sa B. Effect of carboxymethylation on rheological and drug release characteristics of locust bean gum matrix tablets. Carbohydr Polym 2016;144:50–8.

[61] Parvathy KS, Susheelamm NS, Tharanathan RN, Gaonkar AK. A simple non-aqueous method for carboxymethylation of galactomannans. Carbohydr Polym 2005;62:137–41.

[62] Soma PK, Williams PD, Lo YM. Advancements in non-starch polysaccharides research for frozen foods and microencapsulation of probiotics. Front Chem Eng China 2009;3:413–26.

[63] Dakiaa PA, Bleckerb C, Roberta C, Wathaleta B, Paquot M. Composition and physicochemical properties of locust bean gum extracted from whole seeds by acid or water dehulling pre-treatment. Food Hydrocoll 2008;22:807–18.

[64] Maiti S, Chowdhury M, Chakraborty A, Ray S, Sa B. Sulfated locust bean gum hydrogel beads for immediate analgesic effect of tramadol hydrochloride. J Sci Ind Res 2014;73:21–8.

[65] Maiti S, Chowdhury M, Datta R, Ray S, Sa B. Novel gastroulcer protective micro(hydro)gels of sulfated locust bean gum-aluminium complex for immediate release of diclofenac sodium. J Drug Target 2013;21(3):265–76.

[66] Dey P, Sa B, Maiti S. Carboxymethyl ethers of locust bean gum—a review. Int J Pharm Pharm Sci 2011;3:4–7.

[67] Slaughter BV, Khurshid SS, Fisher OZ, Khademhosseini A, Peppas NA. Hydrogels in regenerative medicine. Adv Mater 2009;21:3307.

[68] Maiti S, Banik A, Sa B, Ray S, Kaity S. Tailoring of locust bean gum and development of hydrogel beads for controlled oral delivery of glipizide. Drug Deliv 2010;17(5):288–300.

[69] Sudhakar Y, Kuotsu K, Bandyopadhyay AK. Buccal bioadhesive drug delivery—a promising option for orally less efficient drugs. J Control Release 2006;114:15–40.

[70] Braz L, Grenha A, Corvo MC, Lourenco JP, Ferreira D, Sarmento B, da Costa AMR. Synthesis and characterization of locust bean gum derivatives and their application in the production of nanoparticles. Carbohydr Polym 2018;181:974–85.

[71] Simoesa J, Nunesb FM, Dominguesa MR, Coimbra MA. Demonstration of the presence of acetylation and arabinose branching as structural features of locust bean gum galactomannans. Carbohydr Polym 2011;86:1476–83.

[72] Kaity S, Isaac J, Kumar PM, Bose A, Wong TW, Ghosh A. Microwave assisted synthesis of acrylamide grafted locust bean gum and its application in drug delivery. Carbohydr Polym 2013;98(1):1083–94.

[73] Doyle JP, Giannouli P, Martin EJ, Brooks M, Morris ER. Effect of sugars, galactose content and chain length on freeze–thaw gelation of galactomannans. Carbohydr Polym 2006;64(3):391–401.

[74] Braz L, Grenha A, Ferreira D, Rosa da Costa A, Sarmento B. Locust bean gum derivatives for nanometric drug delivery. Rev Port Farm 2011;52(6 Suppl):127–8.

[75] Dey P, Maiti S, Sa B. Novel etherified locust bean gum-alginate hydrogels for controlled release of glipizide. J Biomater Sci Polym Ed 2013;24(6):663–83.

[76] Samavati V, Razavi SH, Rezaei KA. Intrinsic viscosity of locust bean gum and sweeteners mixture in dilute solutions. Electron J Environ Agric Food Chem 2007;6:1879–89.

[77] Karadag E, Saraydin D, Sahiner N, Guven O. Radiation induced acrylamide/citric acid hydrogels and their swelling behaviors. J Macromol Sci Pure Appl Chem 2001;38(11):1105–21.

[78] Hadinugroho W, Suwaldi M, Achmad F, Sugeng R. Study of a catalyst of citric acid cross-linking on locust bean gum. J Chem Technol Metall 2017;52(6):1086–91.

[79] Hadinugroho W, Martodihardjo S, Fudholi A, Riyanto S. Esterification of citric acid with locust bean gum. Helion 2019;5(8), e02337.

[80] Upadhyay M, Adena SKR, Vardhan H, Pandey S, Mishra B. Development and optimization of locust bean gum and sodium alginate interpenetrating polymeric network of capecitabine. Drug Dev Ind Pharm 2018;44(3):511–21.

[81] Harshal AP, Lalitha KG, Ruckmani K. Alginate beads of captopril using galactomannan containing senna tora gum, guar gum and locust bean gum. Int J Biol Macromol 2015;119–31.

[82] Upadhyay M, Vardhan H, Mishra B. Natural polymers composed mucoadhesive interpenetrating buoyant hydrogel beads of capecitabine: development, characterization and in vivo scintigraphy. J Drug Deliv Sci Technol 2020;55:101480.

[83] Tanaka R, Hatakeyama T, Hatakeyama H. Formation of locust bean gum hydrogel by freezing-thawing. Polym Int 1998;45:118–26.

[84] Turquois T, Doublier J, Taravel F, Rochas C. Synergy of the κ-carrageenan-carob galactomannan blend inferred from rheological studies. Int J Biol Macromol 1994;16:105–7.

[85] Cairns P, Miles MJ, Morris VJ, Brownsey GJ. X-Ray fiber-diffraction studies of synergistic, binary polysaccharide gels. Carbohydr Res 1987;160:411–23.

[86] Wu Y, Li W, Cui W, Eskin NAM, Goff HD. A molecular modeling approach to understand conformation–functionality relationships of galactomannans with different mannose/galactose ratios. Food Hydrocoll 2012;26(2):359–64.

[87] Wu Y, Cui W, Eskin NAM, Goff HD. An investigation of four commercial galactomannans on their emulsion and rheological properties. Food Res Int 2009;42(8):1141–6.

[88] Gadkari PV, Tu S, Chiyarda K, Reaney MJT, Ghosh S. Rheological characterization of fenugreek gum and comparison with other galactomannans. Int J Biol Macromol 2018;119:486–95.

[89] El-Batal H, Hasib A, Ouatmane A, Jaouad A, Naimi M. Rheology and influence factor of locust bean gum solution. Rev Genie Ind 2012;8:55–62.

[90] Lv Y, Pan Z, Song C, Chen Y, Qian X. Locust bean gum/gellan gum double-network hydrogels with superior self–healing and pH-driven shape–memory properties. Soft Matter 2019;30:1–9.

[91] Sandolo C, Coviello T, Matricardi P, Alhaique F. Characterization of polysaccharide hydrogels for modified drug delivery. Eur Biophys J 2007;36:693–700.

[92] Rana V, Kamboj S, Sharma R, Singh K. Modification of gums: synthesis techniques and pharmaceutical benefits. In: Thakur VK, Thakur MK, editors. Handbook of polymers for pharmaceutical technologies: biodegradable polymers. Beverly: Scrivener Publishing; 2015. p. 299–364.

[93] Sharma S, Tiwari S. A review on biomacromolecular hydrogel classification and its applications. Int J Biol Macromol 2020;162:737–47.

[94] Chung HJ, Park TG. Self-assembled and nanostructured hydrogels for drug delivery and tissue engineering. Nano Today 2009;4:429.

[95] Garner J, Park K. Chemically modified natural polysaccharide to form gels. In: Ramawat KG, Merillon JM, editors. Polysaccharides bioactivity and biotechnology. Springer; 2014. p. 1555–85.

[96] Ravat TH, Yardi V, Mallikarjunan N, Jamdar SN. Radiation processing of locust bean gum and assessing its functionality for applications in probiotic and enteral foods. LWT Food Sci Technol 2019;112(108228):1–8.

[97] Yoshida H, Hatakeyama T, Hatakeyama H. Phase transitions of the water-xanthan system. Polymer 1990;31(4):693–8.

[98] Hatakeyama T, Quinn FX, Hatakeyama H. Changes in freezing bound water in water-gellan systems with structure formation. Carbohydr Polym 1996;30(2-3):155–60.

[99] Hatakeyama T, Nakamura K, Yoshida H, Hatakeyama H. Mesomorphic properties of highly concentrated aqueous solutions of polyelectrolytes from saccharides. Food Hydrocoll 1989;3:301–11.

[100] Tanaka R, Hatakeyama T, Hatakeyama H. Differential scanning calorimetry studies on water restrained in hydroxyethylcellulose and hydrophobically modified hydroxyethylcellulose. Macromol Chem Phys 1997;198:883–98.

[101] Hatakeyama T, Yoshida H, Hatakeyama H. The liquid crystalline state of water-sodium cellulose sulphate systems studied by DSC and WAXS. Thermochim Acta 1995;266:343–54.

[102] Sougata J, Kalyan KS. Chitosan—locust bean gum interpenetrating polymeric network nanocomposites for delivery of aceclofenac. Int J Biol Macromol 2017;102:878–84.

[103] Prajapati VD, Jani GK, Moradiya NG, Randeria NP, Maheriya PM, Nagar BJ. Locust bean gum in the development of sustained release mucoadhesive macromolecules of aceclofenac. Carbohydr Polym 2014;113:138–48.

[104] Upadhyay M, Adena SKR, Vardhan H, Yadav SK, Mishra B. Locust bean gum and sodium alginate based interpenetrating polymeric network microbeads encapsulating capecitabine: improved pharmacokinetics, cytotoxicity &in vivo antitumor activity. Mater Sci Eng C Mater Biol Appl 2019;, 109958.

[105] Ganguly S, Das P, Das NC. Chapter 16. Characterization tools and techniques of hydrogels. Hydrogels based on natural polymers. Elsevier; 2020. p. 481–517.

[106] Deya P, Saa B, Maiti S. Impact of gelation period on modified locust bean-alginate interpenetrating beads for oral glipizide delivery. Int J Biol Macromol 2015;76:176–80.

[107] Kulkarni RV, Sa B. Enteric delivery of ketoprofen through functionally modified poly(acrylamide-grafted-xanthan)-based pH-sensitive hydrogel beads: preparation, in vitro and in vivo evaluation. J Drug Target 2008;16(2):167–77.

[108] Alhaique F, Santucci E, Carafa M, Coviello T, Murtas E, Riccieri FM. Gellan in sustained release formulations: preparation of gel capsules and release studies. Biomaterials 1996;17(20):1981–6.

[109] Kikuchi A, Kawabuchi M, Sugihara M, Sakurai Y, Okano T. Pulsed dextran release from calcium-alginate gel beads. J Control Release 1997;47:21–9.

[110] bibek L, Rimpa G, Sabyasachi M, Kalyan KS. Smart karaya-locust bean gum hydrogel particles for the treatment of hypertension: optimization by factorial design and pre-clinical evaluation. Carbohydr Polym 2019;274–88.

[111] Andressa AM, Guilherme LS, Maria RS. Effect of adding galactomannans on some physical and chemical properties of hyaluronic acid. Int J Biol Macromol 2020;527–35.

[112] Fatemeh SM, Rassoul K, Bahareh E, Arash K. Preparation and characterization of tragacanth-locust bean gum edible blend films. Carbohydr Polym 2016;139:20–7.

[113] Yoshinori T, Hideki T, Koichiro N. Molecular dynamics study of polymer–water interaction in hydrogels. 2. Hydrogen-bond dynamics. Macromolecules 1996;29(21):6761–9.

[114] Tarus D, Hachet E, Messager L, Catargi B, Ravaine V, Auzely-Velty R. Readily prepared dynamic hydrogels by combining phenyl boronic acid- and maltose-modified anionic polysaccharides at neutral pH. Macromol Rapid Commun 2014;35:2089–95.

[115] Kennedy JRM, Kent KE, Brown JR. Rheology of dispersions of xanthan gum, locust bean gum and mixed biopolymer gel with silicon dioxide nanoparticles. Mater Sci Eng C 2015;48:347–53.

[116] Malviya R, Sharma PK, Dubey SK. Modification of polysaccharides: pharmaceutical and tissue engineering applications with commercial utility (patents). Mater Sci Eng C 2016;68:929–38.

[117] Chinta M, Obireddy SR, Areti P, Subbarao SMC, Kashayi CR, Rapoli JK. Sodium alginate/locust bean gum-g-methacrylic acid IPN hydrogels for simvastatin drug delivery. J Dispers Sci Technol 2019;0193–2691.

[118] Parikka K, Ansari F, Hietala S, Tenkanen M. Thermally stable hydrogels from enzymatically oxidized polysaccharides. Food Hydrocoll 2012;26:212–20.

[119] Al-Assaf S, Phillips GO, Williams PA, DuPlessis TA. Application of ionizing radiations to produce new polysaccharides and proteins with enhanced functionality. Nucl Inst Methods Phys Res B 2007;265:37–43.

[120] Xiang J, Shena L, Hong Y. Status and future scope of hydrogels in wound healing: synthesis, materials and evaluation. Eur Polym J 2020;130:109609.

[121] Sandolo C, Coviello T, Matricardi P, Alhaique F. Characterization of polysaccharide hydrogels for modified drug delivery. Eur Biophys J 2007;36(7):693–700.

[122] Raghuwanshi VS, Garnier G. Characterisation of hydrogels: linking the nano to the microscale. Adv Colloid Interf Sci 2019;274:102044.

[123] Hanna K, Goutham P, Kevin W, Fadi A. Effects of xanthan-locust bean gum mixtures on the physicochemical properties and oxidative stability of whey protein stabilised oil-in-water emulsions. Food Chem 2015;340–8.

[124] Ngwuluka NC, Choonara YE, Kumar P, du Toit LC, Modi G, Pillay V. A co-blended locust bean gum and polymethacrylate-NaCMC matrix to achieve zero-order release via hydro-erosive modulation. AAPS PharmSciTech 2015;16(6):1377–89.

[125] Harikrishnan V, Madhusudhan S, Santhiagu A. Evaluation of a novel, natural locust bean gum as a sustained release and mucoadhesive component of tizanidine hydrochloride buccal tablets. Asian J Pharm Clin Res 2015;8(6):7–10.

[126] Aydinli M, Tutas M, Bozdemir OA. Mechanical and light transmittance properties of locust bean gum based edible films. Turk J Chem 2004;28:163–71.

[127] Banerjee S, Bhattacharya S. Food gels: gelling process and new applications. Crit Rev Food Sci Nutr 2012;52:334–46.

[128] Bielskis E. Method of increasing cold water solubility of locust bean gum. US3855149; 1972.

[129] Karl CL. Hydroxyalkyl locust bean/xanthomonas hydrophilic colloid blends. US4038206; 1976.

[130] Lin S-L, Pramoda MK. Locust bean gum therapeutic compositions. US4136178A; 1977.

[131] Karl HO, Tiefenthaler N, Erich WK. Phosphated locust bean gums. US4162925; 1978.

[132] Sugden K. Buccal tablet comprising etorphine or a salt thereof. US4829056; 1987.

[133] Baichwal AR, Staniforth JN. Controlled release verapamil tablets. US5169639; 1991.

[134] Benito VJB, Sanchez AD, Viadel MLH, Serrano SA, Picornell JAR. Molecular methods for detecting guar gum additions to locust bean gum. US7037653; 2001.

[135] Gibbs CD, Parry AJ, Rogers SH. Detergent compositions. US7179782; 2004.

[136] Sierakowaski MR, Milas M, Desbrieres J, Rinacedo M. Specific modifications of galactomannans. Carbohydr Polym 2000;42:51–7.

[137] Vijayaraghavan C, Vasanthakumar S, Ramakrishnan A. In-vitro and in-vivo evaluation of locust bean gum and chitosan combination as a carrier for buccal drug delivery. Pharmazie 2008;63:342–7.

[138] Alves AD, Cavaco JS, Guerrero F, Lourenco JP, Costa AMR, Grehna A. Inhalable antitubercular therapy medicated by locust bean gum microparticles. Molecules 2016;, 21060702.

[139] Suzuki S, Lim JK. Microencapsulation with carrageenan-locust bean gum mixture in a multiphase emulsification technique for sustained drug release. J Microencapsul 1994;11(2):197–203.

[140] Perestrelo AR, Grehna A, Rosa da Costa AM, Belo JA. Locust bean gum as an alternative polymeric coating for embryonic stem cell culture. Mater Sci Eng C 2014;336–44.

8

Inulin-based hydrogel

Moumita Das Kirtania[a], Nancy Kahali[b], and Arindam Maity[c]

[a]School of Pharmaceutical Technology, Adamas University, Kolkata, West Bengal, India, [b]Sister Nivedita University, Kolkata, West Bengal, India, [c]Department of Pharmaceutical Technology, JIS University, Kolkata, West Bengal, India

8.1 Introduction

Inulin is a natural polysaccharide that has been discovered about two centuries ago and since then has been widely used in various applications because of its several beneficial properties. It has been found and extracted from various natural sources such as chicory, dandelion root, salisfy, Jerusalem artichoke, and asparagus root and various fruits and vegetables such as banana, wheat, barley, garlic, and onion [1, 2].

Industrially, inulin is produced from plants such as chicory. Besides, dahlia and Jerusalem artichoke are also used (Fig. 8.1) [3]. But most commonly, it is obtained from chicory. Chicory belongs to the family of Asteraceae and is a biennial plant. The chicory plant grows initially when we can see only leaves and roots, which may be fibrous or tap roots. Thereafter, the roots appear as sugar beets, which are small and oblong shaped [4]. Fresh chicory roots generally have about 13%–23% inulin, and dried chicory roots contain about 98% inulin by weight.

Inulin is mainly extracted from chicory roots in a three-step process of extraction, purification, and spray drying to produce fine powder. In the first stage, an extraction is done, and raw syrup is obtained by initial filtration process. In the second stage, the extract is refined further and purified. Finally, by spray drying process, it is converted into a fine powder. Nowadays, production of inulin is done by advanced techniques using ultrasound, simultaneous ultrasonic/microwave supercritical carbon dioxide (CO_2), and pulsed electric field (PEF) to get a higher yield of purified product with less energy consumption [5].

Plant and Algal Hydrogels for Drug Delivery and Regenerative Medicine
https://doi.org/10.1016/B978-0-12-821649-1.00005-2

a   b

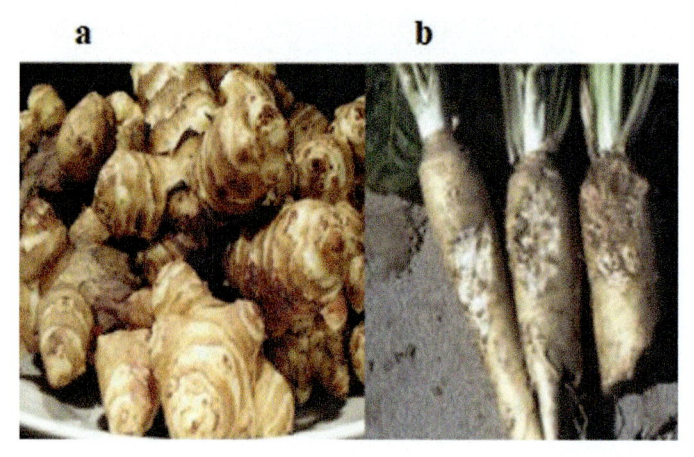

FIG. 8.1 Sources for inulin extraction. (A) Jerusalem artichoke tubers, (B) chicory roots. *Reprinted from Zhu Z, He J, Liu G, Barba FJ, Koubaa M, Ding L, Bals O, Grimi N, Vorobiev E, Recent insights for the green recovery of inulin from plant food materials using nonconventional extraction technologies: a review. Innov Food Sci Emerg Technol 2016;33:1–9, Copyright (2016), with permission from Elsevier.*

8.1.1 Importance of inulin

The polysaccharide has been widely used in various applications related to food, drug delivery, or diagnostics (Fig. 8.2).

The importance of the polysaccharide in various fields can be observed from the discussion further.

1. Inulin has been used as a prebiotic because it is indigestible in the acidic environment of stomach or alkaline environment of small intestine but degraded only in the large intestine by the huge microbial population. Therefore it is also used in colon-targeted drug delivery. About 25% of the bacteria in the gut constitutes of inulinase-producing bifidobacteria, which can cause the breakdown of inulin. Furthermore, the polysaccharide is believed to have bifidogenic activity that causes enhancement of growth of bifidobacteria and, thus, known to be beneficial for health. Bifidobacteria can restrict harmful bacteria to grow in the cecum and, thus, protect the body against them, reducing the chances of infection and decreasing inflammation (Fig. 8.3) [6]. Even the risk of cancer gets reduced in the gut because of the enhancement of cellular immunity. Furthermore, the risk of diabetes, obesity, and heart disease may be reduced because of better metabolism of carbohydrates and fats reducing the amounts of cholesterol, triglycerides, and phospholipids in blood [7].
2. Inulin acts as a dietary fiber and reduces gastric transit time.

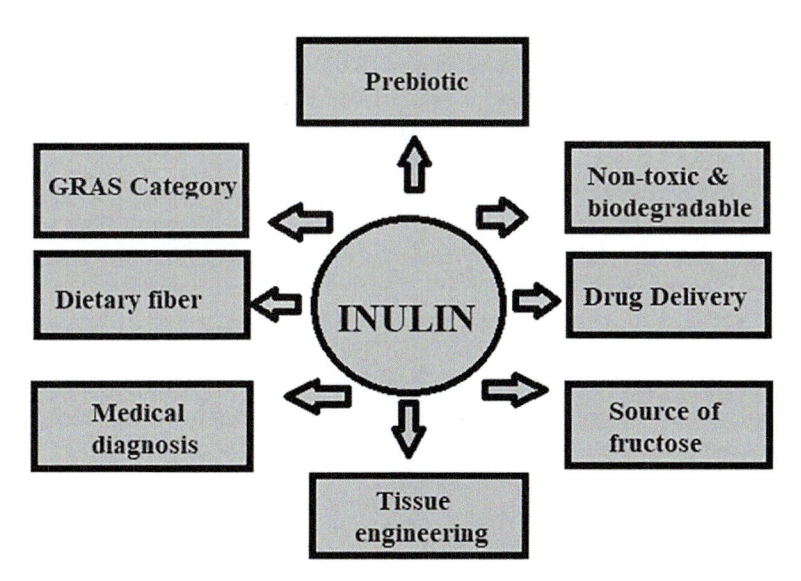

FIG. 8.2 Importance of inulin.

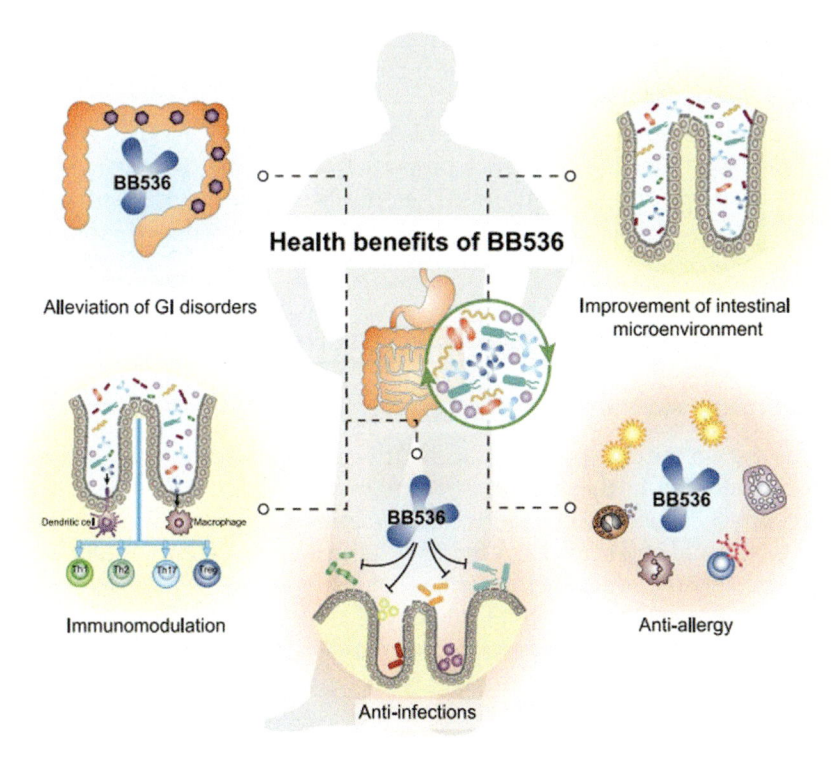

FIG. 8.3 Health benefits of Bifidobacterium BB536. *Reprinted from Wong CB, Odamaki T, Xiao JZ, Beneficial effects of Bifidobacterium longum subsp. longum BB536 on human health: modulation of gut microbiome as the principal action. J Funct Foods 2019;54:506–519, Copyright (2019), with permission from Elsevier.*

3. Traditionally, inulin has found application in drug delivery including solid dispersions, hydrogels, nasal drug delivery systems, parenteral drug delivery systems, colon-targeted delivery systems, intramuscular delivery systems, vaccine formulations, or controlled delivery through inulin complex formation. As research proceeds, newer applications of the polymer in drug delivery are coming into the forefront [1].
4. Inulin also finds application in the food industry as a replacement for fat and sugar. It is a potential source of fructose, which serves as the alternate sweetening agent for sucrose. It has also been used for citric acid, bioethanol, single cell protein synthesis, etc. It is also used in industries dealing with dairy products such as milk, cheese, yogurt, and ice cream and nondairy products such as biscuits, cereals, and meat products. The polysaccharide is approved by the Food and Drug Administration and falls under the generally recognized as safe (GRAS) category [1, 2].
5. It is used to improve organoleptic properties and to increase viscosity of various dosage forms and food products.
6. The polymer has also been used in medical diagnostics for evaluation of filtration through the glomerulus. The test is used for the determination of the filtration efficiency through the glomerulus. Inulin is used in the test because it passes the glomerulus almost completely [1].
7. Inulin is biocompatible, biodegradable, and nontoxic and has good water solubility. Owing to such properties, it is also being explored in tissue engineering as scaffolds. The polysaccharide can be chemically modified with ease because of flexible furanose and hydroxyl groups [8].

8.2 Physicochemical properties

8.2.1 Structure and morphology

Inulin is a natural polysaccharide. It is obtained from natural sources and is included in the fructan family. Chemically, it consists of fructose units attached with $(2 \rightarrow 1)$-β-glycosidic bonds, and a D-glycosyl moiety at the terminal end (Fig. 8.4). Owing to its structural pattern, inulin is not digested in small intestine of human beings but undergoes fermentation in large intestine by intestinal microflora. This nature is because of the presence of β-(2–1) D-frutosyl fructose bonds in between β configuration of anomeric carbon and the fructose units of inulin [9].

It is present in around 45,000 species of plants, fruits, vegetables, and roots [10]. Inulin has been found to produce various shapes of crystals by cooling with Fibruline instant [11]. Furthermore, a fivefold helical structure was observed within the crystal structure of inulin, as found by

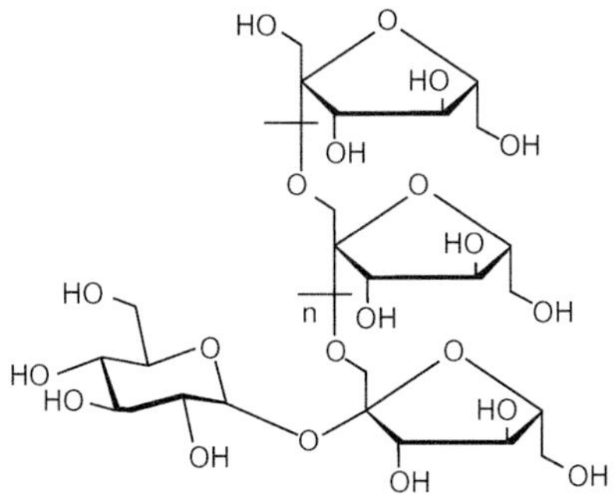

FIG. 8.4 Structure of inulin.

Marchessault et al. [12]. Inulin is marketed mostly in the amorphous form. However, above the glass transition temperature, the molecules become more mobile and change into crystalline structure.

8.2.2 Use in the food industry: Suitable physicochemical properties

Inulin has very high oil-holding capacity and acts as a stabilizer for different high fat-containing materials. Inulin obtained from different sources shows different colors because of variable amounts of phenolic compounds present with different pH (5.53 ± 0.05) [13]. Food materials containing inulin may help to increase mineral absorption in the body [14]. The long-chain inulin can produce microcrystals. When it is mixed with milk or water, a cream-like texture is obtained with fatty properties, and thus it is widely used in replacement of fat- and sugar-containing food products. Few examples include baked items, confectionaries, fillings, spreads, and salad dressings [15].

It also helps in the improvement of texture of yogurt and used as a thickener or bulking agent for mayonnaise, chocolate products, ice cream, and sandwich [16]. Inulin can replace prebiotics in yogurts and pass through the stomach to contribute to colon microflora [17].

Generally, inulin offers no aftertaste and can be used as a dietary fiber having fructose chains from 2 to 60 monomers, for which we get very little sweet taste. However, chicory inulin has around 10% of sweetness level compared with that in sucrose [18].

8.2.3 Solubility

The solubility of inulin is temperature mediated. At 10°C, the solubility is around 6%; however, at 90°C, it is around 35%. Although long-chain inulin is slightly soluble, chicory inulin is moderately dissolved in water [19].

The solubility of inulin gets lowered with increasing molecular weight. The poor solubility of high-molecular weight fraction may improve at high temperatures [20]. Generally, the solubility of polymers decreases with their degree of polymerization [2]. Four polymorphs of crystalline inulin named as α, β, γ, and δ were identified by a group of researchers, which varied in their solubility. The β inulin was soluble at room temperature readily, whereas the other forms dissolved at much higher temperatures. They also varied in stability in the following order: β, α, γ, and δ [21, 22]. Inulin is poorly soluble in ethanol, whereas freely soluble and sparingly soluble in dimethylsulfoxide and isopropanol, respectively [21, 23]. Inulin is insoluble in water at room temperature. However, at 80°C, the water solubility is 280 mg/mL [24].

8.2.4 Degree of polymerization

Inulin has a degree of polymerization (DP) greater than 10, which results in a hydrophobic characteristic of it. The high DP and branching characteristics present different physicochemical and functional properties of inulin, such as glass transition temperature, melting point, gelation properties and gel integrity, which improve the versatility of the applications of inulin [25, 26]. The molecular weights of inulin obtained from various sources were found to vary with the degree of polymerization. Most physicochemical properties of inulin depend on its degree of polymerization [2]. The main difference between naturally sourced and synthetic inulin was in the polydispersity. It was lower for synthetic inulin [27].

8.2.5 Viscosity

The viscosity of inulin depends directly on its solution concentration. It was found that when the concentration of inulin was increased up to 30%, the viscosity also increased simultaneously, but no gelling occured. At temperatures above 80°C, inulin viscosity increased because solubility of the polysaccharide is higher at elevated temperatures [28, 29].

The viscosity of inulin increases with higher molecular weights. The viscosity also increases with the increase in amount of solvent such as dimethylsulfoxide and decreases with the addition of salt [2].

8.2.6 Gelling

Generally, the gel formation of inulin occurs when there is an interaction between the chains of the dissolved polymer. However, inulin gels are also found to contain microcrystals that are not dissolved. These undissolved microcrystals form a network among the other microcrystal particles, the solvent, and inulin particles and increase the strength of the gel [26, 28–32]. Formation of such microcrystals depends on the molecular weight of inulin and temperature, and thus these factors influence the formation of gels. It has been observed that better gels are produced by higher-molecular weight inulins compared with the lower-molecular weight inulins. Thus if the network formed is disturbed by reactions such as hydrolysis, the degree of polymerization decreases and, thus, reduces gel formation [33]. Furthermore, if the concentration of inulin is low, the presence of crystalline inulin is also low, and thus network formation is reduced, resulting in gels of lower mechanical strength [32].

Inulin gels can be produced by applying shear force or by thermal methods of heating and then cooling. Inulin gels formed by the later method were found to be smooth and strong compared with the former one [28, 33]. The factors on which gel formation of inulin depend were found to be temperature, concentration, pH, heating time, or addition of other solvents such as glycerol and ethanol. When other solvents were added, the polarity of the solutions decreased, which resulted in lower inulin–solvent interactions, and strong gel formation occurred faster. The concentration of inulin that is required for gelling was found to be dependent on temperature. It was found that a minimum temperature of 40°C was required for gel formation. But if the temperature was increased above 80°C at pH less than 3, then hydrolysis could occur due to which the gel strength reduced [28]. Furthermore, when the effect of degree of polymerization and concentration of inulin on gel strength was studied, it was observed that gels of higher mechanical strength were produced by higher-molecular weight inulins. The gels with higher-molecular weight inulins were produced at lower concentrations of inulin (Fig. 8.5) [2]. From the figure, it was observed that gels prepared with higher DP values of inulin

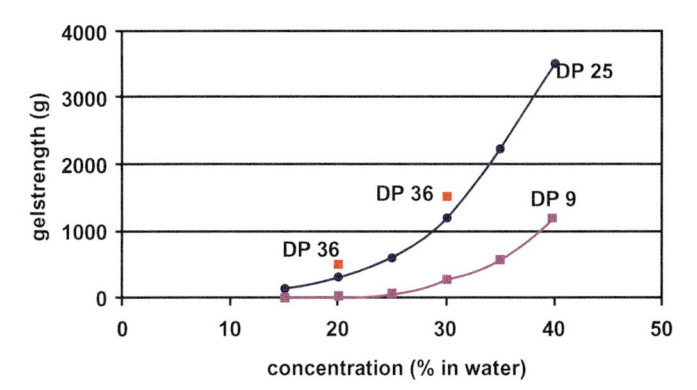

FIG. 8.5 Effect of concentration and degree of polymerization on gel strength. *Reprinted from Mensink, MA, Frijlink, HW, Maarschalk, KV, and Hinrichs WLJ. Inulin, a flexible oligosaccharide I: Review of its physicochemical characteristics. Carbohydr Polym, 2010;130:405–419, Copyright (2010), with permission from Elsevier.*

could be formed at lower concentrations. Furthermore, higher DP inulin hydrogels had more mechanical strength. When the solution concentration is in between the range of 30%–50%, the gelation characteristics are good. This may be because of discontinuous particles available in the solution. At 50% concentration of inulin, the gels become firm and rigid and have the ability to retain fat-like features [34].

It was also observed that by increasing the stress, the smoothness of the inulin gels could be improved. This may be because that at low stress, larger aggregates would have formed, which would be dispersed when stress was increased [28].

Inulin has also been modified to produce derivatives and then cross-linked to produce gels. For example, the methacrylated inulin gels have been used for colonic drug delivery at a controlled rate. Inulin has been modified and suitable side chains have been added, which are then cross-linked by free radical polymerization or other chemical cross-linkers. High mechanical strength and faster rates of formation of the hydrogels were observed because of higher amounts of cross-linking. Swelling of the hydrogels targeted for colon delivery is also critical because higher swelling is required for degradation of hydrogel by colonic bacteria and release of drug, whereas low swelling is required in the upper parts of gastrointestinal tract (GIT) such that drug release is minimum there [35–40].

Overall, the characteristics of inulin are ideal for using this material in hydrogel formation extensively.

8.3 Importance of inulin hydrogels in drug delivery

Hydrogels are polymeric networks that can absorb huge amount of aqueous fluids, usually greater than 20% of dry weight and swell without solubilizing and maintaining their integrity and structure. Hydrogels developed with natural polysaccharides, such as alginate, chitosan, or inulin, are biodegradable and biocompatible formulations, which are degraded enzymatically in the body.

Inulin hydrogels prepared by suitable cross-linking agents can retain their structural integrity in the upper parts of the GIT, mainly in the stomach and small intestine, and are broken down in the lower parts of the GIT because of the release of specific enzymes such as inulinase secreted by microbial flora, especially bifidobacteria. In essence, degradation of the hydrogels depends on the degree of cross-linking of the polymer. The lesser the cross-linking, the higher would be the degradation rate of the hydrogels. Inulin hydrogels have been specially explored for colon-targeted drug delivery because of the favorable characteristics. For colon-targeted delivery, the drug release should be maximized in the large intestine and be insignificant or minimum in the upper parts of the GIT. Drugs targeted for inflammatory bowel disease or cancers in the colon can be loaded onto biodegradable hydrogels like that of inulin for local release and action, which may also act as a safe and nontoxic medium. Inulin hydrogels can also be formulated to be pH sensitive by using suitable cross-linkers and processes [41]. Furthermore, the swelling rates of inulin hydrogels are high, as studied by Vervoort et al. [42]. However, the swelling characteristics may differ based on the method of preparation and inulin derivatives used in the study. A significant advantage of the inulin hydrogels is its biocompatibility. The hydrogels were evaluated as safe during cytotoxicity studies [8]. Furthermore, inulin hydrogels were also studied for tissue engineering applications because they are biocompatible and nontoxic. They can provide the required bulk and mechanical strength due to their swelling characteristics, permit easy diffusion of gases and nutrients required for the growth of cells, and help in cell adhesion. Thus they can be used as biodegradable scaffolds in tissue engineering.

8.4 Preparation of inulin hydrogels

Several formulations have been developed with inulin for various purposes related to drug delivery, including hydrogels, microparticles, micelles, liposomes, or solid dispersions. Inulin hydrogels have been tested for targeted and controlled drug delivery. Hydrogels have cross-linked structure and can absorb large amounts of water and swell in aqueous media. Inulin hydrogels have been developed using different techniques such as cross-linking the polymer with suitable agents called cross-linkers, radical polymerization, and condensation reactions. Some of the methods for preparation of inulin hydrogels are outlined further.

8.4.1 Ionotropic gelation method

Norudin et al. prepared alginate-inulin hydrogel beads using calcium chloride as the cross-linking agent for bovine serum albumin (BSA) delivery in a controlled manner. The hydrogel beads were prepared by dispersing the solution of alginate, inulin, and BSA into calcium chloride solution [43].

8.4.2 Free radical solution polymerization

Free radical polymerization is a method of formation of cross-linked polymers using free radicals generated in chemical reactions. The method is mainly used to synthesize polymers from monomers containing carbon double bonds. The method includes mainly three steps including initiation in which free radicals are generated; propagation in which the generated free radicals are added to the double bonds of the monomer to form polymer chains and termination to end the polymer chain propagation, when the free radicals undergo transfer, and combination of disproportionation reactions [44].

Free radical polymerization was used by Maris et al. to develop inulin-azo hydrogels. For the preparation, inulin was methacrylated (MA-IN) to introduce methacrylic groups in the polymer. MA-IN together with other monomers such as N,N-bis (methacryloylamino) azobenzene (BMAAB), azobisisobutyronitrile (AIBN), methyl methacrylate (MMA), methacrylic acid (MA), or 2-hydroxyethyl methacrylate (HEMA) were dissolved in dimethylformamide (solvent) to prepare solutions. The solutions were placed in cylindrical-shaped polypropylene molds and kept at 60°C for 8 h to produce the hydrogels by free radical polymerization method [40].

In yet another study, methacrylated inulin was synthesized, and their solutions were converted into cross-linked hydrogels by free radical polymerization. The initiator molecules used were ammonium persulfate and N,N,N',N'-tetramethylethylenediamine, which on reacting with methacrylated inulin, dissolved in phosphate buffer pH 6.5, resulted in cross-linked hydrogels [45].

8.4.3 Cross-linking of inulin derivatives with suitable cross-linking agents

Cross-linking of inulin derivatives with suitable cross-linkers can produce hydrogels with improved properties and characteristics. In one such study, oxidized inulin was used as the inulin derivative, which was prepared using sodium periodate that introduced aldehyde groups in the structure. The product was then reacted with adipic acid hydrazide (AAD) to produce the cross-linked hydrogel. The specific advantages were use of aqueous medium (phosphate buffer pH 7.4) instead of organic solvents, reduced time of cross-linking, and suitable erosion properties, which could be monitored effectively by change of cross-linker concentration [8].

Trimethylolpropane tris(3-mercaptopropionate) was used to cross-link inulin derivatives to yield hydrogels that were pH sensitive and compatible on Caco-2 cells and degraded by enzymes such as inulinase and esterase. Thus they were proven to be useful for colon-targeted delivery [46]. Caco-2 cells have been used in research studies as model of epithelial cells found in the intestines. Such cells were derived from colon carcinoma originally [47].

Divinylsulfone and inulin were reacted together to form the divinylsulfone derivative of inulin, which was then reacted with O,O'-bis(2-aminoethyl)poly(ethylene glycol) for cross-linking in phosphate buffer to obtain the hydrogel. Divinylsulfone was added to produce divinylsulfone derivative of inulin, which could be cross-linked [48].

Similarly, inulin-succinic acid derivatives were produced for insertion of carboxyl groups and then dissolved in water maintaining the pH at 6. N-ethyl-N(3-dimethylaminopropyl)-carbodiimidehydrochloride(EDC) and N-hydroxysulfosuccinimide (NHSS) were added, and the reaction was continued at 25°C for 1h. Thereafter, α,β-polyaspartylhydrazide was added for cross-linking. Hydrogels were obtained when the carboxyl groups of the inulin derivative react with hydrazide groups of the cross-linker. The hydrogels gave pH-dependent swelling. Suitable molar concentrations of the various agents were maintained to produce the hydrogels [7]. When inulin-succinic acid derivatives were produced, the resultant hydrogels were resistant to stomach pH and compatible in intestinal conditions [1].

Furthermore, ultraviolet radiation was used to cross-link an inulin derivative produced by reacting with methacrylic and succinic anhydrides to yield a pH-sensitive hydrogel. The cross-linking agent in this study was UV light [35].

8.5 Characterization and evaluation of inulin hydrogels

8.5.1 FTIR studies

Fourier Transform Infrared Spectroscopy studies are used to compare the structure of molecules based on the absorption of the constituent chemical groups. In case of inulin gels, FTIR studies are mainly used to confirm the formation of inulin derivatives during processing. Furthermore, interaction with loaded drugs is also studied. FTIR studies are usually conducted over a wavelength range of $400\text{--}4000\,cm^{-1}$. Samples are ground into fine powder and mixed with KBr and with the help of hydraulic press are pressed into pellets. Afinjuomo et al. oxidized inulin and thereafter cross-linked the oxidized derivative to prepare the hydrogels. FTIR studies were used to detect the structural changes after oxidation. The spectra for the raw inulin and the oxidized ones were similar except for the highly oxidized ones where some extra bands were observed. The positions of the bands changed within the region $1300\text{--}800\,cm^{-1}$. Hemiacetals formation was observed due to which the aldehyde groups were not visible clearly. The spectra for cross-linked hydrogel showed new band at $1550\,cm^{-1}$. Furthermore, drug-loaded hydrogels produced the spectrum with small changes and showed five new bands. A small interaction between the drug, 5-fluorouracil, and inulin hydrogels was observed, resulting in a new peak at 3317 cm. Finally, hydrogen bonding between the hydrogels and the drug caused many peaks of the drug to disappear in the spectrum for the drug-loaded hydrogels [8].

8.5.2 Thermogravimetric analysis and differential scanning calorimetry studies of hydrogels

Thermogravimetric analysis (TGA) studies are mainly done in thermogravimetric analyzer, and the differential scanning calorimetry (DSC) studies are done in differential scanning calorimeter in which the samples are heated over a wide range of temperature, usually in a nitrogen atmosphere passed at a rate of 10°C/min. Thermal degradation studies for inulin were done by Dan et al. In differential thermal analysis (DTA), the endothermic peak for inulin, signifying melting, was observed at 165°C, whereas in TGA studies, around 60% weight loss of the polymer was observed within the range of 225–325°C due to decomposition and gradual combustion of the polymer. In the DSC studies, a distinct peak was observed at 178°C, which leveled off after 180°C. The thermogram for the cooling curve was shaped a shallow concave and was further up from the heating curve. However, on heating above the melting temperature, an irreversible change occurred in the polymer [49]. Afinjuomo et al. performed the thermal degradation studies and compared the data for raw inulin, oxidized inulin, cross-linker, and the hydrogels. It was found that the thermal stability of the cross-linker was highest, and its degradation started at 282°C. Significant amount of weight reduction in inulin was observed between 225°C and 325°C, with onset of degradation from 215°C. However, the degradation for oxidized inulin started at around 192°C, around 25°C less than that for raw inulin, which may be due to damage in the structure of inulin because of oxidation. However, after the oxidized inulin was cross-linked, the thermal stability improved because of formation of hydrazone and hydrogen bonds in the cross-linked structure. The weight loss for the cross-linked inulin hydrogels was observed in three steps, the initial weight loss of around 7% being due to loss of free and bound water and then due to decomposition of inulin and cross-linking agent, respectively. The degradation temperature for the hydrogels increased at higher concentrations of cross-linking agent. Difference of the degradation temperature between the oxidized hydrogels and the cross-linked oxidized hydrogel confirmed the cross-linking reaction. In the DSC studies, the endothermic peaks for oxidized inulin hydrogel and the cross-linking agent were observed at 161.3°C and 183.22°C, respectively. However, the peaks were absent in the cross-linked inulin hydrogels, which were attributed to the formation of highly cross-linked new polymers [8].

8.5.3 Rheological evaluation

It is well observed that the rate of drug release from hydrogels would depend on the measure of viscosity of the hydrogel formulations. At higher levels of viscosity, the drug release from the hydrogels would be slower and controlled compared with hydrogels of low viscosity. Thus measurement of the viscosity of hydrogels is an important parameter during formulation. The viscosity of the hydrogels is usually tested in viscometers, such as the Brookfield viscometer, for evaluation of their viscoelastic characteristics. In a study by Pitaressi et al., methacrylated inulin hydrogels were prepared by UV irradiation with four different cross-linkers, which had an effect on the rate of cross-linking and the elasticity of the hydrogels. Furthermore, it was observed that drug molecules could be loaded onto the hydrogels without having an effect on the rheological properties [50].

8.5.4 Scanning electron microscope analysis

The scanning electron microscope (SEM) studies provide information regarding the surface morphology of the hydrogel formulations including the presence of pores, fissures, channels, or moisture. Afinjuomo et al. performed SEM studies and observed several pores that were connected by irregular channels. Furthermore, the pore size was found to decrease with higher concentrations of cross-linking agent because higher amounts of cross-linker resulted in more cross-linked structure of the hydrogels causing decrease in pore size. A significant observation revealed the increase in pore size when the hydrogels were placed in acetate buffer, pH 5.0, compared with phosphate buffer, pH 7.4, which confirmed hydrolysis of hydrazone bonds in acetate medium causing increase in pore size [8].

8.5.5 Swelling studies

The studies are undertaken to determine the swelling percent and the rate of swelling of the hydrogels. Amount of water absorbed by the hydrogels leading to their swelling is important. The dry hydrogel is weighed and added to water or aqueous buffer solutions and allowed to reach an equilibrium swelling stage, after which the swollen hydrogel is removed, extra water is dried off with tissue paper, and weighed again to determine the amount of water absorbed. The swelling percent is calculated thereafter. Vervoort et al. reported the swelling rates of the prepared inulin hydrogels to be quite high, the swelling times ranging from 0.44 h to 1.12 h. Swelling of the hydrogels was inversely proportional to the degree of substitution in the methycrylated inulin hydrogels. Furthermore, the equilibrium swelling ratios were unaltered in media, mimicking the conditions of the colon-containing enzymes such as esterases and that of small intestine; however, they were affected significantly in gastric medium [42].

8.5.6 Drug release studies

The evaluation of in vitro drug release is important because it give us an idea about the quantity and rate of drug release in GI fluids. Generally, buffer solutions that mimic the conditions in the GIT are prepared, and the hydrogel formulations containing the model drug is added. The release studies are performed in suitable dissolution apparatus. Aliquots or samples are taken at regular time intervals and assayed for quantification of drug that has been released into the medium. Afinjuomo et al. conducted the dissolution studies for cross-linked inulin hydrogels in Falcon tubes of 50 mL capacity, in which was added 10 mL of dissolution media such as sodium acetate buffer (pH 5.0) or phosphate buffer (pH 7.4) at 37°C and 50 rpm. HPLC analysis of the withdrawn samples was performed to determine the drug released [8]. Pitaressi et al. who prepared microparticles from inulin hydrogels dispersed them in 200 mL beakers containing 0.1 N HCl/Polysorbate 80 mixtures for 2 h at 100 rpm and then raised the pH of the medium to 6.8 using 1 M NaOH, in which the drug release studies were continued for 24 h. The drug samples were assayed through HPLC [50]. The drug dissolution data are further fitted into model equations for the first order, zero order, and Higuchi model or Korsmeyer-Peppas model to find out the release mechanism.

For colon-targeted delivery systems, often rat cecal contents or suitable enzymes are added to buffer solution, which mimics the colonic conditions, because the colon harbors diverse microflora and enzymes secreted by cells can degrade the structure of natural polysaccharides. Rat cecal contents have high amount of microorganisms that are present in human colon also, and, thus, would act on natural polymers such as inulin and cause degradation, releasing the drug in higher amounts. In some studies, inulinase enzymes have also been added, which cause the degradation of inulin to break down the hydrogel and release drug. The enzyme is commonly found in the human colon secreted by bifidobacterium, which consists of about 25% of microflora present in the colon. In a particular study, where inulin and shellac was used for film coating on drug-loaded pellets, rat cecal contents were added to phosphate buffer, mimicking colonic conditions. It was found that the drug release increased significantly when rat cecal contents were added to dissolution medium [51]. The degradation of inulin was tested by incubating the hydrogel with buffer media with or without the inulinase enzyme, which can cause degradation of inulin polysaccharide. At regular intervals, the hydrogels were taken out and weighed to determine the degradation of the polymer. Significant reduction of hydrogel weight was observed, which increased with time [8]. Furthermore, in another study by Mooter et al., it was observed that by adding inulinase enzyme to the dissolution medium, the release of BSA from cross-linked inulin hydrogels was enhanced [39].

In certain in vivo studies, the hydrogel formulations are fed in animal model, and after predetermined time interval, the animals are killed to evaluate the therapeutic efficacy of the formulations on the disease, manifested by reduced inflammation in the case of inflammatory bowel diseases or tumor growth in case of cancers. Such studies are conducted to prove that the colon targeting of the hydrogel formulation has been successful in delivering maximum amount of drug in the colonic tract, resulting in better cure and management of the disease. In a study by Pitaressi et al., six male dogs were used for in vivo studies, which were fed with marketed flutamide tablets, and flutamide-loaded inulin hydrogel microparticles and blood samples were collected at regular intervals of time. The bioavailability of drug was increased by twofolds in the case of hydrogel formulations, as observed from the area under the curve (AUC) values. The Tmax value was higher in the case of hydrogel formulation (6h) compared with that in marketed tablet (3h), which showed sustained release and delayed absorption. Furthermore, the half-life of the drug increased by threefold compared with that of marketed tablet [50].

8.5.7 Cytotoxicity assay

Often, the hydrogels with natural polysaccharides are subjected to cytotoxicity assay on human cell lines. The natural polysaccharides such as inulin are biocompatible, safe, and nontoxic, which can be proven with such experiments. The hydrogels with and without drug are tested on the cell lines to determine their toxic potential. Again, in the study by Afinjuomo et al., cytotoxicity of the developed cross-linked inulin hydrogels with or without drug was tested on human colon carcinoma cells HCT116. The cell viability of the inulin hydrogels without any drug was above 85% after 24h of incubation. Thus the inulin hydrogels were proven to be safe and nontoxic [8].

8.6 Research and applications of inulin and inulin-based hydrogels in drug delivery

Inulin and inulin-based hydrogels have been used in food industry, pharmaceutical industry, and for biomedical applications. We shall discuss few research studies with context to drug delivery in the following section.

From earlier researches and reports, it transpires that inulin is a potential carrier used in a number of drug delivery systems such as oral, intranasal/pulmonal, parenteral, intramuscular, intravenous, and subcutaneous drug delivery systems [1]. Inulin does not degrade in the upper GIT and slowly undergoes fermentation in the gut by the action of the microorganisms. For oral delivery, inulin is regarded as a promising candidate [36, 52]. Glomerular filtration rate (GFR) determination is also done by using inulin, especially in recent years. GFR is the estimation of filtration ability through the glomeruli. Inulin is found to be a complete filterable agent through the glomerulus [53, 54]. Inulin increases frequency of stool and enhances mass of bacteria in the gut [55, 56]. In human body, when inulin is taken at a dose of less than 20 g per day basis, it is generally found to be well tolerated. Higher doses may produce GI problems [56, 57]. Some research groups studied that inulin spontaneously reduced the levels of cholesterol and glucose [56, 58]. Nevertheless, inulin is also investigated for its serum cholesterol–lowering effect owing to enhanced excretion of bile acid and neutral steroid, which can lessen the synthesis of cholesterol in the egg laying hens' liver [59].

Inulin being quickly water soluble and stable in gastric or intestinal conditions, while being less friable, has been used widely as a drug delivery constituent by the researchers [60]. The routes through which inulin or its hydrogels are administered are as follows:

8.6.1 Oral drug delivery

One of the most popular routes of drug delivery using inulin-based carriers is the oral route. Drug-loaded inulin has been used more frequently for colon targeting as the site-specific drug delivery system. The major objective of researchers is to shield the drug candidate from the harsh conditions of the upper GIT during the delivery of drug.

The presence of bifidobacteria in colon metabolizes inulin. Bifidobacterium, a gram-positive, immobile, anaerobic bacterium with branched structure is a prevalent endosymbiotic resident of the GIT and one of the prime genera of bacterium, which is found in the colonic flora of mammals. Because inulin can stay longer in gastric juice without any damages, it is found to be an excellent carrier for sensitive drugs. Moreover, inulin imparts protective shield to the walls of the stomach against nonsteroidal antiinflammatory drugs (NSAIDs) [61].

Inulin has also been used to prepare solid dispersions and hydrogels [7, 62]. Furthermore, it is also applied as a formulation coating agent for oral delivery systems [63].

Pitarresi et al. developed cross-linked inulin hydrogels in phosphate buffer pH 7.4 for sustained delivery of flutamide. No toxic solvents were used in the process. Microparticles were prepared from the hydrogel, which had mucoadhesive properties. When flutamide-loaded microparticles were fed to cross-bred dogs, the active metabolite's half-life was found to improve by threefolds, with significant improvement in bioavailability [50].

Inulin methacrylic acid derivatives (INU-MA) were irradiated with UV radiation in the range of 250–364 nm to produce hydrogels, which have high water uptake but partially degraded in stomach pH. Thus inulin derivative was further produced with methacrylic acid and succinic acid (INU-MA-SA), and then hydrogels were produced with the effect of UV light, which was stable and had low swelling in gastric conditions. Ibuprofen was loaded on both types of hydrogels, and the drug release was determined in buffers simulating GI fluids. Drug release from INU-MA hydrogels was faster than that of INU-MA-SA hydrogels that gave controlled pH-dependent release [38].

8.6.2 Colon-targeted drug delivery

The GIT consists of the stomach and the intestines: small and large intestines. There are certain factors that may be used for targeting of drugs to the colon as follows:

1. Residence time: The residence time of food and drugs in the large intestine is much higher than that in small intestine and stomach. Thus colon-targeted delivery systems can obtain sustained release of drug for prolonged periods of time using suitable carriers.
2. Concentration of microbial flora: The GI conditions, including the pH and absence of enzymes, are very suitable for the growth of microbes, and thus the microbial concentration is also high in the large intestine when compared with that in the upper parts of GIT (Fig. 8.6) [64].
3. High diversity of microbial population: The large intestine has a diverse range of microbes that act on various polysaccharides and cause their breakdown, releasing entrapped drugs. Thus natural polysaccharides such as inulin are degraded in the large intestine and may be used for colon-targeted delivery.
4. Viscous fluid in the lumen, which causes sustained release.
5. Low systemic absorption and higher local effect.

Colon-targeted delivery is essential for drugs that treat colonic diseases such as inflammatory bowel diseases or cancers of colon. However, colon targeting is challenging because most of the drugs are absorbed in the stomach or small intestine, and very little concentrations reach the colon. Furthermore, intravenous administered drugs get excreted before reaching the colon. However, natural polysaccharides such as inulin are not absorbed in the upper GIT and can reach the colon where it is broken down by the resident microflora. Hydrogels from inulin and dextran are widely used for colon targeting of drugs [65].

Microflora in the colon is solely responsible for the fermentation of inulin. Vervoort et al. prepared inulin-based hydrogels to target the drugs at the colon, and they also assessed the swelling property of the hydrogels.

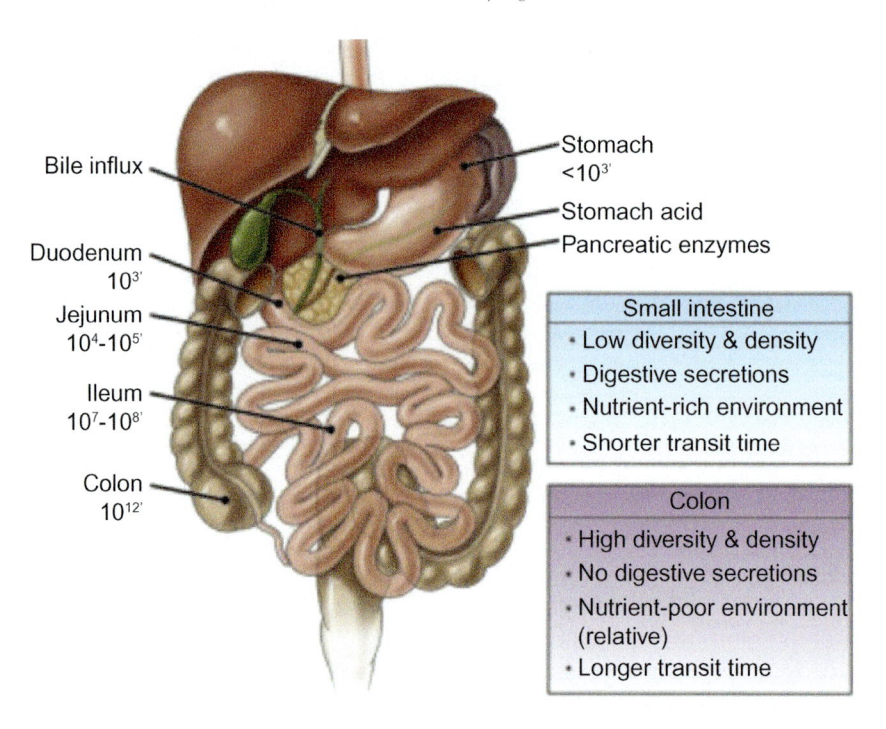

FIG. 8.6 Microbial concentration of different parts of gastrointestinal tract. *Reprinted from KastlJr AJ, Terry NA, DWu G, Albenberg LG, The structure and function of the human small intestinal microbiota: current understanding and future directions. Mol Gastroenterol 2020;9:33–45, Copyright (2020), with permission from Elsevier.*

The authors also investigated the factors affecting the degree of substitution, ionic strength, methacrylated inulin concentration, altered concentrations of the initiator during polymerization process, and swelling characteristics of hydrogel affected by pH [42]. Earlier, Vervoort et al. reported the fermentation of inulin hydrogels by enzymes through in vitro studies, associated with inulinase enzyme obtained from *Aspergillus niger*. After this study, the authors found that inulinase enzyme diffuses into the hydrogels, which leads to degradation of hydrogels [66, 67].

Succinic acid derivatives of inulin were used to prepare hydrogels by different cross-linking agents. FTIR evaluation and swelling studies were conducted on the hydrogels. The hydrogel formulations were degraded in inulinase-added medium. They were also found to be compatible on Caco-2 cells. The potential drugs for inflammatory diseases of colon such as glutathione and oxytocin were encapsulated in the prepared hydrogels and evaluated in GI fluids for drug release studies. The authors concluded that the drug-loaded hydrogels have significant use in the management of inflammatory bowel diseases [7].

Inulin was conjugated with doxorubicin and loaded onto biopolymeric nanoparticles. The developed formulation minimized drug release at low pH and improved drug release in neutral pH conditions. Caco-2 and HT29-MTX cells were used to study the effect of the biopolymers on the tight junctions of the epithelial cells. These cell lines were used because they served as a model of GIT epithelial layer. It was found that low concentrations of the polymers did not disrupt the junctions of the epithelial cells [68].

Various types of inulin-based hydrogels were developed to be used as promising carriers for colonic delivery [1, 69]. Release of Diflunisal, an NSAID (the drug used for the prophylaxis of early morning angina) was evaluated at pH 4.0 and 7.4. Application of inulin protects the dosage forms from the acidic gastric environment, especially for the drugs that can cause side effects in the gastric environment, such as the NSAIDs. Degradation of inulin and release of the drugs took place in the colon by enzymes such as inulinase [35].

Further investigation has already been reported on hydrogels based on methacrylic and succinic acid derivatives of inulin along with α,ß-poly[N-(2-hydroxyethyl)-D,L aspartamide irradiated with UV light. The resultant hydrogel system consisting of polysaccharide/poly (amino acid) was used for protein and peptide drugs delivery to the colon. Proper rate of degradation, bioadhesive character, resistance to water, and strength of hydrogels are the useful parameters attributed by the gels with polysaccharide-polyamino acid moiety, which can be beneficial for targeted drug delivery. Tripodo et al. chose the model drug, immunoglobulin G. The hydrogels prepared with immunoglobulin G were degraded by inulinase, compatible with epithelial layer cells and the antibodies that were released from the formulation, and able to retain their pharmacological activity [70].

In 2008 Pitarresi et al. prepared inulin-based hydrogel. Inulin derivatives were obtained by reaction with divinylsulfone and succinic anhydride and then cross-linked with trimethylolpropane tris. When the hydrogel was complexed with 2-methoxyestradiol, an anticancer drug, an apoptotic effect against Caco-2-cell lines was observed. This gel was also found suitable for colonic drug delivery because it can be degraded by inulinase and esterase enzymes [46].

Pitarresi et al. investigated hydrogels prepared with 5-fluorouracil and methylated inulin (INU-MA) with different cross-linking agents to check the effect of UV irradiation and rheological characteristics. They have produced strong hydrogels with high elasticity, which leads to modified release of drug in the GIT [37].

Afinjuomo et al. prepared pH- and enzyme-augmented colon-specific smart gel cross-linked with pyromelliticdianhydride (PMDA). They also investigated the prepared hydrogels regarding different instrumental analysis, such as FTIR and SEM, and spectrophotometrically. The prepared gels showed better swelling property in water. Moreover, it showed pH dependency because of the presence of carboxylic acid [71].

Palumbo et al. developed and characterized an in situ hydrogel cross-linked with amino derivatives of hyaluronic acid (HA) and divinylsulfone derivative of inulin (INU-DV). They studied two different HA derivatives that produce the portion of pendant ethylenediamine (HA-EDA) as well as both the pendant groups of ethylenediamine and octadecyl (HA-EDA-C_{18}). Here HA-EDA stands for the conjugation of hyaluronic acid and ethylenediamine. Both the groups were reacted with each other for cross-linking, which involved an azo Michael reaction along with INU-DV. They again checked the gelation time and DV consumption rate using 3% w/v HA-EDA and 80/20 w/w ratio of HA-EDA-C_{18} regarding INU-DV cross-linker. The authors concluded that presence of pendant C_{18} chains increases the mechanical performances of hydrogels and reduces the hydrolysis of hyaluronidase during cross-linking. The encapsulated bovine chondrocytes successfully survived and effectively proliferated throughout the 28 days of assay [72].

In 2011 Spizzirri et al. developed antioxidant hydrogels with thermo-sensitive properties. They were prepared by cross-linking inulin with the help of cross-linker and modified/grafted antioxidant and monomer with thermosensitive characteristics. In this study, authors used catechin (an antioxidant) and N-isopropylacrylamide (NIPAAm, thermoresponsive agent) that are incorporated into a polymeric network, applying a redox pair as an environmentally sound radical initiator system. Instrumental analysis such as calorimetric study, FT-IR, UV analysis, and fluorescence test were conducted to verify the formation of covalent bond between inulin–catechin and introduction of bioactive molecules and monomers in the hydrogel. They observed transitional temperature within a range of 31.3–33.1°C of the hydrogels and a temperature dependent affinity toward water. The antioxidant properties of the conjugates were evaluated by determination of radical (2,2′-diphenyl-1-picrylhydrazyl) scavenging activity and total content of flavonoids at different temperatures. Thus the antioxidant hydrogels with thermoresponsive characters ensured the effectiveness of the research approach. It was concluded that the antioxidant–carbohydrate conjugates with thermoresponsive properties hold unique qualities for useful applications in the food industry [73].

Vervoort et al. developed a colon-targeted potent hydrogel as a suitable carrier for drug delivery. The delivery system was supposed to be degraded specifically at the colon by microbial fermentation. Thus the ability of enzymatic digestion of developed hydrogels was analyzed by application of inulinase (capable of degrading inulin network) extracted from *A. niger*. By using anthrone method, the authors quantified the action of inulinase associated with the amount of liberation of fructose from the inulin hydrogel. The hydrogel was assayed on the basis of equilibrium swelling ratio and the mechanical strength with the help of inulinase solutions both preincubation and postincubation. The results confirmed that inulin in the hydrogels was digested enzymatically. The degradation by enzyme was found to be dependent on several factors. It was increased when the degradation time was prolonged or the concentration of enzyme was increased. It was also found to increase when the polymer used had a low degree of substitution, and the concentration of polymer was decreased. Furthermore, when the equilibrium swelling was compared predegradation and postdegradation of the hydrogels, it was found that the swelling enhanced after degradation, which suggested that inulinase was capable of diffusion through the network of inulin hydrogel, resulting in bulk degradation [66].

Maris et al. synthesized and characterized novel colon-targeted hydrogels. Copolymers such as, bis(methacryloylamino)azobenzene (BMAAB) and 2-hydroxyethyl methacrylate (HEMA) or methacrylic acid (MA) were used to prepare the hydrogels along with methacrylated inulin (MA-IN). They assessed the gels on the basis of various parameters such as swelling characteristics. They observed that as the concentration of MA-IN and BMAAB were increased, the water absorbed into the hydrogels was decreased. Furthermore, the amount of water taken up into hydrogels was also found to decrease with greater degree of substitution in the inulin structure. The authors further explained the hydrophobicity and rigidness of the azo agent. They also observed that insertion of the water-soluble monomers (such as HEMA or MA) lessened the equilibrium swelling. They reported that this observation was due to high density of the network formed and presence of hydrogen bonds. They found that water that was absorbed by the hydrogels was maintained by both relaxation as well as diffusion processes, which was explained to be an anomalous behavior. They investigated that the release profile of drug in phosphate buffer medium and found that within initial 3h, the drug release was more than 80% from MA-IN: HEMA hydrogels. When compared with that, the drug release from MA-IN: HEMA: BMAAB hydrogels was less, releasing approximately 50% drug within 5h of the study, which was still high. Similar results were obtained for the hydrogels prepared with MA instead of HEMA. The findings of the study clearly demonstrated the challenges in achieving optimal balance between proper degradation in the colon (requiring high swelling of the gels) and preventing premature release in upper GIT (requiring low swelling of the gels) [40].

Two different azo-polysaccharide hydrogels were produced using dextran and inulin as natural polysaccharides. Azo hydrogels can be degraded only when azo groups are reduced. Thus this study was undertaken to observe and evaluate the azo groups' reduction in the prepared hydrogels and degradation of polysaccharide by action of enzymes. The methycrylated derivatives of the two polysaccharides were cross-linked with N,N'-bis(methacryloylamino)azobenzene (B(MA)AB), and the resultant azo-hydrogels were evaluated for their mechanical characteristics and swelling. When the concentration of cross-linker was increased, denser hydrogels were produced. Dextran hydrogels swelled in water to greater extent than in dimethylformamide, whereas inulin hydrogels shrank in water, which may be because of their hydrophobic character. Degradation studies of the dextran and inulin hydrogels by dextranase and inulinase showed greater extent of hydrogel degradation for dextrose. Furthermore, when rat cecal contents were used in the dissolution medium, the reduction of azo group in azo-inulin hydrogels did not take place [74].

Hydrogels and polymeric micelles are often used for the delivery of soluble and poorly soluble drugs, respectively. Thus both the delivery systems were combined to deliver both hydrophilic and hydrophobic drugs together, as a combination therapy. Hydrogels were developed using methacrylated inulin and vitamin E with the help of UV irradiation. These methacrylated micelles were further subjected to UV light to transform into nanogrids. These were characterized by several studies, including SEM, DSC, and TEM, and release of a hydrophobic drug such as beclomethasone dipropionate and water uptake studies. It was evaluated whether the hydrophobic drug could pass the hydrophilic parts in the formulations and get released [75].

8.6.3 Research studies based on inulin for other routes of administration

Inulin hydrogels have not been studied for pulmonal or parenteral applications. However, inulin, the natural polysaccharide has been thoroughly used in related formulations, some of which are discussed further.

Pulmonal or intranasal route is a desired route for researchers owing to effortless self-administration having an ability to produce both types of immune responses, including local and systemic [76]. Nasal drug delivery provides promising responses with small doses of drugs. Rapid absorption of drugs was obtained through lofty nasal mucosa, which is highly vascularized [77]. Freeze-dried inulin powder in the form of vaccine stabilizer has been analyzed and found to be safe [78, 79]. As a cryoprotectant, Audouy et al. stabilized inactivated virus vaccines by use of inulin and applied it for nasal application and observed very promising effects without any application of adjuvant therapy [79].

Parenteral route of drug delivery through intravenous, intramuscular, and subcutaneous injection was found to be more advantageous over oral or transdermal drug delivery systems. This route offers enhanced bioavailability because there is absence of biological barriers such as the epithelial membrane and stratum corneum for permeation of the drug molecules. Furthermore, the drugs can avoid hepatic first pass metabolism [80].

Intramuscular and subcutaneous routes are found to be the preferred routes for drug delivery using inulin because both routes are generally used for the drugs that are not taken up by the GIT easily. In addition, this route provides rapid and enhanced bioavailability [1]. Conversely, Tripodo et al. produced nanomicelles with inulin and vitamin E in association with curcumin and observed that the formulation was capable of permeation through cellular membrane in a very controlled manner. They also observed promising pharmacokinetic profile after intravenous administration [81].

For intramuscular drug delivery, inulin is applied as a lyoprotectant and as a vaccine adjuvant [78, 82]. To check the fusogenic activity and structural integrity, inulin was evaluated for maintenance during the preservation of influenza virosomes. After analysis of inulin effect on the virosomes, it was preserved for further use in vaccines or for other applications in drug delivery. The assessment confirmed that inulin has two times more capability to protect and stabilize the formulation when compared with another lyoprotectant called the HEPES buffered saline [78].

Humoral and in vivo cellular responses were enhanced in the presence of delta inulin, which is otherwise known as ß-D-[2→1] poly (fructofuranosyl) α-D- glucose, an isomer of inulin (Cooper et al., 2011). A delta inulin adjuvant, AdvaxTM, has been observed to increase the vaccines' immunogenicity. The adjuvant was analyzed for the vaccine named Split-virion H5N1, and improvement was observed with possible protective efficacy by increase in immunogenicity and reduced morbidity [82].

Inulin is found nontoxic and safe in pharmaceutical industries and is used to determine GFR using the intravenous route since long period of time [83, 84]. Shahwar et al. used inulin-based drug delivery associated with polyethylene glycol (PEG) and compared between subcutaneous and intravenous routes. Because it has small-size stays in circulation for long time, inulin has the properties of enhanced permeability and retention effect when the drug is administered subcutaneously [1]. In addition, PEG, considered as an outstanding polysaccharide conjugated with inulin, can modify the immunological and pharmacodynamic properties. In yet another study, Johnston et al. observed the effect of inulin disposition in both solution and gel form after intravenous and intramuscular administration in rats in conjugation with poloxamer 407. Based on their observation, the authors concluded that parallel administration of inulin-poloxamer 407 in the form of gel causes alteration of rat kidney functions by effective removal of inulin through glomerulus filtration [85].

8.7 Commercial applications of inulin

Owing to low crystallization property and high glass transition rate (Tg), inulin has been popularly used by the researchers in preparation of vaccines. Moreover, it has also been used as a lyoprotectant as well as cryopreservative [25, 86]. Inulin is also applied for the preparation of fructose syrup, ice cream, milk products, baked foods, chocolates, etc. [10].

8.8 Inulin in tissue engineering applications

Tissue engineering methods aim to preserve or improve the functions of tissues of bone, cartilage, cardiovascular or nervous system, etc. Furthermore, it also finds applications for replacement and growth of organs and tissues that have been damaged or lost because of injury or disease. Thus it holds a promise to such patients who have lost their organs to grow them back without the use of any artificial organs in a safe and effective way. The common method adopted for tissue engineering includes:

1. Isolation of tissues from body: For isolation of cells from the body, a small biopsy may be conducted to extract suitable amount of cells from the body.
2. Growth of cells: The cells are then grown and harvested in vitro for expanding in number.
3. The cells are then seeded onto suitable scaffolds for delivery.
4. Scaffolds loaded with the growing cells are then transferred at the target areas for them to grow and repair the damaged tissues or organs through direct injection or implantation at the target area by minor surgical procedure (Fig.8.7) [87].

The scaffolds used in the process must be compatible with the target organs extracellular matrices. After transplantation, the cell-loaded scaffolds cause adhesion of delivered cells with the surrounding tissues and promote the transfer of suitable amounts of nutrients, gases, or growth factors to the cells such that they may survive and grow. The scaffolds further ensure minimum toxicity or inflammation at the target site. Biopolymer hydrogels have been popular in tissue engineering to serve as a biocompatible, biomimic, and biodegradable scaffold for delivery of the cells at the target areas.

Hydrogels because of their highly cross-linked structure can swell manifolds and can give the required bulk and mechanical strength to the developing tissue. Furthermore, it permits the easy diffusion of gases and nutrients through its matrices. The adhesion of the delivered cells may be promoted by the peptide groups in the hydrogel structure. It allows immune isolation, and being biocompatible is safe and nontoxic [88].

Examples of some of the hydrogels used in tissue engineering include chondroitin sulfate (CS). Scaffolds based on gelatin-CS-hyaluronan was similar to natural cartilage and promoted the secretion of type II collagen and proteoglycan. The tripolymer combination has also been used for wound healing and nucleus pulposus generation. CS-collagen scaffolds

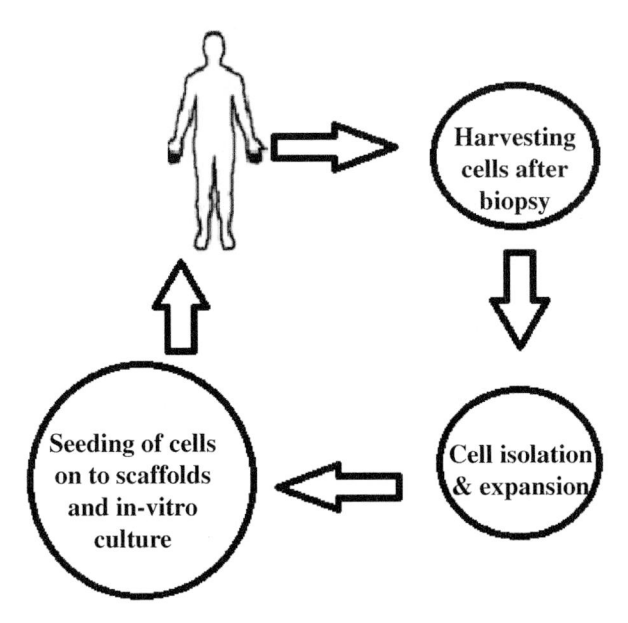

FIG. 8.7 Steps of tissue engineering.

have been used for regeneration of heart and lung tissues and CS-heparin-collagen scaffolds for liver tissues. Chitosan gels in combination with other polymers have been used for bone, cartilage, blood vessels, liver, nerve tissue regeneration, etc. Similarly, cellulose hydrogels have found applications in bone, cartilage, cornea, and nerve tissue generation. Alginate gels have been used for tissue repairs of the blood vessel, bone, bone marrow, cartilage, heart, liver, ligament, etc. Furthermore, hydrogels based on HA, gelatin, elastin, and fibroin have also been used in tissue engineering [89].

8.8.1 Research approaches of inulin-based hydrogel in tissue engineering

The in situ hydrogels based on HA inulin derivatives were also used in a study for regeneration of tissues of cartilage. HA is a natural component of cartilage tissue, and inulin has been used as a biocompatible water-soluble polymer, which has promising biomedical usage. Aminoderivative of HA was used along with divinylsulfone derivative of inulin [72].

In another study, divinyl sulfone derivative of inulin was cross-linked with O'-bis(2-aminoethyl)polyethylene glycol to develop hydrogels in a near-neutral environment. The hydrogels were found to be compatible with Caco-2 cells and suitable for biomedical applications [48].

Inulin was cross-linked with divinylsylfone, and microparticles of cross-linked inulin were developed using microemulsion polymerization process in reverse micelles. Water-in-oil microemulsions were used in the process, and a basic medium was used. The developed microparticles demonstrated beneficial utilization as scaffolds for synthesis of CdS quantum dots in situ and were compatible in fibroblast cell culture. Quantum dots are semiconductor crystals of nano range with several biomedical applications [90]. Furthermore, they were biodegradable in both acidic and alkaline media. When model drugs such as caffeine and gallic acid were encapsulated within the developed microparticles, controlled release of the drugs was obtained [91].

Ding and Fournier determined the transport rates of inulin and oxygen to evaluate vascularization surrounding an implanted bioartificial organ in rat model. Compartment model was used in the study for demonstration of the transport of inulin and oxygen from the cell chamber through the immunoisolation membrane to the neovascularized organ. Blood oxygen partial pressure in the blood capillaries, the fraction of extracellular volume, and residence time of capillary blood were some of the important findings of the study. Bioartificial organs use both living tissues and artificial materials for medicinal purposes such as restoration of lost functions [92].

A hydrogel based on a novel glycopolymer was developed. Inulin scaffold and pendent β-lactosides were used to prepare the glycopolymer. It was observed that the glycopolymer had improved gellation properties compared with inulin and formed firm gels at lower concentrations. Furthermore, specific affinity of the glycopolymer toward lectins was observed [93].

Injectable hydrogels have gained research interest recently for bone and cartilage replacement therapy. Such a process would replace costly and complicated surgeries and help in the regrowth of tissues at the desired location. Various polysaccharides have been used to develop hydrogels for such purposes, synthetic or natural. Some of the polysaccharides that have been used to prepare injectable hydrogels include chitosan, alginate, gelatin, HA, collagen, chondroitin sulfate, heparin, polyethylene glycol, or polyvinyl alcohol (Fig. 8.8) [94].

In yet another study, Palumbo et al. used inulin to produce in situ hydrogels with HA derivatives. The hydrogel-loaded scaffolds were evaluated for tissue engineering purposes. The aminoderivative of HA (HA-EDA) was complexed with oxadiazole (OXA) groups that were fluorinated to produce HA-EDA-OXA which improved the oxygen uptake in scaffolds for survival of the tissues in-vivo. This was proven by dispersing the prepared HA derivatives in water and solubilizing oxygen in the aqueous dispersion. This showed improved oxygen uptake by the aqueous medium. HA-EDA-OXA was used to produce an in situ gel with a vinyl sulfone

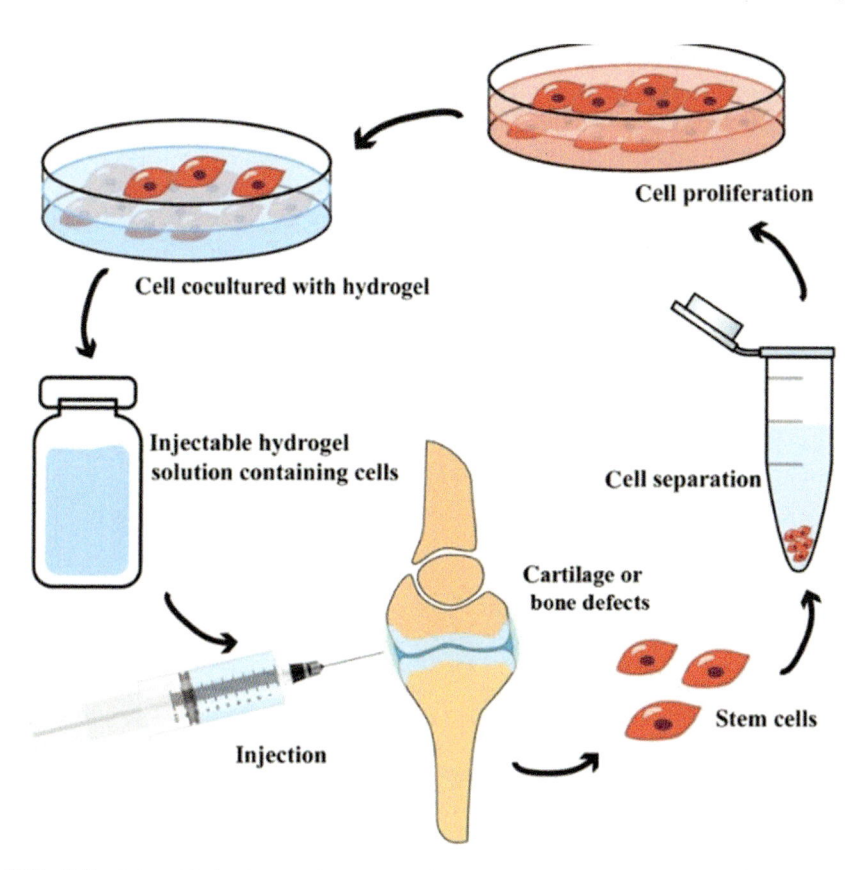

FIG. 8.8   Injectable hydrogels for bone and tissue engineering. *Reprinted from Bone Res, 5, Liu M, Zeng X, Ma C, Yi H, Ali Z, Mou X, Li S, Deng Y, He N, Injectable hydrogels for cartilage and bone tissue engineering, Article number: 17014, Copyright (2017), with permission from Elsevier.*

derivative of inulin. The hydrogel system was tested on fibroblast cells and was proven to promote cell growth even at low oxygen tension [95].

8.9 Conclusions

Natural polysaccharides such as inulin have several benefits compared with synthetic polymers regarding their safety, biocompatibility, and biodegradability. Inulin is already in use as a food supplement or prebiotic. Hydrogels developed from inulin have favorable physicochemical characteristics and have been studied thoroughly for future applications in the pharmaceutical and biomedical industries.

Through this chapter, we not only get an insight into the various applications of inulin and inulin hydrogels but also the latest research-based studies on inulin hydrogels. The chapter also reviews the physicochemical properties of inulin, importance of inulin hydrogels, their preparation, and characterization. We could observe that inulin hydrogels have been used in oral and colon targeted drug delivery extensively. Furthermore, in the past few decades, inulin hydrogels have also been studied for use in tissue engineering scaffolds. Thus we come to understand that inulin hydrogels have tremendous potential for drug delivery and tissue engineering. However, inulin hydrogels can still be explored for parenteral, pulmonal, transdermal, topical, or vaginal drug delivery or use as carriers in bone or cartilage scaffolds, where other hydrogel products have found applications. Thus there is a promising scope for researchers to evaluate new routes and forms of drug delivery with inulin hydrogels.

References

[1] Imran S, Gillis RB, Kok SM, Harding SE, Adams GG. Application and use of inulin as a tool for therapeutic drug delivery. Biotechnol Genet Eng Rev 2012;28:33–46.
[2] Mensink MA, Frijlink HW, Maarschalk KV, Hinrichs WLJ. Inulin, a flexible oligosaccharide I: review of its physicochemical characteristics. Carbohydr Polym 2015;130:405–19.
[3] Zhu Z, He J, Liu G, Barba FJ, Koubaa M, Ding L, Bals O, Grimi N, Vorobiev E. Recent insights for the green recovery of inulin from plant food materials using non-conventional extraction technologies: a review. Innov Food Sci Emerg Technol 2016;33:1–9.
[4] Boeckner LS, Schnepf MI, Tungland BC. Inulin: a review of nutritional and health implications. Adv Food Nutr Res 2001;43:1–63.
[5] Wilson RG, Smith JA, Yonts CD. Chicory root yield and carbohydrate composition is influenced by cultivar selection, planting, and harvest date. Crop Sci 2004;44(3):748–52.
[6] Wong CB, Odamaki T, Xiao JZ. Beneficial effects of *Bifidobacterium longum* subsp. *longum* BB536 on human health: modulation of gut microbiome as the principal action. J Funct Foods 2019;54:506–19.
[7] Mandracchia D, Denora N, Franco M, Pitarresi G, Giammona G, Trapani G. New biodegradable hydrogels based on inulin and α,β-polyaspartylhydrazide designed for colonic drug delivery: in vitro release of glutathione and oxytocin. J Biomater Sci Polym Ed 2011;22(1–3):313–28.
[8] Afinjuomo F, Fouladian P, Parikh A, Barclay TG, Song Y, Garg S. Preparation and characterization of oxidized inulin hydrogel for controlled drug delivery. Pharmaceutics 2019;11:356.
[9] Apolinario AC, de Lima Damasceno BP, de Macedo Beltrao NE, Pessoa A, Converti A, da Silva JA. Inulin-type fructans: a review on different aspects of biochemical and pharmaceutical technology. Carbohydr Polym 2014;101:368–78.
[10] Kaur N, Gupta A. Applications of inulin and oligofructose in health and nutrition. J Biosci 2002;27:703–14.
[11] Lis DG, Preston LA. U.S. Patent No. 5,840,884; 1998. Washington, DC: U.S. Patent and Trademark Office.
[12] Marchessault RH, Bleha T, Deslandes Y, Revol JF. Conformation and crystalline structure of (2→1)-d-fructofuranan (inulin). Can J Chem 1980;58:2415–22.
[13] Lopez-Molina D, Navarro-Martınez MD, Rojas-Melgarejo F, Hiner AN, Chazarra S, Rodrıguez-Lopez JN. Molecular properties and prebiotic effect of inulin obtained from artichoke (*Cynara scolymus* L.). Phytochemistry 2005;66(12):1476–84.

[14] Mudannayake DC, Wimalasiri K, Silva KF, Ajlouni S. Comparison of properties of new sources of partially Purified inulin to those of commercially pure chicory inulin. J Food Sci 2015;80(5):C950–60.

[15] Hidaka H, Adachi T, Hirayama M. Development and benefical effects of fructo-oligosaccharides (neosugar). In: McCleary BV, Prosky L, editors. Advanced dietary fibre technology. Oxford, UK: Blackwell Science Ltd; 2001.

[16] Yi H, Zhang L, Hua C, Sun K, Zhang L. Extraction and enzymatic hydrolysis of inulin from Jerusalem artichoke and their effects on textural and sensorial characteristics of yogurt. Food Bioproc Tech 2010;3(2):315–9.

[17] Graham-Rowe D. How to keep foods bursting with goodness. New Sci 2006;191(2567):24–5.

[18] Valluru R, Van den Ende W. Plant fructans in stress environments: emerging concepts and future prospects. J Exp Bot 2008;59(11):2905–16.

[19] Guggisberg D, Cuthbert-Steven J, Piccinali P, Butikofer U, Eberhard P. Rheological, microstructural and sensory characterization of low-fat and whole milk set yoghurt as influenced by inulin addition. Int Dairy J 2009;19(2):107–15.

[20] Glibowski P. Effect of thermal and mechanical factors on rheological properties of high performance inulin gels and spreads. J Food Eng 2010;99(1):106–13.

[21] Cooper PD, Carter M. Anti-complementary action of polymorphic "solubility forms" of particulate inulin. Mol Immunol 1986;23:895–901.

[22] Cooper PD, Petrovsky N. Delta inulin: a novel, immunologically active, stable packing structure comprising -d-[2→1] poly(fructo-furanosyl) -d-glucose polymers. Glycobiology 2011;21:595–606.

[23] Bouchard A, Jovanovi'c N, Hofland GW, Jiskoot W, Mendes E, DJA C. Supercritical fluid drying of carbohydrates: selection of suitable excipients and process conditions. Eur J Pharm Biopharm 2008;68:781–94.

[24] Anon, https://pubchem.ncbi.nlm.nih.gov/compound/Inulin#section=Experimental-Properties.

[25] Hinrichs WL, Prinsen MG, Frijlink HW. Inulin glasses for the stabilization of therapeutic proteins. Int J Pharm 2001;215:163–74.

[26] Bot A, Erle U, Vreeker R, Agterof WG. Influence of crystallisation conditions on the large deformation rheology of inulin gels. Food Hydrocoll 2004;18(4):547–56.

[27] Wada T, Sugatani J, Terada E, Ohguchi M, Miwa M. Physi-cochemical characterization and biological effects of inulin enzymatically synthesized from sucrose. J Agric Food Chem 2005;53:1246–53.

[28] Kim Y, Faqih M, Wang S. Factors affecting gel formation of inulin. Carbohydr Polym 2001;46:135–45.

[29] Ronkart SN, Paquot M, Deroanne C, Fougnies C, Besbes S, Blecker CS. Development of gelling properties of inulin by microfluidization. Food Hydrocoll 2010;24(4):318–24.

[30] Abou-Arab AA, Talaat H, Abu-Salem F. Physicochemical properties of inulin produced from Jerusalem artichoke tubers on bench and pilot plant scale. Aust J Basic Appl Sci 2011;5(5):1297–309.

[31] Franck A. Technological functionality of inulin and oligofructose. Br J Nutr 2007;87:S287–91.

[32] Van Duynhoven JPM, Kulik AS, Jonker HRA, Haverkamp J. Solid-like components in carbohydrate gels probed by NMR spectroscopy. Carbohydr Polym 1999;40:211–9.

[33] Kim Y, Wang SS. Kinetic study of thermally induced inulin gel. J Food Sci 2001;66:991–7.

[34] Saengthongpinit W, Sajjaanantakul T. Influence of harvest time and storage temperature on characteristics of inulin from Jerusalem artichoke (Helianthus tuberosus L.) tubers. Postharvest Biol Tec 2005;37(1):93–100.

[35] Castelli F, Sarpietro MG, Micieli D, et al. Differential scanning calorimetry study on drug release from an inulin-based hydrogel and its interaction with a biomembrane model: pH and loading effect. Eur J Pharm Sci 2008;35(1–2):76–85.

[36] Fares MM, Salem MS, Khanfar M. Inulin and poly(acrylic acid) grafted inulin for dissolution enhancement and preliminary controlled release of poorly water-soluble Irbesartan drug. Int J Pharm 2011;410:206–11.

[37] Pitarresi G, Giacomazzac D, Triolo D, Giammona G, Luigi P, Biagio S. Rheological characterization and release properties of inulin-based hydrogels. Carbohydr Polym 2012;88(3):1033–40.

[38] Tripodo G, Pitarresi G, Palumbo FS, Craparo EF, Giammona G. UV-photocrosslinking of inulin derivatives to produce hydrogels for drug delivery application. Macromol Biosci 2005;5:1074–84.

[39] Mooter GVD, Vervoort L, Kinget R. Characterization of methacrylated inulin hydrogels designed for colon targeting: in vitro release of BSA. Pharm Res 2003;20(2):303–7.

[40] Maris B, Verheyden L, Van Reeth K, Samyn C, Augustijns P, Kinget R, Van den Mooter G. Synthesis and characterisation of inulin-azo hydrogels designed for colon targeting. Int J Pharm 2001;213(1–2):143–52.

[41] Chiu HC, Hsu YH, Lin PJ. Synthesis of pH-sensitive inulin hydrogels and characterization of their swelling properties. J Biomed Mater Res 2002;61(1):146–52.

[42] Vervoort L, Mooter GVD, Augustijns P, Kinget R. Inulin hydrogels. I. Dynamic and equilibrium swelling properties. Int J Pharm 1998;172:127–35.

[43] Norudin NS, Mohamed HN, Yahya NAM. Controlled released alginate-inulin hydrogel: development and in-vitro characterization. In: Proceedings of the 3rd International Conference on Applied Science and Technology (ICAST'18) AIP Conf. Proc; 2016. 020113-1-020113-6.

[44] Ranganathan N, Joseph Bensingh R, Abdul Kader M, Nayak SK. Synthesis and properties of hydrogels prepared by various polymerization reaction systems. In: Mondal M, editor. Cellulose-based superabsorbent hydrogels. Polymers and polymeric composites: a reference series. Cham: Springer; 2018.

[45] Vervoort L, Van den Mooter G, Augustijns P, Busson R, Toppet S, Kinget R. Inulin hydrogels as carriers for colonic drug targeting: I. Synthesis and characterization of methacrylated inulin and hydrogel formation. Pharm Res 1997;14(12):1730–7.

[46] Pitarresi G, Tripodo G, Calabrese R, Craparo EF, Licciardi M, Giammona G. Hydrogels for potential colon drug release by thiol-ene conjugate addition of a new inulin derivative. Macromol Biosci 2008;8(10):891–902.

[47] Lea T. Caco-2 Cell Line. In: Verhoeckx K, et al., editors. The impact of food bioactives on health. Cham: Springer; 2015.

[48] Pitaressi G, Tripodo G, Triolo D, et al. Inulin vinyl sulfone derivative cross-linked with bis-amino PEG: new materials for biomedical applications. J Drug Deliv Sci Tec 2009;19(6):419–23.

[49] Dan A, Ghosh S, Moulik SP. Physicochemical studies on the Bipolymer inulin: a critical evaluation of its self-aggregation, aggregate- morphology, interaction with water and thermal stability. Biopolymers 2009;91(9):687–99.

[50] Pitarresi G, Triolo D, Giorgi M, Fiorica C, Calascibetta F, Giammona G. Inulin-based hydrogel for Oral delivery of Flutamide: preparation, characterization, and in vivo release studies. Macromol Biosci 2012;12(6):770–8.

[51] Rachmawati H, Mudhakir D, Kusuma J. Combination of inulin-shellac as a unique coating formulation for design of colonic delivery dosage form of ibuprofen. Int J Res Pharm Sci 2012;3(1):17–23.

[52] Kosaraju SL. Colon targeted delivery systems: review of polysaccharides for encapsulation and delivery. Critic Rev Food Nutri 2005;45:251–8.

[53] Kooman JP. Estimation of renal function in patients with chronic kidney disease. J Magnet Res Image 2009;30:1341–6.

[54] Westland R, Abraham Y, Bokenkamp A, Wagner BS, Schreuder MF, Van Wijk JAE. Precision of estimating equations for GFR in children with a solitary functioning kidney: the KIMONO study. Clin J Am Soc Nephrol 2013;8:764–72.

[55] Takemura N, Hagio M, Ishizuka S, Ito H, Morita T. Inulin prolongs survival of Intragastrically administered lactobacillus plantarum no. 14 in the gut of mice fed a high-fat diet. J Nutr 2010;140:1963–9.

[56] Raninen K, Lappi J, Mykkanen H, Poutanen K. Dietary fiber type reflects physiological functionality: comparison of grain fiber, inulin, and polydextrose. Nutr Rev 2011;69:9–21.

[57] Bonnema AL, Kolberg LW, Thomas W, Slavin JL. Gastrointestinal tolerance of chicory inulin products. J Am Diet Assoc 2010;110:865–8.

[58] Bonsu NKA, Johnson CS, Mcleod KM. Can dietary fructans lower serum glucose. J Diabetes 2011;3:58–66.

[59] Shang HM, Hu TM, Lu YJ, Wu HX. Effects of inulin on performance, egg quality, gut microflora and serum and yolk cholesterol in laying hens. Brit Poult Sci 2010;51:791–6.

[60] Akhgari A, Farahmanda F, Garekani HA, Sadeghi F, Vandamme TF. Permeability and swelling studies on free films containing inulin in combination with different polymethacrylates aimed for colonic drug delivery. Eur J Pharm Sci 2006;28:307–14.

[61] Ravi V, Hatna S, Kumar P. Influence of natural polymer coating on novel colon targeting drug delivery system. J Mater Sci Mater Med 2008;19:2131–3155.

[62] Van Drooge DJ, Hinrichs WLJ, Wegman KAM, Visser MR, Eissens AC, Frijlink HW. Solid dispersions based on inulin for the stabilisation and formulation of Δ^9-tetrahydrocannabinol. Eur J Pharm Sci 2004;21:511–8.

[63] Lacorn M, Goerke M, Claus R. Inulin-coated butyrate increases ileal MCT1 expression and affects mucosal morphology in the porcine ileum by reduced apoptosis. J Animal Physio Animal Nutr 2010;94:670–4.

[64] KastlJr AJ, Terry NA, DWu G, Albenberg LG. The structure and function of the human small intestinal microbiota: current understanding and future directions. Cell Mol Gastroenterol 2020;9(1):33–45.

[65] Lopez-Molina D, Chazzara S, How CW, Pruidze N, Navarro-Peran E, Garcia-Canovas F, Garcia-Ruiz PA, Rojas-Melgarejo F, Rodriguez-Lopez JN. Cinnamate of inulin as a vehicle for delivery of colonic drugs. Int J Pharm 2015;479(1):96–102.

[66] Vervoort L, Rombaut P, Mooter GVD, Augustijns P, Kinget R. Inulin hydrogels. II. In vitro degradation study. Int J Pharm 1998;172:137–45.

[67] Rajpurohit H, Sharma P, Sharma S, Bhandari A. Polymers for Colon targeted drug delivery. Indian J Pharm Sci 2010;72:689–96.

[68] Schoener CA, Peppas NA. pH-responsive hydrogels containing PMMA nanoparticles: an analysis of controlled release of a chemotherapeutic conjugate and transport properties. J Biomater Sci Polym Ed 2013;24(9):1027–40.

[69] Jain A, Gupta Y, Jain SK. Perspectives of biodegradable natural polysaccharides for site-specific drug delivery to the Colon. J Pharm Pharm Sci 2007;10:86–128.

[70] Tripodo G, Pitarresi G, Cavallaro G, Palumbo FS, Giammona G. Controlled release of IgG by novel UV induced polysaccharide/poly(amino acid) hydrogels. Macromol Biosci 2009;9:393–401.

[71] Afinjuomo F, Barclay TG, Song Y, Parikh A, Petrovsky A. Synthesis and characterization of a novel inulin hydrogel crosslinked with pyromellitic dianhydride. React Funct Polym 2019;134:104–11.

[72] Palumbo FS, Fiorica C, Di Stefano M, et al. In-situ forming hydrogels of hyaluronic acid inulin derivatives for cartilage regeneration. Carbohydr Polym 2015;122:408–16.

[73] Spizzirri UG, Puoci AF, Parisi OI, Iemma F, Picci N. Innovative antioxidant thermoresponsive hydrogels by radical grafting of catechin on inulin chain. Carbohydr Polym 2011;84:517–23.

[74] Stubbe B, Maris B, Van den Mooter G, De Smedt SC, Demeester J. The in-vitro evaluation of 'azo-containing polysaccharide gels' for colon delivery. J Control Release 2001;75(1–2):103–14.

[75] Mandracchia D, Trapani A, Perteghella S, Di Franco C, Torre MS, Calleri E, Tripodo G. A micellar-hydrogel Nanogrid from a UV crosslinked inulin derivative for the simultaneous delivery of hydrophobic and hydrophilic drugs. Pharmaceutics 2018;10(3):97.

[76] Ishikawa F, Katsura M, Tamai I, Tsuji A. Improved nasal bioavailability of elcatonin by insoluble powder formulation. Int J Pharm 2001;224:105–14.

[77] Turker S, Onur E, Ozer Y. Nasal route and drug delivery systems. Pharm World Sci 2004;26:137–42.

[78] De Jonge J, Amorij JP, Hinrichs WLJ, Wilschut J, Huckriede A, Frijlink HW. Inulin sugar glasses preserve the structural integrity and biological activity of influenza virosomes during freeze-drying and storage. Eur J Pharm Sci 2007;32:33–44.

[79] Audouy SAL, Van der Schaaf G, Hinrichs WLJ, Frijlink HW, Wilschut J, Huckriede A. Development of a dried influenza whole inactivated virus vaccine for pulmonary immunization. Vaccine 2011;29:4345–52.

[80] Bari H. A prolonged release parenteral drug delivery system—an overview. Int J Pharm Sci Rev Res 2010;3:1–11.

[81] Tripodo G, Pasut G, Trapani A, Mero A, Lasorsa FM, Chlapanidas T, Trapani G, Mandracchia D. Inulin-D-α-tocopherol succinate (INVITE) nanomicelles as a platform for effective intravenous administration of curcumin. Biomacromolecules 2015;16:550–7.

[82] Layton RC, Petrovsky N, Gigliotti AP, Pollock Z, Knight J, Donart N, Pyles J, Harrod KS, Gao P, Koster F. Delta inulin polysaccharide adjuvant enhances the ability of split-virion H5N1 vaccine to protect against lethal challenge in ferrets. Vaccine 2011;29:6242–51.

[83] Delanaye P, Souvignet M, Dubourg L, Thibaudin L, Maillard N, Krzesinski JM, Cavalier E, Mariat C. Measurement of inulin: development. Ann Biol Clin 2011;63:273–84.

[84] Nishida M, Uechi M, Kono S, Harada K, Fujiwara M. Estimating glomerular filtration rate in healthy dogs using inulin without urine collection. Res Vet Sci 2012;93:398–403.

[85] Johnston TP, Miller SC. Inulin disposition following intramuscular Administration of an Inulin/Poloxamer gel matrix. J Parenter Sci Technol 1989;49:279–86.

[86] Hinrichs WLJ, Sanders NN, De Smedt SC, Demeester J, Frijlink HW. Inulin is a promising cryo- and lyoprotectant for PEGylatedlipoplexes. J Controlled Rel 2005;103:465–79.

[87] Liu W, Cao Y. Tissue-engineering technology for tissue repair and regeneration. In: Moo-Young M, editor. Comprehensive biotechnology. 2nd ed. Boston: Newnes; 2011. p. 353–75.

[88] El-Sherbiny IM, Yacoub MH. Hydrogel scaffolds for tissue engineering: progress and challenges. Glob Cardiol Sci Pract 2013;2013:316–42.

[89] Vlierberghe SV, Dubruel P, Schacht E. Biopolymer-based hydrogels as scaffolds for tissue engineering applications: a review. Biomacromolecules 2011;12:1387–408.

[90] Mel AD, Oh JT, Ramesh B, Seifalian AM. Biofunctionalized quantum dots for live monitoring of stem cells: applications in regenerative medicine. Regen Med 2012;7:335–47.

[91] Sahiner N, Sagbas S, Yoshida H, Lyon LA. Synthesis and properties of inulin based microgels. Colloid Interfac Sci 2014;2:15–8.

[92] Ding Z, Fournier RL. Oxygen and inulin transport measurements in a planar tissue-engineered bioartificial organ. Tissue Eng 2002;8(1):25–36.

[93] Izawa K, Akiyama K, Abe H, Togashi Y, Hasegawa T. Inulin-based glycopolymer: its preparation, lectin affinity and gellation property. Bioorg Med Chem 2013;21(11):2895–902.

[94] Liu M, Zeng X, Ma C, Yi H, Ali Z, Mou X, Li S, Deng Y, He N. Injectable hydrogels for cartilage and bone tissue engineering. Bone Res 2017;5. Article number: 17014.

[95] Palumbo FS, Di Stefano M, Piccionello AP, Florica C, Pitarresi G, Pibiri I, Buscemi S, Giammona G. Perfluorocarbon functionalized hyaluronic acid derivatives as oxygenating systems for cell culture. RSC Adv 2014;4:22894–901.

9

Hydrogels based on carrageenan

Reshma Joy, P.N. Vigneshkumar, Franklin John, and Jinu George

Biotechnology Laboratory, Department of Chemistry, Sacred Heart College, Kochi, India

9.1 Introduction

Scientists are constantly searching for novel systems with enhanced drug delivery and tissue engineering potential. Tremendous investment is made in this field by researches because a suitable drug carrier is an inevitable component for the efficient delivery of potential drugs in the target site. Tissue engineering, on the other hand, also requires a suitable material for the delivery of cells and engineering the damaged tissue. A lot of candidates are so far identified and developed for the same purpose. An extensive variety of carrier platforms comprising various materials such as lipids, polymers, and inorganic materials have been proposed in the biomedical field. The resulting delivery systems, depending on their physicochemical properties, are suitable for different applications [1]. However, the above materials are found to have some flaws that restrict them to be an ideal delivery platform. Drug delivery system (DDS) developed from natural polysaccharides offers better scope to overcome the flaws regarding the application of therapeutic molecules on the biological target. Natural polysaccharides or polymers that are used for drug delivery applications such as carrageenan, alginate, agarose, and chitosan have much acceptability due to their performance inside the biological system. Advanced safety and economically and biologically stable factors are the need of this scenario, and biopolymers unveil plentiful benefits that reflect the aptness for this purpose [2]. Biocompatibility and low cytotoxicity offered by these biopolymers always make them superior over other delivery platforms. In addition, the efficient extraction procedures facilitate the scaling up of these materials for commercial purposes.

Among these biopolymers, carrageenan—a renewable anionic sulfated polysaccharide derived from red marine algae of Rhodophyceae class—parades excellent behavior for medicinal practices. Carrageenan was first extracted in 1837, and it has been used in the food industry for a very long time due to its excellent gelling and thickening properties along with its stabilizing and emulsifying capabilities. These properties are used in the processing and manufacture of puddings, desserts, cottage cheese, hamburgers, and sausages [3]. Besides, the application of carrageenan can also be found in shoe polish, air freshener gels, toothpaste, shampoo, and cosmetic creams [4]. In the past two decades, the versatile biopolymer carrageenan has been explored for its biomedical applications. High robustness, high biocompatibility, and persistent viscoelasticity of carrageenan make it assuring excipient for biomedical uses [5]. Carrageenan found its application in pharmaceuticals as anticancer, anticoagulant, immunomodulatory, and antihyperlipidemic agents [6]. The study by Girond et al. on the ability of carrageenan in inhibiting the hepatitis A virus replication and the study by Buck et al. on carrageenan as a potent inhibitor for infections caused by sexually transmitted human papillomavirus revealed the antiviral effects of carrageenan [7, 8]. Various formulations of carrageenan have been developed, including tablets, microcapsules, microspheres, nanoparticles, and hydrogel beads. Different applications of carrageenan in the biomedical field are illustrated in Fig. 9.1.

In pharmaceuticals, hydrogels based on carrageenan are found to have better consideration compared with other carrageenan formulations.

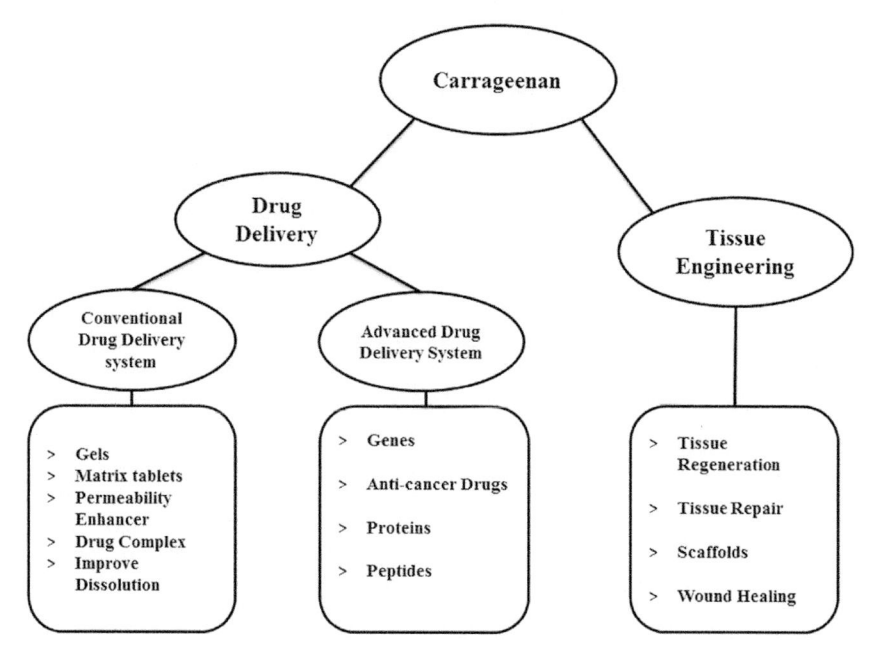

FIG. 9.1   Biomedical applications of carrageenan.

Hydrogel beads based on carrageenan are reported more extensively because of their viscoelastic properties, easy gelling, and thermoreversibility of the gel network [9]. Hydrogels that are hydrophilic polymer chain network with 90%–99% water content have gained considerable attention among researchers. Their high biocompatibility, low cytotoxicity and immunogenicity, tunable physicochemical properties, and ease of functionalization have garnered unprecedented applications in the field of tissue engineering and drug delivery [10]. They have already proved their ability to act as an excellent substrate for cell transplantation, differentiation, and endogenous regeneration [11, 12]. The three-dimensional (3D) network system of hydrogels can provide in vivo niche-like conditions for cell survival by mimicking the microarchitecture of native tissue extracellular matrix (ECM) [13, 14]. The versatility of hydrogels as a candidate for the application of drug delivery and tissue engineering is well known and incorporating the same with the biopolymer carrageenan provides a lot of scope for research to explore the potential of this amazing combination.

This chapter discusses in detail the various structural features of carrageenan hydrogels that facilitate its potential functions and the recent progress that is made in the abovementioned fields.

9.2 Carrageenan—General properties

9.2.1 Source and production

Carrageenan—a renewable anionic sulfated polysaccharide derived from red marine algae of Rhodophyceae class. Gigartina, Furcellaria, Ahnfeltia, Gynmogongrus, Phyllophora, Iridaea, Meristotheca, Anatheca, and Hypnea represent common sources of carrageenan [15]. *Chondrus crispus* was the most common source for the extraction of carrageenan in the 1960s, and later, it got replaced by red algal species such as *Eucheuma denticulatum* and *Kappaphycus alvarezii* [16]. The cell wall of these species contains 30%–80% (dry weight basis) of carrageenan [17]. Variation in algal species, growth condition, and seasonal variations can alter the concentration of carrageenan in the cell wall.

The process of extraction of carrageenan from the seaweed requires special attention, and various companies have developed efficient methods for obtaining maximum yield and high purity. However, the extraction process can be discussed in a general way because all the methods almost follow a similar pattern. Initially, to get rid of degradation, the seaweed is well dried. The drying also helps in its preservation for long-distance shipping. After that, the seaweed is repeatedly washed to get rid of any impurities such as salts, sand, and other small marine life forms. The release of carrageenan from the cells is facilitated by the hot alkali extraction process. Once carrageenan gets in the hot solution, it undergoes clarification and gets converted into a powder form [18]. Various parameters of extraction such as pH, temperature, and the duration of

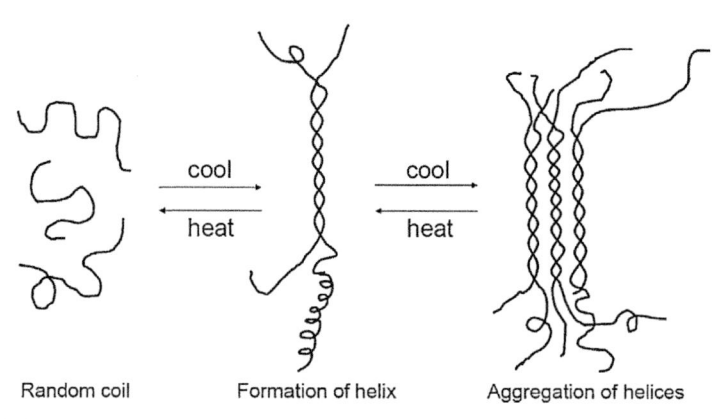

Random coil   Formation of helix   Aggregation of helices

FIG. 9.3   Representation of the gelling mechanism of carrageenan.From Liu J, Zhan X, Wan J, Wang Y, Wang C. Review for carrageenan-based pharmaceutical biomaterials: favorable physical features versus adverse biological effects. Carbohydr Polym 2015;121:27–36, Copyright (2015), with permission from Elsevier.

made possible with the help of trivalent ions [25]. Their study could raise lambda-carrageenan to the level of other types, and its gelling properties opened more applications. Gelling property of carrageenan is an important parameter, and developing strategies for the regulation of gelation and viscoelastic properties can increase its range of application. Several studies have been done in this regard. In 2006, Kara et al. showed that stronger kappa-carrageenan gels can be obtained with KCl when compared with other salts [26].

9.2.3 Chemical modifications

Various physicochemical properties associated with carrageenan can be modulated with chemical modification. The multifarious functional groups present in carrageenan such as hydroxyl groups and sulfate groups make a lot more scope for chemical modifications [21]. Several modifications are reported to date that successfully made desired changes in the carrageenan properties. In 1978, Guiseley et al. reported that the extent of syneresis could effectively be reduced when the gels are formulated from derivatives of hydroxyalkyl kappa-carrageenan [27]. Their synthesis widened the application of this polysaccharide.

Hydrogel based on kappa-carrageenan with very high absorptivity was synthesized by Hosseinzadeh et al. in 2005. The hydrogel was prepared through the cross-linking of polyacrylamide followed by alkaline hydrolysis [28]. Further studies on the same revealed that the swelling behavior of these hydrogels can be modified using γ-irradiation as the initiator and cross-linking agent simultaneously [29]. Biodegradable hydrogels

physicochemical features   **applications**

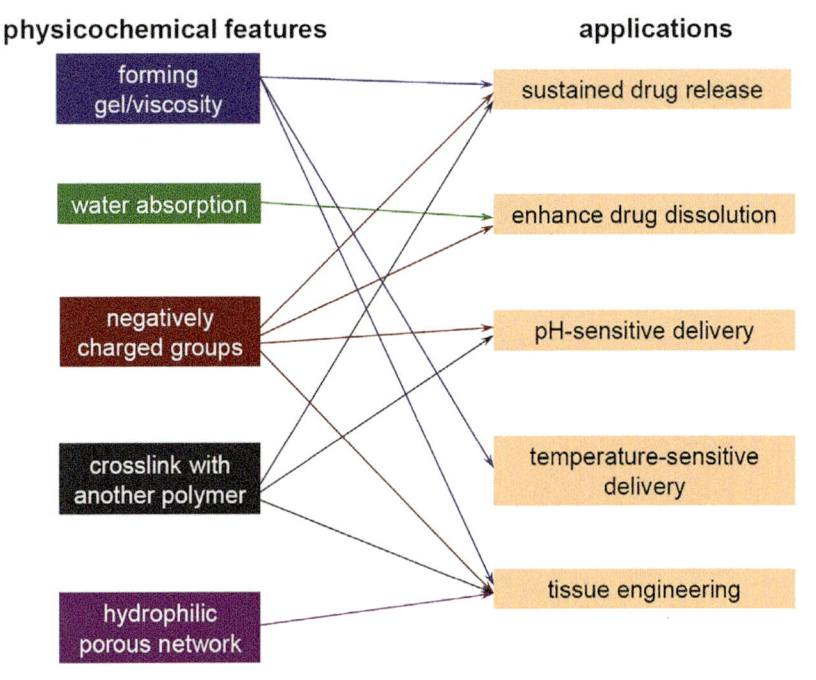

FIG. 9.4 Various physiochemical properties of carrageenan and its application.From Liu J, Zhan X, Wan J, Wang Y, Wang C. Review for carrageenan-based pharmaceutical biomaterials: favorable physical features versus adverse biological effects. Carbohydr Polym 2015;121:27–36, Copyright (2015), with permission from Elsevier.

with the potential to be used as novel delivery platforms are prepared through the copolymerization of kappa-carrageenan with 2-acrylamido-2-methylpropanesulfonic acid and acrylic acid [30].

Generally, the carrageenan-based hydrogels are brittle in nature with poor mechanical stability and high swelling ratios [31]. Chemically modifying the polymeric backbone of carrageenan is an effective strategy to overcome these drawbacks. The various influence of chemical modification on biomedical applications due to the modulation in physicochemical properties is represented in Fig. 9.4.

9.3 Carrageenan-based hydrogels

Carrageenan-based hydrogels are generally prepared by the methods of thermoreversible gelation, ionic cross-linking, ultraviolet (UV) cross-linking, and dual cross-linking. Various forms of carrageenan-based hydrogels can be obtained using these methods (Fig. 9.5). Different forms of carrageenan-based hydrogels are discussed further.

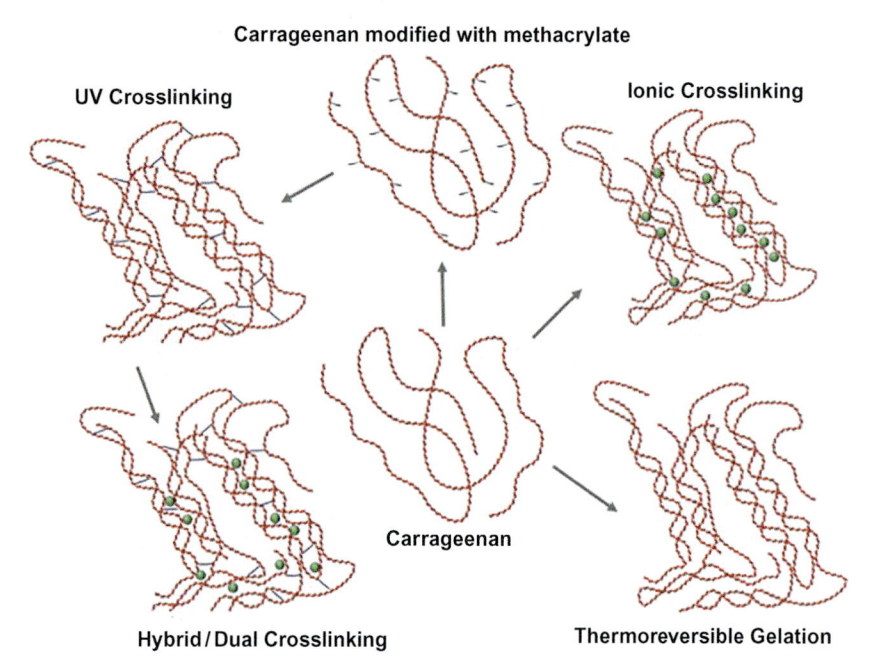

FIG. 9.5   Various cross-linking mechanisms for developing hydrogels based on carra-geenan.From Yegappan R, Selvaprithiviraj V, Amirthalingam S, Jayakumar R. Carrageenan based hydrogels for drug delivery, tissue engineering and wound healing. Carbohydr Polym 2018;198:385–400, Copyright (2018), with permission from Elsevier.

9.3.1 Photo-cross-linking hydrogels

A widely used method for the formulation of hydrogels is photo-cross-linking. The formation of brittle hydrogels by cross-linking through ionic interactions in the presence of Ca^{2+} and K^+ was a major hurdle [32, 33]. Photo-cross-linking emerged as a successful solution to this problem. Chemical modifications are made in the kappa-carrageenan backbone by the incorporation of photo-cross-linking moieties such as methacrylate. This modified carrageenan when undergoing UV cross-linking in the presence of chemical photoinitiators produces effi-cient photo-cross-linking hydrogels. Adding methacrylate groups have a considerable effect on the viscosity of kappa-carrageenan. Interaction between the side chains gets limited because of the methacrylate modifi-cation, and this can decrease the viscosity. Modified kappa-carrageenan with specific properties can be formulated through the replacement of the hydroxyl group with varying degrees of methacrylation. The method of cross-linking also affects the properties of hydrogel formed. It is found that the physically cross-linked modified kappa-carrageenan exhibits a lower swelling ratio compared with its chemically cross-linked version. Considering water retention capabilities, higher performance is offered by chemically cross-linked hydrogels that result in a more flexible hydrogel network. The degree of methacrylation decides the pore size distribution in the hydrogel. Interconnected pores have resulted from a lower degree of methacrylation, whereas the higher degree of methacrylation offers lower pore size distribution. Although the methacrylate groups, photoinitiators, and UV exposure determine the swelling ratio and pore size, the cell viability seems to be unaffected by these factors [34]. All these results, thus, finally conclude that dual cross-linking of methacrylated kappacarrageenan offers enhanced stability than physical cross-linking, thereby hindering the ion exchange in the dissolution media.

9.3.2 Gradient hydrogels

Gradient hydrogels find their application mainly in the field of tissue engineering. Gradient hydrogels can mimic interfaces, such as bone cartilage, which have a gradient in physical, structural, and chemical properties. Gradient hydrogels demonstrate gradient in any of the physical properties of the material that can be tuned to mimic the native tissue interface [35]. Smooth transitions between various tissue regions similar to the native tissue environment provided by these hydrogels offer great advantages over the conventional ones [36]. Multilayered gradient hydrogels can be easily prepared using the polymeric capillary flow [37]. There are also other techniques such as microfluidics, electrospinning, and gradient makers, which can be effectively used for the preparation [38]. However, compared with the polymeric capillary flow, the latter are more complex. Cross et al. in their work fabricated hydrogels based on methacrylated gelatin and carrageenan by a technique that makes use of the natural flow property of the material (Fig. 9.6) [39]. An increase in compressive moduli and strength along with shear-thinning property without affecting the gelation time was observed when nanosilicates were incorporated into these hydrogels. They also observed the change in pore structure across gelatin toward the carrageenan region in the scanning electron microscopy (SEM) microstructure analysis. This revealed the role of nanosilicates in the distribution of the pore area. In the gradient hydrogel, human mesenchymal stem cells (hMSCs) encapsulated into the gelatin region exhibited elongated morphology, which is the osteoblast's characteristic feature, whereas cells in carrageenan region exhibited rounded morphology, which is the characteristic feature of chondrocytes. In addition, the interface region displayed the presence of cells of both morphologies. Thus they could infer the potential of gradient hydrogels to modulate the cell fate.

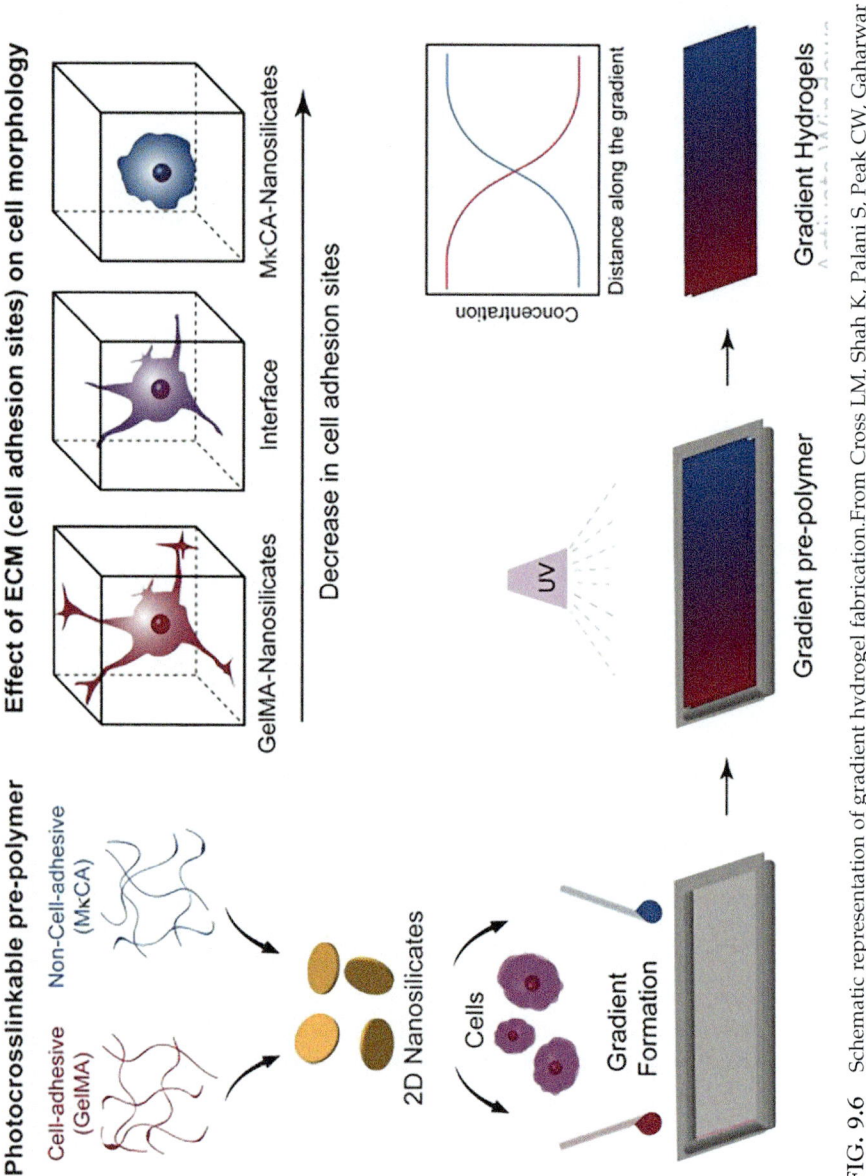

FIG. 9.6 Schematic representation of gradient hydrogel fabrication. From Cross LM, Shah K, Palani S, Peak CW, Gaharwar AK. Gradient nanocomposite hydrogels for interface tissue engineering. Nanomedicine 2007;14(7):2465–74, Copyright (2007), with permission from Elsevier.

9.3.3 Micropatterned hydrogels

To control the cellular microenvironment, microscale patterns are designed for the in vitro cell culture substrate using a micropatterning technique [40, 41]. Most of the techniques used for micropatterning are expensive, often tedious, and cannot be extended to a large class of biopolymers. Recently, Vignesh et al. formulated a template based on a micropatterned wax module that can be effectively used for the formulation of micropatterned hydrogels [42]. The template was able to design micropatterns of various sizes and shapes. Chondrogenesis is favored by these micropatterned hydrogels, and they are comparable with stiffer gels regarding their gel strength [43]. The biodegradable nature of these hydrogels made them suitable for the transplantation of stem cells and their differentiation. Considering the above results and similar studies revealed that the effect of physical signals of the microenvironment on the fate of stem cells can be studied with micropatterned kappa-carrageenan hydrogels.

9.3.4 Floating hydrogels

The ability to stay afloat in the stomach and the controlled drug release property shown by floating hydrogels gained the recent attention of researchers. These hydrogels can absorb the fluid in a controlled manner from their immediate environment and undergo swelling. Hence they achieve the ability to float over the gastric fluids [44]. Selvakumaran et al. studied the kappa-carrageenan–based floating hydrogel for their drug delivery efficacy and the effect of pore-forming agents [45, 46]. The pore-forming agents $NaHCO_3$ and $CaCO_3$ are incorporated in the synthesis of the kappa-carrageenan–based floating agent. They observed the increase in porosity with an increase in the concentration of pore-forming agents. But higher concentrations of pore-forming agents cause a reduction in the gel strength. Another major drawback with the use of a higher concentration of pore-forming agents is poor entrapment efficiency. Nevertheless, controlled drug release offered by these hydrogels compensated the other flaws. Their studies, thus, revealed the role of pore-forming agents and cross-linkers in improving the gastrosensitive properties and controlled drug delivery efficiency of kappa-carrageenan–based hydrogels.

9.3.5 Nanogels

The stability of biomolecule that is encapsulated by the delivery system is always a concern that is to be dealt properly while designing a drug carrier. Nanogels can be considered as a better solution for this problem [47]. Using the technique of spray drying, nanogels can be prepared by complexing carrageenan with low-density lipoproteins [48]. Various studies revealed that nanogels are temperature sensitive. They undergo thermal-stimulated reversible volume transition at a temperature range of 37–45°C. Their thermosensitive nature helps to develop smart drug delivery platforms where the controlled and sustained drug delivery can be achieved with controlled temperature [49]. Proper optimization of the concentration of carrageenan can result in the formation of nanogels with desired characteristics, including size, thermal behavior, swelling ratio, and drug release kinetics.

9.3.6 Interpenetrating polymer network hydrogels

The issues such as slow swelling response and weak mechanical properties of conventional hydrogels can be mitigated to a great extent by using interpenetrating polymer network (IPN) hydrogels. IPNs are basically polymer alloys, without forming a covalent bond; one of the polymers got synthesized and cross-linked within the presence of the other. The formed network remains unless the chemical bonds are broken [50]. Simultaneous and sequential IPNs are the two classes of IPN hydrogels based on the chemistry of their preparation. When the precursors of both networks are mixed and the synthesis of two networks take place simultaneously, they belong to simultaneous IPN. On the other hand, sequential IPNs are prepared by swelling single network hydrogel into a mixture containing initiator, activator, and monomer, with or without the cross-linker. A fully interpenetrating polymer network is formed in the presence of a cross-linker, and a semiinterpenetrating polymer network with linear polymers embedded in the first network is formed when the cross-linker is absent [51]. Factors including gelation time, polymer ratio, and amount of cross-linker influence the IPN formation and drug encapsulation efficiency.

IPNs are a great option for tissue engineering applications especially for the spinal disk regeneration because they can mimic the natural mechanics of intervertebral disk pulposus region [52]. Dual cross-linking mechanisms for the IPN hydrogel preparation have significance on its swelling ratio. In 2014, Wen et al. formulated IPN hydrogels through enzymatic and ionic cross-linking [53]. They cross-linked gelatin with microbial transglutaminase (mTG), making it more flexible by increasing the swelling. It is then followed by the ionic cross-linking of kappa-carrageenan that reduces its flexibility and water retention. This suggested the possibility of the synthesis of IPN hydrogels with tunable swelling ratio and degradation. Several studies also revealed that smaller bead size and rigid structure can be achieved by a higher concentration of cross-linker. In addition, higher cross-linker concentration resulted in high drug encapsulation efficiency and improved sustained drug release.

Chen et al. in 2009 developed a stimuli-responsive kappa-carrageenan semi-IPA hydrogel [54]. The hydrogel was sensitive to both temperature and pH. They synthesized a semiinterpenetrating polymer network hydrogel of kappa-carrageenan-g-poly(methacrylic acid)/poly(N,N-diethylacrylamide) using ammonium persulfate as an initiator and N,N,N',N'-tetramethylethylenediamide as an accelerator. A temperature-dependent deswelling was observed when the lower critical solution temperature was increased. Breaking of hydrogen bonds is considered to be the reason for deswelling. In addition, the protonation of carboxylic acid groups occurs because of the increase in pH, which consequently increased swelling ratio. This increase in the swelling ratio made the chains more flexible.

9.3.7 Hydrogel scaffolds

For tissue engineering applications, scaffolds based on hydrogels that can mimic the native ECM have gained considerable attention, and various methods have been used so far for their development [55]. The concentration of carrageenan in making the scaffolds plays a significant role in the pore size. The higher concentration of carrageenan offers scaffolds with large pore size, whereas lower concentration leads to small pore size and lower distribution. In addition, higher carrageenan concentration is associated with a higher swelling ratio. However, considering the compressive property, higher carrageenan concentration leads to lower compressive moduli. An investigation by Chopra et al. concluded that iota-carrageenan blended with poly(vinyl alcohol) of various ratios is an efficient scaffold for cryopreservation of cells [56]. They prepared hydrogels with various poly(vinyl alcohol) ratios and carrageenan followed by lyophilization for obtaining the scaffold. The scaffolds were found highly biocompatible and highly compatible with hemoglobin. They proposed that the ratios 7:3 and 8:2 provide ideal features for tissue engineering and cryopreservation of cells. Formation of evenly distributed pores at the particular ratios made them ideal candidates. Pore size and distribution, the fluid-retaining ability of pores, and polymer hydrophilicity play a vital role in the water uptake in the scaffolds [57].

9.3.8 Bioink for 3D bioprinting

3D printing has evolved as one of the breakthroughs in scientific advancement. Extending its application to bioprinting has opened several applications, especially in the area of tissue engineering. Choosing a perfect bioink is an essential part of successful bioprinting, and amazingly, the thermoresponsive kappa-carrageenan is a perfect fit. Gel formation in various shapes achieved through the fibrillary networks of kappa-carrageenan made it an excellent choice for the preparation of biomaterial scaffolds. As mentioned earlier, the hydrogels formed directly from kappa-carrageenan are brittle in nature, which makes them unsuitable in this application. However, making favorable chemical modification can effectively address this problem. Studies have opened various methods for the improvement of the toughness of the hydrogel [58]. Ionic-covalent entanglement (ICE) gels represent one of the tough hydrogel categories. Bakarich et al. fabricated printed ICE hydrogels based on carrageenan and epoxy amine [59]. In ICE hydrogels, among the interpenetrating polymer networks, one polymer is cross-linked with covalent bonds and the other cross-linked with metal cations [60]. Epoxy amine polymer network is synthesized through an epoxy-amine addition reaction between the two polymers poly(oxyalkylene amine) and poly(ethylene glycol)diglycidylether. The final bioink was obtained through the one-pot synthesis method by mixing the kappa-carrageenan with the synthesized epoxy amine solution in the presence of $CaCl_2$ solution. Through the process of thermal gelation transition, the biopolymer forms a polymer network. On the other hand, the synthetic polymer forms a covalent polymer network through the epoxy-amine addition mechanism. A significant mechanical performance was observed in the bioprinted hydrogel.

Recently, Li et al. developed a 3D printed hydrogel structure based on kappa-carrageenan and gelatin and studied the interfacial bonding in them (Fig. 9.7) [61]. Kappa-carrageenan being anionic and gelatin being cationic exhibit strong electrostatic interaction at their interface. The study proposed the efficiency of gelatin as a bioink medium for the loading of cells. The bonding strength is found significantly higher at the interface between kappa-carrageenan and gelatin compared with that of the bilayers formed by kappa-carrageenan and bilayers formed by gelatin. High cell viability and good structural stability are also offered by the bioprinted structure.

9.4 Application of carrageenan hydrogel in drug delivery

Originally, the word carrageenan is developed from carrageen, an Irish name that denotes the colloquial name of Rhodophyta, which means "small rock" [21]. Marine-derived carragcenan possesses versatile properties as a better constituent or participant in drug delivery. Nowadays, the importance of controlled and site-specific delivery urges keen attention, and carrageenan as a natural polysaccharide gives more possibilities to the controlled drug delivery field as well as in the medicinal field. Ideality of carrageenan as delivery vehicle includes its viscoelastic properties, thermoreversible gelation, biocompatibility, biodegradability, low cost of production, the comfort of physicochemical modifications, and simple gelation mechanism.

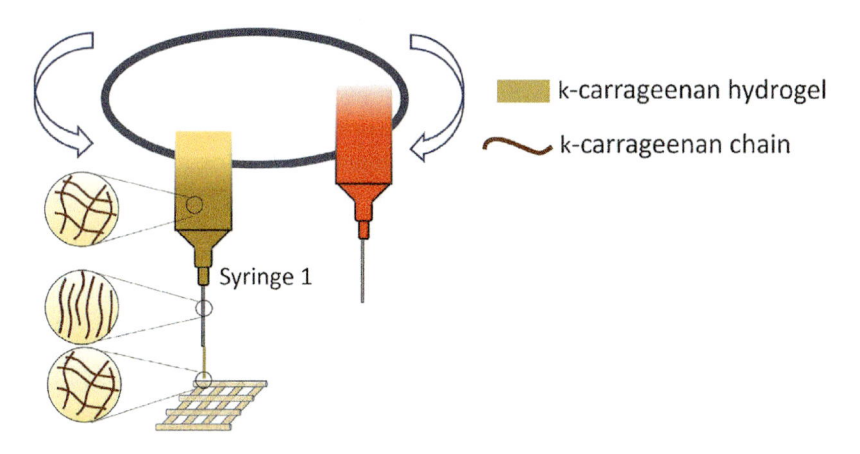

k-carrageenan hydrogel

k-carrageenan chain

Syringe 1

Syringe 1 for k-carrageenan hydrogel printing

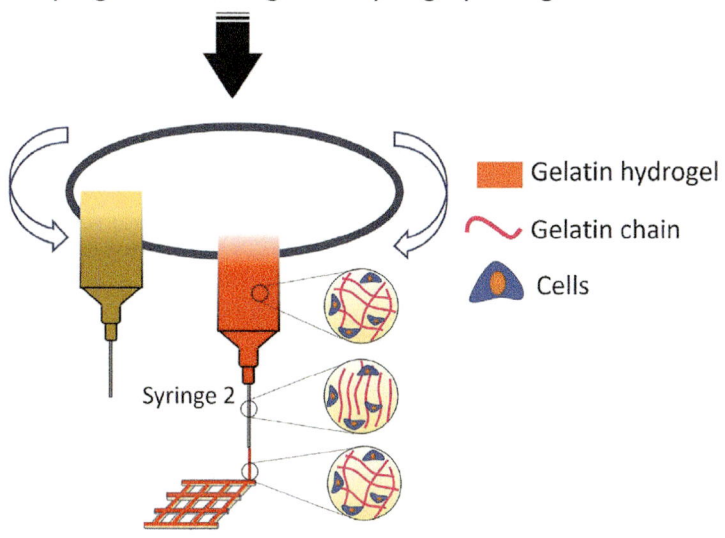

Gelatin hydrogel

Gelatin chain

Cells

Syringe 2

Syringe 2 for cell-laden Gelatin hydrogel printing

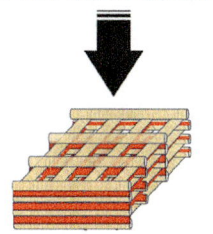

Layered k-carrageenan-Gelatin
hydrogel construct with live cells

FIG. 9.7 A schematic representation of the process of bioprinting. From Li H, Tan YJ, Li L. A strategy for strong interface bonding by 3D bioprinting of oppositely charged κ-carrageenan and gelatin hydrogels. Carbohydr Polym 2018;198:261–9, Copyright (2018), with permission from Elsevier.

9.4.1 Carrageenan hydrogel for oral drug delivery

The application of biopolymers that are biodegradable in nature is increasing due to their degradable nature in the internal physiological condition. The nontoxic degraded products that they form, which can be readily excreted from the body, made these biodegradable hydrogels a suitable choice to administrated through oral route for the drug delivery on to the gastrointestinal (GI) tract [62, 63].

Metal nanoparticles are extensively studied for their wide application in the biomedical fields [64]. Their antibacterial effect and drug delivery applications can be combined with carrageenan hydrogels for the formulation of novel drug delivery platforms with properties of both [65]. Hezaveh et al. studied modified kappa-carrageenan nanocomposite hydrogel and the effect of nanoparticles in their drug release profile in the GI tract [66]. A modified kappa-carrageenan nanocomposite was prepared by blending the kappa-carrageenan with sodium carboxymethyl cellulose (NaCMC). The incorporation of NaCMC increases the swelling property of carrageenan, and it was found that the blend of kappa-carrageenan/NaCMC shows most swelling at the 80:20 blend ratio. The modified carrageenan is then formulated into silver/carrageenan nanocomposite and magnetic/carrageenan nanocomposite. They were loaded with methylene blue and are studied for their drug delivery efficiency in the GI tract. The drug release profile varied in different parts of the GI tract. Considering the overall performance, Ag nanocomposite hydrogel shows maximum drug release of 90.86%, whereas the magnetic nanocomposite shows only 63.69% drug release. However, the performance of the two composites varies across different parts of the tract. The silver nanocomposite shows the highest performance in the stomach, whereas in duodenum and intestine, the magnetic nanocomposite performed well. The results also showed that the increase in nanoparticle concentration can improve the release profile in both silver and magnetic nanocomposite hydrogels. The study revealed the possibility of controlled drug delivery that can be rendered by metallic nanoparticles in hydrogels. The same group has also studied the effect of MgO in pH-sensitive hydrogels in oral drug delivery of methylene blue [67]. The results were similar to the previous study and again confirmed the potential of metal oxides in hydrogels for controlled drug release. In the study, they also used the compound genipin that can reduce the drug release at the stomach and increase the drug release at the intestine. More control over the release profile was achieved.

Clay nanoparticles are another category that has gained their attention in recent years. With their high surface area, absorption capabilities, drug-loading ability, and amazing biological properties, they have been widely studied in the medical field [68]. Halloysite nanotube (HNT), a member of that clay family, is one of the most important ones, with its hollow tubular network and characteristic strength. The positive charge on the inner surface and the negative charge on the outer surface of HNT provide space for forming electrostatic interactions with various drugs and other charged molecules. The hollow structure and porosity of HNT made it a suitable drug carrier, and in the work by Sharifzadeh et al., they incorporated this HNT with kappa-carrageenan [69]. They have studied the effect of HNT in various physicochemical properties of kappa-carrageenan. Orange G and rhodamine B were used as the model drugs. The composite hydrogel was prepared by physical cross-linking. Enhanced thermal stability, high swelling behavior, and enhanced drug loading and release profile were observed with the incorporation of HNT. The in vitro cytotoxicity analysis revealed the safety and biocompatibility of the hydrogel. Another observation was that the release performance of the cationic drug rhodamine B was higher than the anionic drug orange G. The whole study, thus, revealed the potential of the HNT/kappa-carrageenan composite to act as a drug delivery platform.

A very similar investigation was recently conducted by Akrami-Hasan-Kohal et al. again by incorporating HNT [70]. But in this study, instead of kappa-carrageenan, they have used aldehyde-modified kappa-carrageenan/gelatin film, which was incorporated into HNT. The overall improvement in various parameters was observed, which ensure the compatibility of the system to be used for biomedical applications.

Metal-organic frameworks (MOFs) always had the special attention of scientists with their various characteristics, including high surface area, large pore volume, and tunable pore size [71, 72]. The high drug-loading capability and rooms for chemical modification for the enhancement of performance throws special attention to MOF-based drug delivery platforms. Among various MOFs, the high chemical, mechanical, and thermal stabilities together with the high porosity of UiO-66 gave them prominent attention as a drug delivery platform [73]. Combining such an efficient nanoencapsulating agent with a biopolymer can be effectively used to obtain the desired drug delivery and release profile. Such an approach was used by Javanbakht et al. [74]. They developed tramadol (Tr)-loaded biopolymeric system of kappa-carrageenan in combination with UiO-66 as a unique oral DDS (Fig. 9.8). The drug release controllability was improved under GI tract conditions by the incorporation of the kappa-carrageenan hydrogel. Another important observation about this study was that this biopolymeric composite had cytocompatible nature against human colon cells and stomach pH.

9.4.2 Carrageenan hydrogel for ocular drug delivery

Even though several therapeutic formulations are developed for ocular drug delivery applications, several barriers in the eye, including low corneal penetration, lacrimation, and blinking, necessitated novel efficient

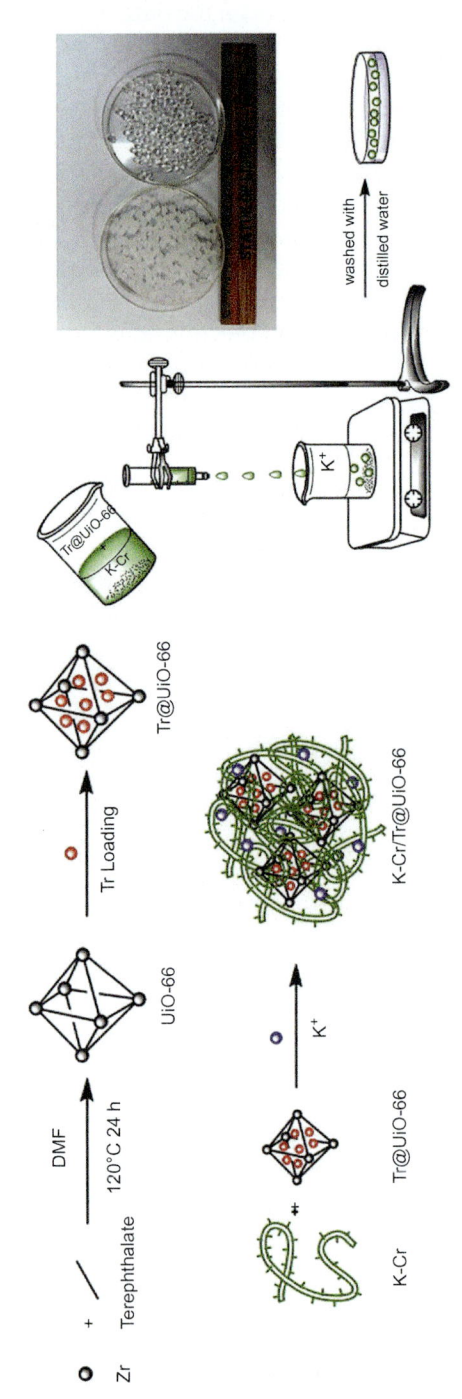

FIG. 9.8 Schematic representation of tramadol (Tr)-loaded biopolymeric system of kappa-carrageenan in combination with UiO-66. From Javanbakht S, Shadi M, Mohammadian R, Shaabani A, Amini MM, Pooresmaeil M, Salehi R. Facile preparation of pH-responsive k-carrageenan/tramadol loaded UiO-66 bio-nanocomposite hydrogel beads as a nontoxic oral delivery vehicle. J Drug Deliv Sci Technol 2019;54:1–7, Copyright (2019), with permission from Elsevier.

drug delivery platforms [75]. Besides colloids and polymeric implants, sustained drug delivery is offered by hydrogels [76].

The residence time of the drug in the eye surface is a significant parameter affecting the efficiency of a drug. Various formulations have been proposed as a solution for this. However, stimuli-sensitive delivery platforms based on hydrogels have gained their prominence in recent times [77]. Stimuli-sensitive hydrogels, especially the ion-sensitive hydrogels, evolved as a breakthrough because the stimuli can cause sol-gel transition leading in situ hydrogel formation. These can further facilitate prolonged drug release [78]. Fernández-Ferreiro et al. reported an ion-sensitive hydrogel formulation that is based on kappa-carrageenan and gellan gum [79]. The hydrogel was prepared using kappa-carrageenan and gellan gum, and two radiotracers, Technetium-99m (^{99m}Tc) and ^{99m}Tc pentatate [diethylene triamine pentaacetic acid] (^{99m}Tc-DTPA) were incorporated for radiolabeling. The radiotracer loss from ion-sensitive hydrogel in the presence of simulated tear fluid (STF) was analyzed. The analysis revealed the prolonged retention of radiotracers in the hydrogel due to the rapid gelation of the hydrogel in contact with STF. The scintigraphy studies in rats on the ocular residence time shows a significant increase in it.

9.4.3 Carrageenan hydrogel for pulmonary drug delivery

Hydrogels have gained their prominence in nasal drug delivery due to their characteristic phase of matter. Rapid clearance of solutions from the nasal cavity and incomplete wetting of solid inserts have become the barriers for effective drug delivery [80]. Li et al. reported their formulation of hydrogel based on poloxamer 407 and carrageenan for the delivery of antiinflammatory drug ketorolac tromethamine through the intranasal route [81]. The concentration of potassium ion is observed to have a significant effect on the erosion characteristics of the system. Higher potassium ion concentration can lead to a lower erosion rate. Approximately 15% of the drug when incorporated into the drug delivery hydrogel system showed a sustained drug release profile and suitable gelation temperature near to 35°C. The nasal ciliotoxicity was evaluated using in situ toad palate model, and the observed results revealed safety of the hydrogel system.

9.4.4 Carrageenan hydrogel for vaginal drug delivery

Carrageenan has been reported as a potential candidate for its application in vaginal drug delivery [82]. Carrageenan-based hydrogels have more advantages over other gel systems such as gelatin, and they can overcome severe drawbacks of other DDSs. Zoonotic infection risks, incompatibility with tropical climate due to instability with heat during storage, and lack of accessibility by vegetarians were some drawbacks of gelatin. Carrageenan could effectively overcome these drawbacks, and the antiviral effect of carrageenan reported open rooms for more of its applications [83].

Zaveri et al. investigated carrageenan-based hydrogel for drug delivery toward HIV treatment [84]. AIDS and other sexually transmitted diseases were reduced significantly with the act of educating people about reproductive health and by the development of efficient protective methods [85]. However, the number cannot have been reduced to a negligible value, which makes it essential to develop efficient strategies for the prevention of its transmission [86]. One successful category is the microbicides that have the capability to prevent HIV transmission [87]. Before intercourse, they are inserted in the vagina in the form of foam, sponge, gel, or cream. Tenofovir, the antiretroviral drug is a microbicide that has been studied for its prevention of HIV transmission and herpes simplex virus-2 transmission [88]. As mentioned earlier, carrageenan is suitable to be administrated in the vagina for the delivery of tenofovir. The group developed prototypes of microbicides prepared from carrageenan and evaluated their physical properties for better adherence and acceptability. Drug delivery efficacy of carrageenan loaded with tenofovir is analyzed through in vitro dissolution studies conducted in three fluids such as water, semen simulant fluid (SSF), and vaginal simulant fluid (VSF). IN SSF and VSF, the loaded drug is released through diffusion out of the matrix, whereas in case of water, the drug release is by both diffusion and matrix erosion. Rapid drug release is observed initially, which is followed by a slow-release curve over the first 24 hours.

Liu et al. explored how the drug release profile of poloxamer 407–based gel is affected by the incorporation of carrageenan into it [89]. Various characteristic properties such as availability, ease of gel preparation, drug compatibility, and excellent drug-loading capacity make poloxamer 407 a suitable choice for pharmaceutical applications [90]. Composite gel systems with enhanced sustained drug release profile can be obtained by incorporating carrageenan and other natural macromolecules into poloxamer 407 [91]. The team used acyclovir as the model drug for the study. Acyclovir, which is chemically 9-(2-hydroxyethoxymethyl)guanine, is an antiviral drug widely used for the treatment of herpes viruses [92]. The composite gel was prepared through the cold method. A significant decrease in the acyclovir release rate, concentration-dependent gel erosion, and retarded poloxamer 407 dissolutions were observed with the addition of carrageenan in in vitro release experiments. In addition, prolonged local drug residence of acyclovir and enhanced bioadhesive effect was observed in the in vivo experiments. All the results together concluded the enhanced efficiency of carrageenan-incorporated poloxamer 407 for in situ vaginal drug delivery.

Another vaginal drug delivery platform for the delivery of acyclovir was developed by Sánchez-Sánchez et al. in 2015 [93]. The chitosan and kappa-carrageenan–based formulation were developed for the prevention of herpes simplex virus transmitted through sexual intercourse. Cellulose-derived polymer formulations such as hydroxyl-ethyl-cellulose and methylcellulose are well known for their applications in the vagina [94, 95]. In this work, the group developed a novel formulation by combining the cellulose-derived polymer hydroxyl-propyl-methyl-cellulose (HPMC) with kappa-carrageenan or chitosan. Both the polymers are excellent in drug delivery applications, and combining the two will help to exploit the benefits of two. The formulation with kappa-carrageenan shows the complete release of acyclovir drug. In addition, the time required for 100% of the drug release from the formulation seems to depend on the kappa-carrageenan/HPMC ratio. The drug release profile investigation was conducted in both SVF and SVF/SSF mixture. In addition, biovine vaginal mucosa was used as the substrate for the ex vivo determination of bioadhesion characteristics. The in vitro cellular toxicity assays, thus, revealed that acyclovir drug and the drug carrier are safe.

9.4.5 Carrageenan hydrogel for transdermal drug delivery

The largest organ in the human body, skin, is a site for the delivery of many supplements. The diffusion of contents form the hydrogel is facilitated by the keratinocytes surface of the skin. Several potential systems have been developed for the purposes of delivering active ingredients on the epidermis, water retention, skin temperature regulation, and hydration [96].

Yee et al. formulated a hydrogel based on carrageenan for the sustained release of tocotrienol-rich palm-based vitamin E [97]. Exposure to UV radiation can cause severe damage to the skin. An active ingredient used in cosmetic products to protect skin from damage caused by UV radiation is tocotrienol-rich palm-based vitamin E (TRPE) [98]. Hydrogels were rarely reported as the delivery vehicles for TRPE due to their hydrophobic nature. However, further studies revealed the possibility of entrapment of TRPE in hydrogels through the formation of oil-in-water emulsions by the preparation of semiinterpenetrating networks and surfactant incorporation. As mentioned earlier, the properties of carrageenan can be improved by incorporating various units. The team incorporated locust bean gum (LBG) and guar gum (GG) with carrageenan for the development of the hydrogel composite. LBG has been extensively studied, and it has already been reported that LBG incorporation with carrageenan exhibits excellent synergism and leads to the formation of strong hydrogels with enhanced viscoelastic properties [99]. By forming more sites for hydrogen bonding, LBG contributed significantly to the bioadhesive effects of the hydrogel to which it is associated [100]. Modified carrageenan shows enhanced flexibility and strength with the incorporation of guar gum, glycerin, and potassium citrate. The in vitro skin irritation test revealed its nonirritating character. A mixture of PEG-40 hydrogenated castor oil when included with TRPE has improved the bioavailability of TRPE. All the above results with a special focus on the enhanced bioavailability find the delivery system suitable for skincare applications.

9.5 Application of carrageenan hydrogel in tissue engineering

Tissue engineering includes cartilage and bone tissue reconstruction, repair, and regeneration. Hence this approach draws a lot of clinical interest as the replacement with a biocompatible material, thus permanently repairing the damaged cartilage has a vital role in medicine. Owing to its high similarity with the ECM, hydrogels have widely been used as scaffolds in tissue engineering.

9.5.1 Carrageenan hydrogel for bone tissue regeneration

Carrageenan is efficient for bone tissue engineering applications because a bone-like apatite layer is induced by the carrageenan, which is highly desirable for scaffolding [101]. Feng et al. synthesized and studied collagen-hydroxyapatite/kappa-carrageenan composite [102]. The study revealed how the composite microstructure and collagen-hydroxyapatite bond formation are influenced by composite preparation conditions. Using various characterization techniques, they concluded that a significant increase in compressive strength can be achieved by incorporating kappa-carrageenan on the collagen-hydroxyapatite composite gel and making it a potential bone repair material. A lot of injectable bone substitutes are commercially available in the market. Along with the efficiency of the substitute, optimum injectability is also of utmost importance. Substitutes based on carrageenan with hydroxyapatite nanorods were investigated for their injectability by González and Ossa [103]. The results revealed the excellent injectability of carrageenan-based substitutes. In 2017, Goonoo et al. reported their novel electrospun material for the application of bone tissue engineering [104]. Biodegradable polyhydroxybutyrate (PHB) or polyhydroxybutyrate valerate (PHBV) is blended with the kappa-carrageenan in varying ratios. In the PHBV/kappa-carrageenan blend, preferential localization of kappa-carrageenan at the fiber surface is observed, whereas the carrageenan is found within the fiber in case of PHB/kappa-carrageenan blend. Fast apatite formation and nanosized apatite crystal deposition were observed. Their study concluded that the biomineralization as well as the osteogenic differentiation of PHB and PHBV can be enhanced with kappa-carrageenan. Similarly, hydrogels developed from hydrolyzed collagen and iota-carrageenan in aqueous mixtures containing $CaCl_2$ and H_3PO_4 were used to fabricate biomembranes. They exhibited excellent activity for bone regeneration by stimulating biological reactions essential to promote bone development. In an aqueous mixture containing $CaCl_2$ and H_3PO_4, hydrolyzed collagen and iota-carrageenan is dissolved. Mineral precipitation in hydrogels was observed with a rise in pH by exposure to ammonia gas. Using solvent casting, membranes were fabricated. The mechanical behavior of membrane is found to depend on the carrageenan content and controlled degradability in membranes were obtained with higher polysaccharide concentration. Collagen was released from these membranes in physiological conditions. The work revealed the potential of the hydrogel system to be considered as a temporary guided tissue regeneration membrane [105].

Cross et al. fabricated gradient scaffolds making use of kappa-carrageenan, gelatin, and nanosilicates in a simple microfabrication method [39]. To mimic the native tissue interface, two-dimensional nanosilicates were used to reinforce the gradient scaffold fabricated with the two polymers methacrylated kappa-carrageenan and gelatin methacryloyl. The inclusion of the nanosilicates explicitly raised the compressive moduli and endurance of the kappa-carrageenan and gelatin-based hydrogels. The strength of the matrix found to increase up to sevenfold with a small number of nanosilicate addition due to the shear-thinning characteristics, whereas the strength of the hydrogels rose approximately threefold at the same concentration. This simple method could be explored for the reconstruction of the bone-cartilage interface.

Mandible distraction osteogenesis is always concerned with the injury of the inferior alveolar nerve (IAN). The study by Wang et al. in a rabbit model of mandible distraction osteogenesis confirmed the significant enhancement in the regeneration and development of IAN with local repeated injections of human nerve growth factor β (NGF-β) [106]. Further studies led to the development of collagen/nanohydroxyapatite/kappa-carrageenan gel that can deliver human NGF-β effectively, which resulted in accelerated IAN recovery. The study was conducted in four groups in which human NGF-β in gel, human NGF-β in saline, gel alone, and saline alone were considered for groups 1, 2, 3, and 4 respectively. Injections were given at the end of the distraction period, and histologic and histomorphometric analyses were performed after 14 days, suggesting the abundant regeneration of IAN fibers in human NGF-β in the gel than in other groups [107].

In 2014, Mihaila et al. proposed microsized hydrogel fibers based on chitosan-coated kappa-carrageenan for scalable and flexible 3D systems [108]. These 3D systems can act as building blocks for the formulation of hydrogel constructs for vascularized bone tissue engineering applications

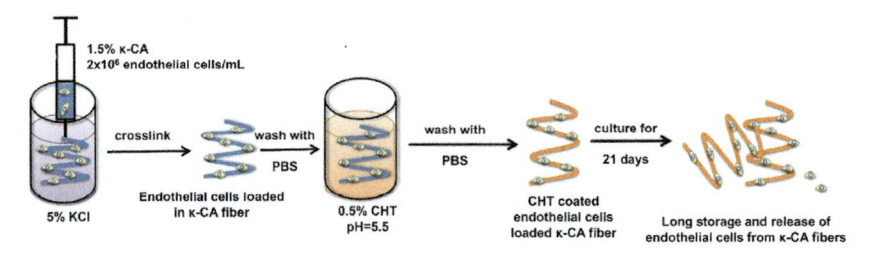

FIG. 9.9   Schematic representation of the experimental set up for the encapsulation of endothelial cells into kappa-carrageenan fibers.From Mihaila SM, Popa EG, Reis RL, Marques AP, Gomes ME, Fabrication of endothelial cell-laden carrageenan microfibers for microvascularized bone tissue engineering applications. Biomacromolecules 2014;15(8):2849–60, Copyright (2014), with permission from American Chemical Society.

(Fig. 9.9). Evaluation of various parameters, including swelling behavior, stability, endothelial cell carrying and releasing profiles, and ability to assemble cell-laden fibers within the matrix of the hydrogel, thus proved the suitability of the fibers. This is a multifaceted approach to study the various interactions between different cell types in a controlled setting. This also opens the door for mimicking the complexity of tissues using 3D in vitro culture techniques.

9.5.2 Carrageenan hydrogel for cartilage tissue regeneration

The inability of spontaneous regeneration of cartilage tissues made it essential the requirement of a platform for the efficient delivery of cells and other factors to the area with a defect. Pereira et al. reported a novel injectable hydrogel system for human articular chondrocytes [109]. A carrageenan/fibrin/hyaluronic acid-based hydrogel system with gelling properties in situ was developed. Kappa-carrageenan, which has the sulfate groups in the backbone has the characteristics to mimic sulfated glycosaminoglycans, which are naturally occurring in the ECM of cartilage. On the other hand, hyaluronic acid with its rapid degradation and characteristic biological properties came out to be a candidate for the fabrication of new biomaterials. In addition, hyaluronic acid represents one of the major constituents of ECM. Carrageenan/fibrin/hyaluronic acid–based hydrogel is first seeded with chondrogenic cells and is then cultured for 3 weeks. A significant increase in the cell number, the formation of cartilage-specific ECM, and maintenance of cell viability was observed. Thus they showed the potential of injectable hydrogels that are seeded with human articular chondrocytes in repairing and regenerating defective cartilage tissues.

A study was conducted by Rocha et al. where the human adipose stem cells (ADSCs) were encapsulated in carrageenan together with transforming growth factor-$\beta 1$ (TGF-$\beta 1$) [110]. The investigation mainly focuses on evaluating the cytotoxicity along with the influence of biopolymers on cell proliferation and viability. Enhanced cartilage differentiation of human ADSCs was observed with the incorporation of TGF-$\beta 1$. A similar study by Popa et al. developed another injectable kappa-carrageenan–based hydrogel with chondrogenic potential that can encapsulate adipose stem cells [43]. Hydrogels were prepared by encapsulating human ADSCs in the kappa-carrageenan solution through the ionotropic gelation method. The viability, proliferation, and chondrogenic differentiation properties of the carrageenan-encapsulated human adipose stem cells were analyzed after being cultured for up to 21 days. They also observed enhanced viscoelastic properties and increased stiffness of the system that made them conclude that kappa-carrageenan exhibits properties that facilitate the in vitro functionality of the encapsulated adipose stem cells. The same group also reported the freeze-thawing stability of carrageenan and the maintenance of the structural integrity of the cryopreservation-thawing process [111].

There were studies related to kappa-carrageenan incorporated into magnetic nanoparticles for developing magnetically responsive hydrogels. The studies revealed that the incorporation of magnetic nanoparticles makes considerable influence in the efficacy of hydrogel, and the concentration of magnetic nanoparticle enhanced the cell content, cell viability, and metabolic activity of the human ADSCs. The most promising outcomes were obtained in 5% nanoparticle-carrageenan matrices [112].

Thakur et al. proposed a kappa-carrageenan hydrogel reinforced with 2D nanosilicate for cellular delivery in cartilage tissue regeneration [113]. Kappa-carrageenan is chemically modified by methacrylation, and it is then incorporated with 2D nanosilicate, resulting in characteristics such as shear-thinning, enhanced mechanical stiffness, elastomeric properties, and physiological stability. The system shows high cell viability with human mesenchymal stem cell delivery.

9.5.3 Carrageenan hydrogel for wound healing

For patients suffering from burn injuries and other medical conditions that can cause severe tissue damage, wound healing remains a major challenge. Dressing of wounds using the conventional gauzes and bandages provide a dry environment. However, studies have shown that a moist environment is most favorable for fast healing [114]. Wound healing is an intricate process that involves the reorientation of damaged tissues in a process comprising several steps such as hemostasis, swelling, proliferation, and tissue remodeling [115]. Because wounds are not guarded against microbial attack, deciding on the perfect wound filling substance is highly vital. The perfect wound filling substance should have incorporated properties such as prevention of microbial attack, regeneration of tissues, diminishing blemishes, and reconstructing skin homeostasis [116]. However, hydrogels are reported as the best options among all dressing forms because of their dominance over other conventional modes. The only drawback of hydrogels is their poor mechanical stability at the swollen state. By incorporating more than one polymer in the system significantly addresses this disadvantage. Demonstrated that the addition of poly(vinylpyrrolidone) (PVP) and silk powder improved the mechanical properties of membranes significantly in a PVA-PVP-kappa-carrageenan-silk powder hydrogel membrane. They affirmed that these membranes are nontoxic, which supported its use for accelerated wound and burn to heal [117].

Nair et al. synthesized cyclic β-$(1 \rightarrow 3)(1 \rightarrow 6)$ glucan/carrageenan hydrogels (CBG/Car) and reported its potential in encapsulating ciprofloxacin, a hydrophobic drug [118]. The wound healing efficacy of the system is studied in rats. Chemical modification on carrageenan by incorporating CBG shown to have improved wound healing efficiency with enhanced cell attachment and proliferation. A recent study by Jaiswal et al. found the excellent wound healing effect shown by kappa-carrageenan hydrogel incorporated into chitosan-capped sulfur nanoparticles and grapefruit seed extract [119]. Along with the wound healing effect, it also shows the antibacterial effect that destroyed *Escherichia coli* and *Staphylococcus epidermis* within 3 hours of incubation. In 2018 Lokhande et al. reported a nanoengineered injectable hydrogel system with synthetic 2D nanosilicates loaded on kappa-carrageenan [120]. The tunable stiffness of the hydrogel by varying the ration between carrageenan and nanosilicate provides an extra advantage. The highly porous interconnected networks and high mechanical stiffness resulted in increased platelet binding, enhanced cell adhesion and spreading, and reduced clotting time of blood. Silva et al. developed a hydrogel based on kappa-carrageenan together with PVP and PEG by γ-irradiation [121]. The hydrogel developed is suitable for the Sri Lankan tropical condition. The hydrogel system has advantages of affordable cost and long shelf life.

For accelerating the wound healing process, incorporating antibacterial agents into the hydrogel emerged as an effective strategy. An antistaphylococcal and neutrophil chemotactic injectable kappa-carrageenan hydrogel was developed especially for infectious wound healing. The kappa-carrageenan hydrogel is developed by incorporating 0.01% (v/v) octenidine dihydrochloride (Oct) and 0.5% (w/w) chitosan-treated serum (CTS). The antiseptic action of Oct and neutrophilic attractant properties of CTS enabled the system to act as a solution infected with *Staphylococcus aureus*. The sustained release of Oct and CST from the hydrogel causes the migration of fibroblast and polymorphonuclear neutrophils and shows excellent antibacterial efficacy together facilitating the tissue regeneration at the wound site [122]. Azizi et al. fabricated a bionanocomposite hydrogel by incorporating biosynthesized silver nanoparticles with kappa-carrageenan [123]. *Citrullus colocynthis* seed extract was used for the synthesis of Ag nanoparticles. The swelling behavior observed was comparatively lower. It shows excellent antimicrobial effect against *S. aureus*, methicillin-resistant *S. aureus*, *E. coli*, and *Pseudomonas aeruginosa*. The study also concluded that the hydrogel system is safe at a concentration below 1000 μg/mL. In 2013 a novel biodegradable hydrogel of silver nanocomposite was reported [124]. The silver nanocomposite was prepared using *Azadirachta indica* leaf extract. The hydrogel was prepared by the green process. They showed antibacterial activity against *Bacillus* and *E. coli*.

9.6 Conclusion

Carrageenan is an amazing natural polysaccharide derived from the red algae, and it possesses numerous biomedical properties. The characteristic physical properties and the presence of functional groups that enable further fabrication in its structure for purposeful actions made the biopolymer carrageenan a promising candidate for diverse biomedical applications such as tissue engineering and drug delivery. A variety of methods were applicable to synthesize useful carrageenan-based hydrogels, which gives us a better platform to achieve good medicinal practices in tissue engineering, drug delivery, and regenerative medicines. Although the biopolymer faces some drawbacks in certain fields of application, being an active topic in the research field, further studies could mitigate the flaws and bring the polymer to new heights. Incorporating other polymers, molecules, and making chemical modification in the structure of carrageenan enhanced its various properties, and the synergistic effects because of the combinations successfully resulted in novel formulations with amazing potentials.

Further research and detailed investigation on carrageenan-based hydrogels can reveal more secrets about the wonder polymer. Incorporation of new structures into carrageenan can open the doors for the formulation of novel systems with characteristic properties that can address various problems in the list.

Acknowledgments

We thank KSCSTE for KSCSTE/5130/2017-SRSPS grant and Sacred Heart College for the Major research grant to JG (2020).

References

[1] Allen TM, Cullis PR. Drug delivery systems: entering the mainstream. Science 2004;303(5665):1818–22.
[2] Singh AV. Biopolymers in drug delivery: a review. Pharmacologyonline 2011;1:666–74.
[3] Van de Velde F, Knutsen SH, Usov AI, Rollema HS, Cerezo AS. 1H, and 13C high resolution NMR spectroscopy of carrageenans: application in research and industry. Trends Food Sci Technol 2002;13(3):73–92.

[4] Necas J, Bartosikova L. Carrageenan: a review. Vet Med 2013;58(4):187–205.

[5] Bhardwaj TR, Kanwar M, Lal R, Gupta A. Natural gums and modified natural gums as sustained-release carriers. Drug Dev Ind Pharm 2000;26(10):1025–38.

[6] Wijesekara I, Pangestuti R, Kim SK. Biological activities and potential health benefits of sulfated polysaccharides derived from marine algae. Carbohydr Polym 2011;84(1):14–21.

[7] Girond S, Crance JM, Van Cuyck-Gandre H, Renaudet J, Deloince R. Antiviral activity of carrageenan on hepatitis A virus replication in cell culture. Res Virol 1991;142(4):261–70.

[8] Buck CB, Thompson CD, Roberts JN, Müller M, Lowy DR, Schiller JT. Carrageenan is a potent inhibitor of papillomavirus infection. PLoS Pathog 2006;2(7), e69.

[9] Hezaveh H, Muhamad II, Noshadi I, Shu Fen L, Ngadi N. Swelling behaviour and controlled drug release from cross-linked κ-carrageenan/NaCMC hydrogel by diffusion mechanism. J Microencapsul 2012;29(4):368–79.

[10] Hoffman AS. Hydrogels for biomedical applications. Adv Drug Deliv Rev 2012;64:18–23.

[11] Williams DF. Hydrogels in regenerative medicine. In: Principles of regenerative medicine. Academic Press; 2019. p. 627–50.

[12] Anitha A, Sowmya S, Kumar PS, Deepthi S, Chennazhi KP, Ehrlich H, Tsurkan M, Jayakumar R. Chitin and chitosan in selected biomedical applications. Prog Polym Sci 2014;39(9):1644–67.

[13] Geckil H, Xu F, Zhang X, Moon S, Demirci U. Engineering hydrogels as extracellular matrix mimics. Nanomedicine 2010;5(3):469–84.

[14] Tibbitt MW, Anseth KS. Hydrogels as extracellular matrix mimics for 3D cell culture. Biotechnol Bioeng 2009;103(4):655–63.

[15] Stanley N. Production, properties and uses of carrageenan. Production and utilization of products from commercial seaweeds. FAO Fish Tech Pap 1987;288:116–46.

[16] Imeson AP, Phillips G, Williams P. Carrageenan, furcellaran and other seaweed-derived products. In: Handbook of hydrocolloids. 2nd ed. Woodhead Publishing series in food science. Sawston, Cambridge, UK: Woodhead Publishing; 2009. p. 87–101.

[17] Whistler RL, BeMiller JN. Carrageenans. Carbohydrate chemistry for food scientists. 3rd. Elsevier; 2019. p. 279–91.

[18] Rowe RC, Sheskey PJ, Quinn ME. Handbook of pharmaceutical excipients. London: Pharmaceutical Press; 2009.

[19] Hilliou L, Larotonda FD, Abreu P, Ramos AM, Sereno AM, Gonçalves MP. Effect of extraction parameters on the chemical structure and gel properties of κ/ι-hybrid carrageenans obtained from Mastocarpus stellatus. Biomol Eng 2006;23(4):201–8.

[20] McHugh DJ. Production and utilization of products from commercial seaweeds. FAO; 1987.

[21] Campo VL, Kawano DF, da Silva Jr DB, Carvalho I. Carrageenans: biological properties, chemical modifications and structural analysis–a review. Carbohydr Polym 2009;77(2):167–80.

[22] Nanaki S, Karavas E, Kalantzi L, Bikiaris D. Miscibility study of carrageenan blends and evaluation of their effectiveness as sustained release carriers. Carbohydr Polym 2010;79(4):1157–67.

[23] Cunha L, Grenha A. Sulfated seaweed polysaccharides as multifunctional materials in drug delivery applications. Mar Drugs 2016;14(3):42.

[24] Stone AK, Nickerson MT. Formation and functionality of whey protein isolate–(kappa-, iota-, and lambda-type) carrageenan electrostatic complexes. Food Hydrocoll 2012;27(2):271–7.

[25] Running CA, Falshaw R, Janaswamy S. Trivalent iron induced gelation in lambda-carrageenan. Carbohydr Polym 2012;87(4):2735–9.

[26] Kara S, Arda E, Kavzak B, Pekcan Ö. Phase transitions of κ-carrageenan gels in various types of salts. J Appl Polym 2006;102(3):3008–16.

[27] Guiseley KB, inventor; FMC Corp, assignee. Modified kappa-carrageenan. United States patent US 4,096,327; 1978.

[28] Hosseinzadeh H, Pourjavadi A, Mahdavinia GR, Zohuriaan-Mehr MJ. Modified carrageenan. 1. H-CarragPAM, a novel biopolymer-based superabsorbent hydrogel. J Bioact Compat Polym 2005;20(5):475–90.

[29] Bardajee GR, Pourjavadi A, Sheikh N, Amini-Fazl MS. Grafting of acrylamide onto kappa-carrageenan via γ-irradiation: optimization and swelling behavior. Radiat Phys Chem 2008;77(2):131–7.

[30] Pourjavadi A, Barzegar S, Zeidabadi F. Synthesis and properties of biodegradable hydrogels of κ-carrageenan grafted acrylic acid-co-2-acrylamido-2-methylpropanesulfonic acid as candidates for drug delivery systems. React Funct Polym 2007;67(7):644–54.

[31] Thakur R, Saberi B, Pristijono P, Golding J, Stathopoulos C, Scarlett C, Bowyer M, Vuong Q. Characterization of rice starch-ι-carrageenan biodegradable edible film. Effect of stearic acid on the film properties. Int J Biol Macromol 2016;93:952–60.

[32] Chronakis IS, Doublier JL, Piculell L. Viscoelastic properties for kappa-and iota-carrageenan in aqueous NaI from the liquid-like to the solid-like behaviour. Int J Biol Macromol 2000;28(1):1–4.

[33] Mangione MR, Giacomazza D, Bulone D, Martorana V, Cavallaro G, San Biagio PL. K + and Na + effects on the gelation properties of κ-carrageenan. Biophys Chem 2005;113(2):129–35.

[34] Zhang H, Patel A, Gaharwar AK, Mihaila SM, Iviglia G, Mukundan S, Bae H, Yang H, Khademhosseini A. Hyperbranched polyester hydrogels with controlled drug release and cell adhesion properties. Biomacromolecules 2013;14(5):1299–310.

[35] Genzer J, Bhat RR. Surface-bound soft matter gradients. Langmuir 2008;24(6):2294–317.

[36] Khanarian NT, Haney NM, Burga RA, Lu HH. A functional agarose-hydroxyapatite scaffold for osteochondral interface regeneration. Biomaterials 2012;33(21):5247–58.

[37] Piraino F, Camci-Unal G, Hancock MJ, Rasponi M, Khademhosseini A. Multi-gradient hydrogels produced layer by layer with capillary flow and crosslinking in open microchannels. Lab Chip 2012;12(3):659–61.

[38] Seidi A, Ramalingam M, Elloumi-Hannachi I, Ostrovidov S, Khademhosseini A. Gradient biomaterials for soft-to-hard interface tissue engineering. Acta Biomater 2011;7(4):1441–51.

[39] Cross LM, Shah K, Palani S, Peak CW, Gaharwar AK. Gradient nanocomposite hydrogels for interface tissue engineering. Nanomedicine 2018;14(7):2465–74.

[40] Griffin MF, Butler PE, Seifalian AM, Kalaskar DM. Control of stem cell fate by engineering their micro and nanoenvironment. World J Stem Cells 2015;7(1):37.

[41] Lee LH, Peerani R, Ungrin M, Joshi C, Kumacheva E, Zandstra P. Micropatterning of human embryonic stem cells dissects the mesoderm and endoderm lineages. Stem Cell Res 2009;2(2):155–62.

[42] Vignesh S, Gopalakrishnan A, Poorna MR, Nair SV, Jayakumar R, Mony U. Fabrication of micropatterned alginate-gelatin and k-carrageenan hydrogels of defined shapes using simple wax mould method as a platform for stem cell/induced pluripotent stem cells (iPSC) culture. Int J Biol Macromol 2018;112:737–44.

[43] Popa EG, Caridade SG, Mano JF, Reis RL, Gomes ME. Chondrogenic potential of injectable κ-carrageenan hydrogel with encapsulated adipose stem cells for cartilage tissue-engineering applications. J Tissue Eng Regen Med 2015;9(5):550–63.

[44] Mayavanshi AV, Gajjar SS. Floating drug delivery systems to increase gastric retention of drugs: a review. Res J Pharm Technol 2008;1(4):345–8.

[45] Selvakumaran S, Muhamad II, Abd Razak SI. Evaluation of kappa carrageenan as potential carrier for floating drug delivery system: effect of pore forming agents. Carbohydr Polym 2016;135:207–14.

[46] Selvakumaran S, Muhamad II. Evaluation of kappa carrageenan as potential carrier for floating drug delivery system: effect of cross linker. Int J Pharm 2015;496(2):323–31.

[47] Neamtu I, Rusu AG, Diaconu A, Nita LE, Chiriac AP. Basic concepts and recent advances in nanogels as carriers for medical applications. Drug Deliv 2017;24(1):539–57.

[48] Zhou M, Wang T, Hu Q, Luo Y. Low density lipoprotein/pectin complex nanogels as potential oral delivery vehicles for curcumin. Food Hydrocoll 2016;57:20–9.

[49] Daniel-da-Silva AL, Ferreira L, Gil AM, Trindade T. Synthesis and swelling behavior of temperature responsive κ-carrageenan nanogels. J Colloid Interface Sci 2011;355(2):512–7.

[50] Myung D, Waters D, Wiseman M, Duhamel PE, Noolandi J, Ta CN, Frank CW. Progress in the development of interpenetrating polymer network hydrogels. Polym Adv Technol 2008;19(6):647–57.

[51] Sperling LH. Interpenetrating polymer networks: an overview. In: Klempner D, Sperling LH, Utracki LA, editors. Interpenetrating polymer networks. Washington: ACS; 1994. p. 3–38.

[52] Chan AH, Boughton PC, Ruys AJ, Oyen ML. An interpenetrating network composite for a regenerative spinal disc application. J Mech Behav Biomed Mater 2017;65:842–8.

[53] Wen C, Lu L, Li X. Enzymatic and ionic crosslinked gelatin/K-carrageenan IPN hydrogels as potential biomaterials. J Appl Polym Sci 2014;131(21).

[54] Chen J, Liu M, Chen S. Synthesis and characterization of thermo-and pH-sensitive kappa-carrageenan-g-poly (methacrylic acid)/poly (N, N-diethylacrylamide) semi-IPN hydrogel. Mater Chem Phys 2009;115(1):339–46.

[55] Bose S, Roy M, Bandyopadhyay A. Recent advances in bone tissue engineering scaffolds. Trends Biotechnol 2012;30(10):546–54.

[56] Chopra P, Nayak D, Nanda A, Ashe S, Rauta PR, Nayak B. Fabrication of poly (vinyl alcohol)-carrageenan scaffolds for cryopreservation: effect of composition on cell viability. Carbohydr Polym 2016;147:509–16.

[57] Araujo JV, Davidenko N, Danner M, Cameron RE, Best SM. Novel porous scaffolds of pH responsive chitosan/carrageenan-based polyelectrolyte complexes for tissue engineering. J Biomed Mater Res 2014;102(12):4415–26.

[58] Zhao X. Multi-scale multi-mechanism design of tough hydrogels: building dissipation into stretchy networks. Soft Matter 2014;10(5):672–87.

[59] Bakarich SE, Balding P, Gorkin III R, Spinks GM. Printed ionic-covalent entanglement hydrogels from carrageenan and an epoxy amine. RSC Adv 2014;4(72):38088–92.

[60] Bakarich SE, Pidcock GC, Balding P, Stevens L, Calvert P. Recovery from applied strain in interpenetrating polymer network hydrogels with ionic and covalent cross-links. Soft Matter 2012;8(39):9985–8.

[61] Li H, Tan YJ, Li L. A strategy for strong interface bonding by 3D bioprinting of oppositely charged κ-carrageenan and gelatin hydrogels. Carbohydr Polym 2018;198:261–9.

[62] Tan ML, Choong PF, Dass CR. Recent developments in liposomes, microparticles and nanoparticles for protein and peptide drug delivery. Peptides 2010;31(1):184–93.

[63] Kakinoki S, Taguchi T, Saito H, Tanaka J, Tateishi T. Injectable in situ forming drug delivery system for cancer chemotherapy using a novel tissue adhesive: characterization and in vitro evaluation. Eur J Pharm Biopharm 2007;66(3):383–90.

[64] Hezaveh H, Fazlali A, Noshadi I. Synthesis, rheological properties and magnetoviscos effect of Fe_2O_3/paraffin ferrofluids. J Taiwan Inst Chem Eng 2012;43(1):159–64.

[65] Xiang Y, Chen D. Preparation of a novel pH-responsive silver nanoparticle/poly (HEMA–PEGMA–MAA) composite hydrogel. Eur Polym J 2007;43(10):4178–87.

[66] Hezaveh H, Muhamad II. The effect of nanoparticles on gastrointestinal release from modified κ-carrageenan nanocomposite hydrogels. Carbohydr Polym 2012;89(1):138–45.

[67] Hezaveh H, Muhamad II. Impact of metal oxide nanoparticles on oral release properties of pH-sensitive hydrogel nanocomposites. Int J Biol Macromol 2012;50(5):1334–40.

[68] Ruiz-Hitzky E, Darder M, Fernandes FM, Wicklein B, Alcântara AC, Aranda P. Fibrous clays based bionanocomposites. Prog Polym Sci 2013;38(10 − 11):1392–414.

[69] Sharifzadeh G, Wahit MU, Soheilmoghaddam M, Whye WT, Pasbakhsh P. Kappa-carrageenan/halloysite nanocomposite hydrogels as potential drug delivery systems. J Taiwan Inst Chem Eng 2016;67:426–34.

[70] Akrami-Hasan-Kohal M, Ghorbani M, Mahmoodzadeh F, Nikzad B. Development of reinforced aldehyde-modified kappa-carrageenan/gelatin film by incorporation of halloysite nanotubes for biomedical applications. Int J Biol Macromol 2020;160:669–76.

[71] Wang HS. Metal–organic frameworks for biosensing and bioimaging applications. Coord Chem Rev 2017;349:139–55.

[72] Giménez-Marqués M, Hidalgo T, Serre C, Horcajada PJ. Nanostructured metal–organic frameworks and their bio-related applications. Coord Chem Rev 2016;307:342–60.

[73] Lázaro IA, Haddad S, Sacca S, Orellana-Tavra C, Fairen-Jimenez D, Forgan RS. Selective surface PEGylation of UiO-66 nanoparticles for enhanced stability, cell uptake, and pH-responsive drug delivery. Chem 2017;2(4):561–78.

[74] Javanbakht S, Shadi M, Mohammadian R, Shaabani A, Amini MM, Pooresmaeil M, Salehi R. Facile preparation of pH-responsive k-carrageenan/tramadol loaded UiO-66 bio-nanocomposite hydrogel beads as a nontoxic oral delivery vehicle. J Drug Deliv Sci Technol 2019;54:101311.

[75] Farkouh A, Frigo P, Czejka M. Systemic side effects of eye drops: a pharmacokinetic perspective. Clin Ophthalmol 2016;10:2433.

[76] Kirchhof S, Goepferich AM, Brandl FP. Hydrogels in ophthalmic applications. Eur J Pharm Biopharm 2015;95:227–38.

[77] Kushwaha SK, Saxena P, Rai AK. Stimuli sensitive hydrogels for ophthalmic drug delivery: a review. Int J Pharm Investig 2012;2(2):54.

[78] Zhu L, Ao J, Li P. A novel in situ gel base of deacetylase gellan gum for sustained ophthalmic drug delivery of ketotifen: in vitro and in vivo evaluation. Drug Des Devel Ther 2015;9:3943.

[79] Fernández-Ferreiro A, Silva-Rodríguez J, Otero-Espinar FJ, González-Barcia M, Lamas MJ, Ruibal A, Luaces-Rodríguez A, Vieites-Prado A, Lema I, Herranz M, Gómez-Lado N. In vivo eye surface residence determination by high-resolution scintigraphy of a novel ion-sensitive hydrogel based on gellan gum and kappa-carrageenan. Eur J Pharm Biopharm 2017;114:317–23.

[80] Bertram U, Bodmeier R. In situ gelling, bioadhesive nasal inserts for extended drug delivery: in vitro characterization of a new nasal dosage form. Eur J Pharm Sci 2006;27(1):62–71.

[81] Li C, Li C, Liu Z, Li Q, Yan X, Liu Y, Lu W. Enhancement in bioavailability of ketorolac tromethamine via intranasal in situ hydrogel based on poloxamer 407 and carrageenan. Int J Pharm 2014;474(1–2):123–33.

[82] Zacharopoulos VR, Phillips DM. Vaginal formulations of carrageenan protect mice from herpes simplex virus infection. J Clin Diagn Res 1997;4(4):465–8.

[83] Gonzalez ME, Alarcón B, Carrasco L. Polysaccharides as antiviral agents: antiviral activity of carrageenan. Antimicrob Agents Chemother 1987;31(9):1388–93.

[84] Zaveri T, Hayes JE, Ziegler GR. Release of tenofovir from carrageenan-based vaginal suppositories. Pharmaceutics 2014;6(3):366–77.

[85] Alfonsi GA, Shlay JC. The effectiveness of condoms for the prevention of sexually transmitted diseases. Curr Womens Health Rev 2005;1(2):151–9.

[86] Prejean J, Song R, Hernandez A, Ziebell R, Green T, Walker F, Lin LS, An Q, Mermin J, Lansky A, Hall HI. Estimated HIV incidence in the United States, 2006–2009. PLoS ONE 2011;6(8), e17502.

[87] Stone A. Microbicides: a new approach to preventing HIV and other sexually transmitted infections. Nat Rev Drug Discov 2002;1(12):977–85.

[88] Karim QA, Karim SS, Frohlich JA, Grobler AC, Baxter C, Mansoor LE, Kharsany AB, Sibeko S, Mlisana KP, Omar Z, Gengiah TN. Effectiveness and safety of tenofovir gel, an antiretroviral microbicide, for the prevention of HIV infection in women. Science 2010;329(5996):1168–74.

[89] Liu Y, Zhu YY, Wei G, Lu WY. Effect of carrageenan on poloxamer-based in situ gel for vaginal use: improved in vitro and in vivo sustained-release properties. Eur J Pharm Sci 2009;37(3–4):306–12.

[90] Koffi AA, Agnely F, Ponchel G, Grossiord JL. Modulation of the rheological and mucoadhesive properties of thermosensitive poloxamer-based hydrogels intended for the rectal administration of quinine. Eur J Pharm Sci 2006;27(4):328–35.

[91] Paavola A, Yliruusi J, Rosenberg P. Controlled release and dura mater permeability of lidocaine and ibuprofen from injectable poloxamer-based gels. J Control Release 1998;52(1–2):169–78.

[92] Baker DA. The use of antiviral medications in the treatment of herpes simplex virus infections of women. Int J Fertil Womens Med 1999;44(5):227.

[93] Sánchez-Sánchez MP, Martín-Illana A, Ruiz-Caro R, Bermejo P, Abad MJ, Carro R, Bedoya LM, Tamayo A, Rubio J, Fernández-Ferreiro A, Otero-Espinar F. Chitosan and kappa-carrageenan vaginal acyclovir formulations for prevention of genital herpes. In vitro and ex vivo evaluation. Mar Drugs 2015;13(9):5976–92.

[94] Yang S, Chen Y, Gu K, Dash A, Sayre CL, Davies NM, Ho EA. Novel intravaginal nanomedicine for the targeted delivery of saquinavir to CD4 + immune cells. Int J Nanomedicine 2013;8:2847.

[95] Li N, Yu M, Deng L, Yang J, Dong A. Thermosensitive hydrogel of hydrophobically-modified methylcellulose for intravaginal drug delivery. J Mater Sci Mater Med 2012;23(8):1913–9.

[96] Tsujihata S, inventor; Fujifilm Corp, assignee. Gel sheet and cosmetic preparation in sheet form using the same. United States patent application US 12/740,629; 2010.

[97] Yee CM, Hasan ZA, Ahmad N, Hazimah AH. Development of carrageenan hydrogel as a sustained release matrix containing tocotrienol-rich palm-based vitamin E. J Oil Palm Res 2016;28(3):373–86.

[98] Hasan ZA, Ismail R, Ahmad S. Does the palm tocotrienol-rich fraction induce irritant contact dermatitis? J Oil Palm Res 2008;20:508–15.

[99] Imeson AP. Carrageenan. In: Handbook of hydrocolloids. Woodhead Publishing; 2000. p. 87–102.

[100] Kianfar F, Antonijevic MD, Chowdhry BZ, Boateng JS. Formulation development of a carrageenan based delivery system for buccal drug delivery using ibuprofen as a model drug. J Biomater Nanobiotechnol 2011;2(05A):582–95.

[101] Daniel-da-Silva AL, Lopes AB, Gil AM, Correia RN. Synthesis and characterization of porous κ-carrageenan/calcium phosphate nanocomposite scaffolds. J Mater Sci 2007;42(20):8581–91.

[102] Feng W, Feng S, Tang K, He X, Jing A, Liang G. A novel composite of collagen-hydroxyapatite/kappa-carrageenan. J Alloys Compd 2017;693:482–9.

[103] González JI, Ossa CP. Injectability evaluation of bone-graft substitutes based on carrageenan and hydroxyapatite nanorods. In: Proceedings of the 3rd Pan American materials congress. Cham: Springer; 2017. p. 33–46.

[104] Goonoo N, Khanbabaee B, Steuber M, Bhaw-Luximon A, Jonas U, Pietsch U, Jhurry D, Schönherr H. κ-Carrageenan enhances the biomineralization and osteogenic differentiation of electrospun polyhydroxybutyrate and polyhydroxybutyrate valerate fibers. Biomacromolecules 2017;18(5):1563–73.

[105] Nogueira LF, Maniglia BC, Blácido DR, Ramos AP. Organic–inorganic collagen/iota-carrageenan/hydroxyapatite hybrid membranes are bioactive materials for bone regeneration. J Appl Polym Sci 2019;136(39):48004.

[106] Wang L, Zhou S, Liu B, Lei D, Zhao Y, Lu C, Tan A. Locally applied nerve growth factor enhances bone consolidation in a rabbit model of mandibular distraction osteogenesis. J Orthop Res 2006;24(12):2238–45.

[107] Wang L, Cao J, Lei DL, Cheng XB, Yang YW, Hou R, Zhao YH, Cui FZ. Effects of nerve growth factor delivery via a gel to inferior alveolar nerve in mandibular distraction osteogenesis. J Craniofac Surg 2009;20(6):2188–92.

[108] Mihaila SM, Popa EG, Reis RL, Marques AP, Gomes ME. Fabrication of endothelial cell-laden carrageenan microfibers for microvascularized bone tissue engineering applications. Biomacromolecules 2014;15(8):2849–60.

[109] Pereira RC, Scaranari M, Castagnola P, Grandizio M, Azevedo HS, Reis RL, Cancedda R, Gentili C. Novel injectable gel (system) as a vehicle for human articular chondrocytes in cartilage tissue regeneration. J Tissue Eng Regen Med 2009;3(2):97–106.

[110] Rocha PM, Santo VE, Gomes ME, Reis RL, Mano JF. Encapsulation of adipose-derived stem cells and transforming growth factor-β1 in carrageenan-based hydrogels for cartilage tissue engineering. J Bioact Compat Polym 2011;26(5):493–507.

[111] Popa EG, Rodrigues MT, Coutinho DF, Oliveira MB, Mano JF, Reis RL, Gomes ME. Cryopreservation of cell laden natural origin hydrogels for cartilage regeneration strategies. Soft Matter 2013;9(3):875–85.

[112] Popa EG, Santo VE, Rodrigues MT, Gomes ME. Magnetically-responsive hydrogels for modulation of chondrogenic commitment of human adipose-derived stem cells. Polymers 2016;8(2):28.

[113] Thakur A, Jaiswal MK, Peak CW, Carrow JK, Gentry J, Dolatshahi-Pirouz A, Gaharwar AK. Injectable shear-thinning nanoengineered hydrogels for stem cell delivery. Nanoscale 2016;8(24):12362–72.

[114] Boateng JS, Matthews KH, Stevens HN, Eccleston GM. Wound healing dressings and drug delivery systems: a review. J Pharm Sci 2008;97(8):2892–923.

[115] Li J, Mooney DJ. Designing hydrogels for controlled drug delivery. Nat Rev Mater 2016;1(12):1–7.

[116] Gómez-mascaraque LG, Llavata-cabrero B, Martínez-sanz M, Fabra MJ. Self-assembled gelatin-i-carrageenan encapsulation structures for intestinal-targeted release applications. J Colloid Interface Sci 2018;517:113–23.

[117] Wu M, Bao M, Yoshii F, Makuuchi K. Irradiation of crosslinked, poly (vinyl alcohol) blended hydrogel for wound dressing. J Radioanal Nucl Chem 2001;250(2):391–5.

[118] Nair AV, Raman M, Doble M. Cyclic β-(1 → 3)(1 → 6) glucan/carrageenan hydrogels for wound healing applications. RSC Adv 2016;6(100):98545–53.

[119] Jaiswal L, Shankar S, Rhim JW. Carrageenan-based functional hydrogel film reinforced with sulfur nanoparticles and grapefruit seed extract for wound healing application. Carbohydr Polym 2019;224:115191.

[120] Lokhande G, Carrow JK, Thakur T, Xavier JR, Parani M, Bayless KJ, Gaharwar AK. Nanoengineered injectable hydrogels for wound healing application. Acta Biomater 2018;70:35–47.

[121] De Silva DA, Hettiarachchi BU, Nayanajith LD, Milani MY, Motha JT. Development of a PVP/kappa-carrageenan/PEG hydrogel dressing for wound healing applications in Sri Lanka. J Natl Sci Found Sri Lanka 2011;39(1):25–33.

[122] Muthuswamy S, Viswanathan A, Yegappan R, Selvaprithiviraj V, Vasudevan AK, Biswas R, Jayakumar R. Antistaphylococcal and neutrophil chemotactic injectable κ-carrageenan hydrogel for infectious wound healing. ACS Appl Bio Mater 2018;2(1):378–87.

[123] Azizi S, Mohamad R, Rahim RA, Mohammadinejad R, Ariff AB. Hydrogel beads bio-nanocomposite based on kappa-carrageenan and green synthesized silver nanoparticles for biomedical applications. Int J Biol Macromol 2017;104:423–31.

[124] Jayaramudu T, Raghavendra GM, Varaprasad K, Sadiku R, Ramam K, Raju KM. Iota-carrageenan-based biodegradable Ag0 nanocomposite hydrogels for the inactivation of bacteria. Carbohydr Polym 2013;95(1):188–94.

10

Hydrogels based on gum ghatti

Falguni Patra[a], Madhumita Dey[b], and Tapan Kumar Giri[c]

[a]School of Pharmacy, Techno India University, Kolkata, West Bengal, India, [b]Hemraj Blood Bank, Katwa Sub-divisional Hospital, Purba Bardhaman, West Bengal, India, [c]Department of Pharmaceutical Technology, Jadavpur University, Kolkata, West Bengal, India

10.1 Introduction

Gum ghatti is mainly isolated from *Anogeissus latifolia* species that belongs to Combretaceae family and known as Indian gum. It is a natural polysaccharide and exists as a salt of calcium and magnesium. The powder is reddish gray, and the lump is light to dark brown. Gum ghatti contains L-arabinose, D-xylose, D-galactose, D-glucuronic acid, and D-mannose in 10:1:6:2:2 molar ratios. Moreover, it contains traces of 6-deoxyhexose and huge amounts of tannin. Recently, a new product of gum ghatti named gatifolia is produced by spray-drying process. Spray-drying procedure gives a satisfactory product that has desirable quality, resistance to acid, tolerance to salt, and improved rheological properties [1–3]. As per USFDA, gum ghatti is considered as a safe substance in food additives in view of the toxicity, teratogenicity, or mutagenicity.

Gum ghatti is used as an excipient in a variety of dosage forms such as creams, chewing gums, syrups, and emulsions [4, 5]. It is also used as an additive, a preservative, and a thickening agent in food industry. Gum ghatti is degraded enzymatically by microflora present in gastrointestinal tract (GIT), and the degraded product is used as an energy source by beneficial bacteria present in the GIT [6]. Gum ghatti can be given during chemotherapy because it reduces the side effects and strengthens the immune system [7]. Gum ghatti is very efficient for the treatment of diabetes, diarrhea, and hypolipidemia [8].

In recent times, the application of polysaccharide hydrogels is extensively used in industry and biomedical areas for their biocompatibility, biodegradability, and high water content [9–11]. Hydrogel is the cross-linked three-dimensional (3D) network of polymers that have the capability of absorbing a huge quantity of fluids owing to the existence of $-SO_3H$, $-OH$, $-CONH_2$, $-COOH$, and $-CONH-$ hydrophilic functional groups [12–14]. Hydrogels have numerous advantages and have extensive application in different fields such as drug delivery, regenerative madicine, and environmental bioremediation [15–17].

Recently, numerous researchers have investigated gum ghatti hydrogel for drug delivery, regenerative medicine, and removal of toxic materials from the environment. Gum ghatti-based hydrogels showed pH- and temperature-responsive behavior. Gum ghatti-grafted poly (acrylamide-co-acrylonitrile) hydrogels with responsive (pH, salt, and temperature) properties were developed [18]. Rani et al. prepared the gum ghatti hydrogel that can be used as a flocculant for environmental remediation [19]. Acrylamide-grafted gum ghatti-based responsive (electrical, pH, and temperature) hydrogels were developed [20]. Gum ghatti-based hydrogels have also been used in environmental remediation for the recovery of crude oil and waste water treatment [21]. Sharma et al. synthesized gum ghatti hydrogels that act as conductive carriers for colonic delivery [22]. Gum ghatti hydrogel can be used in heavy metal removal because it can reduce hexavalent chromium ion to a greater extent than any polysaccharide [23].

10.2 Structure, properties, and application of gum ghatti

10.2.1 Structure

The backbone of gum ghatti contains galactopyranosyl units with some L-arabinofuranosyl units, glucopyranosyluronic acid units, and mannopyranosyl units (Fig. 10.1) [24]. It also contains neutral sugar (Galp, Araf, and Arap) and GlcA connected to a molecular core through alteration of -d-GlcA (linking through O-4) and d-Man residues (linking through O-2). The 1–6 linked glycosidic bonds were accountable for the excellent solubility of gum ghatti [25, 26].

10.2.2 Physicochemical properties

Gum ghatti is obtainable in numerous grades depending on solubility and viscosity. The powder is reddish gray, and the lump is light to dark brown. It is not entirely water soluble at more than 5% concentration but produces colloidal dispersions.

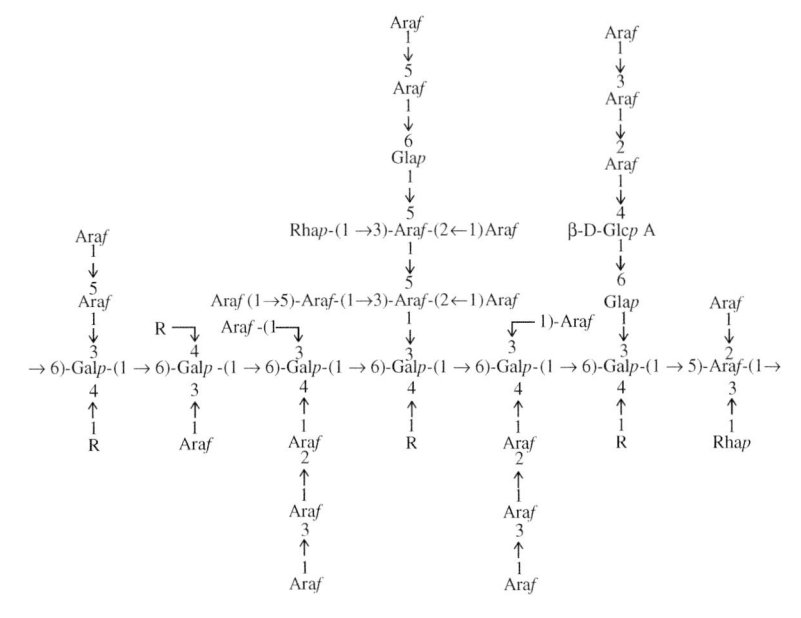

R can be represented by the following groups:

→2,3-Man*p*1→, →3,4-Glc*p*1 →, →4-Gal*p*1 →, T-α-L-Ara*f* 1→, T-Glc*p* A1→, T-Gal*p*→ and T-L-Ara*p* 1→ ,

All the galactose are in -β-D form, all the arabinose and rhamnose are in α-L form

FIG. 10.1 Chemical structure of gum ghatti. *Reprinted from Kang J, Cui SW, Phillips GO, Chen J, Guo Q, Wang Q. New studies on gum ghatti (Anogeissus latifolia). Part III: structure characterization of a globular polysaccharide fraction by 1D, 2D NMR spectroscopy, and methylation analysis, Food Hydrocoll 2011;25:1999–2007, Copyright (2011), with permission from Elsevier.*

10.2.3 Toxicity

The micronucleus/Comet assays were performed to assess the capability of gum ghatti to induce the damage of DNA [27]. Gum ghatti was given to rats through gavages for 4 days at 1000, 1500, and 2000 mg/kg per day. After 4 h of final dosing, the samples were collected. In peripheral blood, the effect of gum ghatti on the frequency of micronucleated reticulocyte was not observed. Moreover, no damage of DNA was observed in liver or blood leukocytes. A 90-day toxicity study of gum ghatti in rats was conducted according to OECD guideline #408 [28]. Up to 5% of gum ghatti in the diet was given to rats for minimum 90 days. There was a predictable augment in cecum weight, and the results were consistent with other reported gums. The enlarged cecum exhibited no unambiguous morphological changes.

10.2.4 Applications

Gum ghatti exhibited outstanding emulsification property owing to the presence of proteinous components in the molecule. It is used as a stabilizer and emulsifier in beverages. For many years, polysaccharides attracted researchers owing to the development of solid oral dosage forms. Joshi et al. developed diltiazem hydrochloride-loaded matrix tablets using gum ghatti as a release modifier [29]. Incorporation of gum ghatti modified the release of drug. The gum was used as an adsorbent in barium sulfate suspensions [30]. In photoelectric determinations, gum ghatti is used to stabilize the Prussian blue color [31]. A salt of gum ghatti was used as a light-sensitive paper, pigment, and fungicide [32].

10.3 Preparation of gum ghatti hydrogel

10.3.1 By grafting

Graft copolymer is a long chain of backbone polymer with one or more other polymer branches [33, 34]. The synthesis of graft copolymer was started from preformed polymer. The free radical sites were created on polymer backbone by an external agent. However, the external agent should not destroy the polymer backbone. The free radical sites were created on backbone polymer, and then monomer was added resulting in the creation of grafted chains. The numerous process parameters, including concentration of monomer, initiator type, initiator concentration, reaction time, and reaction temperature, influence the efficiency of grafting and percent of grafting [35–38].

Moreover, synthesized graft copolymer properties are usually controlled by the side chain characteristics such as number, length, and molecular structure. Numerous methods of grafting are available to synthesize graft copolymers such as chemical grafting (free radical or ionic), living polymerization grafting, photochemical grafting, enzymatic grafting, plasma radiation grafting, and radiation grafting. The responsibility of initiator is extremely imperative in chemical grafting technique because it determines the grafting path. In free radical technique, the initiator produces free radicals and reacts with monomer to synthesize graft copolymer. In ionic grafting technique, grafting process can occur through ionic interaction between cationic (alkaline metal salts are used) and anionic (alkoxide of alkali metals are used) compounds. In living polymerization, living polymers retain their capability to propagate for extended time with maximum size while termination degree is still negligible. In photochemical grafting technique, photochemical radiations are used to start the process of grafting. Photochemical radiations dissociate the chromophore to free radicals reactive sites. The photochemical grafting method proceeds in two ways such as with or devoid of sensitizer. In devoid of sensitizer mechanism, free radicals are generated on backbones that react with monomer to produce graft copolymer. Conversely, with sensitizer mechanism, the free radicals are produced by sensitizer and are diffused. The diffused free radicals abstract hydrogen atoms from polymer backbone and create radical sites requisite for grafting. In enzymatic grafting process, enzymes were used in the grafting reaction. Enzymatic grafting process was a green process because it eliminates the use of reactive reagents. Grafting of polymers by plasma radiations offered equal grafting efficiency as ionizing radiation. The electron-induced excitation, ionization, and dissociation were the main steps in plasma radiations grafting. Plasma radiations produced high energy that accelerated electrons to induce the breakdown of polymeric chemical bonds that consequently created macromolecule radicals and initiated grafting. In radiation grafting, high-energy radiation was used to create free radical sites that served as grafting site for propagation.

Biodegradable hydrogels of gum ghatti using acrylamide monomer were prepared through graft copolymerization technique [39]. The initiators ascorbic acid and potassium persulfate as redox pair and MBA as a cross-linker were used for the synthesis of graft copolymer. The effects of different parameters on graft copolymerization were studied. The percent grafting augmented considerably with augment in reaction time; after 90 min, reached an utmost value of 83% (Fig. 10.2A) and then diminished percent grafting. The interaction between substrate and *OH was augmented with augment in reaction time and created active sites on gum ghatti and acrylamide chain resulting in high grafting reaction with enhanced percent grafting. However, grafting decreased at long reaction time due to diminished concentration of radicals and acrylamide and formation of homopolymer. In addition, the reaction medium was viscous due to the formation of homopolymers that hinder free radical movement to reach in active sites. The percent grafting was augmented with augment in temperature and reaches an utmost value at 50°C (Fig. 10.2B). The rate of creation of initiators and active sites amount was augmented with increase in temperature. The active site formation was increased with increase in temperature and consequently speeding up the propagation reactions. In addition, the free volume of gum ghatti augmented with exposure of all active sites. Maximum percent grafting was observed at 1:1 molar ratio of potassium persulfate (KPS): ascorbic acid (ABC) (Fig. 10.2C) and then diminished with further augment in molar ratio. Initially, percent grafting augmented with augment in the concentration of acrylamide and reached an utmost value at 0.7042 mol/L and then diminished with further increase in acrylamide concentration (Fig. 10.2D). Maximum percent of grafting was exhibited at 0.0974 mol/L of MBA (Fig. 10.2E). But further augment in the concentration of MBA resulted in the diminished

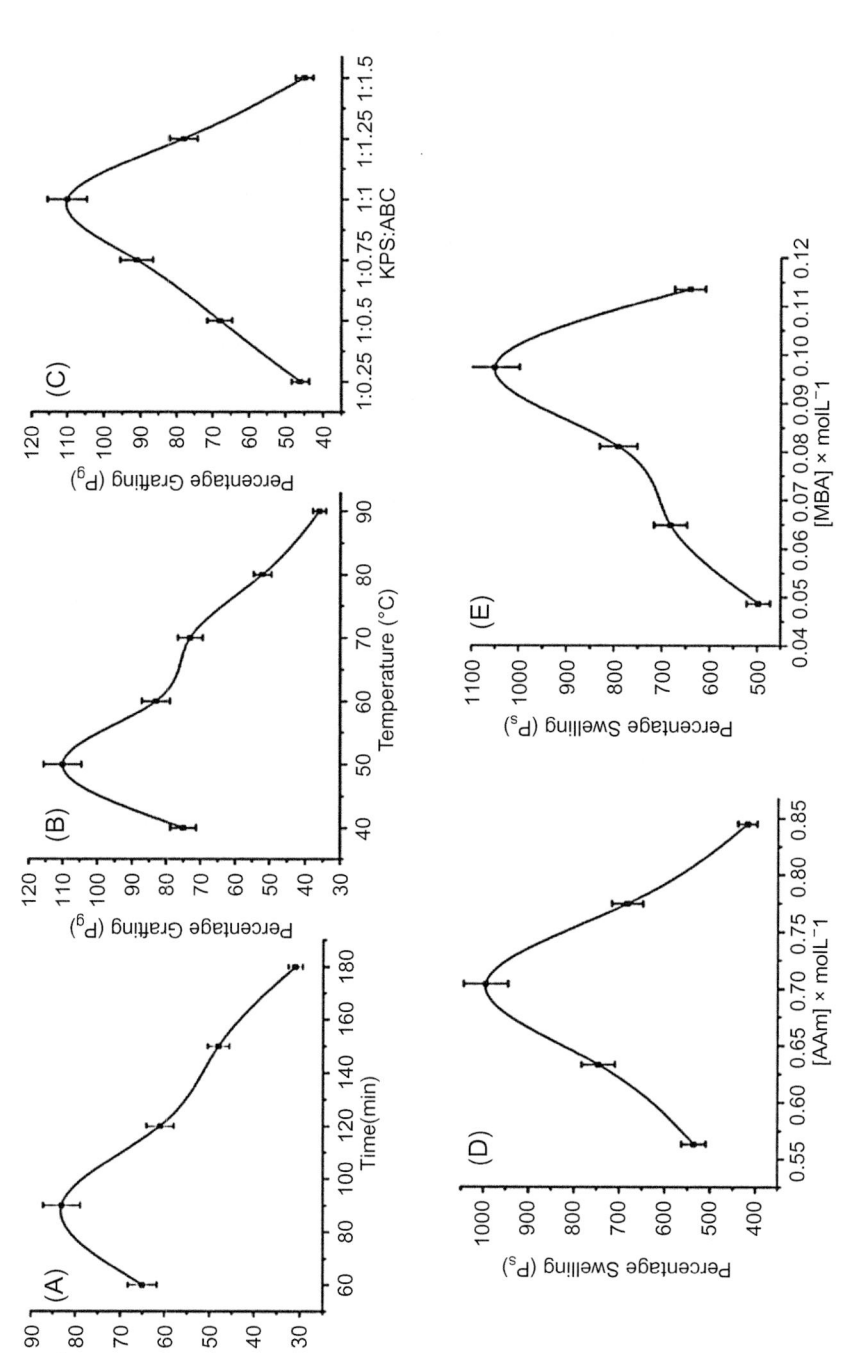

FIG. 10.2 Effect of (A) time on percent grafting, (B) temperature on percent grafting, (C) KPS: ABC ratio on percent grafting, (D) concentration of AAm on percent grafting, and (E) concentration of MBA on percent grafting. *Reprinted from Mittal H, Mishra SB, Mishra AK, Kaith BS, Jindal R, Flocculation characteristics and biodegradation studies of Gum ghatti-based hydrogels, Int J Biol Macromol 2013;58:37–46, Copyright (2013), with permission from Elsevier.*

percent grafting. Initial augment in percent grafting was owing to augmented surface area of the polymer. However, the cross-link density was augmented with further increase in the concentration of MBA concentration away from maximum value and led to the reduction of pore size along with desorption.

Gum ghatti grafted poly (methacrylic acid) was synthesized using ammonium persulfate as initiator and MBA as cross-linking agent [40]. The modification of the synthesized hydrogel was performed through the irradiation of Au^{8+} and Ni^{9+} ion beams. The reduction in transmittance value was observed in FTIR spectrum, which attributed to scissioning of chain and cross-linking of the bands. The X-ray diffractogram showed reduced peaks of grafted copolymer. This may be due to nonalignment of chain orientations resulting in diminished crystallinity.

Grafted gum ghatti was synthesized using acrylic acid and acrylamide by microwave method [41]. Hydrogels were formulated by using a mixture of redox initiators named potassium persulfate and ascorbic acid and MBA as a cross-linking agent (Fig. 10.3). At first, the reaction of ascorbic acid and potassium persulfate took place and SO_4^{-*} was formed, and later, OH^* radical was generated when it reacted with water. Then the active site of gum ghatti was generated for graft copolymerization.

The thermal stability of gum ghatti hydrogel was enhanced because of cross-linking. The developed hydrogel showed very good swelling in water of approximately 2547% at the temperature of 50°C. Gum ghatti hydrogels were prepared using acrylamide and methacrylic acid by the technique of microwave graft copolymerization [42]. Grafting was proved by FTIR. The synthesized hydrogel exhibited exceptional capacities to remove methyl violet and methylene blue from water. The surface area of the developed hydrogel was increased due to graft copolymerization, and subsequently, dye adsorption was enhanced. The pH of the aqueous solution influenced the adsorption of both the dyes, and maximum adsorption occurred at neutral pH. In addition, the synthesized hydrogel was fully biodegradable within 50 days.

Gum ghatti-grafted poly (methacrylic acid) was synthesized using MBA as a cross-linking agent in a vacuum oven [43]. After that, these samples were irradiated using gamma radiation at room temperature. After irradiation, it was noticed that significant changes were present in structural as well as in morphological properties. From the XRD study, it was revealed that the peak intensity was decreased gradually when the peak intensity of ion fluence was increased. From that, it can be concluded that after irradiation, crystallinity was lost to some extent. On the other side, FTIR spectra reveal a reduction in the intensity at the higher fluence of the typical bands.

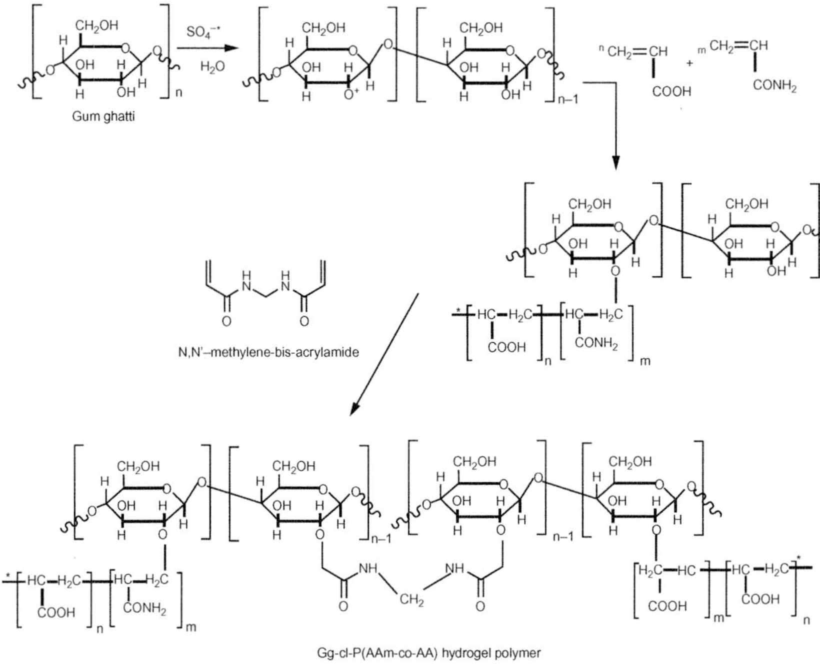

FIG. 10.3 Synthesis of gum ghatti-grafted acrylic acid and acrylamide. *Reprinted from Mittal H, Maity A, Ray SS, Gum ghatti and poly (acrylamide-co-acrylic acid)-based biodegradable hydrogel—evaluation of the flocculation and adsorption properties, Polym Degrad Stab 2015;120:42–52, Copyright (2015), with permission from Elsevier].*

10.3.2 Through interpenetrating polymer network

Two or more cross-linked polymers are interconnected to form polymer composites called interpenetrating polymer networks (IPNs). The polymers cannot be alienated because they do not have any covalent bonding, but they can be separated through chemical bonds breakdown. They can be categorized as sequential, semiinterpenetrating polymer networks, and simultaneous polymer networks. In sequential IPN, the first network is formed by the polymerization/cross-linking using monomer, cross-linker, and initiator. Then the second monomer, cross-linker, and initiator were dissolved in the first network, resulting in the polymerization/cross-link of second network, and IPN was formed. It was easily synthesized. In the synthesis of simultaneous IPN, the two different monomers and cross-linking agent were polymerized/cross-linked in one step. In semi-IPN hydrogel, one polymer is cross-linked and another polymer interpenetrated into polymer network linearly. They have more benefits than cross-linked polymers or polymer blends [44]. As interpenetrating polymer networks hydrogels are greatly approved by the scientific community and have various applications, including delivery of drug molecules, environmental remediation, and remedial medicine.

IPN hydrogels were developed using alginate and grafted gum ghatti [45]. At first, the gum ghatti-grafted polyacrylamides were prepared by microwave technique. The microwave irradiation and initiator (ceric ammonium nitrate) were used to create free radical sites on gum ghatti backbone. Ceric ammonium nitrate ceases the electrons from –OH groups present in gum ghatti, and Ce-O bond was formed. The Ce-O bond was more polar in comparison with O-H bond and can be broken by the simple exposure of microwave irradiation method and leads to the creation of free radical on gum ghatti backbone, which assists in the growth of graft chains. The synthesis of grafted gum ghatti is represented in Fig. 10.4. Then the sodium hydroxide was used to hydrolyze the graft polymer to produce pH-sensitive carrier (Fig. 10.4A). The graft polymer solution that was hydrolyzed dipped into calcium chloride solution, and then the cross-linking was formed between two strands of sodium alginate by the method of ionic cross-linking. After treating the cross-linked microbeads with glutaraldehyde, an acetal structure was made between the glutaraldehyde aldehyde groups and alginate hydroxyl groups (Fig. 10.4B).

Another hydrogel was prepared based on gum ghatti-polymethacrylic acid-polyaniline with an interpenetrated network structure by two-step aqueous polymerization method [46]. At the initial stage, polymethacrylic acid was cross-linked with gum ghatti using MBA as a cross-linking agent and ammonium persulfate as an initiator. The semiinterpenetrating network was changed into an interpenetrating polymer network through interaction with aniline. The synthesized hydrogel exhibited good electrical conductivity. In addition, the synthesized hydrogel was sensitive toward pH and temperature.

Biodegradable interpenetrated network hydrogels were synthesized using gum ghatti, aniline, and acrylic acid [47]. It was completed by a two-step method. Gum ghatti-grafted acrylic acid was synthesized by the technique of polymerization using MBA as a cross-linker, which was gamma rays induced (Fig. 10.5). First, water molecules dissociated to produce OH* radicals in the presence of gamma rays. Then OH* radicals created free radical sites on gum ghatti and acrylic acid. Then the acrylic acid chains get integrated onto active sites of the backbone throughout propagation reaction. Finally, gum ghatti-grafted acrylic acid was cross-linked with MBA to form gum ghatti-grafted acrylic acid cross-linked hydrogel. Next, cross-linked hydrogels were treated with aniline. Then interpenetrated polymer network hydrogel was formed when polyaniline chains got interpenetrated in the semiinterpenetrated polymer network moiety (Fig. 10.6).

The prepared hydrogel has efficiently absorbed water in a large quantity and the retained water remain for a very long time. The advantage

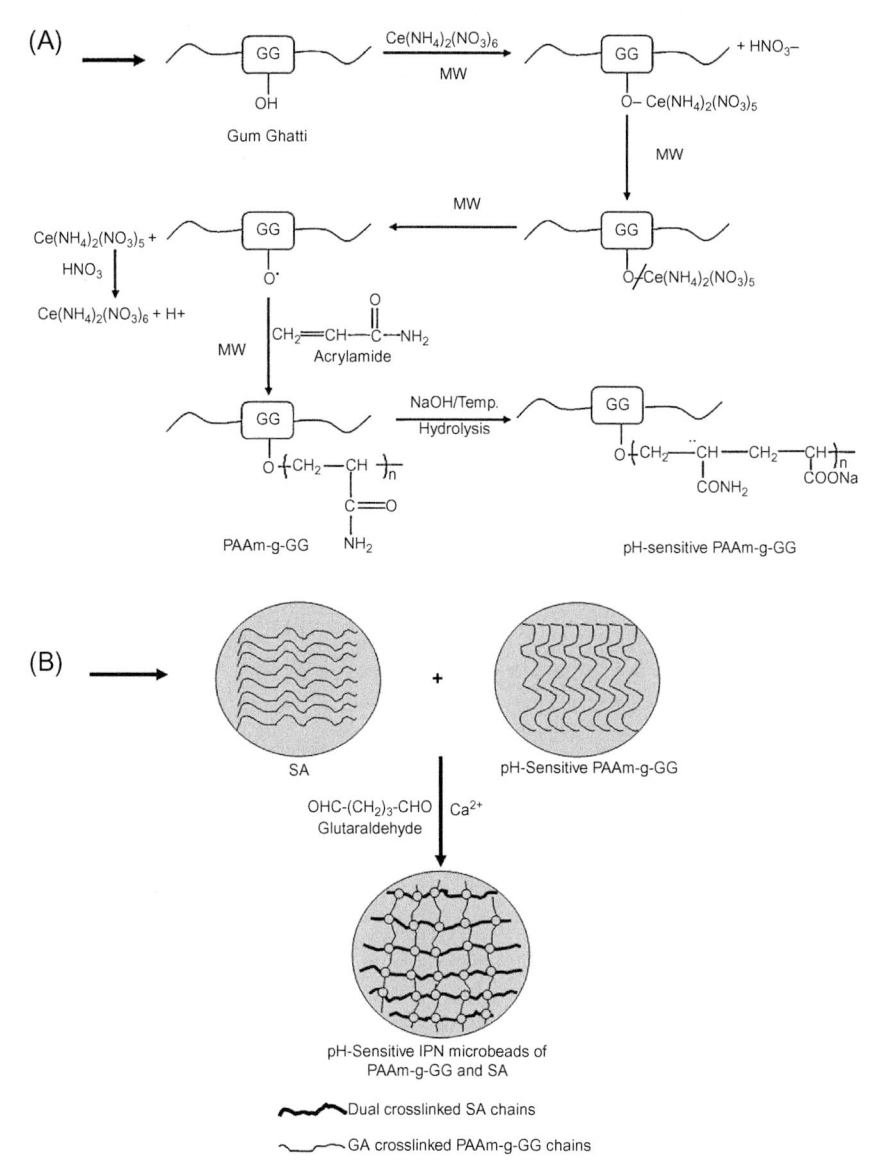

FIG. 10.4 (A) Synthesis of graft copolymer. (B) Preparation of interpenetrating polymer network microbeads. *Reprinted from Boppana R, Mohan GK, Nayak U, Mutalik S, Sa B, Kulkarni RV, Novel pH-sensitive IPNs of polyacrylamide-g-gum ghatti and sodium alginate for gastroprotective drug delivery, Int J Biol Macromol 2015;75:133–143, Copyright (2015), with permission from Elsevier.*

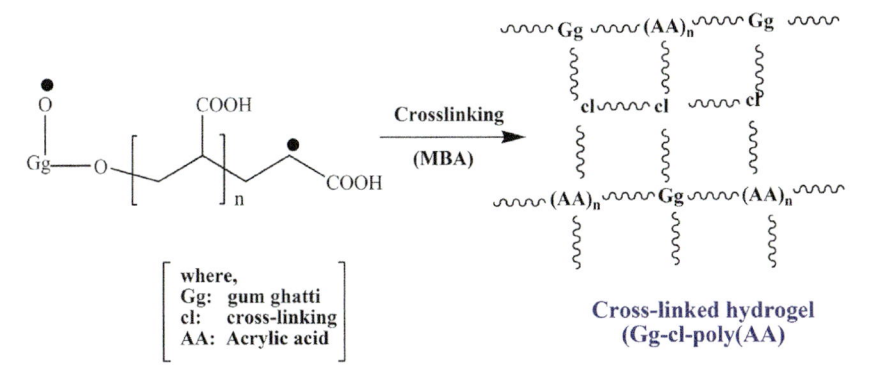

FIG. 10.5 Synthesis mechanism of gum ghatti-grafted poly acrylic acid. *Reprinted from Sharma K, Kumar V, Kaith BS, Kumar V, Som S, Kalia S, Swart HC, Synthesis, characterization, and water retention study of biodegradable Gum ghatti-poly (acrylic acideaniline) hydrogels, Polym Degrad Stab 2015;111:20–31, Copyright (2015), with permission from Elsevier.*

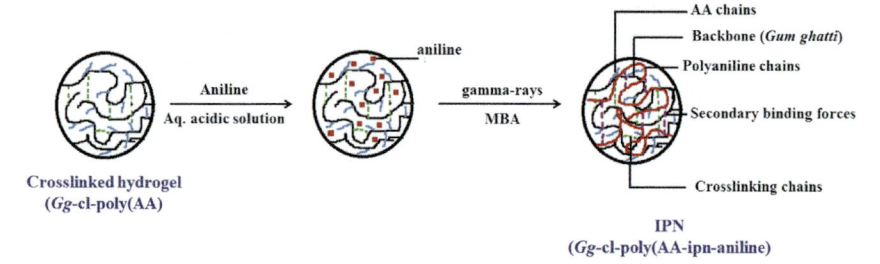

FIG. 10.6 Synthesis of IPN hydrogel. *Reprinted from Sharma K, Kumar V, Kaith BS, Kumar V, Som S, Kalia S, Swart HC, Synthesis, characterization, and water retention study of biodegradable Gum ghatti-poly (acrylic acideaniline) hydrogels, Polym Degrad Stab 2015;111:20–31, Copyright (2015), with permission from Elsevier.*

of interpenetrated polymer network hydrogel over semiinterpenetrated polymer network hydrogel is that the interpenetrated polymer network hydrogel has more thermal stability than the other one. Degradation study by composting soil method was conducted, and the degradation rate of interpenetrated polymer network hydrogel was more than the semiinterpenetrated polymer network hydrogel.

IPN hydrogel was synthesized using grafted ghatti gum and poly (aniline) by gamma irradiation method [48]. Initially, grafted gum ghatti was synthesized using gum ghatti and acrylamide (Fig. 10.7). Then the grafted gum ghatti was swelled in aniline solution at room temperature for 16h. The aniline monomer was adsorbed in the grafted network and swollen sample was formed. Next, the swollen sample was irradiated with gamma

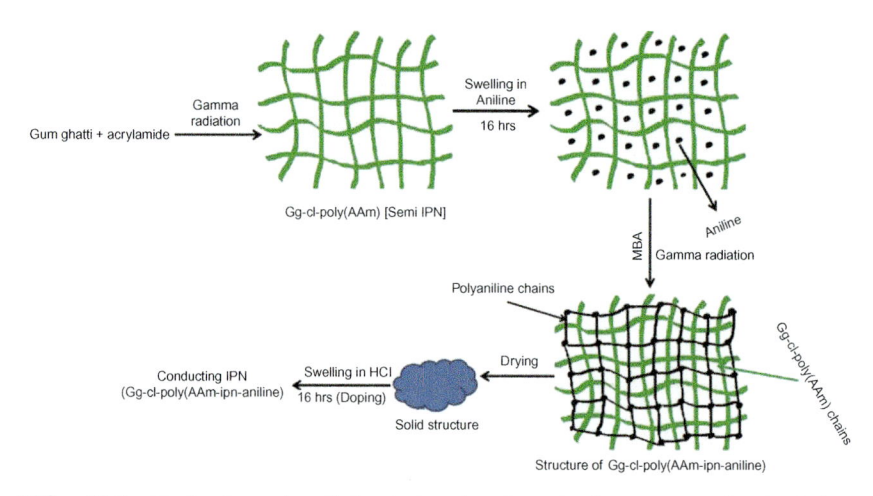

FIG. 10.7 Mechanism of radiation-induced polymerization process. *Reprinted from Sharma K, Kaith BS, Kumar V, Kalia S, Kumar V, Swart HC, Synthesis and biodegradation studies of gamma-irradiated electrically conductive hydrogels, Polym Degrad Stab 2014;107:166–177, Copyright (2014), with permission from Elsevier.*

rays using MBA as cross-linking agent to produce poly (acrylamide-aniline)- grafted gum ghatti interpenetrating polymer network hydrogel. Then the homopolemer was separated from cross-linked polymer by washing with 1-methyl-2-pyrrolidone solution. Lastly, the IPN hydrogel was kept in a vacuum oven at 50°C and dried.

Grafting degree enhanced very fast to 361.7% with radiation dose up to 1.5 kGy and then diminished with augmenting of radiation dose. Initially, grafting was augmenting with augmenting radiation dose due to enhancement of the hydroxyl radical density that can augment the gum ghatti active sites. With further augment in radiation dose, the amount of homopolymer augmented and diminished the efficiency of grafting. The grafting degree was increased with an increase in solvent amount up to 10 mL and then decreased with further increase in amount of solvent. The concentration of hydroxyl radicals was increased with augment in solvent amount, which were used in copolymerization reaction, resulting in augment in percent grafting. With further augment in the amount of solvent, the percent grafting was decreased due to reduction of monomer radicals per unit volume. The formed hydrogels are biodegradable, and they may be used as a flocculent in case of treatment of waste water.

10.3.3 Through polyelectrolyte complexation

Polyelectrolyte complexes stand for unique compounds containing polyions that are oppositely charged (cationic or anionic). They are hydrophilic and water soluble because of their charges and are used in different applications such as in drug delivery, in preparation of shampoos, a coating polymer, and in water treatment as a flocculating agent. No chemical cross-linking agent is used in the formation of polyelectrolyte complexes, so the side effect is less than other complexes. The complex is very useful in various dosage forms. A mixture of many polymers is used in the formation of polyelectrolyte complex [49]. Gum ghatti hydrogel nanoparticles with chitosan were formulated by using polyelectrolyte complexation method [50]. The complex is prepared through the interaction between chitosan (cationic) and gum ghatti (anionic). The chitosan was solubilized in acetic acid, and gum ghatti was dissolved in water. Then by using spray gun, the dispersion of gum ghatti was sprayed in the chitosan solution, and the complex was formed.

10.4 Application

10.4.1 Gum ghatti hydrogel for drug delivery

The natural polysaccharides have a significant role in drug delivery system owing to biocompatibility, nontoxicity, biodegradability, and flexibity for chemical modification [51, 52]. These biopolymers are used to develop pH-sensitive microsphere, hydrogel beads, and nanocomposite hydrogels. The biodegradable polymers are used as vehicles in drug delivery system such as controlled release systems, so that there is no need to remove these polymers because they are biocompatible. Gum ghatti has emulsification property with high viscosity. Researchers have interest to prepare sustained release dosage form where gum ghatti controlled the release of encapsulated drug.

10.4.1.1 *Intragastric drug delivery*

There are various affords in the research and development for oral sustained release of drug to conquer short gastric emptying and residence times. There are many intra- and intersubject variability of stomach physiology such as gastric pH and gastric motility, which significantly affect the gastric retention time and performance of drug delivery. Thus the stomach-specific delivery of drug can solve these problems. The delivery of "narrow absorption window" drugs will be possible by this delivery system. There are numerous approaches that are recently used in the gastric residence time prolongation as well as modified release systems, including bioadhesive systems, floating systems, high-density systems, swelling systems, etc. [53].

The composite matrix was formulated for the delivery of flurbiprofen by intragastric route with two mechanisms, including mucoadhesion and floating [54]. The composite matrix was developed by coating Arabic gum-alginate gel membrane with montomorillonite-modified gum ghatti-alginate. The percent buoyancy was 72%–90% of uncoated matrices at 8 h. The percent buoyancy was decreased when the alginate concentration and cross-linking agent were increased. There is a formation of numerous pores caused by the alginate matrices decrosslinked in the acidic medium as the extraction of Ca^{2+} ions occurs. This initiates more imbibitions of water and matrices sink. The formulations that were coated floated more time than the uncoated ones. The coated formulations remained buoyant. Coated matrices have greater floating ability because their densities were very low and an air compartment is present between the coating membrane and the core matrices. The uncoated matrices showed sustained release of drug release in acidic pH for more than 8 h. In the beginning, the drug was deintercalated from interlayer of the uncoated matrices, and then the drug molecules moved into the dissolution medium from the rigid polymer matrices; thus the drug diffusion path got increased, and consequently, controlled release was observed. The enhancement of mass fraction of alginate to the polymer blend increases the drug release rate. The Ca^{2+} ion cross-linked alginate was transformed to alginic acid in acidic condition, which results in a significant decline in the gel strength, resulting in enhancement of the drug release. On the contrary, the matrices that contain more amount of gum ghatti could combine with the water molecules more tightly for the formation of a viscous gel structure because of great hydrophilicity. This leads to blockade of the pores on the matrix surfaces, and ultimately, it helps to sustain the release of drug. Moreover, high amount of gum ghatti promotes greater tortuosity to the matrices, which delay the drug transport. The coated matrix showed slow release of drug compared with uncoated matrix. Coating might help to delay the drug release from the core matrix because it could act as a further diffusion barrier. Moreover, the coating might block the pores of the matrix surfaces, resulting in slower drug elution rate through the micropores.

Sustained release paracetamol tablets that are delivered by intragastric route were formulated by using xanthum gum, gum ghatti, as well as chitosan [55]. In the acidic dissolution medium, the hydratable polymers of those tablets swell, and a gel was formed. A cross-linking occurs between cationic polymer chitosan and anionic polymer xanthan gum or else gum ghatti. Chitosan-xanthan gum layer or chitosan-gum ghatti layer of polyelectrolyte complex is created at the tablet surface in coacervate (layer of hydrogel) form. The release of drug was retarded because of slow drug flux from the tablet by the hydrogel barrier. The hydrogel layer acts as a hindrance barrier to the drug release. The ionic interaction between chitosańs NH_3^+ and COO^- of gum ghatti and xanthan gum was confirmed by FT-IR and DSC. The polyelectrolyte complex formed by the above interaction helped in the sustained delivery of paracetamol. Moreover, the diluents such as starch and lactose were incorporated into tablet, and a release study was conducted. It was exhibited that the release of drug was faster from tablet prepared with lactose in comparison with tablet prepared with starch.

Novel stomach-specific mucoadhesive microspheres were developed to deliver ranitidine HCl [56]. The IPN network hydrogel was prepared using gum ghatti and polyvinyl alcohol. The different formulations were developed by using varying amount of ghatti gum and polyvinyl alcohols as well as cross-linking duration to optimize the entrapment efficiency and drug release rate. FTIR study was performed to determine the stability of entrapped ranitidine HCl and to confirm the creation of interpenetrating network. The developed microspheres were spherical in shape, and particle size ranged between 17.17 and 35.48 µm. The maximum entrapment efficiency of the drug was observed as 87.80%. The release of drug in pH 1.2 media depended on both duration of cross-linking and ratio of gum ghatti and polyvinyl alcohols.

Floating tablet was developed using gum ghatti to deliver diltiazem hydrochloride [57]. The tablets were developed using various amount of gum ghatti, hydroxypropyl methyl cellulose, and sodium bicarbonate by direct compression method. Sodium bicarbonate was used in the tablet formulation for the production of carbon dioxide that gives buoyancy.

It was observed that the developed formulation exhibited minimum floating lag time and floated constantly for a longer time. The releases of drug from the tablets were decreased with increase in the amount of gum ghatti. Moreover, floating ability of the tablets was improved by the incorporation of hydroxypropyl methyl cellulose.

Domperidone-loaded mucoadhesive matrix-sustained release tablet was developed using gum ghatti and hydroxypropyl methyl cellulose by direct compression method to extend the gastrointestinal residence time [58]. Gum ghatti and hydroxypropyl methyl cellulose as mucoadhesive polymers are more effectual in combination in comparison with alone for gastric retention and drug release. Ex vivo mucoadhesion study was performed using rat stomach mucosa, and more than 24 h mucoadhesion time was observed.

10.4.1.2 Sustained intestinal delivery

Drug absorption mainly occurs in the small intestine because it has larger surface area, and it also consists of villi and microvilli, which enhance the area of absorption by many folds. The duodenum and jejunum have greater surface area than ileum because villi and microvilli are located there in more numbers. The pharmaceutical formulations have a goal to present the drug at a specific rate that is needed for the body and to deliver the active ingredient to action site. The transit time is very short and less variable in small intestine than colon, which is also a great advantage for delivering drugs. The transit time is not only short but also less variable in comparison with colon. Short transit time, targetability, and high surface area are benefits of delivery of drugs to the small intestine.

Gum ghatti was transformed into sodium carboxymethyl gum ghatti by the process called carboxymethylation, and again it was cross-linked with Al^{3+} ion for the formulation of hydrogel beads to deliver ropinirole hydrochloride in a controlled manner [59]. Dissolution study was conducted in acidic (pH 1.2) and basic (pH 6.8) buffer solutions. It was observed that the release of drug was quicker in acidic solution compared with basic solution. The release rate does not only depend on pH of the medium but also was varied with the cross-linking agent (Al^{3+} ion) concentration (Fig. 10.8). When the concentration of aluminium ion increased, a tight rigid structure formed, which inhibits the drug release, so drug release rate was reduced. Moreover, the increased concentration of aluminium ion combined with each binding site of sodium carboxymethyl gum ghatti and a rigid structure formed, which can regulate the diffusivity of drug to the dissolution medium. At the other side, the rate of drug release reduced when the concentration of polymer was increased (Fig. 10.9). Adequate numbers of binding sites were presented for the attachment with Al^{3+} ions at higher concentration of sodium carboxymethyl gum ghatti and formed a rigid structure, resulting in decrease in drug release rate.

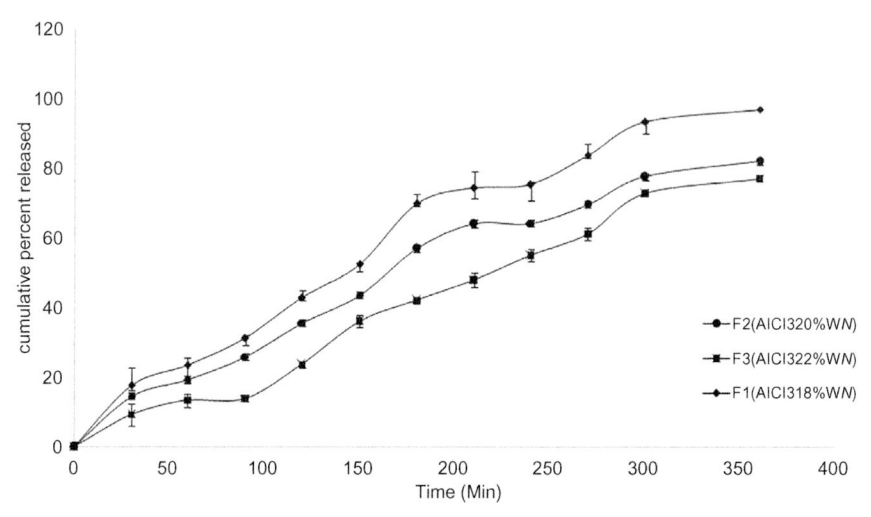

FIG. 10.8 Effect of aluminum chloride concentration on in vitro drug release in pH 6.8. *Reprinted from Ray S, Roy G, Maiti S, Bhattacharyya UK, Sil A, Mitra R, Development of smart hydrogels of etherified gum ghatti for sustained oral delivery of ropinirole hydrochloride, Int J Biol Macromol 2017;103:347–354, Copyright (2017), with permission from Elsevier.*

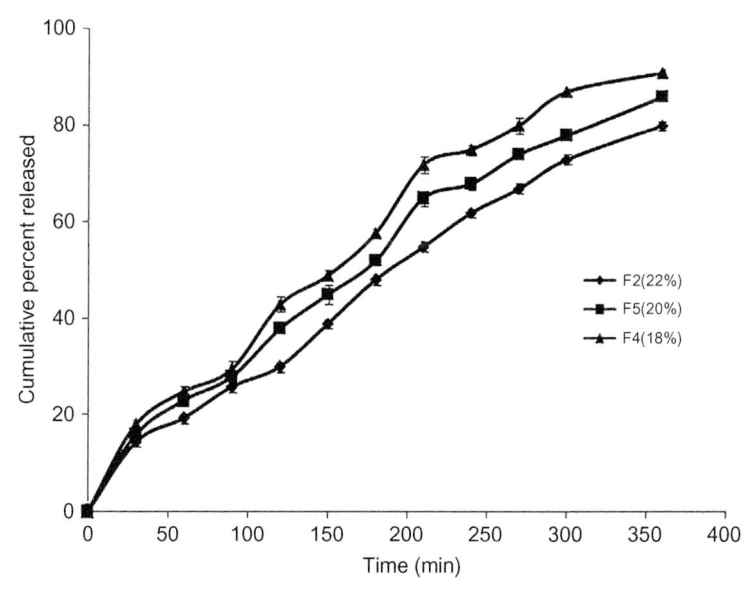

FIG. 10.9 Effect of polymer concentration on in vitro drug release in pH 6.8. *Reprinted from Ray S, Roy G, Maiti S, Bhattacharyya UK, Sil A, Mitra R, Development of smart hydrogels of etherified gum ghatti for sustained oral delivery of ropinirole hydrochloride, Int J Biol Macromol 2017;103:347–354, Copyright (2017), with permission from Elsevier].*

Matrix tablets were prepared using gum ghatti and karaya gum for sustained diclofenac sodium delivery [60]. The release of drug from different formulations varies between 61.88% and 100.96% in 12 h. The different formulations showed nonlinear release pattern. The drug release was diminished when the concentration of polymer blend increased. The release of drug was also diminished with augment in concentration of karaya gum and gum ghatti. The viscosity of the gel layer around the tablet enhanced with augment in concentration of gum, which inhibits the drug release. The gel formation occurs when the media penetrates the matrix consisting of closely packed swollen particles.

A polyelectrolyte nanoparticle was prepared through interaction of gum ghatti and chitosan for ofloxacin delivery [50]. The encapsulation efficiency was diminished with increase in gum ghatti concentration. The solution viscosity was increased with an augment in gum ghatti concentration, and larger size droplets were formed when sprayed by spray gun, resulting in reduced interaction between gum ghatti and chitosan. Owing to this reason, ofloxacin was not trapped properly and leached out from matrix, and the percent encapsulation efficiency decreased. It is necessary to increase the concentration of chitosan, which will help to increase the extent of drug entrapment because chitosan can interact with gum ghatti. A comparative antibacterial study was performed for the optimized formulation. No significant differences in results were observed for optimized formulation and ofloxacin aqueous solution. It was observed that the formulation has sustained release property because only 27% of the drug was released in 12 h. So it can be concluded that gum ghatti-chitosan polyelectrolyte complex has good sustained release property.

The hydrogel beads were prepared using gum ghatti-grafted polyacrylamide and sodium alginate for oral sustained delivery of ketoprofen [45]. Dissolution study was performed in pH 1.2 and pH 7.4 buffer solutions (Fig. 10.10). The release of drug was fast when hydrogel beads were prepared using only sodium alginate. Approximately 47% of drug was released within 2 h in acidic solution (pH 1.2), and in basic solution (pH 7.4), the released drug was 90% within 6 h. However, hydrogel beads were prepared using sodium alginate, and graft copolymer exhibited a pH-responsive behavior with sustained drug release up to 12 h. The pH-responsive release of drug up to 12 h may be owing to superior mechanical strength because of interpenetrating polymer network structure and existence of huge number of COO^- groups in the graft copolymer. The release of drug was slow in acidic buffer solution compared with basic media. This may be due to higher swelling of hydrogel in basic media. The drug release was decreased with augmented amount of graft copolymer (Fig. 10.10A). This result may be due to the enhanced diffusional path length with augmented concentration of polymer. Furthermore, the drug release was diminished with increase in the concentration of Ca^{2+} (Fig. 10.10B). Free volume of

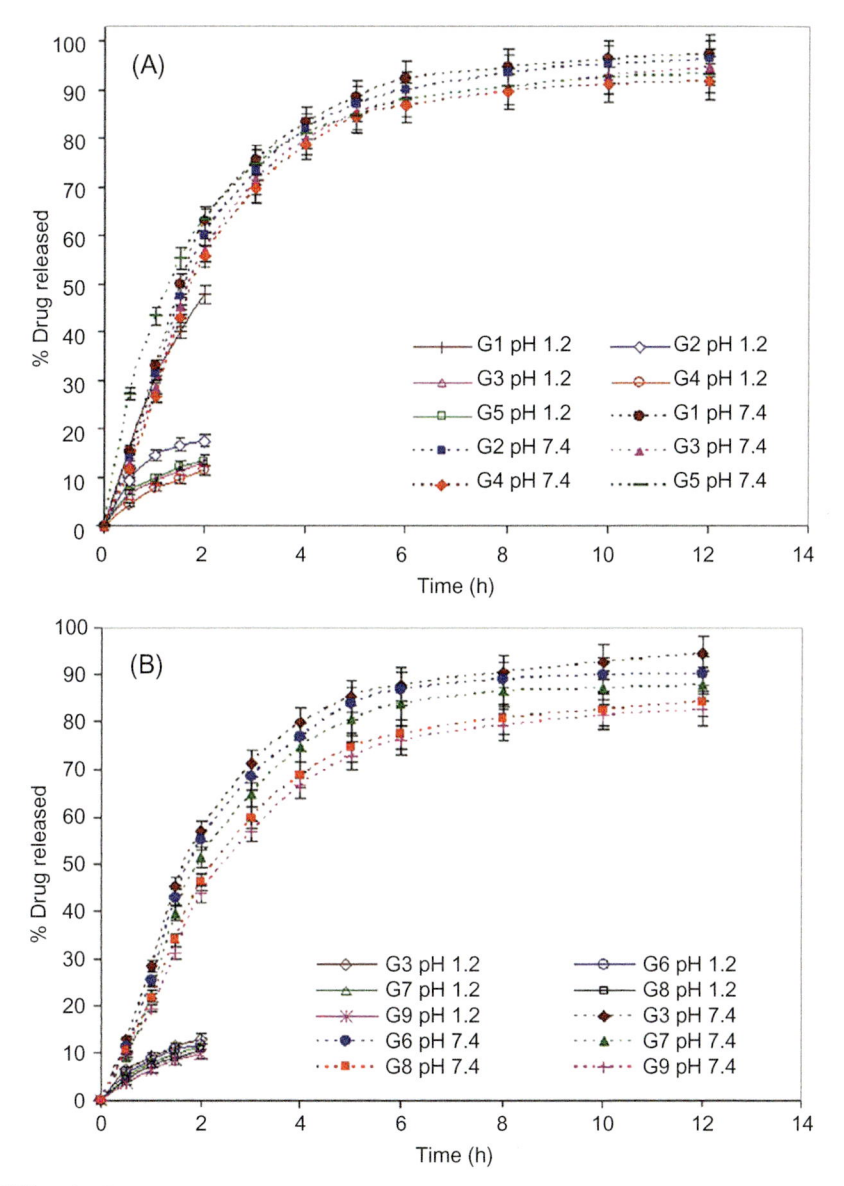

FIG. 10.10 In vitro release of drug from pH-sensitive interpenetrating polymer network microbeads. Effect of the concentration of graft copolymer (A) and cross-linking agents (B). *Reprinted from Boppana R, Mohan GK, Nayak U, Mutalik S, Sa B, Kulkarni RV, Novel pH-sensitive IPNs of polyacrylamide-g-gum ghatti and sodium alginate for gastro-protective drug delivery, Int J Biol Macromol 2015;75:133–143, Copyright (2015), with permission from Elsevier.*

matrix diminished at higher cross-linking density, and consequently, slow diffusion of drug through hydrogel beads was observed.

The in vivo study of the developed hydrogels was conducted on rats (Fig. 10.11). The developed hydrogel beads showed higher AUC compared with pure drug, indicating enhanced bioavailability of ketoprofen from hydrogel beads (Fig. 10.11A). This result may be owing to sustained drug release from the developed beads up to 10 hours. It was observed that the pure drug exhibited rapid augment in plasma drug concentration of drug administered through oral route and declining after 1.5–2 h. The developed hydrogel beads showed lower plasma concentration of

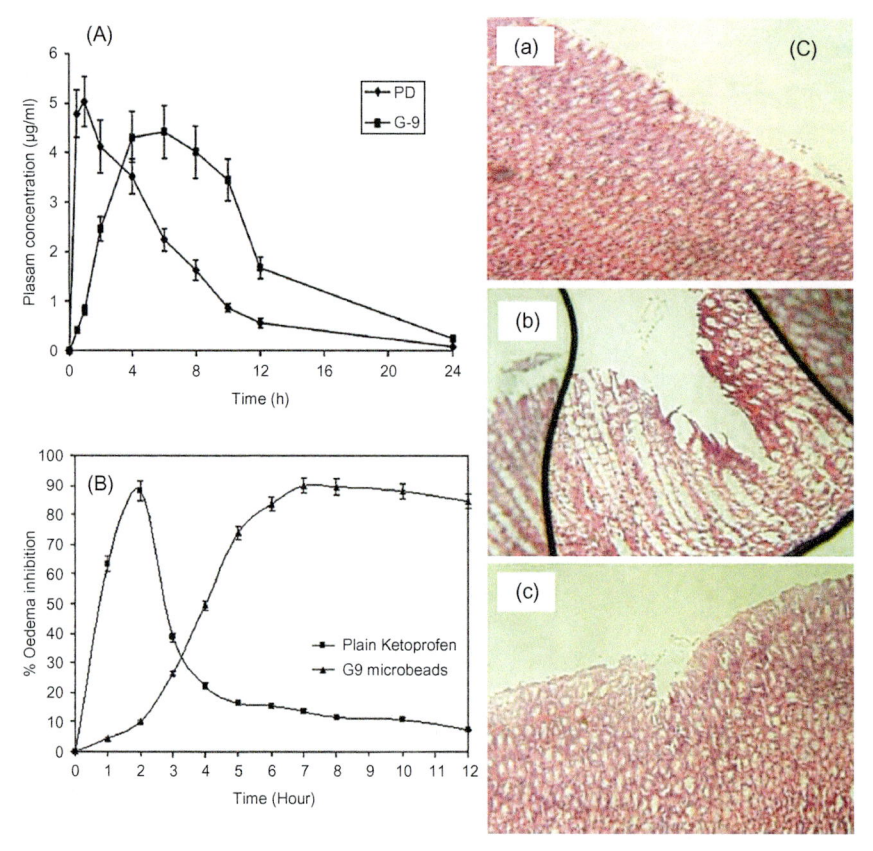

FIG. 10.11   (A) Plasma pristine ketoprofen (PD) concentration and G9 interpenetrating polymer network microbeads after oral administration in rats. (B) Antiinflammatory activity of PD and G9 interpenetrating polymer network microbeads in carrageenan-induced rat paw edema. (C) Stomach histopathology of control rats (a), PD treated rats (b), and G9 interpenetrating polymer network microbeads-treated rats (c). *Reprinted from Boppana R, Mohan GK, Nayak U, Mutalik S, Sa B, Kulkarni RV, Novel pH-sensitive IPNs of polyacrylamide-g-gum ghatti and sodium alginate for gastro-protective drug delivery, Int J Biol Macromol 2015;75:133–143, Copyright (2015), with permission from Elsevier.*

drug up to 2h in comparison with pure ketoprofen. The result indicated that the fast absorption of drug and quick emergence in plasma within 2h from oral administration of pure drug than fast elimination. However, pH-responsive hydrogel beads release the drug in acidic milieu of stomach, which was low because hydrogel bead was unionized with lowest swelling and release of drug. When the hydrogel beads reached the intestine, they were ionized with utmost swelling and release of drug.

The antiinflammatory action of pure drug exhibited paw edema inhibition of 88.6% within 2h and then decreased. A 7.21% paw edema inhibition was noted at the end of 12h (Fig. 10.11B). The result indicated maximum activity of drug within 2h because it was eliminated from the blood after 2h. pH-responsive hydrogel beads exhibited 10.23% of edema inhibition within 2h and then gradually enhanced to 90.23% within 7h. After 7h, the inhibition of edema was decreased, and at the end of 12h, 84.4% of inhibition was observed. In stomach milieu, the release amount of drug was small, but in the intestinal milieu, maximum amount of drug was released.

Stomach histopathologies of rats were studied and represented in Fig. 10.11C. Control rat groups (vehicle treated) exhibited no signs of hemorrhages/ulcer, and normal layers of mucosa were found. The gastric glands and epithelium surface seemed to be undamaged and unchanged. Pure ketoprofe-treated rat groups exhibited hemorrhages and ulcers. Moreover, erosion of mucosa was observed with perforations, congestion, and edema. It was also observed that the gastric glands were not intact, and epithelium surface was not normal. Small-size ulcers were observed with very mild mucosal erosions, congestion, and hemorrhage in the rat groups treated with interpenetrating network hydrogel beads. The normal gastric glands exhibited no signs of necrosis, perforation, and edema. This result indicated that the adverse effects of ketoprofen such as mucosal erosion, ulcers, and hemorrhage were diminished when drug was formulated as pH-responsive hydrogel beads.

10.4.1.3 Colon-specific delivery

Delivery of drug to the colon is extremely advantageous to treat local diseases, including amebiosis, ulcerative colitis, colonic cancer, and Crohn's disease [61–64]. The colon-targeted delivery system protected the drug during transit through the upper part of the GIT and released the drug on reaching the colon. The colon is an appropriate site for protein and peptide delivery because of less number of digestive enzymes and low proteolytic activity of colon mucosa. The absorption duration of drug from colon is high, which is up to 5 days [65].

Poly (acrylic acid)-grafted gum ghatti and poly (acrylic acid-aniline)-grafted gum ghatti were synthesized through grafting to deliver amoxicillin trihydrate to the colon [66]. The drug was entrapped into the hydrogel through absorption of drug by dissolving the cross-linked hydrogel in the solution of drug. The releases of drug from synthesized hydrogel at different pH are represented in Figs. 10.12 and 10.13. A fast drug release (70%–80%) was observed from synthesized hydrogel during the first 6 h. After 6 h, the release of drug was slow and extended up to 14 h. The release of drug from hydrogel matrix was highest at pH 9.2 and lowest at 2.2 and pH 7. The utmost release of drug at basic pH may be due to amoxicillin trihydrate dissociation constant. The solubility of drug in alkaline pH was more in comparison with neutral or acidic media. Moreover, at low pH, the carboxylate groups of hydrogel matrix were in unionized form and matrix in collapsed state, resulting in slow drug release. The carboxylate groups of hydrogel matrix were ionized at higher pH, and repulsion of the polymer chains occurred, resulting in increased absorption of water and higher diffusion of drug.

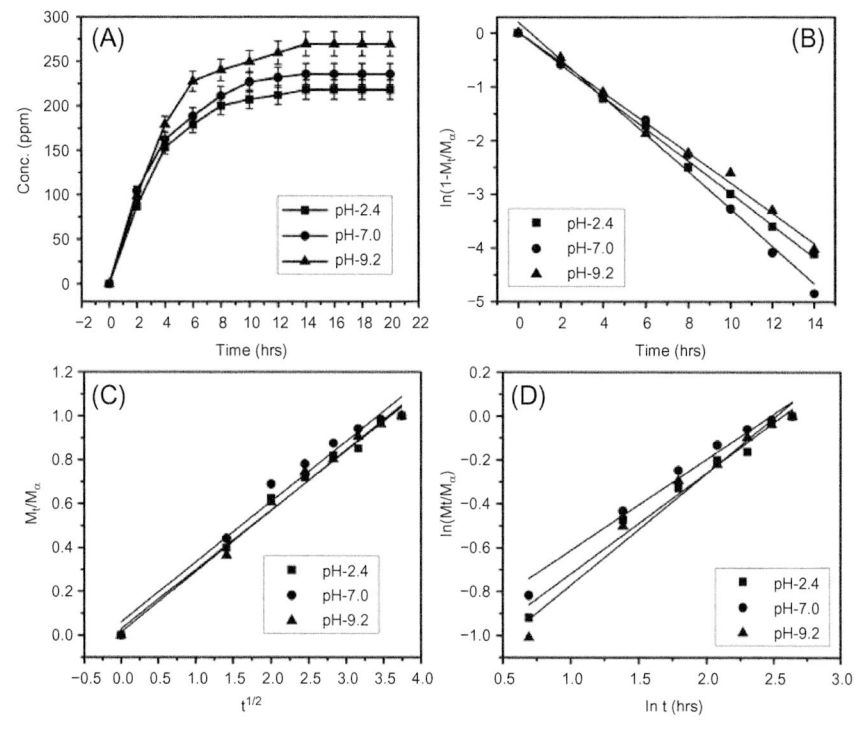

FIG. 10.12   Effect of pH on drug release through poly (acrylic acid)-grafted gum ghatti (A) Concentration versus time, (B) $\ln(1 - Mt/M\infty)$ versus time, (C) $Mt/M\infty$ versus $t1/2$, (D) $\ln Mt/M_\alpha$ versus $\ln t$. *Reprinted from Sharma K, Kumar V, Chaudhary B, Kaith BS, Kalia S, Swart HC, Application of biodegradable superabsorbent hydrogel composite based on Gum ghatti-co-poly (acrylic acid-aniline) for controlled drug delivery, Polym Degrad Stab 2016;124:101–111, Copyright (2016), with permission from Elsevier.*

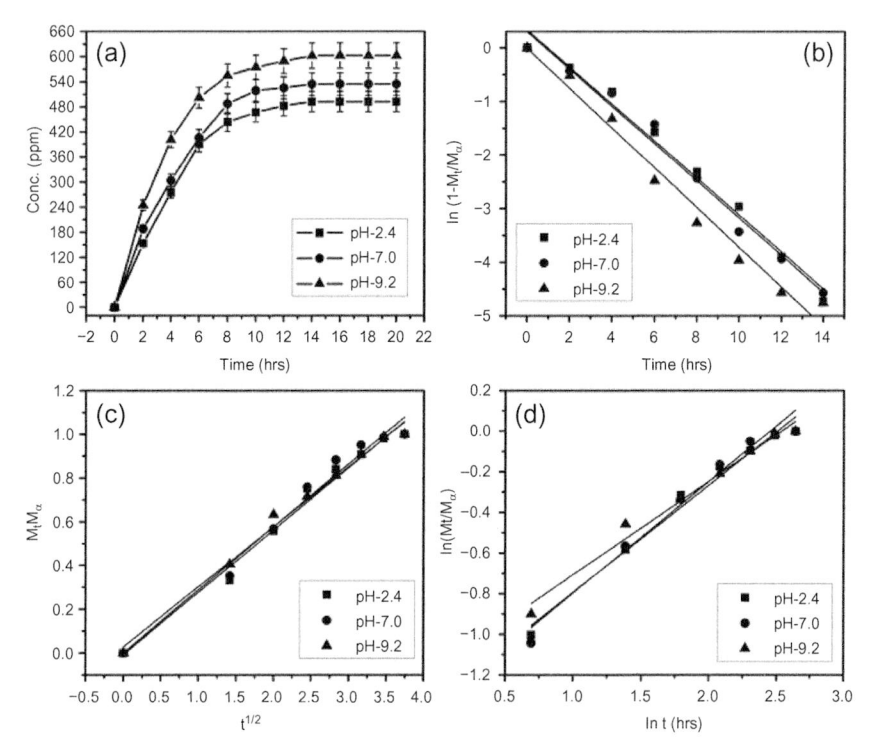

FIG. 10.13 Effect of pH on drug release through poly (acrylic acid-aniline)-grafted gum ghatti (A) Concentration versus time, (B) ln(1 − $Mt/M∞$) versus time, (C) $Mt/M_∞$ versus $t1/2$, and (D) ln$Mt/M_∞$ versus ln$t$. *Reprinted from Sharma K, Kumar V, Chaudhary B, Kaith BS, Kalia S, Swart HC, Application of biodegradable superabsorbent hydrogel composite based on Gum ghatti-copoly (acrylic acid-aniline) for controlled drug delivery, Polym Degrad Stab 2016;124:101– 111, Copyright (2016), with permission from Elsevier.*

pH-responsive hydrogel beads were developed using gum ghatti-grafted polyacrylamide by ionotropic gelation method for diclofenac sodium enteric delivery [67]. Grafted copolymer was synthesized by microwave technique. The synthesized graft copolymer was nontoxic and biodegradable. The synthesized graft copolymer showed pH-responsive swelling behavior. Approximately 20% of drugs was released in pH 1.2– 5.5 in 3h and 80% of drugs was released in pH 6.8–7.4 in 8h from the hydrogel beads.

Diclofenac sodium-loaded interpenetrating polymer network microparticles were synthesized using chitosan and gum ghatti as polymer for sustained delivery [68]. The particle sizes of the developed microparticles were in the range of 294–366 μm. The drug encapsulation efficiency of the developed microparticulate hydrogel was 84.09%–96.81%. The drug release was extended up to 12h and depended on the amount of chitosan and gum ghatti present in the microparticles. Metoprolol succinate-loaded controlled release tablets were developed using gum ghatti as a rate controlling polymer [69]. Dissolution was performed in acidic solution (pH 1.2) for 2 h and in basic solution (pH 7.2) for 12 h. The release of drug was sustained up to 12 h. The stability data showed that there was no considerable difference in release mechanism and drug content during the storage of 3 months.

Interpenetrating polymer network hydrogel beads were prepared using gum ghatti and povinyl alcohol for the controlled delivery of glipizide [70]. The maximum entrapment efficiency of the drug was 92.85%. The release of drug was extended up to 7 h by changing the cross-linking agent concentration. In vivo antidiabetic activity study was conducted using alloxane-induced diabetic rats. Initial blood glucose reduction was slow up to 3 h in comparison with pure drug, but after 6 h, 90% blood glucose reduction was observed, indicating controlled release of glipizide from the developed hydrogel beads.

10.4.1.4 Transdermal drug delivery

In transdermal delivery, the drug was delivered through the skin in a specific and controlled rate. It has several advantages compared with oral and injectable dosage forms. Transdermal delivery of drug is used when the drug is metabolized in GIT and liver. It also has advantages over injectable dosage forms that are invasive, painful, and transmitted disease through reuse of needle [71]. In addition, transdermal drug delivery systems are noninvasive, inexpensive, improve patient compliance, provide controlled release of drug up to 1 week, and can be self-administered [72, 73].

Electric stimulus triggered transdermal delivery of quetiapine fumerate was developed using gum ghatti-grafted polyacrylamide [74]. Gum ghatti-grafted polyacrylamide was prepared by free radical polymerization method. Then hydrolysis was performed in alkaline condition to convert gum ghatti-grafted polyacrylamide – $CONH_2$ groups to –COOH groups resulting electrically-responsive copolymer. Rat abdominal skin was used to conduct the permeation study. The drug permeation was lower without electrical stimulus in comparison with electrical stimulus. The developed formulation exhibited an utmost of 9.41% drug permeation at the end of 4 h without electrical stimulus. The permeation of drug was diminished with enhanced concentration of graft copolymer, which may be owing to the enhanced viscosity of the formulation. The permeation of drug in the existence of electric stimulus was improved in comparison with that in devoid of electric stimulus. The drug permeation was enhanced twofold when electric current was applied. Moreover, the permeation of drug was enhanced when the strength of electric current was enhanced from 2 to 8 mA. The developed formulations exhibited the flux values of 0.0407 to 0.0495 mg/cm^2 per hour. The permeation study of drug was also performed under on-off electric stimuli. The drug was permeated more rapidly in on condition, and slowed down when the electric current was in off condition.

10.4.2 Gum ghatti hydrogel for tissue engineering

The tissue engineering looks forward to patients with organ failure or injuries. Presently, organs are transplanted to the patients with injured or diseased organs. The number of organ failure cases increases day by day, but there is a lack of donor organs. The scientists of tissue engineering field are currently applying the basic principles of life science, material science, bioengineering, and transplantation of cell to make natural substitutes for the repairs of injured and diseased organs [75–77]. Biomaterials play a significant role in tissue engineering. It provides a 3D structure where cells are attach, grow, and form a new tissue with suitable configuration and function. Biomaterials also delivered the cells, growth factors, and peptides for cell adhesion to preferred location in the body [78, 79]. It can give a mechanical support in response to in vivo forces during tissue development and should be biodegradable and bioresorbable. Recently, biomaterial-based scaffolds are extensively used to repair and regenerate damaged tissue. Hydrogels are polymeric 3D network structures and are proficient to entrap huge amount of water owing to the existence of hydrophilic functional groups [80–82]. They share similar features with natural living environment due to high water content and are highly biocompatible. Moreover, proteins, oxygen, and other biomolecules are easily transported through the hydrogels to support the entrapped cells [83, 84]. Natural and synthetic polymers are used for the construction of hydrogel scaffolds [85–87]. Hydrogels prepared from synthetic polymer exhibited tunable properties but have drawbacks such as lack of the bioactive amino acid sequences requisite for attachment, expansion, and maturation of the entrapped cells [88, 89]. Accordingly, hydrogels prepared from natural polymer are widely used in tissue engineering.

Lett et al. prepared porous hydroxyapatite scaffolds using gum ghatti as a natural binding agent by template-assisted polymer sponge replication method for repair and regeneration of bone [90]. It was observed that the 15 wt% gum ghatti was suitable for the preparation of stable scaffold. Moreover, developed scaffolds retain 70% free space for blood vessels circulation. The in vivo study of the developed scaffold exhibited the complete colonization of phosphate and calcium ions and traces of magnesium ions on porous scaffold surface. The stability of the developed scaffold for the use of bone tissue regeneration was established by in vitro degradation studies. The nontoxicity of the developed scaffold was studied by MTT assay and established the nontoxicity.

10.5 Conclussion

Gum ghatti is a polysaccharide having high viscosity, nontoxicity, and biocompatibility with emulsifying property. In recent times, several researchers synthesized gum ghatti-based hydrogel through different methods such as graft copolymerization, interpenetrating polymer network, and polyelectrolyte complexation. Gum ghatti-based hydrogels were comprehensively used in drug delivery and regeneration of tissue. It retards the drug release, which is an important criterion to develop the sustained release dosage forms. Primarily, hydrogels based on gum ghatti were extensively used in intragastric drug delivery, sustained intestinal delivery, as well as in colon-specific delivery. Enough attention and investigation concerning applications in pharmaceutical field are necessary for this natural exudate gum.

References

[1] Al-Assaf S, Amar V, Phillips G. Characterization of gum ghatti and comparison with gum arabic. In: Williams PA, Phillips GO, editors. Gums and stabilisers for the food industry. Cambridge: Royal Society of Chemistry Publishing; 2008. p. 280–90.
[2] Ido T, Ogasawara T, Katayama T, Sasaki Y, Al-Assaf S, Phillips GO. Emulsification properties of GATIFOLIA (gum ghatti) used for emulsions in food products. Foods Food Ingred J 2008;213:365–70.
[3] Al-Assaf S, Amar V, Phillips G. Gum ghatti. In: Handbook of hydrocolloids. Cambridge: CRC Press; 2009. p. 477–94.
[4] Amar V, Al-Assaf S, Phillips G, Amar V, Phillips GO. An introduction to gum ghatti, another proteinceous gum. Foods Food Ingred J 2006;211(3):275–80.
[5] Kaur L, Singh J, Singh H. Characterization of gum ghatti (Anogeissus latifolia), a structural and rheological approach. J Food Sci 2009;74(6):E328–32.
[6] Kora AJ, Beedu SR, Jayaraman A. Size-controlled green synthesis of silver nanoparticles mediated by gum ghatti (Anogeissus latifolia) and its biological activity. Org Med Chem Lett 2012;2(1):17.
[7] Aspinall GO. Chemistry of cell wall polysaccharides. In: Preiss J, editor. The biochemistry of plants. New York: Academic Press; 1980. p. 473–500.
[8] Parvathi KMM, Ramesh CK, Krishna V, Paramesha M, Kuppast IJ. Hypolipidemic activity of gum ghatti of Anogeissus latifolia. Pharmacogn Mag 2009;5(19):11.
[9] Giri TK, Bhowmick S, Maity S. Entrapment of capsaicin loaded nanoliposome in pH responsive hydrogel beads for colonic delivery. J Drug Deliv Sci Technol 2017;39:417–22.
[10] Giri TK, Dey B, Maity S. Preparation and characterization of nanoemulsome entrapped in enteric coated hydrogel beads for the controlled delivery of capsaicin to the colon. Curr Drug Ther 2018;13:98–105.
[11] Dey M, Das M, Chowhan A, Giri TK. Breaking the barricade of oral chemotherapy through polysaccharide nanocarrier. Int J Biol Macromol 2019;130:34–49.
[12] Giri TK, Verma D, Badwaik HR. Effect of aluminium chloride concentration on diltiazem hydrochloride release from pH-sentive hydrogel beads composed of hydrolyzed grafted k-carrageenan and sodium alginate. Curr Chem Biol 2017;11:44–9.
[13] Giri TK, Thakur A, Tripathi DK. Biodegradable hydrogel bead of casein and modified xanthan gum for controlled delivery of theophylline. Curr Drug Ther 2016;11:150–62.

[14] Peppas NA, Khare AR. Preparation, structure and diffusional behavior of hydrogels in controlled release. Adv Drug Deliv Rev 1993;11:1–35.

[15] Kaith BS, Saruchi RJ, Manprret SB. Screening and RSM optimization for synthesis of a gum tragacantheacrylic acid based device for in situ controlled cetirizine dihydrochloride release. Soft Matter 2012;8:2286–93.

[16] Feil H, Bae YH, Feijen J, Kim SW. Molecular separation by thermosensitive hydrogel membranes. J Membr Sci 1992;64:283–94.

[17] Hoare TR, Kohane DS. Hydrogels in drug delivery: progress and challenges. Polymer 2008;49:1993–2007.

[18] Kaith BS, Jindal R, Mittal H. Superabsorbent hydrogels from poly(acrylamide-co-acrylonitrile) grafted Gum ghatti with salt, pH and temperature responsive properties. Der Chem Sin 2010;1(2):92–103.

[19] Rani P, Sen G, Mishra S, Jha U. Microwave assisted synthesis of polyacrylamide grafted gum ghatti and its application as flocculant. Carbohydr Polym 2012;89:275–81.

[20] Kaith BS, Jindal R, Mittal H, Kumar K. Temperature, pH and electric stimulus responsive hydrogels from gum ghatti and polyacrylamide synthesis, characterization and swelling studies. Der Chem Sin 2010;1(2):44–54.

[21] Kaith BS, Jindal R, Mittal H, Kumar K. Synthesis, characterization and swelling behavior evaluation of Gum ghatti and acrylamide based hydrogel for selective absorption of saline from different petroleum fraction-saline emulsions. J Appl Polym Sci 2011;124:2037–47.

[22] Sharma K, Kaith BS, Kalia S, Kumar V, Swart H. Gum ghatti based biodegradable and conductive carriers for colon-specific drug delivery. Colloid Polym Sci 2015;293:1181–90.

[23] Jorge FS, Santos TM, de Jesus JP, Banks WB. Reactions between Cr(VI) and wood and its model compounds—part 1: a qualitative kinetic study of the reduction of hexavalent chromium. Wood Sci Technol 1999;33(6):487–99.

[24] Whistler LR. Exudate gums. In: Whistler LR, BeMiller JN, editors. Industrial gums polysaccharide and their derivatives. San Diego, California: Academic Press, Inc; 1993. p. 326–9.

[25] Guo MQ, Hu X, Wang C, Ai L. Polysaccharides: structure and solubility. In: Xu Z, editor. Solubility of polysaccharides. China: Intechopen; 2017. p. 7–20.

[26] Kang J, Cui SW, Phillips GO, Chen J, Guo Q, Wang Q. New studies on gum ghatti (Anogeissus latifolia). Part III: structure char-acterization of a globular polysaccharide fraction by 1D, 2D NMR spectroscopy and methylation analysis. Food Hydrocoll 2011;25(8):1999–2007.

[27] Hobbs CA, Swartz C, Maronpot R, Davis J, Recio L, Hayashi SM. Evaluation of the genotoxicity of the food additive, gum ghatti. Food Chem Toxicol 2012;50(3-4):854–60.

[28] Maronpot RR, Davis J, Moser G, Giri DK, Hayashi SM. Evaluation of 90-day oral rat toxicity studies on the food additive, gum ghatti. Food Chem Toxicol 2013;51:215–24.

[29] Joshi MG, Setty CM, Deshmukh AS, Bhatt YA. Gum ghatti: a new release modifier for zero order release in 3-layered tablets of diltiazem hydrochloride. Indian J Pharm Educ 2010;44(1):78–85.

[30] Williams PA. Adsorption of polyelectrolytes onto barium sulphate. PhD Thesis, University of Salford; 1982.

[31] Nussenbaum S, Hassid WZ. Estimation of molecular weight of starch polysaccharides. Anal Chem 1952;24:501–3.

[32] Kang KS, Pettitt DJ. Xanthan, gellan, welan, and rhamsan. In: JN BM, Whistle RL, editors. Industrial gums: polysaccharides and their derivatives. 3rd ed. San Diego, California: Academic Press, Inc; 1993. p. 346.

[33] Giri TK, Vishwas S, Tripathi DK. Synthesis of grafted locust bean gum using vinyl monomer and studies of physicochemical properties and acute toxicity. Nat Prod J 2016;6:1–9.

[34] Giri TK, Yadav BK, Badwaik H. Synthesis and characterization of gellan gum based bioadsorbent for wastewater treatment. Curr Microwave Chem 2018;5(2):84–96.

[35] Giri TK, Verma P, Tripathi DK. Grafting of vinyl monomer onto gellan gum using microwave: synthesis and characterization of grafted copolymer. Adv Compos Mater 2015;24:531–43.

[36] Giri TK, Pure S, Tripathi DK. Synthesis of graft copolymers of acrylamide for locust bean gum using microwave energy: swelling behavior, flocculation characteristics and acute toxicity study. Polimeros 2015;25:168–74.

[37] Giri TK, Verma D, Tripathi DK. Effect of adsorption parameters on biosorption of Pb++ ions from aqueous solution by poly (acrylamide)-grafted kappa-carrageenan. Polym Bull 2015;72:1625–46.

[38] Giri TK, Pradhan M, Tripathi DK. Synthesis of graft copolymer of kappa-carrageenan using microwave energy and studies of swelling capacity, flocculation properties, and preliminary acute toxicity. Turk J Chem 2016;40:283–95.

[39] Mittal H, Mishra SB, Mishra AK, Kaith BS, Jindal R. Flocculation characteristics and biodegradation studies of Gum ghatti based hydrogels. Int J Biol Macromol 2013;58:37–46.

[40] Sharma K, Kaith BS, Kumar V, Kumar V, Kalia S, Kapur BK, Swart HC. A comparative study of the effect of Ni^{9+} and Au^{8+} ion beams on the properties of poly (methacrylic acid) grafted gum ghatti films. Radiat Phys Chem 2014;97:253–61.

[41] Mittal H, Maity A, Ray SS. Gum ghatti and poly (acrylamide-co-acrylic acid) based biodegradable hydrogel-evaluation of the flocculation and adsorption properties. Polym Degrad Stab 2015;120:42–52.

[42] Mittal H, Maity A, Ray SS. Effective removal of cationic dyes from aqueous solution using gum ghatti-based biodegradable hydrogel. Int J Biol Macromol 2015;79:8–20.

[43] Kaith BS, Sharma K, Kumar V, Kumar V, Swart HC, Kalia S. Effects of swift heavy ion beam irradiation on the structural and morphological properties of poly(methacrylic acid) cross-linked gum ghatti films. Vacuum 2014;101:166–70.

[44] Karabanova LV, Mikhalovsky SV, Lloyd AW, Boiteux G, Sergeeva LM, Novikova TI, Lutsyk ED, Meikle S. Gradient semi-interpenetrating polymer networks based on polyurethane and poly(vinyl pyrrolidone). J Mater Chem 2005;15:499–507.

[45] Boppana R, Mohan GK, Nayak U, Mutalik S, Sa B, Kulkarni RV. Novel pH-sensitive IPNs of polyacrylamide-g-gum ghatti and sodium alginate for gastro-protective drug delivery. Int J Biol Macromol 2015;75:133–43.

[46] Kaith BS, Sharma K, Kumar V, Kaliad S, Swart HC. Fabrication and characterization of gum ghatti-polymethacrylic acid based electrically conductive hydrogels. Synth Met 2014;187:61–7.

[47] Sharma K, Kumar V, Kaith BS, Kumar V, Som S, Kalia S, Swart HC. Synthesis, characterization and water retention study of biodegradable Gum ghatti-poly (acrylic acide-aniline) hydrogels. Polym Degrad Stab 2015;111:20–31.

[48] Sharma K, Kaith BS, Kumar V, Kalia S, Kumar V, Swart HC. Synthesis and biodegradation studies of gamma irradiated electrically conductive hydrogels. Polym Degrad Stab 2014;107:166–77.

[49] Verma A, Verma A. Polyelectrolyte Complex- An Overview. Int J Pharm Sci Res 2013;4:1684–91.

[50] Shelly AM, Kumar A. Gum ghatti–chitosan polyelectrolyte nanoparticles: preparation and characterization. Int J Biol Macromol 2013;61:41–415.

[51] Chowhan A, Giri TK. Polysaccharide as renewable responsive biopolymer for in situ gel in the delivery of drug through ocular route. Int J Biol Macromol 2020;150:559–72.

[52] Das M, Giri TK. Hydrogels based on gellan gum in cell delivery and drug delivery. J Drug Deliv Sci Technol 2020;56(Part A), 101586.

[53] Shah SH, Patel JK, Patel NV. Stomach specific floating drug delivery system: a review. Int J Pharm Tech Res 2009;1(3):623–33.

[54] Bera H, Ippagunta SR, Kumar S, Vangala P. Core-shell alginate-ghatti gum modified montmorillonite composite matrices for stomach-specific flurbiprofen delivery. Mater Sci Eng C 2017;76:715–26.

[55] Lal N, Dubey J, Gaur P, Verma N, Verma A. Chitosan based in situ forming polyelectrolyte complexes: a potential sustained drug delivery polymeric carrier for high dose drugs. Mater Sci Eng C 2017;79:491–8.

[56] Jain N, Banik A. Novel interpenetrating polymer network mucoadhesive microspheres of gum ghatti and poly(vinyl alcohol) for the delivery of ranitidine HCl. Asian J Pharm Clin Res 2013;6:119–23.

[57] Ravi V, Kumar P, Hatna S. Investigation of ghatti gum as a carrier to develop sustained release floating tablets of diltiazem hydrochloride. Thai J Pharm Sci 2012;36(4):155–64.

[58] Arora G, Malik K, Rana V, Singh I. Gum Ghatti—a pharmaceutical excipient: development, evaluation and optimization of sustained release mucoadhesive matrix tablets of domperidone. Acta Pol Pharm 2012;69(4):725–37.

[59] Ray S, Roy G, Maiti S, Bhattacharyya UK, Sil A, Mitra R. Development of smart hydrogels of etherified gum ghatti for sustained oral delivery of ropinirole hydrochloride. Int J Biol Macromol 2017;103:347–54.

[60] Reddy SC, Shivakumar HG, Megha Shyam M, Narendra C, Moin A. Karaya and ghatti gum as a novel polymer blend in preparation of extended release tablets: optimization by factorial design. J Drug Deliv Sci Technol 2014;24:525–32.

[61] Antonin KH, Rak R, Beick PR, Schenker U, Hastewell J, Fox R. The absorption of human calcitonin from the transverse colon of man. Int J Pharm 1996;130:33–9.

[62] Tozaki H, Komoike J, Tada C, Maruyama T, Terabe A, Suzuki T, Yamamoto A, Muranishi S. Chitosan capsules for colon specific drug delivery: improvement of insulin absorption from the rat colon. J Pharm Sci 1997;86:1016–21.

[63] Giri TK, Alexander A, Ajazuddin BTK, Maity S. Infringement of the barriers of cancer via dietary phytoconstituents capsaicin through novel drug delivery system. Curr Drug Deliv 2016;13:27–39.

[64] Bera S, Maity S, Ghosh B, Ghosh A, Giri TK. Development and characterization of solid dispersion system for enhancing the solubility and cytotoxicity of dietary capsaicin. Curr Drug Ther 2020;15:143–51.

[65] Philip AK, Philip B. Colon targeted drug delivery systems: a review on primary and novel approaches. Oman Med J 2010;25(2):79–87.

[66] Sharma K, Kumar V, Chaudhary B, Kaith BS, Kalia S, Swart HC. Application of biodegradable superabsorbent hydrogel composite based on Gum ghatti-co-poly (acrylic acid-aniline) for controlled drug delivery. Polym Degrad Stab 2016;124:101–11.

[67] Moin A, Hussain T, Gowda DV. Enteric delivery of diclofenac sodium through functionally modified poly (acrylamide-grafted-ghatti gum)-based pH-sensitive hydrogel beads: development, formulation and evaluation. J Young Pharm 2017;9(4):525–36.

[68] Reddy J, Nagashubha B, Reddy M, Moin A, Shivakumar HG. Novel interpenetrating polymer matrix network microparticles for intestinal drug delivery. Curr Drug Deliv 2014;11(2):191–9.

[69] Ravi V, Kumar P, Hatna S. Ghatti gum based matrix tablets for oral sustained delivery of metoprolol succinate. Int J Pharm Pharm Sci 2012;4:210–6.

[70] Ray S, Bera M, Bhattacharyya UK, Das S, Seth S, Pal PK, Aziz A. pH Sensitive interpenetrating network bio containers of gum ghatti for sustained release of glipizide. Curr Drug Deliv 2019;16(9):849–61.

[71] Miller MA, Pisani E. The cost of unsafe injections. Bull World Health Organ 1999;77:808–11.

[72] Thakre S, Shinde M. Approaches for transdermal drug delivery system: a review. Asian J Pharm Res Develop 2014;2:1–12.

[73] Nanda S, Saroha K, Sharma B. Formulation, evaluation and optimization of transdermal gel of ketorolac tromethamine using face centered central composite design. Int J Pharm Pharm Sci 2014;6:133–9.

[74] Birajda RP, Patil SB, Alange VV, Kulkarni RV. Electro-responsive polyacrylamide-grafted-gum ghatti copolymer for transdermal drug delivery application. J Macromol Sci A 2019;56:306–15.

[75] Mikos AG, Lyman MD, Freed LE, Langer R. Wetting of poly (L-lactic acid) and poly (DL-lactic-co-glycolic acid) foams for tissue culture. Biomaterials 1994;15:55–8.

[76] Choi JS, Lee SJ, Christ GJ, Atala A, Yoo JJ. The influence of electrospun aligned poly (epsilon-caprolactone)/collagen nanofiber meshes on the formation of self-aligned skeletal muscle myotubes. Biomaterials 2008;29:2899–906.

[77] Lee SJ, Liu J, Oh SH, Soker S, Atala A, Yoo JJ. Development of a composite vascular scaffolding system that withstands physiological vascular conditions. Biomaterials 2008;29:2891–8.

[78] Kim BS, Mooney DJ. Development of biocompatible synthetic extracellular matrices for tissue engineering. Trends Biotechnol 1998;16:224–30.

[79] Freeman MR, Yoo JJ, Raab G, Soker S, Adam RM, Schneck FX, Renshaw AA, Klagsbrun M, Atala A. Heparin-binding EGF-like growth factor is an autocrine growth factor for human urothelial cells and is synthesized by epithelial and smooth muscle cells in the human bladder. J Clin Invest 1997;99:1028–36.

[80] Kushwaha SK, Saxena P, Rai A. Stimuli sensitive hydrogels for ophthalmic drug delivery: a review. Int J Pharm Investig 2012;2(2):54–60.

[81] Gong C, Qi T, Wei X, Qu Y, Wu Q, Luo F, Qian Z. Thermosensitive polymeric hydrogels as drug delivery systems. Curr Med Chem 2013;20(1):79–94.

[82] Zhang XZ, Xu XD, Cheng SX, Zhuo RX. Strategies to improve the response rate of thermosensitive PNIPAAm hydrogels. Soft Matter 2008;4:385–91.

[83] Pereira TA, Ramos DN, Lopez RF. Hydrogel increases localized transport regions and skin permeability during low frequency ultrasound treatment. Sci Rep 2017;7:44236.

[84] Fan C, Wang DA. Effects of permeability and living space on cell fate and neo-tissue development in hydrogel-based scaffolds: a study with cartilaginous model. Macromol Biosci 2015;15:535–45.

[85] Aurora A, Wrice N, Walters TJ, Christy RJ, Natesan S. A PEGylated platelet free plasma hydrogel based composite scaffold enables stable vascularization and targeted cell delivery for volumetric muscle loss. Acta Biomater 2018;65:150–62.

[86] Ekaputra AK, Prestwich GD, Cool SM, Hutmacher DW. The three-dimensional vascularization of growth factor-releasing hybrid scaffold of poly (epsilon-caprolactone)/collagen fibers and hyaluronic acid hydrogel. Biomaterials 2011;32:8108–17.

[87] Ziv K, Nuhn H, Ben-Haim Y, Sasportas LS, Kempen PJ, Niedringhaus TP, Hrynyk M, Sinclair R, Barron AE, Gambhir SS. A tunable silk-alginate hydrogel scaffold for stem cell culture and transplantation. Biomaterials 2014;35:3736–43.

[88] Patel D, Sharma S, Screen HRC, Bryant SJ. Effects of cell adhesion motif, fiber stiffness, and cyclic strain on tenocyte gene expression in a tendon mimetic fiber composite hydrogel. Biochem Biophys Res Commun 2018;499:642–7.

[89] Komatsu M, Konagaya S, Egawa EY, Iwata H. Maturation of human iPS cell-derived dopamine neuron precursors in alginate-Ca^{2+} hydrogel. Biochim Biophys Acta 1850;2015:1669–75.

[90] Lett JA, Sagadevan S, Shahnavaz Z, Latha MB, Alagarswamy K, Hossain MAM, Mohammad F, Johan MR. Exploration of gum ghatti-modified porous scaffolds for bone tissue engineering applications. New J Chem 2020;44:2389–401.

11

Alginate-based hydrogels

Kasula Nagaraja[a], Kummara Madhusudana Rao[b], and Kummari S.V. Krishna Rao[a]

[a]Polymer Biomaterial Design and Synthesis Laboratory, Department of Chemistry, Yogi Vemana University, Kadapa, Andhra Pradesh, India, [b]School of Chemical Engineering, Yeungnam University, Gyeongsan, Gyeongbuk, South Korea

11.1 Introduction

11.1.1 Overview/objective

Alginate is a natural anionic polymer extracted from the brown seaweed, which comprises β-D-mannuronic acid (M) and α-L-glucuronic acid (G) units (Fig. 11.1); these are arranged in a linear manner either by homogeneous (GG/MM) or heterogeneous (GM/MG) units through $1 \rightarrow 4$ glycosidic linkages [1] (Fig. 11.2). The genus of brown seaweed includes the *Saccharina japonica, Laminaria hyperborean, Macrocystis pyrifera, Ascophyllum nodosum*, etc. [2]. In addition, alginate can be produced in a laboratory scale by bacteria *Azotobacter vinelandii* and *Pseudomonas* spp. [3]. It was first discovered by Stanford ECC in 1881 [4]; however, the industrial commercialization of this polymer has taken place after 100 years, especially in Europe, the United States, and Japan. The hydroxyl (−OH) and carboxyl (−COOH) functional groups of alginate are responsible for its potential physicochemical properties. Hence it has been widely used in various applications such as drug delivery, tissue engineering (TE), agriculture, food industry, cosmetics, water purification, wound dressings, and electrical devices (Fig. 11.3). In addition, these properties are significantly influenced by alginate production parameters such as molecular weight, acetylation degree, the arrangement of uronate units, and M/G ratio [5].

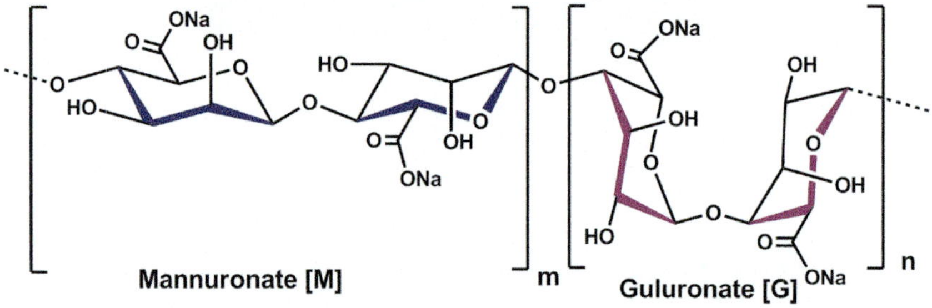

FIG. 11.1　Schematic representation of alginate chemical structure.

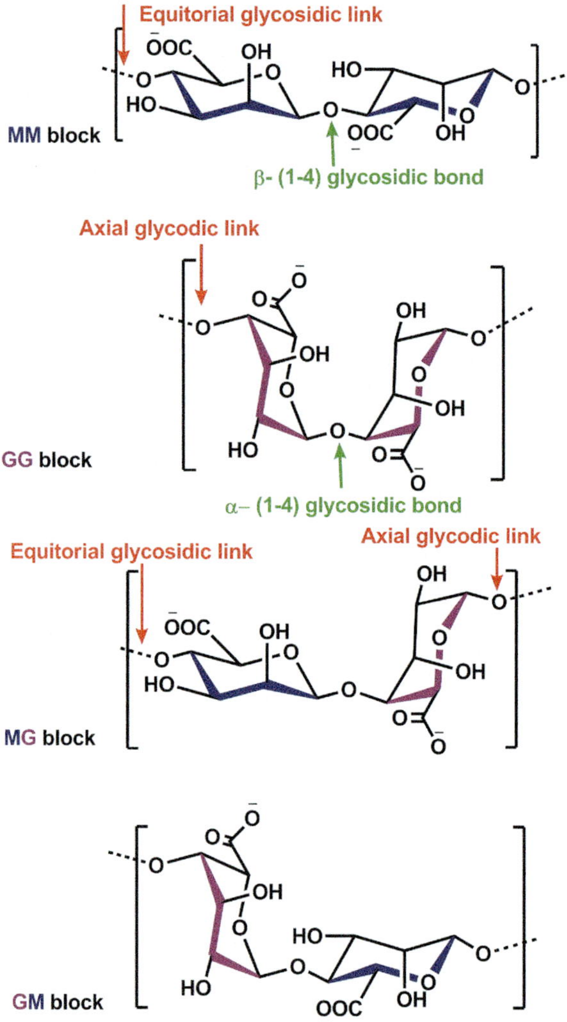

FIG. 11.2　Chemical structures of sodium alginate containing α-L-guluronate (G) and β-D-mannuronate block polymers (possible arrangement of G and M blocks).

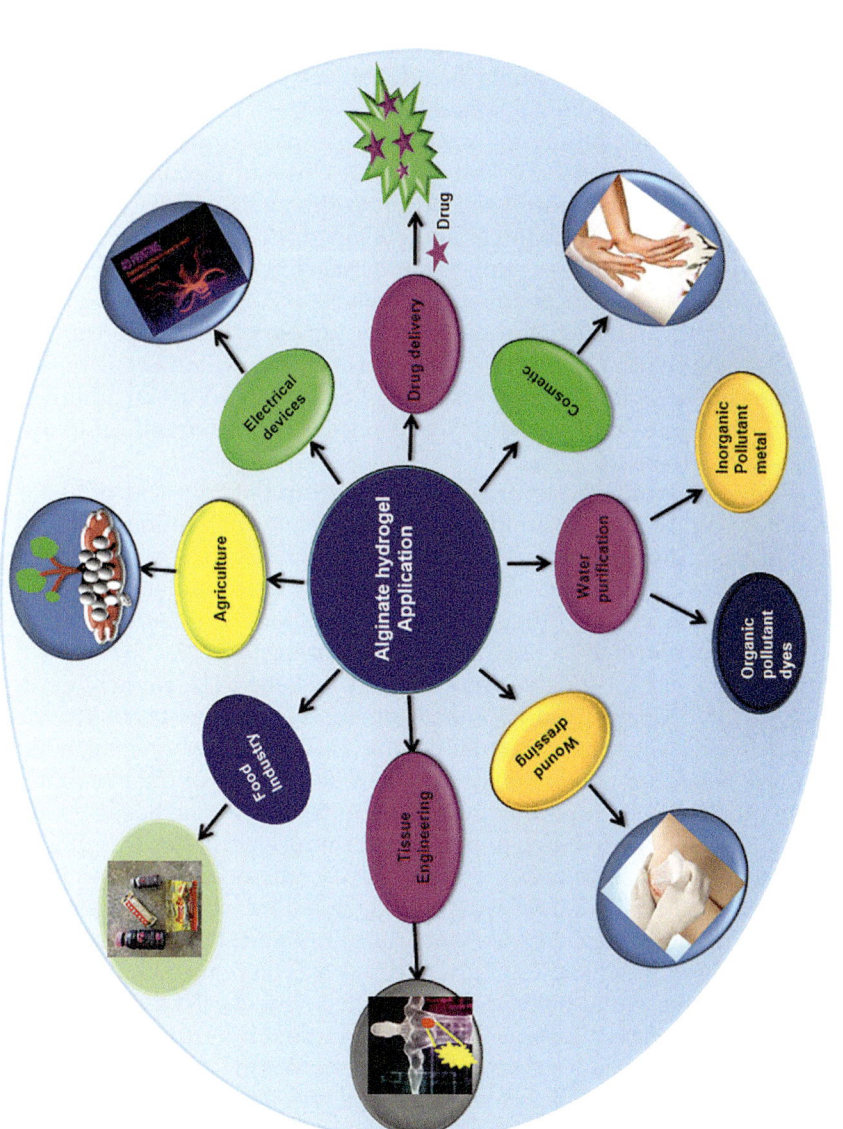

FIG. 11.3 Application sodium alginate hydrogels in various fields.

11.2 Alginate-based biomedical devices: A historical prospective

Alginate has been paid much attention to the fabrication of biomaterials in combinations with other biodegradable and biocompatible synthetic or natural polymer. Biomaterials include tablets, pellets, sol-gel formulations, beads, hydrogels, microspheres, nanospheres, and polyelectrolyte complexes. Initially, sodium alginate (SA) was used to prepare the oral mucosa bioadhesive tablets by mixing with chitosan through compression method for controlled release of diltiazem, and the release was extended up to 6 h [6]. Hodsdon et al. developed SA-based matrix tablets by blending SA with lactose and low amounts of magnesium stearate for controlled release of chlorpheniramine maleate [7]. Yuk et al. designed a pH-sensitive semiinterpenetrating polymer network (semi-IPN) capsule from SA and poly(acrylic acid) for hydrocortisone [8]. Murata et al. developed the chondroitin sulfate and chitosan beads with SA (as an additive) for controlled release of diclofenac, and release has enhanced up to approximately 3 h [9].

Aslani et al. fabricated hydrated of alginate and alginic acid films for controlled diffusion of acetaminophen. However, the acetaminophen was diffused from the alginate gels in the order alginic acid > acid-exposed alginic acid > divalent alginate [10]. Kimura et al. formulated the medium molecular weight SA-based dietary fibers for cholesterol excretion and glucose absorption in rats. The results demonstrate that this type of formulation is useful for the prevention of diabetes [11]. Kikuchi et al. developed the physically cross-linked calcium alginate gel beads for the pulsatile release of macromolecular dextran (MW 145,000) and concluded that these beads are good enough for controlled release of the macromolecular substances such as proteins and peptides. [12]. Cohen et al. developed pilocarpine-loaded SA based in situ, forming a gel in the eye without using any external cross-linker, and the pilocarpine released slowly over the period of 24 h [13]. Takka et al. investigated a factorial design on SA-based gels for the controlled release of nicardipine and studied the effect of polymer (SA), cross-linker ($CaCl_2$), and drug/polymer ratio [14]. Kulkarni et al. fabricated glutaraldehyde cross-linked (chemical cross-link) SA beads for controlled release of diclofenac sodium [15]. In addition, they developed the chemically cross-linked SA beads for the controlled release of liquid pesticide (*Azadirachta indica* A. Juss.) for agriculture application [16]. Gåserød et al. developed microcapsules from the SA-chitosan blends using the two-stage procedure method for permeation of hemoglobin and immunoglobulin G [17].

Miyazaki et al. designed orally administered aqueous solutions of SA containing Ca^{2+} ions, which form gelation in the stomach for sustained release of theophylline [18]. In addition, SA-based liquid formulations were used for the controlled release of cimetidine [19]. González-Rodríguez et al. fabricated SA (1.5% w/v)-based microspheres by using aqueous solutions of Ca^{2+} and Al^{3+} (1.3% w/v) along with chitosan solution, these microspheres are used for controlled release of diclofenac by escaping gastric mucosa in the stomach [20]. Xing et al. developed colon-specific drug delivery gel beads using calcium alginate. These are successfully used for entrapment of bee venom peptide and liposome; the same was examined to analyze the entrapped material by γ-scintigraphy technique [21]. Holte et al. prepared tablets from SA (four different grades) by compression method for sustained release of acetylsalicylic acid (water-soluble drug) [22]. Lai et al. prepared sponges from SA and chitosan blends in three ratios (3:1, 1:1, and 1:3) by freeze-drying method for paracetamol release [23].

Kubo et al. formulated aqueous solutions of deacetylated gellan gum (1.0% w/v) or SA with paracetamol for oral sustained drug delivery applications [24]. Lee et al. designed heparin- and chitosan-reinforced SA hydrogel for sustained release of angiogenic growth factor (vascular endothelial growth factor, VEGF), this could act as vessel formation in vivo [25]. Chatchawalsaisin et al. prepared spherical pellets from chitosan and SA alone and in combination by extrusion/spheronization method. The statistical design was used for the controlled release of paracetamol, and drug release behavior was controlled by the diffusion of the polymers [26]. Rousseau et al. developed calcium alginate particles for the release of macromolecule (sodium polystyrene sulfonate). The release of macromolecule from the Ca^{2+} ions affects the particles and molecular weight of SA and the ratio of M/G ratio of SA [27]. Hurteaux et al. fabricated human serum albumin–coated calcium alginate microspheres (~ 60 μm) by transacylation method for microencapsulation of the peptide (lysine-arginine-phenylalanine-lysine) to improve osteointegration [28]. Bučko et al. developed polyelectrolyte complexes from SA (polyanion) and cellulose sulfate-poly(methyle-*co*-guanidine) (polycation). These polyelectrolyte complexes are used as capsules for encapsulation of "*Nocardia tartaricans* bacterial cells with *cis*-epoxysuccinate" [29]. Puttipipatkhachorn et al. prepared calcium alginate beads reinforced with sodium starch glycolate (SSG) and magnesium aluminum silicate (MAS). The molecular interaction of calcium alginate and SSG/MAS was evaluated and correlated with the effect of SSG and MAS on diclofenac drug release studies [30].

Yoo et al. prepared SA microcapsules for microencapsulation of α-tocopherol; the resulted microcapsules were able to release the nutrient at mild alkali conditions [31]. Krishna Rao et al. developed $CaCl_2$ cross-linked blend beads of SA and hydroxyethyl cellulose for controlled release of hydrophilic (diclofenac sodium) and hydrophobic (ibuprofen) drugs. Percentage encapsulation efficiency and drug release from the blend beads were varied with varying ratios of blend composition, $CaCl_2$ concentration, and amount of drug present in the beads. In addition to this, drug release characteristics were analyzed for concentrations profiles of the beads by mathematical modeling using the Fick's diffusion Eq. [32]. Ramesh Babu et al. developed interpenetrating polymer network (IPN)-type microgels from SA-grafted acrylic acid by water-in-oil emulsion method for the controlled release of ibuprofen. Owing to the acrylic acid grafting on to the SA, IPN microgels were able to retain in a low-pH environment for more than 12 h [33]. Sangeetha et al. formulated nanospheres (~ 4519.6 $\pm$ 0.28 nm) from SA polymer and amphotericin-B by a simple gellification technique. SA-encapsulated amphotericin B has shown better antifungal activity when compared with the pristine amphotericin B [34]. Wells et al. fabricated SA microspheres (700 $\pm$ 120 μm) for site-specific long-term drug delivery applications. In this study, SA microspheres are encapsulated with albumin, lysozyme, and chymotrypsin; release of these model proteins is enhanced over 2000 h in 0.15% NaCl solution. However, the release of proteins from SA microspheres is explained by the mechanism that swelling, charge interaction, diffusion, and bulk erosion (hydrolysis) [35].

Sriamornsak et al. prepared microcrystalline cellulose-contained SA pellet formulations by extrusion and spheronization for the controlled release of theophylline. In this study, SA pellets are examined for size, shape, and drug release patterns based on the SA content and type of calcium salts. Approximately, 75%–85% of theophylline is released within 60 min, and release patterns are fitted with Higuchi and Korsmeyer-Peppas model [36]. Ciofani et al. fabricated calcium alginate microspheres (r = 1.12 $\pm$ 0.12 mm), films (r = 2.0 $\pm$ 0.2 mm and a thickness of h = 0.51 $\pm$ 0.12 mm), and fibers (r = 0.43 $\pm$ 0.08 mm and a length of l = 1.5 $\pm$ 0.1 cm) for in vivo evaluation of *Wisteria floribunda* agglutinin in rats [37]. Kim et al. developed SA/poly(vinyl alcohol) blend hydrogels by freeze-thaw method for wound care application. These hydrogels are encapsulated with nitrofurazone, and significant in vitro release, proteins adsorption, and in vivo wound healing (for artificial wounds in rats) characteristics are observed [38].

Taha et al. formulated sodium lauryl sulfate (SLS) and xanthan gum–modified zinc cross-linked SA beads for chlorpheniramine maleate release application. The results indicated that SLS could be able to control the release patterns of the chlorpheniramine maleate; hence these beads are helpful for finely tunable drug release applications [39]. Liu et al. prepared the core-shell type SA microspheres (colloidosome beads) by water-in-sunflower oil method to study the release behavior of brilliant blue (a model drug) [40]. Builders et al. formulated microspheres from mucinated SA by diffusion filling of insulin; these were used for in vitro release of insulin. However, the results indicate that the dissolution time of insulin from SA, mucin, mucinated SA, mucin:SA ratios 1:1, 3:1, and 1:3 is varied from 11.21 $\pm$ 0.75 to 3.3 $\pm$ 0.42 min. In addition, among five formulations, mucinated SA has shown better release characteristics; hence it was suggested as the best oral insulin delivery system [41]. Reddy et al. fabricated pH- and temperature-responsive semi-IPN type microgels by water-in-oil emulsion method from poly(N-isopropyl acrylamide) (PNIPA) and SA for controlled release of the chemotherapeutic agent (5-fluorouracil). Swelling characteristics of semi-IPN microgels were supported by the prolonged drug delivery of 5-fluorouracil due to the presence of PNIPA [42]. Li et al. developed composite type microcapsules (150 nm) of chitosan, SA, and ZnS by water-in-oil-in-water (W/O/W) emulsion method (chemical cross-link) for in vitro release of aspirin. ZnS nanoparticles (NPs) significantly decreased the release rates of aspirin from the microcapsules when compared with the microcapsules without ZnS. In addition, aspirin-release behavior from microcapsules was well fitted with the Higuchi model [43]. Lee et al. developed SA-collagen composite microgels and collagen microgels-inserted SA gels to control and monitor the Glial cell line-derived neurotrophic factor (GDNF) from HEK 293 cells. In this study, the presence of SA in the gels helped to prevent cell leakage and controlled release of GDNF from HEK 293 cells [44]. Chunmei et al. synthesized SA *grafted* poly((2-dimethyl amino)ethyl methacrylate) (SA-g-PDMAEMA) for the fabrication of SA-based hydrogel beads using $CaCl_2$ for controlled release of bovine serum albumin (BSA). The release studies of BSA from SA-g-PDMAEMA gel seem to be a potential protein release system for oral drug delivery applications [45].

11.3 Method of preparation of SA-based matrices (beads, gels, fibers, and in situ gelling formulations)

In general, SA matrices can be prepared by either physical or chemical/covalent cross-linking methods. For physical cross-linking (ionic cross-linking), SA or SA blend solution extruded as droplets using a syringe into bivalent ion (i.e., Ca^{2+}, Ba^{2+}, Sr^{2+}, Pb^{2+}, Cu^{2+}, Co^{2+}, Ni^{2+}, Zn^{2+}, Fe^{2+}, and Mn^{2+}) solution or strong positively charged solution [32, 46, 47]. But the binding capacity of these bivalent metal ions with SA has order that $Mn^{2+} < Zn^{2+}, Ni^{2+}, Co^{2+} < Fe^{2+} < Ca^{2+} < Sr^{2+} < Cd^{2+} < Cu^{2+} < Pb^{2+}$ [48]. In this process, monovalent ions (Na^+) of SA are replaced by the above said bivalent ions; hence gelation occurs through the ion exchange mechanism. However, chemical cross-linking of SA matrices was generally prepared by cross-linking with dialdehydes (i.e., glutaraldehyde, SA aldehyde, etc.) and diamines (i.e., ethylenediamine, dodecyl amine, poly(ethylene glycol)-diamines, poly(allylamine), etc.) by acetal and amide linkage, respectively [33, 42, 49–53]. In addition, SA matrices can be prepared by thermo gelation/in situ gelling method and cell cross-linking. Thermo gelation/in situ gelling can be achieved by adjusting lower critical solution temperature of the SA formulations; for this, SA should be functionally modified or blended with thermoresponsive polymers such as poly(N-isopropyl acrylamide) and poly(ethylene glycol)-co-poly(ε-caprolactone). [42, 54–57]. However, in situ gelation properties of alginate were first reported by M.G. Blaine in 1947 [54]. In the case of cell cross-linked SA gels, SA gels are obtained by simple, specific receptor-ligand interactions; to this, SA is modified with cell adhesion ligands.

Based (> 1 mm in diameter) on the requirement, SA-based gel formulations can be prepared in various sizes such as films/membranes, beads, gels, fibers, and in situ gelling systems [46, 47, 50, 58]. Membranes/films can be prepared by solution casting method using 4%–5% (w/v) [59]. Beads can be prepared by extruding sufficient viscous solution (aqueous) of SA with pipette and needle of syringe [32] (Fig. 11.4). But microbeads or

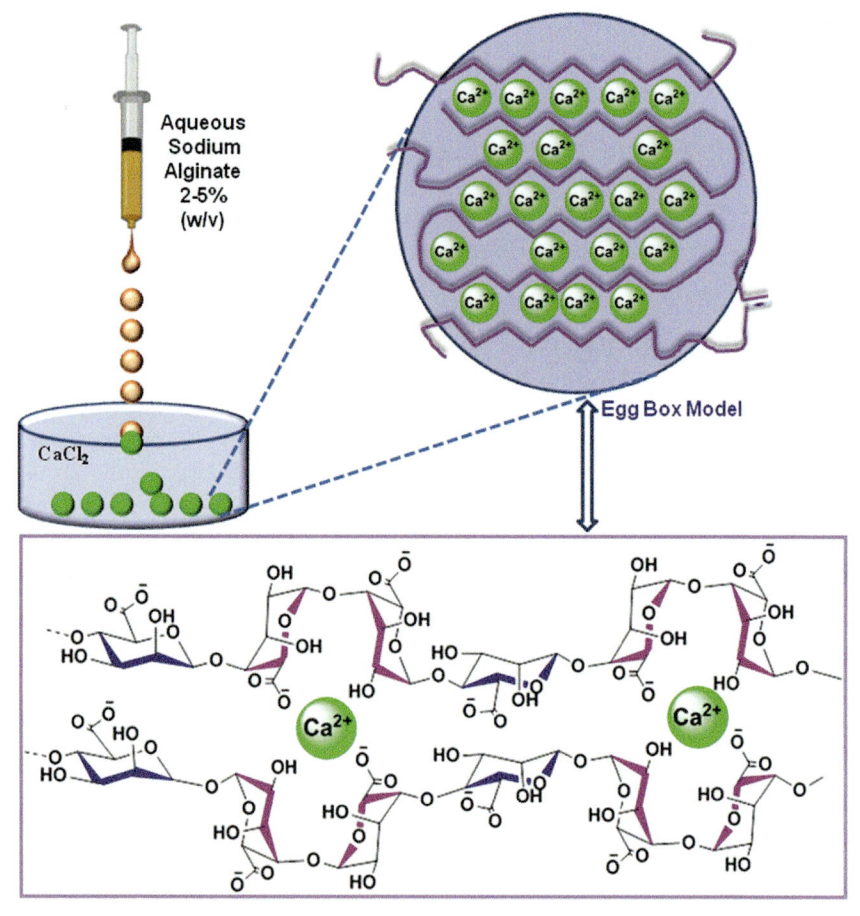

FIG. 11.4 Schematic representation of calcium alginate beads preparation (egg box model) from sodium alginate aqueous solution.

gels (< 0.2 mm in diameter) can be prepared by atomization or spraying method, where the device has small orifice and water in oil emulsification methods [33, 42]. In addition, SA-based NPs are prepared by emulsification using the external gelation method [60, 61]. However, SA-based hydrogels can be prepared by both ionic or covalent cross-linking methods [32, 33, 42, 62–65]; however, here the hydrogel formation, dimension, size, and mechanical properties are entirely dependent on the ratio of copolymer/graft copolymer or blended polymer.

11.4 Recent developments of SA-based hydrogels for drug delivery

The recent development of SA-based hydrogels for various potential applications has been reviewed by various authors [5, 66–81]. However, only drug delivery and tissue engineering fields are emphasised.

Madhusudana Rao et al. [82] prepared semi-IPN hydrogels from natural polymer NaAlg with acryal amide (Am) and DMAEMA and using cross-linker MBA by radical redox polymerization. In this study, in situ generations of silver NPs (AgNPs) by reduction of Ag ions to AgNPs into semi-IPN hydrogel networks were achieved using $NaBH_4$ as a reducing agent. The developed Ag nanocomposite (NC) hydrogel exhibited good antibacterial activity when tested with both gram-positive (*Staphylococcus aureus*) and gram-negative (*Escherichia coli*) bacteria. The developed semi-IPN hydrogels were cytocompatible and biodegradable.

Rama Subba Reddy et al. [65] fabricated NaAlg-based dual responsive Ag NC hydrogels for controlled release of 5-fluorouracil (5-FU) and antimicrobial application. The Ag NC fabrication, drug loading, and drug release at various conditions are shown in a schematic sketch. The fabricated hydrogels and Ag NCs are potential in the enhancement of 5-FU release up to 1400 min; in addition, they are able to inhibit the growth of *E. coli* and *Bacillus* spp. Azhar et al. [83] prepared NaAlg-CS/montmorillonite NC systems for in vitro delivery of 5-FU studied at pH 7.4 buffer medium. Wang et al. [84] developed pH-responsive KGM/NaAlg and KGM/NaAlg/graphene oxide (GO) hydrogels for the cumulative release of 5-FU at pH 1.2 and 6.8 buffers. In this work, the release amount of 5-FU loaded into KGM/NaAlg/GO-3 hydrogels were about 38.02% at pH 1.2 and 84.19% at pH 6.8 after 6 h and 12 h, respectively. Basu et al. [85] synthesized nanosilver composite hydrogel by a free radical polymerization reaction in the presence of NaAlg and Am using *Dolichos biflorus* Linn used as both reducing agent and stabilizing for AgNPs. In this experiment, in vitro drug release studies were performed in pH 7.4 medium, and 60% of drug release was found to be up to 24 h due to the presence of ionizable acidic groups.

Sadeghi et al. synthesized the superabsorbent hydrogel from SA grafted acrylic acid by free radical polymerization for controlled release of BSA. In vitro release of BSA was examined at pH 7.4 and 1.2 at 37°C; the results indicate that electrostatic repulsive forces of carboxylate functionalities helped to release more BSA at pH 7.4 when compared with pH 1.2 [86]. Bhutani et al. synthesized SA/gelatin hydrogels by blending of PEG (2000, 4000, and 6000) using glutaraldehyde as a cross-linker for controlled release of piperine, a hydrophobic drug. The amount of PEG played a crucial role in encapsulation and release of piperine from hydrogels. PEG 4000 showed better encapsulation of drugs and helped burst release at pH 1.2 [87]. Zhang et al. prepared injectable hydrogels from oxidized SA and thiol/hydrazide-modified hyaluronic acid to evaluate drug delivery profiles by using BSA as a model drug. The developed hydrogels are successfully evaluated for gelling time, rheology, morphology, swelling, and degradability studies. The authors concluded that the results of this study help to use these hydrogels for drug delivery, cell encapsulation, TE, and regenerative medicine [88]. Fan et al. synthesized hydrogels from SA and functionally modified GO through an amide linkage. GO was functionalized with adipic acid dihydrazide introduced the amine group. Amine-functionalized GO is covalently conjugated with SA by amide bond formation. These hydrogels are encapsulated with doxorubicin hydrochloride, a chemotherapeutic agent. In vitro DOX release studies were performed in pH 5.0, 6.5, and 7.4 at 37°C; the results demonstrate that 11.6% of DOX was released in 96 h in pH 7.4, and at the same time, 40% was released in pH 5. In addition, these hydrogels were used for in vitro anticancer activity against the Hela cells [89].

Jabeen et al. composed SA-based sol-gel type formulations with cetyltrimethylammonium bromide (CTAB) and butanediyl-1-4-bis(dimethylcetylammonium bromide) (BCTAB) in aqueous media in the presence of K_2CO_3 for controlled release of ibuprofen. BCTAB-based formulations have shown the better release of the ibuprofen from the gel due to the strong hydrophilic and hydrophobic interactions resulting in the formation of the reduced free void spaces [90]. In addition, SA-based pH responsive composite hydrogels were developed with acrylic acid polyethylene oxide and cyclodextrin at various pH solutions. Ibuprofen was successfully loaded into the composite hydrogels with encapsulation capacity range from 45.76% to 54.73%. At higher pH 1.2, a prepared hydrogel is a better one for the encapsulation of drug as well as for the drug release studies [91].

Cong et al. developed mixed matrix-type pH-responsive hydrogels by incorporation of emodin-loaded chitosan-glycerol 2-phosphate disodium micelles in SA hydrogels. The percent of encapsulation efficiency of the drug was 85.26 ± 1.13, with the drug-loading capacity of 0.696 ± 0.037. However, the mixed matrix hydrogels have a better ability to enhance the drug release (~ 9 h) when compared with the pure chitosan micelles (2 h). Hence the developed hydrogel system would be a tunable drug release carrier for colon due to the low release profiles in low pH (1.2) and high release profile at higher pH (7.4) [92] (Fig. 11.5). Lima et al. developed vinylated SA macromonomer-based pH-sensitive hydrogel with N-vinyl-pyrrolidone monomer by simple free radical polymerization method. These hydrogels were used for BSA delivery for that hydrogels are evaluated for cytotoxicity, swelling, and drug delivery studies both in an acidic and basic environment. Cytotoxicity results demonstrate that these hydrogels are cell compatible, and drug release profiles followed pseudo-Fickian mechanism in basic medium and anomalous mechanism in the acidic medium [93]. Rezk et al. synthesized dopamine-grafted alginate (DGA) to develop calcium ion free pH-responsive hydrogel from DGA and bortezomib (BTZ) through conjugation of dopamine (catechol group) and BTZ (boronic acid group). Drug release was performed at pH 5, 6.5, and 7.4 at 37°C; BTZ has released (84%) up to 72 h in low at pH 5, and these results indicate that catechol-conjugated drug delivery systems are pH-dependent [94].

Taleb et al. synthesized NC hydrogels from SA and chitosan with hydroxyapatite (HAP) by ^{60}Co gamma radiation (6 kGy doses with a dose rate of 2.86 Gy/s) for oral drug delivery. The NC hydrogels were encapsulated with doxorubicin (DOX) (for liver cancer), and in-vitro drug release studies were performed at pH 7.4 and 5 at 37°C for 24 h. The DOX released 95% at pH 5 and 60% at pH 7.4; these results follow the Fickian type. The two pH values are selected because DOX drug might be exposed to those pH conditions while moving through the blood liver cancer cells. The higher DOX release at lower pH, and behavior attributed to the fast dissolution of drug released increases results in quick diffusion of the drug concentration within the NC hydrogels [95].

Lin et al. fabricated biocompatible dual (pH and temperature)-responsive hydrogels from SA and poly(N-isopropyl acrylamide) (PNIPA) using EDC/NHC as initiators. These gels are encapsulated with oxytetracycline (OTC); these OTC formulations play a significant role in reduced cytotoxicity against human umbilical vein endothelial cells and potentiality in better antimicrobial activity against E. coli BL21. SA/PNIPA hydrogels are degraded at pH 1.2 during the 156 h, but at pH 7.4, gels are slightly degraded; however, degradation rates of hydrogels are slightly increased with the time. OTC drug release studies demonstrated that to be slow in pH at 1.2 and prolonged release at pH 7.4 at 37°C [96]. Treenate et al. developed polyelectrolyte complex hydrogels from SA and hydroxyethylacryl chitosan by using different bivalent metal ions (Ca^{2+}, Zn^{2+}, and Cu^{2+}) for drug delivery application using paracetamol as a model drug. The developed hydrogel could be able to control the drug release at acidic medium, but maximum drug release was observed at pH 7.4 at 37°C. Among all

11. Alginate-based hydrogels

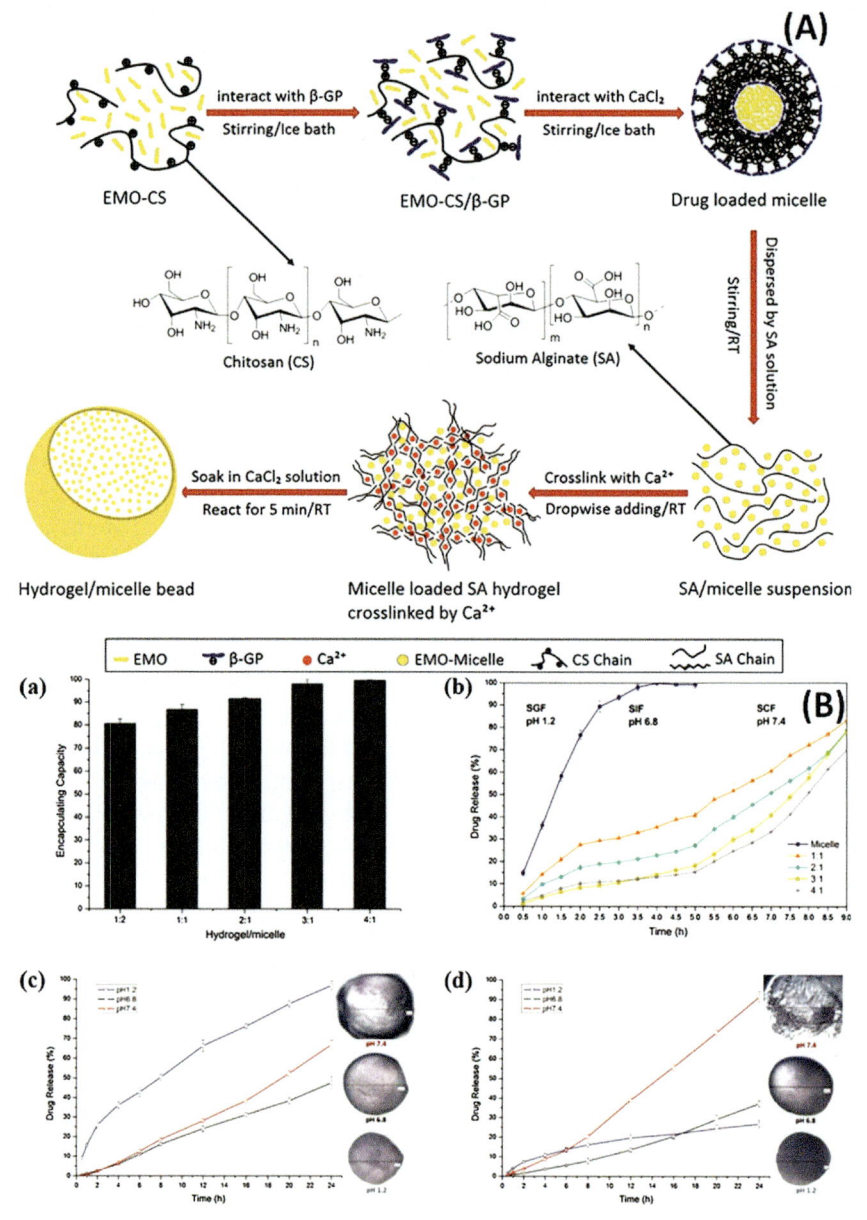

FIG. 11.5 (A) Schematic representation for the preparation of drug loaded micelle and hydrogel/micelle bead. (B) (a) The encapsulating capacity of different hydrogel/micelle systems. (b) In vitro drug release profiles of micelles and different hydrogel/micelle systems (all samples, $P < .05$ in SGF, SIF and SCF). The drug release profiles of (c) hydrogel/micelle = 1:1 and (d) hydrogel/micelle = 3:1 systems in SGF, SIF and SCF individually. Reproduced from Cong Z, Shi Y, Wang Y, Wang Y, Chen N, Xue H. A novel controlled drug delivery system based on alginate hydrogel/chitosan micelle composites. Int J Biol Macromol 2018;107:855–64, Copyright (2018), with permission from Elsevier.

formulations, calcium cross-linked hydrogel (HC75SA25) showed better performance in the drug delivery of paracetamol at the intestine [97].

Wang et al. developed SA composite hydrogels (SA-KG-GO) with the konjac glucomannan/GO for controlled release of 5-fluorouracil, where GO acted as the drug-binding effecter. 5-FU entrapment efficiencies of SA-KG-GO composite hydrogels were between 10.29% and 32.04%. 5-FU release from the SA-KG-GO hydrogels at pH 1.2 was 98% and at pH 6.8100%, which is better compared with that from pure SA hydrogels [84]. Martínez-Gómez et al. prepared pH- and temperature-responsive hydrogels from the blends of SA and polyvinyl alcohol by freeze-thaw method (6, 9, and 10 cycles), a green and low-cost method. The hydrogels were used to encapsulate metformin and studied swelling ratio values in double distilled water. The drug release studies were conducted in various pH conditions at 37°C—pH 1.2, 6.5, and 8.0; the results demonstrate that about 40% drug was released. However, the drug release was increased with higher SA content in the matrix. At pH 1.2, SA/PVA hydrogel showed very low liberation capacities, whereas an increase in pH afforded an increase in the percent of drug release; higher drug release (55%) was obtained after 6 h at pH 8.0 at 37°C (15) [98].

Bahadori et al. developed core-shell type nanogels from $CaCl_2$ cross-linked SA with functionally modified inulin. These nanogels are successfully encapsulated with 5-aminosalicylic acid (ASA), an antiinflammatory drug, by the solution diffusion method. In addition, these nanogels provide high drug-loading capacity, and excellent stability in outer shell can be hydrophobically functionalized with specific functional groups about the location where the drug releases. The drug release studies were conducted in two different pH conditions; drug release assay was conducted for 72 h and different hours measured. The synthesized nanogels showed fast release in the initial 6 h, probably due to burst release of drug absorbed in the nanodrug delivery systems (NDDSs) sore surface [99].

Babu et al. synthesized the dual (pH and temperature) responsiveness of hydrogels (SAPA-NIPA) from SA-g-N-acryloyl-L-phenylalanine and poly(N-isopropyl acrylamide) by using N,N-methylene bis acrylamide as a cross-linker and ammonium persulfate as an initiator through simple free radical polymerization tourniquet. SAPA-NIPA hydrogels were encapsulated with an imatinib mesylate drug with excellent encapsulation efficiency, that is, a maximum of 79%. In-vitro drug release studies were conducted in two different pH conditions: pH 1.2 and pH 7.4 at 37°C and 25°C. The imatinib mesylate–loaded SAPA-NIPA hydrogels have shown higher drug release in pH 7.4 compared with that in pH 1.2. This can be explained that more acidic groups present in the NaAlg-APA backbone of the polymer are more sensitive to the pH changes; at pH 7.4, more COOH functional groups, easily ionizable feature, and repulsion among the carboxylate ion result in the polymer chain drug molecules easily leached from the hydrogel network [100]. Zhao et al. developed SA hydrogels reinforced with cellulose nanocrystals (CNCs) by suspension. Composite hydrogels were cross-linked with $CaCl_2$, and swelling kinetics were analyzed by a power law and Schott's second-order kinetic equation. These SA-CNC hydrogels modulated as "rinsed" and "soaked" to remove the excess of the Ca^{2+} ions were encapsulated with a model drug chloramphenicol; in this study, both rinsed and soaked samples had the highest drug loading. SA-CNC hydrogels exhibited fast drug release initially, followed by sustained release. However, rinsed SA-CNC hydrogels released higher rates of chloramphenicol than soaked hydrogels with the same composition of hydrogels [101].

Silva et al. developed hydrogels from SA and carboxymethyl cellulose (CMC) by cross-linking with bismuth(III) citrate, Bi(III), and calcium chloride for controlled release of furazolidone (FZ). These hydrogels are used to eradicate *Helicobacter pylori* through the synergistic effect of FZ and Bi(III). These hydrogels are successfully encapsulated with FZ and Bi(III), encapsulation efficiencies around 71%–76%, and 88%, respectively. The drug-loaded hydrogels were performed FZ drug release pattern in different pH cumulative drug release at 37°C. The results demonstrate that these hydrogels are more resistant to the degradation in the acidic medium than neutral medium; it observed greater drug release in medium buffer pH 7.4 than compared with that in pH 1.2 [102].

El-Ghaffar et al. synthesized the pH-responsive SA-grafted polyglycidal methacrylate hydrogels (SAPGM) by emulsion free radical polymerization method with $CaCl_2$ for controlled release of riboflavin. Riboflavin encapsulation efficiency SAPGM hydrogels varied in the range of 80%–97.7%. But the SAPGM hydrogels have a better ability to enhance the drug release when compared with the pure SA hydrogels. Hence the developed hydrogel system would be a tunable drug release carrier for colon due to the low release profiles in low pH (1.2) and high release profile at higher pH (7.4) [103].

Chang et al. synthesized pH-responsive hydrogels from SA and starch-*g*-poly(acrylic acid) (SASPC) hydrogels by simple free radical polymerization for controlled release of diclofenac sodium. These gels were synthesized using *N*,*N*-methylene bis acrylamide as cross-linker, and ammonium persulfate as a cross-linker. Diclofenac sodium encapsulation efficiency SAPGM hydrogels were varied in the range of 48%–72.11%. The results demonstrate that SAPGM hydrogels are successful in intestinal tract drug delivery [104]. Min Liu et al. formulated injectable hydrogels form the SA-*g*-poly(*N*-isopropyl acrylamide) by self-assembly method at 37°C for controlled release of doxorubicin hydrochloride. Copolymers were synthesized by the atom transfer radical polymerization (ATRP) to get the narrow size distribution. Three formulations are prepared (Alg-PN

31%–77%, Alg-PN 48%–72%, and Alg-PN 46%–81%) based on the degree of polymerization and %PNIPA present in the copolymer. Only two copolymers formed gels at 37°C and were loaded with drugs to achieve slow and stained drug delivery [105].

Rudhrabatla et al. synthesized the semi-IPN type hydrogels (SAPEGHA) from SA and its copolymers poly(acryloylphenylalanine) and poly(ethylene glycol vinyl ether) poly(hydroxyethyl acrylate) by simple redox polymerization method. SAPEGHA hydrogels were loaded with curcumin, as a model drug, and encapsulation efficiency was achieved in the range of 40%–75%. SAPEGHA hydrogels released high drug content at pH 7.4 compared with that at pH 1.2. The release patterns were followed by non-Fickian diffusion, and curcumin molecules released from the polymer network through both diffusion and relaxation of polymer network [106]. Xie et al. developed pH-sensitive hydrogels (SACMCS) from SA and carboxymethyl chitosan sodium salt blends, which were cross-linked by EDC and hydroxy succinimide. SACMCS hydrogels were loaded with BSA, a model drug; in vitro release studies of BSA were performed in simulated GIT conditions at 37°C. BSA drug released from the hydrogels at pH 1.2 was found to be lower than that released at pH 7.4. In addition, all results, that is, swelling, BSA release, and cytotoxicity studies against the L-929 cells, are influenced by the SA content present in the hydrogels [107].

Gao et al. fabricated functionally rich SA-based potential hydrogels by incorporation of polydopamine particles in dopamine-functionalized SA through self-gelation. In vitro release of gatifloxacin studied from various SA hydrogel formulations, 98% Gatifloxacin released from SA hydrogels, but the release of the drug was extremely fast within 2 h (45%), and 25% was continuously released in the next 22 h [108]. Yun et al. fabricated electro- and pH-responsive hydrogel (SA-GO) from SA with GO; Ca^{2+} used as a cross-linker, and the reaction performed at 48 formed SA-GO hydrogels were centrifugally separated. The prepared SA-GO hydrogels were encapsulated with methotrexate (MTX) in aqueous media. The drug release medium was performed in various pH-responsive conditions. The cumulative release of MTX was higher at pH 7.4 compare with that at pH 6.0; in addition, MTX release was significantly enhanced with the increase of external electrical stimuli [109].

Xie et al. fabricated pH-sensitive hydrogels (SA-PVA) form the blend of SA and PVA by freeze–thaw method; in addition, calcium chloride was used as a cross-linker. These hydrogels are encapsulated with chloramphenicol drug. Loading efficiency and encapsulated into SA/PVA hydrogel network, the investigated drug release medium was in two different pH conditions. The chloramphenicol drug release behavior of SA-PVA hydrogels was maximum at pH 7.4 (intestinal) and minimum at pH 1.2 (gastric). In addition, all results, that is, swelling, chloramphenicol encapsulation, and release studies, are influenced by the freeze-thaw cycles, calcium chloride, and SA content present in the SA-PVA hydrogels [110].

Jahanban et al. fabricated novel bioinspired magnetic hydrogels (Alg-Gel) oxidized alginate and amine groups of gelatine through the Schiff base formation. In addition, Fe_3O_4 NPs were synthesized by in situ method using Alg-Gel hydrogel networks (Alg-Gel/Fe_3O_4) by using the chemical coprecipitation method. The fabricated Alg-Gel/Fe_3O_4 hydrogels were encapsulated with DOX drug, and drug release behavior was studied at various pH conditions. The drug encapsulation efficiency and loading ability of Alg-Gel-DOX hydrogel was 59% and Alg-Gel/Fe_3O_4-DOX hydrogel 47%. The fabricated Alg-Gel-DOX and Alg-Gel/Fe_3O_4-DOX hydrogels samples examined in invitro release studied were pH 4.0 and pH 7.4 (physiological condition) at 37°C. The higher amount of drug released for Alg-Gel-DOX compared with that for Alg-Gel/Fe_3O_4-DOX at similar conditions arises from its higher drug-loading ability. The drug-loaded Alg-Gel/Fe_3O_4 hydrogels exhibit higher drug release medium acidic regions than physiological conditions [111].

Rasool et al. developed biopolymer-based hydrogels from SA and carrageenan with different molecular weights polyethylene glycol (PEG) by using 3-(aminopropyl)triethoxysilane as cross-linker. These hydrogels are used for drug delivery applications by choosing lidocaine as a model drug. The lidocaine-loaded hydrogel samples were examined in phosphate-buffered saline (PBS) solution for in vitro drug delivery studies. The 20.16% drug released from GAP 60 (the sample consisting of PEG-6000) in PBS during the first 2 h. The sustained drug release amount of lidocaine has been released; it became a constant amount right after 6 h. The pH-responsive hydrogels are prominent and illustrated distension around higher release at pH 10 and low swelling behavior in acidic region [112] (Fig. 11.6).

Afshar et al. fabricated composite-type hydrogel with double network from the blends of SA and PVA hydrogels with various mass variations polymer concentration by solvent costing method. The SA/PVA composite hydrogel was embedded with rosuvastatin-loaded chitosan NPs for controlled drug delivery application. In vitro release studies of rosuvastatin from composite hydrogel (3% drug-loaded chitosan NPs) were performed by using a dialysis bag in PBS at 37°C. The cumulative drug release profile of rosuvastatin drug from the fabricated SA-PVA composite hydrogel indicates that 13% rosuvastatin released in the first 4 h and 67% released within the next four 4 h from the composite hydrogel due to drug release rate was higher corresponding to the gradual dissolving of the drug from the surface area of the chitosan NPs. SA-PVA composite hydrogel showed only drug release rate to be slower, only about 20% was released between 8 and 24 h [113].

Singh et al. fabricated biopolymer matrix films by SA and sterculia gum with PVA by radiation-induced polymerization method using the ^{60}Co gamma chamber at 0.49 kGy/h dose. Biopolymer matrix films were

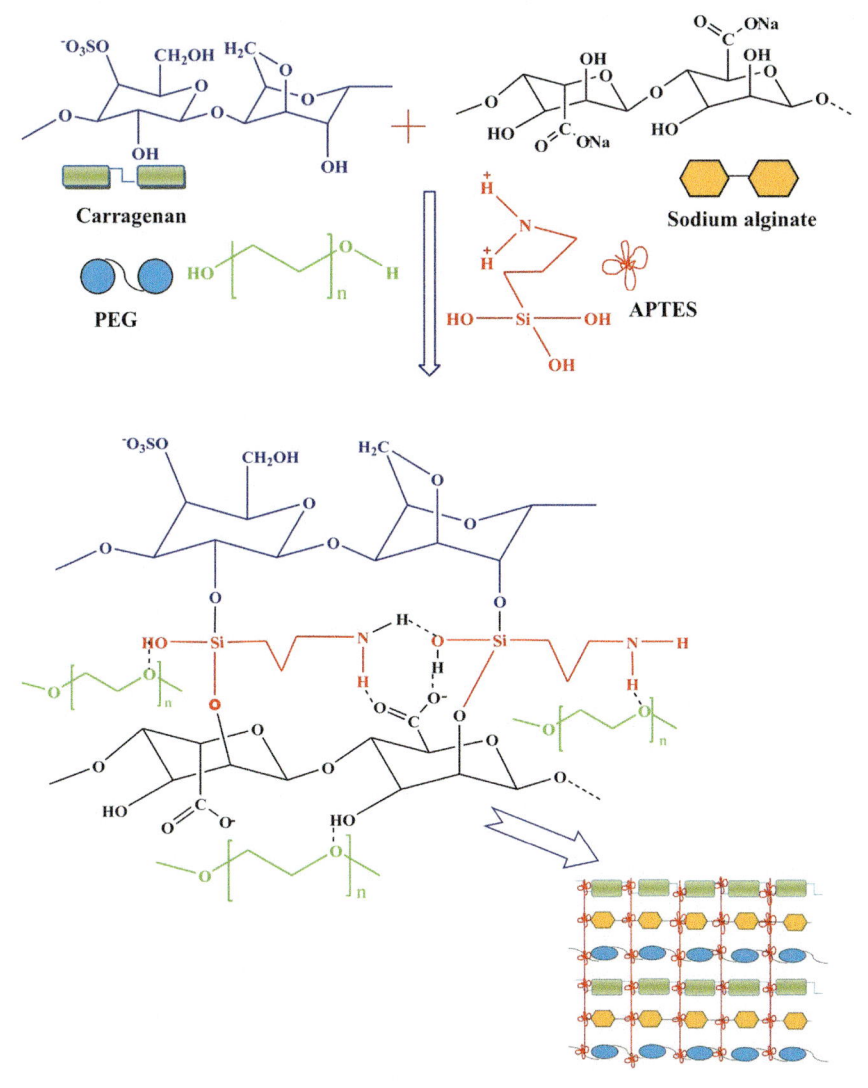

FIG. 11.6 The formation of chemical cross links and proposed physical interactions present in synthesized blend hydrogel. Reproduced from Rasool A, Ata S, Islam A, Rizwan M, Azeem MK, Mehmood A, Khan RU, Mahmood HA. Kinetics and controlled release of lidocaine from novel carrageenan and alginate-based blend hydrogels. Int J Biol Macromol 2020;147:67–78, Copyright (2020), with permission from Elsevier.

loaded (loading capacity 40% ± 0.8%) with the model drug citicoline, a nerve regenerating agent. It exerts beneficial effects in different CNS injury and neurodegenerative diseases in humans. The loaded drug into biopolymer matrix films was released by 40%. The drug diffusion was best fitted in the first-order kinetic model; these kinetic parameters are dependent on the drug concentration within the drug-loaded polymer. However, the drug release of citicoline as a nerve-generating agent from biopolymer matrix films occurred in a slow manner without burst effect and followed Fickian type of mechanism with best-fit first-order kinetic model [114].

11.5 Tissue engineering application of SA hydrogels

According to Langer and Vacanti, TE is "an interdisciplinary field of research that applies the principles of engineering and life science to develop, replace or enhance biological substitutes that restore, enhance or improve the function of tissue" [115]. TE aims to replace diseased/ damaged substances by combining cells with biomimetic materials that provide good patterns to stimulate the growth of new content to revive components, just similar to the natural tissues [115]. In recent decades, many reports have published the potential of biodegradable hydrogels as a basis for TE application to a wide variety of organs such as the liver, heart valve, muscle, skin, eyes, and bone. Besides, the essential characteristics of a comprehensive framework fulfill the following vital requirements in TE: (1) biocompatibility, (2) bioactivity, and (3) biodegradability. The autonomous polymeric biomaterials have their own merits and demerits for the regeneration of the tissue.

Moreover, the biomaterials applied in TE need a mix of various properties such as mechanical properties, cell biocompatibility, biodegradability, histocompatibility, and cell adhesion. These multiple polymers elucidate many properties applied for TE. Numerous strategies have been used to construct tissues, which depend on using a material hydrogel. The hydrogels serves as temporary extracellular matrix (ECM) to support the growth of cells under external stimuli conditions which favor the formation of tissue [116]. Depending on the specific targeted tissue, the fabrication of hydrogel requires specific materials and processing methods. The strength and properties of hydrogels depend on cross-links formed between polymer chains through various chemical bonds and physical interactions. Hydrogels used in TE applications are degradable, can be fabricated under mild conditions, and have excellent mechanical properties as similar to native tissues.

Although many biopolymers have already been used in TE applications, SA is also a well-known biopolymer used in TE because of its excellent biocompatibility, biodegradability, low cost, and simple gelation with various divalent cations. SA can quickly form a hydrogel with Ca^{2+} that can deliver cells and growth factors for TE [5]. Moreover, the use of ionically cross-linked SA hydrogels can be applied at the desired tissue site to integrate with tissue without affecting any toxicity [117].

To date, ionically (Ca^{2+}) cross-linked SA-based hydrogels have been prepared for the transplantation of hepatocytes, islets of Langerhans, and chondrocytes to treat diabetes. Despite the advantages of SA hydrogels, Ca^{2+} cross-linked SA hydrogels may not be ideal because the hydrogels rapidly degrade through the dissolution of Ca^{2+} ions into the medium. Therefore the covalent cross-linking with different cross-linking densities has been used to precisely control the physicochemical properties of SA hydrogels [118]. In addition to that, the molecular weights of many SA are typically above the renal clearance threshold of the kidney. The physicochemical properties of hydrogels (chemistry, surface charge, stiffness, and roughness) can affect the cell phenotype function. In general, the cell adhesion between cells and hydrogels depends on the wettability of hydrogels [119]. Owing to a lack of cellular interactions, the SA can be modified with bioactive molecules to regulate cell behaviors (proliferation, adhesion, migration, and differentiation) [120–122]. Therefore SA has been modified with an RGD peptide (arginine-glycine-aspartic acid) to accelerate the cellular functions, for example, the chondrogenic differentiation of chondrocyte cells [123]. In addition to that, the cell adhesive molecules are also introduced for cell/tissue adhesion for TE applications [124]. In this book, the chapter highlights the SA-based hydrogels with various factors such as mechanical, swelling, morphology, and biodegradation that can regulate the cell functions such as adhesion, cell adhesion, cell proliferation, and cell differentiation for various TE applications.

Diaz-Rodriguez et al. developed mineralized SA hydrogels reinforced with $CaCO_3$ fillers originated from marine-derived farmed mussels (MS) and oysters (OY) [125]. The compression modulus and Young's modulus of SA hydrogels reinforced with MS or OY were significantly improved for different SA-127 and SA-155, whereas the compressive strength of SA hydrogel was decreased for SA-150. The cell culture results confirmed that the osteoblasts cell adhesion and proliferation depend on the SA types. Therefore the cell viability was decreased for SA-150 (M/G 0.51) hydrogels when compared with that for SA-127 (M/G 0.61) hydrogels because of high G content that resulted in high immunogenic by in vivo [126]. As shown in Fig. 11.7 extracellular mineral was deposited on mineralized SA hydrogel seeded with osteoblasts cells for a 5-day incubation period. The results confirmed that the hydrogels reinforced with MS and OY particles (7 mg/mL) could accelerate the ECM mineralization. However, SA 155 hydrogels with OY (7 mg/mL) particles could promote the osteogenic differentiation of hMSCs [125].

Injectable, biodegradable hydrogels can provide the uniform cell distribution to mimic the native ECM. Dhanya et al. reported biocompatible and biodegradable hydrogels with a comparative study of blends of SA/O O-carboxymethyl chitosan (OCMC) (SA/OCMC) and SA/PVA loaded with fibrin NPs and were cross-linked with Ca^{2+} [127]. SA/OCMC hydrogels showed excellent stability than SA/PVA because of more efficient cross-linking

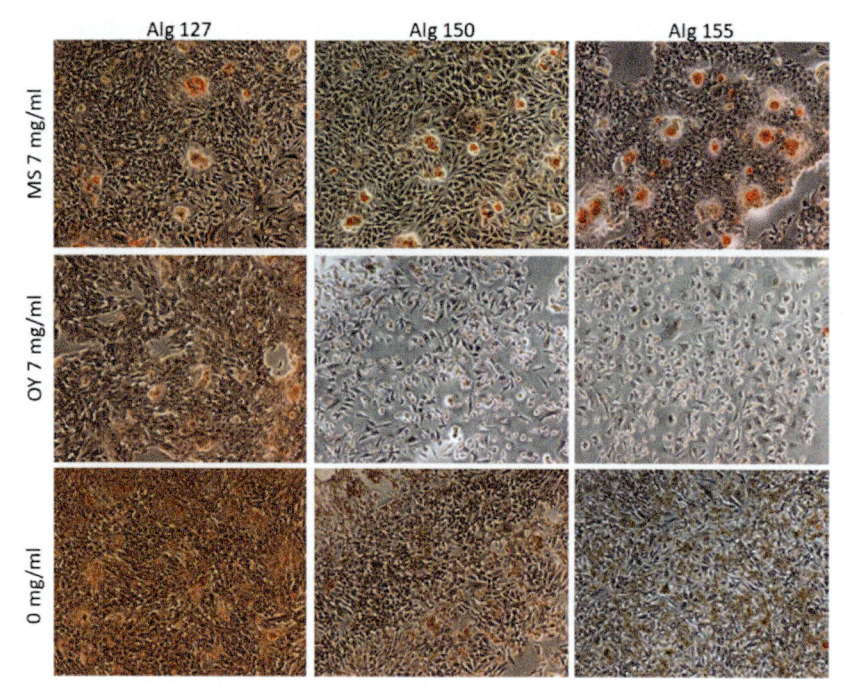

FIG. 11.7 Alizarin red staining of bone ECM mineralization observed after 5 days of os-teoblasts cell culture on SA hydrogels. Reproduced from Díaz-Rodríguez P, Garcia-Triñanes P, López ME, Santoveña A, Landin M. Mineralized alginate hydrogels using marine carbonates for bone tissue engineering applications. Adv Drug Deliv Rev 2018;195:235–42, Copyright (2018), with permission from Elsevier.

of Ca^{2+} with SA/OCMC blend. In addition to stability, the hydrogels maintained viscoelastic nature with elastic modulus is approximately 2 kPa, which is closer to adipose tissue. The in vitro performance of human adipose stem cells (ADSCs) cultured on SA/OCMC hydrogels supported the growth when compared with ADSCs cultured on SA/PVA hydrogels. Moreover, the incorporation of fibrin NPs further improved cell adhesion and proliferation. The results confirmed the fibrin NPs–embedded SA/OCMC injectable hydrogels can have the potential for soft TE applications.

Sarker et al. synthesized SA-gelatin (GT) cross-linked hydrogel (SA-ADA/GT) by covalent cross-linking of SA-di-aldehyde (ADA) and GT [128]. The hydrogels encapsulated with osteoblast-like MG-63 cells showed the highest degree of cell adhesion, spreading, migration, and proliferation, as well as a faster degradation rate than individual polymer hydrogels.

Stress relaxation of viscoelastic hydrogels plays a significant impact on the improving the cell functions (proliferation, spreading, and differentiation). Stress relaxation of hydrogels depends on the cross-linking of polymers [129]. SA shows stress relaxation through cross-linking with the ionic cross-linker. To achieve better stress relaxation of SA-based hydrogels, Sungmin et al. reported simple stress relaxed hydrogels composed of SA-PEG through grafting of PEG-NH$_2$ (amino groups) on to SA (–COOH) using carbodiimide reaction [130]. The hydrogels were prepared by the incorporation of PEG into ionically (Ca^{2+}) cross-linked SA matrix. As shown in Fig. 11.8, SA chains are grafted with different molecular weights of PEG and then cross-linked with Ca^{2+}. The incorporation of higher molecular weight with high concentration of PEG into SA hydrogel resulted in rapid stress relaxation than low molecular weight because PEG acts as steric spacing of the cross-linking zone in hydrogels. RGD-coupled SA-PEG hydrogels show the improved growth of fibroblast cells as well as osteogenic differentiation of mesenchymal stem cells (MSCs). Therefore this approach resulted in tuning stress relaxation in SA hydrogels for 3D cell culture models for TE.

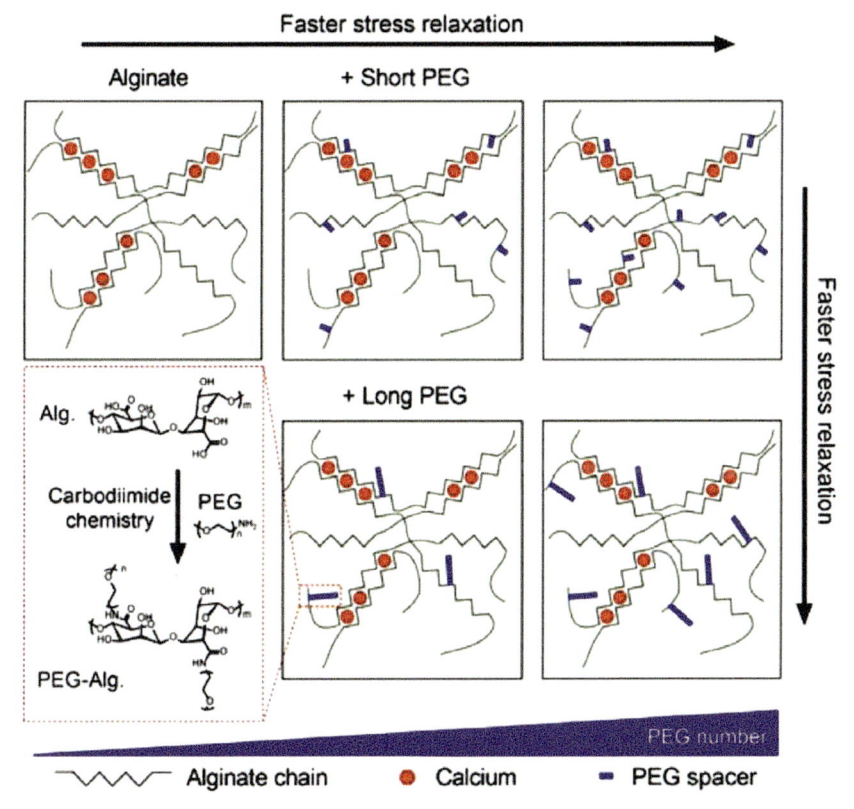

FIG. 11.8 Schematic representation of stress-relaxation of SA-PEG hydrogels with varying molecular weights of PEG. Reproduced from Nam S, Stowers R, Lou J, Xia Y, Chaudhuri O. Varying PEG density to control stress relaxation in alginate-PEG hydrogels for 3D cell culture studies. Biomaterials 2019;200:15–24, Copyright (2019), with permission from Elsevier.

Polyelectrolyte complexation (PEC) of SA with cationic polymers produces mechanically weak hydrogels. For this, Maduru et al. developed hydrogels by the incorporation of PEC into PAM covalent networks. The mixing of SA with cationic biopolymers leads to fast gelation [131]. In this report, the PEC was formed in the PAM hydrogel networks during the polymerization by the addition of GDL (Fig. 11.9). The formation of PEC between SA with CS improved the mechanical performance with controlling porosity. Moreover, the fibrous structures formed in the hydrogels further provide the apatite formation and enhanced hFOB1.19 bone cell functions (growth, biocompatibility, and adhesion). Thus the PEC hydrogels have potential for bone TE.

Recently, NC hydrogels have been used in TE applications because they provide excellent mechanical properties. So far, various nanofillers such as GO, chitin whiskers (CWs), carbon nanotubes (CNTs), and cellulose nanostructures (CNs) have been used in TE [132]. The reinforcement of nanofillers not only improved the mechanical performance of hydrogels but also improve the cell functions. Kumar et al. synthesized cellulose nanocrystals (CNCs) that reinforced PAM/SA/silica glass hybrid hydrogels for bone TE [133]. The incorporation of CNCs (2.5–10.0 wt%) into hydrogels improved the mechanical performance of hydrogels. Owing to the presence of functional groups such as carboxylate (–COO–) and the inorganic phase silanol (Si-OH), the hydrogels produced globular-shaped structures of hydroxyapatite in SBF solutions. The bioactive hydrogels

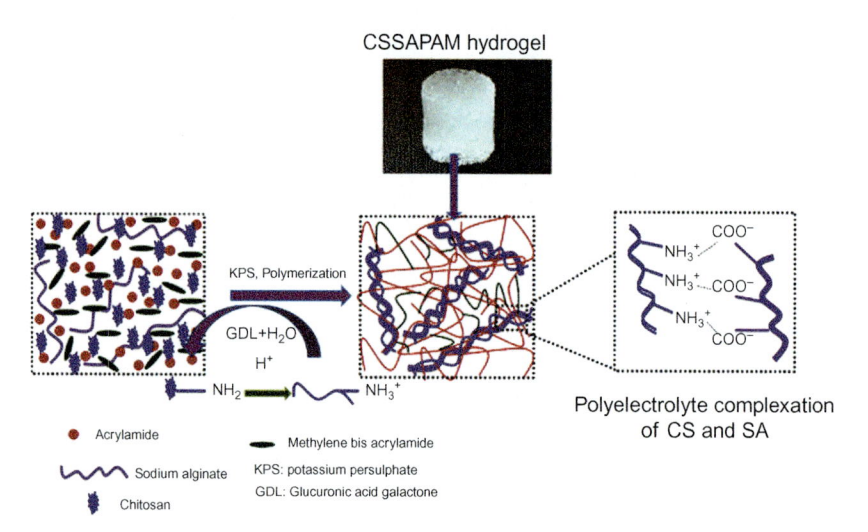

FIG. 11.9   Schematic representation of chemistry of PEC formed in PAM hydrogel networks. Reproduced from Suneetha M, Rao KM, Han SS. Mechanically improved porous hydrogels with polysaccharides via polyelectrolyte complexation for bone tissue engineering. Int J Biol Macromol 2020;144:160–9, Copyright (2020), with permission from Elsevier.

yielded well in in vitro MC3T3-E1 cell adhesion and proliferation onto the hybrid hydrogels. In clinical applications, it is necessary to know how fabrication methods can influence the properties of hydrogels for tissue regeneration. It is well known that cross-linking and sterilization methods can affect the microstructure and mechanical properties of hydrogels. Sabah et al. developed the hydrogels composed of plant-derived cellulose nanostructures (CNs) (fibrils, crystals, and/or blend) and SA cross-linked with Ca^+ [134]. The use of simple cross-linking and sterilization has shown excellent mechanical properties of hydrogels. In general, SA cross-linked with Ca^{2+} had organized and uniform pore size distribution. The incorporation of CNs with various forms into SA resulted in irregular pore distribution and pore connectivity. The swelling capacity and the mechanical properties of the CNs-based hydrogels were also affected by the amount of cross-linker. In addition to the cross-linking of hydrogels, the use of different sterilization methods (physical, thermal, and chemical) showed significant striking decreases in average pore size. At the same time, porosity was maintained in the hydrogels due to the rearrangement of CNs in the hydrogels. The hydrogels have an optimized environment for growth and adhesion of human nasoseptal chondrocytes cells.

Huang et al. developed NC hydrogels based on PEC of SA and CWs with mean length and width of 300 and 20 nm subsequently cross-linked with Ca^{2+} [135]. The mechanical performance of hydrogels significantly improved when compared with that of SA hydrogels. The properties of hydrogels are similar to the structure of native ECM because hydrogels exhibited crystallinity and hierarchical structure incorporation of CWs. The integration of chitin whiskers (CWs) remarkably enhanced the cell proliferation and adhesion of MC3T3-E1 osteoblast cells to the nanocomposite (NC) hydrogels further potentiality in bone tissue engineering (TE).

Marrella et al. developed GO nanosheets incorporated SA-based cell-laden hydrogels for articular TE applications [136]. The incorporation of 2 wt% GO into SA hydrogels show a significant improvement in the mechanical properties with compressive modulus values approximately 300 kPa (six times higher stiffness) than other SA hydrogels. Interestingly, the hydrogel provides a 3D environment for improvement in the viability of fibroblasts cells. The findings of this study are important for the biochemical requirements of hydrogels, in particular TE.

Binata Joddar et al. developed hydrogels from multiwalled carbon nanotubes (MWCNTs; 1–3 mg/mL) reinforced with SA through ionically cross-linked with Ca^{2+} [137]. The strength of the hydrogel depends on the bonding between SA, MWCNT (–COOH functionalization), and Ca^{2+}. The addition of 1 mg/mL of MWCNT (8% of –COOH functionalization)-reinforced SA hydrogel had a high elastic modulus with low mechanical strength. However, the extent –COOH functionalization of MWCNT (> 8%) showed enhanced mechanical strength because the bonding strength has been increased. The hydrogels also maintained porous structures with higher stiffness. The in vitro cell studies of HeLa cells seeded on hydrogels confirmed the formation of cell clusters with ECM protein deposition when compared with SA hydrogel alone. The results provide the fundamental concepts on the development of mechanically improved SA-based hydrogels to be used for TE applications.

Homaeigoha et al. developed SA hydrogels reinforced with graphite nanofilaments (GNFs) functionalized with citric acid (CA) (CAGNFs) for enhancing the mechanical, electrical and biological properties for neural TE [138]. The modification of GNFs with CA is simple for introducing hydrophilic functional groups, which thereby improved the uniform distribution in SA matrix gel. The hydrogels show improved durability, less degradation rate, and conductive properties, which provide the intercellular signaling of neural cell activities. The hydrogels provide the 3D matrix with growth and proliferation of PC12 cells. The in vitro of PC12 cells cultured on hydrogels are biocompatible. The hydrogels are implantable within the body, and results confirmed the no inflammatory and side effects after 14 days of exposure in the body. The electroactive hydrogels have the capability for successful regeneration of nerve tissue.

Conventional cross-linking techniques have disadvantageous for TE due to noninvasive manner. Recently, rapid UV-cross-linking method has been used to solve the problems associated with conventional cross-linking techniques to construct hydrogel networks for TE. From this technique, the cells/bioactive growth factors were mixed with macromere aqueous suspensions. They can be injected into damaged/diseased tissue, followed by rapid cross-linking under the exposure of ultraviolet (UV) light. Moreover, the UV light did not influence the toxic effect on the cells. The viability of cells maintained 80%–90% after exposure to UV light [139]. Lewandowska et al. synthesized photo-cross-linkable hybrid hydrogels composed of SA-methacrylate, GT-methacrylamide, and silica particles [140]. The addition of silica particles (SiO_2-S1: 210 $\pm$ 0.9 nm and SiO_2-S2: 438 $\pm$ 4.8 nm) does not affect the efficiency of photo-cross-linking within the hydrogel networks. The addition of silica particles influenced the hydrogel swelling (> 700%) and mechanical and physicochemical properties. The results confirmed that the hydrogels are stiffer. Furthermore, the XTT assay test confirmed that the incorporation of silica particles did not influence the toxicity for both and osteoblast-like cells, mouse embryonic fibroblasts (MEFs), and MG-63. The MG-63 cells adhered well with flattened morphology on the surfaces of hydrogel networks, whereas osteoblast cells were quite spread in the hydrogels. Owing to the presence of silica particles, the hydrogels show excellent in vitro biomineralization capacity and are suitable candidates for hydrogels in TE.

In TE, the selection of synthetic ECMs could be critical to control the cell-cell interactions for undifferentiated stem cells. Lee et al. developed

SA hydrogels modified with low-density lipoprotein (5(LRP5)) [141]. In this study, 5(LRP5)-SA hydrogels showed the cell-cell interactions through N-cadherin. The in vitro results confirmed that the 5(LRP5)-SA hydrogels induce enhanced chondrogenic differentiation and cell aggregation of D1 stem cells when compared with RGD-SA hydrogels. The improvement of chondrogenic differentiation stem cells (D1) in hydrogels at low densities have the potential for cartilage TE purposes when compared with the cells used for conventional regeneration of cartilage (> 10^7 cells/mL). The engineering of LRP5-SA hydrogels as ECMs can find applications in TE for the treatment of osteochondral defects. Park et al. synthesized hydrogels composed of low-molecular weight hyaluronate (HA) (20,000 g/mol) grafted with SA modified with ethylenediamine as liker through carbodiimide chemistry, followed by cross-linking with Ca^{2+} [142]. The physicochemical properties depend on the weight ratio of SA and HA. The hydrogel stiffness (G′) was significantly increased from 3.2 + 0.7 to 9.1 + 0.7 kPa because weight ratio (SA-g-HA) increased (from 0.1 to 1) in the hydrogels due to increase in viscosity of SA-g-HA. However, the hydrogel stiffness was decreased with increasing the weight ratio from 1 to 2 because of a reduction in carboxylic functional groups in the hydrogels, which reduces the cross-linking density of hydrogels. HA, a main component of ECM glycosaminoglycans, provide interactions with chondrocytes through CD44. Thus the SA-g-HA hydrogels promoted the chondrogenic differentiation of ATDC5 cells than SA hydrogels alone. The optimized hydrogels were considered to be prominent for chondrogenic differentiation due to the high stiffness of hydrogels (weight ratio of SA-g-HA from 0.5 to 1.0). To promote the regulation of phenotype of the chondrogenic potential of chondrocytes, the SA-g-HA was modified with RGD peptide. The RGD modified hydrogels can enhance cartilage regeneration in vivo. Ghosh et al. developed injectable SA-peptide hydrogels for bone TE applications [143]. In this work, self-assembly of fluorenyl methoxycarbonyl diphenylalanine (FmocFF) peptide in SA produced a rigid and injectable hydrogel without using any cross-linker. The hydrogel exhibits thixotropic behavior with nanofibrous structures and a high storage modulus of approximately 10 kPa. The in vitro performance of hydrogel with MC3T3-E1 preosteoblast cells demonstrated good cell viability and adhesion to the hydrogel fibers. In addition to that, the hydrogel promoted osteogenic differentiation and calcium mineralization deposition. Therefore the hydrogel structures mimic the native bone structures and provide 3D environment for bone TE.

Mussel-inspired polydopamine (PDA) hydrogels have attractable considerable interest in TE applications because of self-adhesion to various tissues. Moreover, the PDA can promote cell proliferation and cell adhesion. However, the integration of a single hydrogel with multiple properties remains a challenge. Lee et al. developed bioinspired calcium-free

SA hydrogels using SA conjugated with DA through oxidative cross-linking [144]. The hydrogels had interconnected porous structures with average pore size, which were 37.7 $\pm$ 7.4 and 29.1 $\pm$ 1.9 μ for the 2% and 4% SA-DA, respectively. The hydrogels are completely swellable within 3 days. The hydrogels also showed consistency storage modulus or loss modulus when compared with SA hydrogels cross-linked with Ca^{2+}. The degradation of SA-DA hydrogels did not produce any significant mass loss for 2–4 weeks. The hydrogels are biocompatible toward various cell types (99%–100%), such as hADSC, Neuro-2a, and Huh-7, similar to SA hydrogels cross-linked with Ca^{2+}. Therefore the introduction of catechol moieties can create biological functions of hydrogels with improved therapeutic efficacy for cell transplantation. Although the SA-DA hydrogels have excellent biological performance, they would require toughness and flexibility for TE applications. Bai et al. developed tough and tissue adhesive hydrogels using polyacrylamide (PAM), collagen (CL), and oxidized-SA for wound dressing applications [145]. The oxidized-SA is having aldehyde functional groups interacting with amide ($-CO-NH_2$) of CL and amino ($-NH_2$) of covalently cross-linked PAM, thereby forming double network (DN) to yield toughness and flexibility of hydrogels. Thus the incorporation of oxidized SA into hydrogels significantly improved the mechanical properties. The presence of catechol moieties in the hydrogels promoted the growth and adhesion of L929 fibroblasts in vitro. Furthermore, in vivo study of wound healing results of PAM-COL-COA hydrogel also promoted wound healing. Therefore the presence of catechol moieties with toughness and flexibility of hydrogels have the potential for wound healing applications. In another work, Maduru et al. synthesized mussel-inspired hydrogels based on SA, PAM, and PDA through alkali-induced polymerization and redox polymerization methods [146]. The incorporation of PDA-SA chains in the hydrogel networks influenced their physicochemical properties. The hydrogels showed good elastic property with a compressive stress about 0.24 MPa. The hydrogel are highly swellable and biodegradable. The hydrogels also show good adhesion to various substrates (glass, plastic, skin computer screens, and leaves). Moreover, the adhesive strength of the hydrogel to porcine skin is about 24.5 kPa. The hydrogels significantly enhanced the functional expression of keratinocytes and skin fibroblast cells due to adhesive component of PDA-SA chains. The hydrogels also showed hemostatic properties and have potential for skin TE applications.

Recently, 3D printing has shown promise in TE applications because it can provide a rapid and robust approach to assemble functional tissue in vitro. This technique produces 3D structures and provides a suitable microenvironment for cells to induce the cell proliferation and differentiation toward the functional tissue [147]. There are two types of 3D printing models that have been used in TE. One is 3D scaffolds cultured with specifically targeted cells by in vitro after fabrication. Another one is 3D bioprinting hydrogels where the cells are combined within the bioinks. More recently, 3D bioprinting provides the cell-to-cell interaction, which allows the printed cells to assemble with polymer matrix and enable the growth and functional expression of cells similar to native tissues [148].

Conventional hydrogels composed of SA with other biopolymers are not suitable for TE due to the lack of mechanical properties. Pan et al. manufactured 3D hydrogel scaffolds layer-by-layer deposition of SA and gelatine (GT) polymers using a Bioplotter device [149]. Postprocessing method is used to improve the physicochemical properties such as mechanical properties and pore architectures of 3D hydrogel scaffolds using two cross-linkers such as Ca^{2+} and glutaraldehyde (GA). As shown in Fig. 11.10, fluorescence images of hydrogels visible as fibers were deposited layer by layer using FITC-labeled polymers with the deposition angle 60 degrees (A–D) with different GA ratio and 90 degrees (E) with 0.25% GA at constant Ca^{2+} concentration. The diameter and spacing between fibers are about approximately 500 μm and approximately 300 μm, respectively. The concentration of GA did not influence the structure and shape of 3D hydrogel scaffolds. In general, SA hydrogels alone do not support cell attachment [150]. In this work, the presence of GT improved the cell attachment, growth, and viability of mBMSCs [149]. Based on physicochemical and excellent biocompatibility of hydrogels are the potential for TE applications.

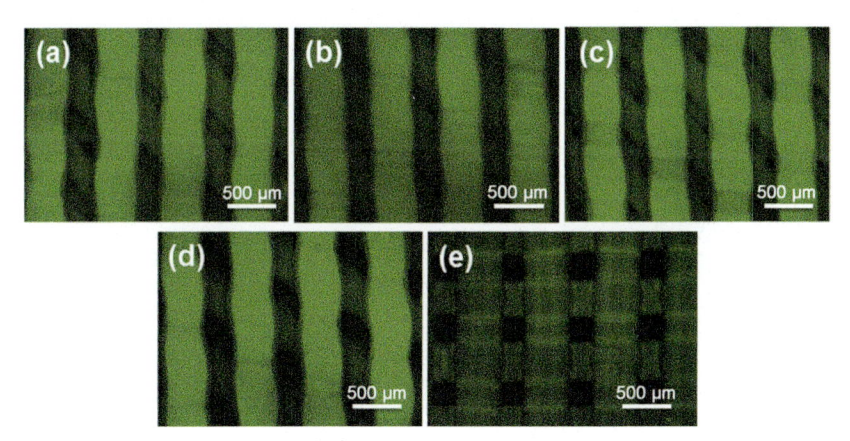

FIG. 11.10 Fluorescent images of wet scaffolds treated with different crosslinking processes: (A) $CaCl_2$; (B) $CaCl_2$ + 0.25% GTA; (C) $CaCl_2$ + 1% GTA; (D) $CaCl_2$ + 2.5% GTA; (E) $CaCl_2$ + 0.25% GTA – 90 degrees. Reproduced from Pan T, Song W, Cao X, Wang Y. 3D bioplotting of gelatin/alginate scaffolds for tissue engineering: influence of crosslinking degree and pore architecture on physicochemical properties. J Mater Sci Technol 2016;32:889–900, Copyright (2016), with permission from Elsevier.

The hydrogels prepared from SA could not provide cell attachment and adhesion because SA-based bioinks are inert hydrogels. The incorporation of other biopolymers such as collagen (CL) contains RGD sequences that can facilitate cell growth, proliferation, and differentiation of cell types [151]. Yang et al. developed 3D printed hydrogels of chondrocytes-incorporated collagen type I (COL) or agarose (AG) mixed with SA as bioink for cartilage TE [152]. As shown in Fig. 11.11A, porous hydrogel scaffolds were printed as six layers (size of 2 × 2 cm) using a 3D bioprinter. The optimal

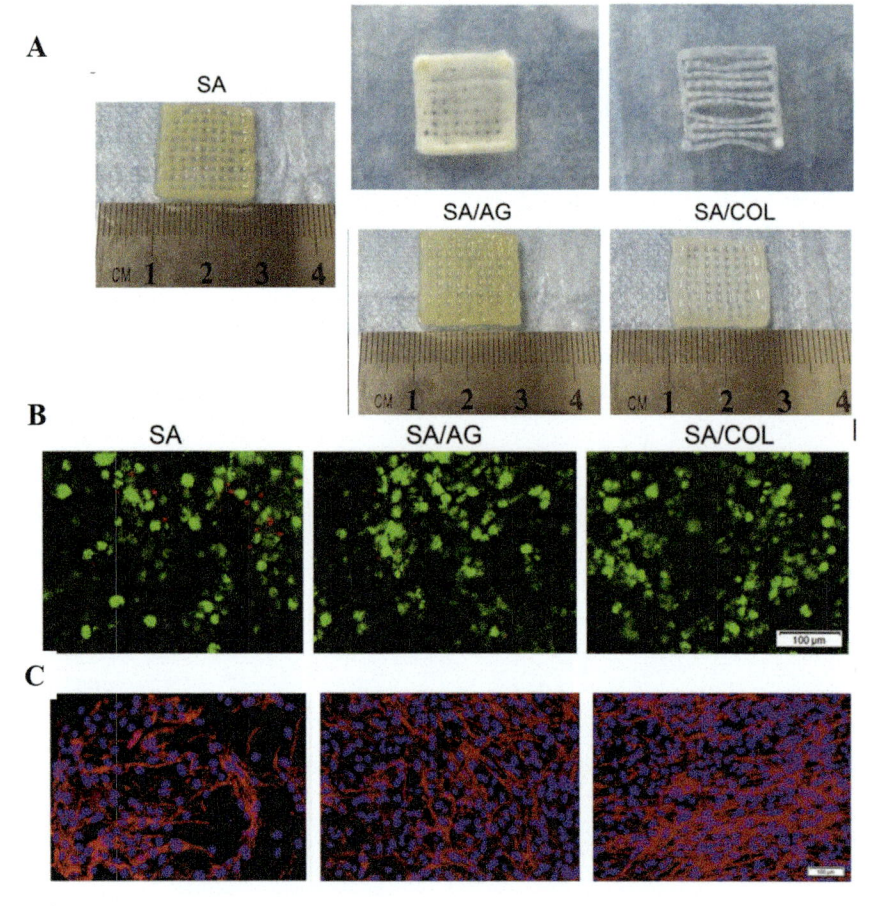

FIG. 11.11   (A) 3D bioprinting of SA/AG (3:1), SA/COL (3:1), SA, SA/AG (4:1), and SA/COL (4:1) hydrogels seeded with chondrocytes, (B) live/dead fluorescence images of chondrocytes cells in the 3D-bioprinted hydrogels, and (C) chondrocytes cell morphology in 3D-printed hydrogels stained with rhodamine-phalloidin/Hoechst. Reproduced from Yang X, Lu Z, Wu H, Li W, Zheng L, Zhao J. Collagen-alginate as bioink for three-dimensional (3D) cell printing based cartilage tissue engineering. Mater Sci Eng C 2018;83:195–201, Copyright (2018), with permission from Elsevier.

blend compositions of SA/COL or SA/AG (3:1 and 4:1) were used for 3D bioprinting. The 3D printed scaffold of SA/AG (4:1) showed reproducible construct based on diameter and distance of pores within 3D hydrogel scaffold. The combination of SA/AG and SA/COL 3D printed hydrogel decreased swelling capacity when compared with SA alone. However, the tensile strength of hydrogels improved with excellent toughness (124.48% and 162.08% for SA/COL and SA/AG, respectively) when compared with SA alone. The live/dead results indicate that the viability of chondrocytes cells that were grown in SA/COL hydrogel scaffold is higher than pristine SA and SA/AG hydrogel scaffolds for 14 days of incubation (Fig. 11.11B). Furthermore, the cytoskeleton morphology confirmed that the intensive polymerized actin filaments of chondrocytes were observed for SA/AG and SA/COL groups than SA hydrogels (Fig. 11.11C). The chondrocyte phenotype was maintained in the 3D hydrogel scaffold (SA/COL) based on cartilage specific genes acceleration, followed by decrease in Col1a1 expression. The results shows the combination of SA/COL 3D bioprinting bioinks have the potential for the application in cartilage TE.

11.6 Conclusion

SA-based hydrogels have demonstrated great potential as versatile materials for many applications. However, they have played significant role in biomedical field, particularly as drug delivery device and TE material. Alginate-based formulations were used for drug delivery in various forms such as gels, injectable gels, beads, microparticle, and NPs. Based on the need, these formulations could be used for drug delivery. In addition, alginate 3D scaffolds were successfully used for TE applications with various combinations of other synthetic and natural polymers. Hence this review will help to understand the medical and pharmaceutical specification of alginate-based biomaterials.

References

[1] Brownlee IA, Allen A, Pearson JP, Dettmar PW, Havler ME, Atherton MR, Onsoyen E. Alginate as a source of dietary fiber. Crit Rev Food Sci Nutr 2005;45:497–510.

[2] Gomez CG, Perez Lambrecht MV, Lozano JE, Rinaudo M, Villar MA. Influence of the extraction-purification conditions on final properties of alginates obtained from brown algae (*Macrocystis pyrifera*). Int J Biol Macromol 2009;44:365–71.

[3] Skjaak-Brae G, Grasdalen H, Larsen B. Monomer sequence and acetylation pattern in some bacterial alginates. Carbohydr Res 1986;154:239–50.

[4] MCC Stanford. Elliptic Curve Cryptography (E.C.C). British Patent 142; 1881.

[5] Lee KY, Mooney DJ. Alginate: properties and biomedical applications. Prog Polym Sci 2012;37(1):106–26.

[6] Miyazaki S, Nakayama A, Oda M, Takada M, Attwood D. Drug release from oral mucosal adhesive tablets of chitosan and sodium alginate. Int J Pharm 1995;118(2):257–63.

[7] Hodsdon AC, Mitchell JR, Davies MC, Melia CD. Structure and behaviour in hydrophilic matrix sustained release dosage forms: the influence of pH on the sustained-release performance and internal gel structure of sodium alginate matrices. J Control Release 1995;33(1):143–52.

[8] Yuk SH, Cho SH, Lee HB. pH-sensitive drug delivery system using O/W emulsion. J Control Release 1995;37(1–2):69–74.

[9] Murata Y, Miyamoto E, Kawashima S. Additive effect of chondroitin sulfate and chitosan on drug release from calcium-induced alginate gel beads. J Control Release 1996;38(2–3):101–8.

[10] Aslani P, Kennedy RA. Studies on diffusion in alginate gels. I. Effect of crosslinking with calcium or zinc ions on diffusion of acetaminophen. J Control Release 1996;42(1):75–82.

[11] Kimura Y, Watanabe K, Okuda H. Effects of soluble sodium alginate on cholesterol excretion and glucose tolerance in rats. J Ethnopharmacol 1996;54(1):47–54.

[12] Kikuchi A, Kawabuchi M, Sugihara M, Sakurai Y, Okano T. Pulsed dextran release from calcium-alginate gel beads. J Control Release 1997;47(1):21–9.

[13] Cohen S, Lobel E, Trevgoda A, Peled Y. A novel in situ-forming ophthalmic drug delivery system from alginates undergoing gelation in the eye. J Control Release 1997;44(2–3):201–8.

[14] Takka S, Ocak ÖH, Acartürk F. Formulation and investigation of nicardipine HCl–alginate gel beads with factorial design-based studies. Eur J Pharm Sci 1998;6(3):241–6.

[15] Kulkarni AR, Soppimath KS, Aminabhavi TM. Controlled release of diclofenac sodium from sodium alginate beads crosslinked with glutaraldehyde. Pharm Acta Helv 1999;74(1):29–36.

[16] Kulkarni AR, Soppimath KS, Aminabhavi TM, Dave AM, Mehta MH. Glutaraldehyde crosslinked sodium alginate beads containing liquid pesticide for soil application. J Control Release 2000;63:97–105.

[17] Gåserød O, Sannes A, Skjåk-Bræk G. Microcapsules of alginate-chitosan. II. A study of capsule stability and permeability. Biomaterials 1999;20(8):773–83.

[18] Miyazaki S, Kubo W, Attwood D. Oral sustained delivery of theophylline using in-situ gelation of sodium alginate. J Control Release 2000;67:275–80.

[19] Miyazaki S, Kawasaki N, Kubo W, Endo K, Attwood D. Comparison of in situ gelling formulations for the oral delivery of cimetidine. Int J Pharm 2001;220:161–8.

[20] González-Rodrıguez ML, Holgado MA, Sanchez-Lafuente C, Rabasco AM, Fini A. Alginate/chitosan particulate systems for sodium diclofenac release. Int J Pharm 2002;232:225–34.

[21] Xing L, Dawei C, Liping X, Rongqing Z. Oral colon-specific drug delivery for bee venom peptide: development of a coated calcium alginate gel beads-entrapped liposome. J Control Release 2003;93(3):293–300.

[22] Holte Ø, Onsøyen E, Myrvold R, Karlsen J. Sustained release of water-soluble drug from directly compressed alginate tablets. Eur J Pharm Sci 2003;20:403–7.

[23] Lai HL, Abu'Khalil A, Craig DQ. The preparation and characterisation of drug-loaded alginate and chitosan sponges. Int J Pharm 2003;251:175–81.

[24] Kubo W, Miyazaki S, Attwood D. Oral sustained delivery of paracetamol from in situ-gelling gellan and sodium alginate formulations. Int J Pharm 2003;258(1–2):55–64.

[25] Lee KW, Yoon JJ, Lee JH, Kim SY, Jung HJ, Kim SJ, Joh JW, Lee HH, Lee DS, Lee SK. Sustained release of vascular endothelial growth factor from calcium-induced alginate hydrogels reinforced by heparin and chitosan. Transplant Proc 2004;36:2464–5.

[26] Chatchawalsaisin J, Podczeck F, Newton JM. The influence of chitosan and sodium alginate and formulation variables on the formation and drug release from pellets prepared by extrusion/spheronisation. Int J Pharm 2004;275:41–60.

[27] Rousseau I, Le Cerf D, Picton L, Argillier JF, Muller G. Entrapment and release of sodium polystyrene sulfonate (SPS) from calcium alginate gel beads. Eur Polym J 2004;40(12):2709–15.

[28] Hurteaux R, Edwards-Lévy F, Laurent-Maquin D, Lévy MC. Coating alginate microspheres with a serum albumin-alginate membrane: application to the encapsulation of a peptide. Eur J Pharm Sci 2005;24:187–97.

[29] Bučko M, Vikartovská A, Lacík I, Kolláriková G, Gemeiner P, Pätoprstý V, Brygin M. Immobilization of a whole-cell epoxide-hydrolyzing biocatalyst in sodium alginate-cellulose sulfate-poly (methylene-co-guanidine) capsules using a controlled encapsulation process. Enzym Microb Technol 2005;36:118–26.

[30] Puttipipatkhachorn S, Pongjanyakul T, Priprem A. Molecular interaction in alginate beads reinforced with sodium starch glycolate or magnesium aluminum silicate, and their physical characteristics. Int J Pharm 2005;293:51–62.

[31] Yoo SH, Song YB, Chang PS, Lee HG. Microencapsulation of α-tocopherol using sodium alginate and its controlled release properties. Int J Biol Macromol 2006;38(1):25–30.

[32] Rao KK, Subha MCS, Naidu BV, Sairam M, Mallikarjuna N, Aminabhavi TM. Controlled release of diclofenac sodium and ibuprofen through beads of sodium alginate and hydroxy ethyl cellulose blends. J Appl Polym Sci 2006;102(6):5708–18.

[33] Ramesh Babu V, Krishna Rao KSV, Sairam M, Naidu BV, Hosamani KM, Aminabhavi TM. pH sensitive interpenetrating network microgels of sodium alginate-acrylic acid for the controlled release of ibuprofen. J Appl Polym Sci 2006;99(5):2671–8.

[34] Sangeetha S, Venkatesh DN, Adhiyaman R, Santhi K, Suresh B. Formulation of sodium alginate nanospheres containing amphotericin B for the treatment of systemic candidiasis. Trop J Pharm Res 2007;6(1):653–9.

[35] Wells LA, Sheardown H. Extended release of high pI proteins from alginate microspheres via a novel encapsulation technique. Eur J Pharm Biopharm 2007;65(3):329–35.

[36] Sriamornsak P, Nunthanid J, Luangtana-Anan M, Weerapol Y, Puttipipatkhachorn S. Alginate-based pellets prepared by extrusion/spheronization: effect of the amount and type of sodium alginate and calcium salts. Eur J Pharm Biopharm 2008;69(1):274–84.

[37] Raffa GV, Pizzorusso T, Menciassi A, Dario P. Characterization of an alginate-based drug delivery system for neurological applications. Med Eng Phys 2008;30(7):848–55.

[38] Kim JO, Park JK, Kim JH, Jin SG, Yong CS, Li DX, Choi JY, Woo JS, Yoo BK, Lyoo WS, Kim JA. Development of polyvinyl alcohol–sodium alginate gel-matrix-based wound dressing system containing nitrofurazone. Int J Pharm 2008;359(1–2):79–86.

[39] Taha MO, Nasser W, Ardakani A, AlKhatib HS. Sodium lauryl sulfate impedes drug release from zinc-crosslinked alginate beads: switching from enteric coating release into biphasic profiles. Int J Pharm 2008;350(1–2):291–300.

[40] Liu H, Wang C, Gao Q, Liu X, Tong Z. Fabrication of novel core-shell hybrid alginate hydrogel beads. Int J Pharm 2008;351(1–2):104–12.

[41] Builders PF, Kunle O, Okpaku LC, Builders MI, Attama AA, Adikwu MU. Preparation and evaluation of mucinated sodium alginate microparticles for oral delivery of insulin. Eur J Pharm Biopharm 2008;70(3):777–83.

[42] Mallikarjuna Reddy K, Ramesh Babu V, Krishna Rao KSV, Subha MCS, Chowdoji Rao K, Sairam M, Aminabhavi TM. Temperature sensitive semi-IPN microspheres from sodium alginate and N-isopropylacrylamide for controlled release of 5-fluorouracil. J Appl Polym Sci 2008;107(5):2820–9.

[43] Li Z, Chen P, Xu X, Ye X, Wang J. Preparation of chitosan–sodium alginate microcapsules containing ZnS nanoparticles and its effect on the drug release. Mater Sci Eng C 2009;7(29):2250–3.

[44] Lee M, Lo AC, Cheung PT, Wong D, Chan BP. Drug carrier systems based on collagen-alginate composite structures for improving the performance of GDNF-secreting HEK293 cells. Biomaterials 2009;30:1214–21.

[45] Gao C, Liu M, Chen S, Jin S, Chen J. Preparation of oxidized sodium alginate-graft-poly((2-dimethylamino) ethyl methacrylate) gel beads and in vitro controlled release behavior of BSA. Int J Pharm 2009;371:16–24.

[46] Crow BB, Nelson KD. Release of bovine serum albumin from a hydrogel-cored biodegradable polymer fiber. Biopolymers 2006;81(6):419–27.

[47] Kuo CK, Ma PX. Ionically crosslinked alginate hydrogels as scaffolds for tissue engineering: Part 1. Structure, gelation rate and mechanical properties. Biomaterials 2001;22(6):511–21.

[48] Mørch ÝA, Donati I, Strand BL, Skjåk-Bræk G. Effect of Ca2 +, Ba2 +, and Sr2 + on alginate microbeads. Biomacromolecules 2006;7(5):1471–80.

[49] Vallée F, Müller C, Durand A, Schimchowitsch S, Dellacherie E, Kelche C, Leonard M. Synthesis and rheological properties of hydrogels based on amphiphilic alginate-amide derivatives. Carbohydr Res 2009;344(2):223–8.

[50] Eiselt P, Lee KY, Mooney DJ. Rigidity of two-component hydrogels prepared from alginate and poly(ethylene glycol)-diamines. Macromolecules 1999;32(17):5561–6.

[51] Lu MZ, Lan HL, Wang FF, Chang SJ, Wang YJ. Cell encapsulation with alginate and α-phenoxycinnamylidene-acetylated poly(allylamine). Biotechnol Bioeng 2000;70(5):479–83.

[52] Hashimoto T, Suzuki Y, Suzuki K, Nakashima T, Tanihara M, Ide C. Review peripheral nerve regeneration using non-tubular alginate gel crosslinked with covalent bonds. J Mater Sci Mater Med 2005;16(6):503–9.

[53] Sanchez-Moran H, Ahmadi A, Vogler B, Roh KH. Oxime cross-linked alginate hydrogels with tunable stress relaxation. Biomacromolecules 2019;20(12):4419–29.

[54] Blaine G. Experimental observations on absorbable alginate products in surgery: gel, film, gauze and foam. Ann Surg 1947;125(1):102.

[55] Reddy NS, Rao KK. Polymeric hydrogels: recent advances in toxic metal ion removal and anticancer drug delivery applications. Int J Adv Chem Sci 2016;4(2):214–34.

[56] Eswaramma S, Rao KK, Zhong Q, Rao KM. Carbohydrate based hydrogels for controlled release of cancer therapeutics. In: Functional Hydrogels in Drug Delivery. CRC Press; 2017. p. 113–53.

[57] Rao KM, Rao KSV, Ha CS. Functional stimuli-responsive polymeric network nanogels as cargo systems for targeted drug delivery and gene delivery in cancer cells. In: Design of Nanostructures for Theranostics Applications. William Andrew Publishing; 2018. p. 243–75.

[58] Lee KY, Bouhadir KH, Mooney DJ. Controlled degradation of hydrogels using multi-functional cross-linking molecules. Biomaterials 2004;25(13):2461–6.

[59] Rao KK, Naidu BV, Subha MCS, Sairam M, Mallikarjuna NN, Aminabahvi TM. Novel carbohydrate polymeric blend membranes in pervaporation dehydration of acetic acid. Carbohydr Polym 2006;66(3):345–51.

[60] De Castro SC, Da Silva de Bastiani FMW, Biagini Lopes L, Ishida K. Alginate nanoparticles as non-toxic delivery system for miltefosine in the treatment of candidiasis and cryptococcosis. Int J Nanomed 2019;14:5187.

[61] Hong JS, Vreeland WN, DePaoli Lacerda SH, Locascio LE, Gaitan M, Raghavan SR. Liposome-templated supramolecular assembly of responsive alginate nanogels. Langmuir 2008;24(8):4092–6.

[62] Rao KM, Rao KK, Sudhakar P, Rao KC, Subha MCS. Synthesis and characterization of biodegradable poly (vinyl caprolactam) grafted on to sodium alginate and its microgels for controlled release studies of an anticancer drug. J Appl Pharm Sci 2013;3(06):061–9.

[63] Sekhar EC, Rao KM, Eswaramma S, Rao KK, Raju RR. Development of sodium alginate/(lignosulfonicacid-g-acrylamide) IPN micro beads for controlled release of an anti-malarial drug. Indian J Adv Chem Sci 2014;4:7.

[64] Reddy CL, Rao KK, Reddy PR, Subha MC. Sodium alginate-g-acrylamide and PEG blend beads: development and controlled release of enalapril maleate. Indian J Adv Chem Sci 2014;2(3):182–9.

[65] Reddy PR, Rao KM, Rao KK, Shchipunov Y, Ha CS. Synthesis of alginate based silver nanocomposite hydrogels for biomedical applications. Macromol Res 2014;22(8):832–42.

[66] Pawar SN, Edgar KJ. Alginate derivatization: a review of chemistry, properties and applications. Biomaterials 2012;33(11):3279–305.

[67] Sosnik A. Alginate particles as platform for drug delivery by the oral route: state-of-the-art. ISRN Pharm 2014;, 926157.

[68] Prajapati BG. Alginate: a natural polymer in wound management. Int J Green Pharm 2007;1(1):5–6.

[69] Madhavan SA. Review on hydrocolloids-agar and alginate. J Pharm Sci Res 2015;7(9):704–7.

[70] Szekalska M, Puciłowska A, Szymańska E, Ciosek P, Winnicka K. Alginate: current use and future perspectives in pharmaceutical and biomedical applications. Int J Polym Sci 2016;, 697031.

[71] Nagarajan A, Shanmugam A, Zackaria A. Mini review on alginate: scope and future perspectives. J Algal Biomass Util 2016;7(1):45–55.

[72] Qin Y, Deng Y, Hao Y, Zhang N, Shang X. Marine bioactive fibers: alginate and chitosan fibers—a critical review. J Text Eng Fash Technol 2017;1(6):228–31.

[73] Ching SH, Bansal N, Bhandari B. Alginate gel particles—a review of production techniques and physical properties. Crit Rev Food Sci Nutr 2017;57(6):1133–52.

[74] Zarif ME. A review of chitosan-alginate-and gelatin-based bio composites for bone tissue engineering. Biomater Tissue Eng Bull 2018;5:97–109.

[75] Nandini VV, Venkatesh KV, Nair KC. Alginate impressions: a practical perspective. J Conserv Dent 2008;11(1):37.

[76] Reshma T, Preetham PN. Alginate impression material—a review. Drug Invent Today 2018;10:3556–61.

[77] De Castro SC, Da Silva de Bastiani FMW, Biagini Lopes L, Ishida K. Alginate nanoparticles as non-toxic delivery system for miltefosine in the treatment of candidiasis and cryptococcosis. Int J Nanomed 2019;14:5187–99.

[78] Chowdhury S, Chowdhury IR, Kabir F, Mazumder MA, Zahir MH, Alhooshani K. Alginate-based biotechnology: a review on the arsenic removal technologies and future possibilities. J Water Supply Res Technol 2019;68(6):369–89.

[79] Rastogi P, Kandasubramanian B. Review of alginate-based hydrogel bioprinting for application in tissue engineering. Biofabrication 2019;11(4):042001.

[80] Liu J, Yang S, Li X, Yan Q, Reaney MJ, Jiang Z. Alginate oligosaccharides: production, biological activities and potential applications. Compr Rev Food Sci Food Saf 2019;18(6):1859–81.

[81] Mărțău GA, Mihai M, Vodnar DC. The use of chitosan, alginate, and pectin in the biomedical and food sector-biocompatibility, bioadhesiveness, and biodegradability. Polymers 2019;11(11):1837.

[82] Madhusudana Rao K, Krishna Rao KSV, Ramanjaneyulu G, Chowdoji Rao K, Subha MCS, Ha CS. Biodegradable sodium alginate-based semi-interpenetrating polymer network hydrogels for antibacterial application. J Biomed Mater Res 2014;102(9):3196–206.

[83] Azhar FF, Olad A. A study on sustained release formulations for oral delivery of 5-fluorouracil based on alginate-chitosan/montmorillonite nanocomposite systems. Appl Caly Sci 2014;101:288–96.

[84] Wang J, Liu C, Shuai Y, Cui X, Nie L. Controlled release of anticancer drug using graphene oxide as a drug-binding effector in konjac glucomannan/sodium alginate hydrogels. Colloids Surf B: Biointerfaces 2014;113:223–9.

[85] Basu S, Samanta HS, Ganguly J. Green synthesis and swelling behavior of agnanocomposite semi-IPN hydrogels & its drug delivery using Dolichos biflorus Linn. Soft Mater 2017;16:7–19.

[86] Sadeghi M, Shafiei F, Esmat Mohammadinasab MJ, Khodabakhshi LM. Crosslinking of graft-co-polymerization alginate with acrylic acid for releasing drugs. Int J Biosci 2014;4(6):185–9.

[87] Bhutani U, Laha A, Mitra K, Majumdar S. Sodium alginate and gelatin hydrogels: viscosity effect on hydrophobic drug release. Mater Lett 2016;164:76–9.

[88] Zhang Y, Li X, Zhong N, Huang Y, He K, Ye X. Injectable in situ dual-crosslinking hyaluronic acid and sodium alginate based hydrogels for drug release. J Biomater Sci Polym Ed 2019;30(12):995–1007.

[89] Fan L, Ge H, Zou S, Xiao Y, Wen H, Li Y, Feng H, Nie M. Sodium alginate conjugated graphene oxide as a new carrier for drug delivery system. Int J Biol Macromol 2016;93:582–90.

[90] Jabeen S, Chat OA, Maswal M, Ashraf U, Rather GM, Dar AA. Hydrogels of sodium alginate in cationic surfactants: surfactant dependent modulation of encapsulation/release toward ibuprofen. Carbohydr Polym 2015;133:144–53.

[91] Jabeen S, Maswal M, Chat OA, Rather GM, Dar AA. Rheological behavior and ibuprofen delivery applications of pH responsive composite alginate hydrogels. Colloids Surf B: Biointerfaces 2016;139:211–8.

[92] Cong Z, Shi Y, Wang Y, Wang Y, Chen N, Xue H. A novel controlled drug delivery system based on alginate hydrogel/chitosan micelle composites. Int J Biol Macromol 2018;107:855–64.

[93] Lima DS, Tenório-Neto ET, Lima-Tenório MK, Guilherme MR, Scariot DB, Nakamura CV, Muniz EC, Rubira AF. pH-responsive alginate-based hydrogels for protein delivery. J Mol Liq 2018;262:29–36.

[94] Rezk Abdelrahman I, Francis O, Ghizlane C, Park CH, Kim CS. Drug release and kinetic models of anticancer drug (BTZ) from a pH-responsive alginate polydopamine hydrogel: towards cancer chemotherapy. Int J Biol Macromol 2019;141:388–400.

[95] Taleb MF, Alkahtani A, Mohamed SK. Radiation synthesis and characterization of sodium alginate/chitosan/hydroxyapatite nanocomposite hydrogels: a drug delivery system for liver cancer. Polym Bull 2015;72(4):725–42.

[96] Lin X, Ma Q, Su J, Wang C, Kankala RK, Zeng M, Lin H, Zhou SF. Dual-responsive alginate hydrogels for controlled release of therapeutics. Molecules 2019;24(11):2089.

[97] Treenate P, Monvisade P. In vitro drug release profiles of pH-sensitive hydroxyethylacryl chitosan/sodium alginate hydrogels using paracetamol as a soluble model drug. Int J Biol Macromol 2017;99:71–8.

[98] Martínez-Gómez F, Guerrero J, Matsuhiro B, Pavez J. In vitro release of metformin hydrochloride from sodium alginate/polyvinyl alcohol hydrogels. Carbohydr Polym 2017;155:182–91.

[99] Bahadori F, Buse SA, Akyıl S, Eroğlu MS. Synthesis and engineering of sodium alginate/inulin core-shell nano-hydrogels for controlled-release oral delivery of 5-ASA. Org Commun 2019;12(3):142.

[100] Jalababu R, Satya Veni S, Suresh Reddy KVN. Synthesis and characterization of dual responsive sodium alginate-g-acryloyl phenylalanine-poly N-isopropyl acrylamide smart hydrogels for the controlled release of anticancer drug. J Drug Deliv Sci Technol 2018;44:190–204.

[101] Zhao J, Li S, Zhao Y, Peng Z. Effects of cellulose nanocrystal polymorphs and initial state of hydrogels on swelling and drug release behavior of alginate-based hydrogels. Polym Bull 2019;1–6.

[102] Silva KM, de Carvalho DÉ, Valente VM, Rubio JC, Faria PE, Silva-Caldeira PP. Concomitant and controlled release of furazolidone and bismuth (III) incorporated in a cross-linked sodium alginate-carboxymethyl cellulose hydrogel. Int J Biol Macromol 2019;126:359–66.

[103] El-Ghaffar MA, Hashem MS, El-Awady MK, Rabie AM. pH-sensitive sodium alginate hydrogels for riboflavin controlled release. Carbohydr Polym 2012;89(2):667–75.

[104] Chang A. pH-sensitive starch-g-poly (acrylic acid)/sodium alginate hydrogels for controlled release of diclofenac sodium. Iran Polym J 2015;24(2):161–9.

[105] Liu M, Song X, Wen Y, Zhu J-L, Li J. Injectable thermoresponsive hydrogel formed by alginate-g-poly (N-isopropylacrylamide) that releases doxorubicin-encapsulated micelles as a smart drug delivery system. ACS Appl Mater Interfaces 2017;41(9):35673–82.

[106] Rudhrabatla VSAP, Jalababu R, Krishna Rao KSV, Suresh Reddy KVN. Fabrication and characterisation of curcumin loaded pH dependent sodium alginate-g-poly (acryloyl phenylalanine)-cl-ethylene glycol vinyl ether-co-hydroxyethyl acrylate hydrogels and their in-vitro, in-vivo and toxicological evaluation studies. J Drug Deliv Sci Technol 2019;51:438–53.

[107] Xie CX, Tian TC, Yu ST, Li L. pH sensitive hydrogel based on carboxymethyl chitosan/sodium alginate and its application for drug delivery. J Appl Polym Sci 2019;136(1):46911.

[108] Gao B, Chen L, Zhao Y, Yan X, Wang X, Zhou C, Shi Y, Xue W. Methods to prepare dopamine/polydopamine modified alginate hydrogels and their special improved properties for drug delivery. Eur Polym J 2019;110:192–201.

[109] Yun Y, Hongwei W, Gao J, Dai W, Linhong D, Ouyang D, Yong K. Facile synthesis of Ca^{2+}-crosslinked sodium alginate/graphene oxide hybrids as electro-and pH-responsive drug carrier. Mater Sci Eng 2020;108:110380.

[110] Xie L, Wei H, Kou L, Ren L, Zhou J. Antibiotic drug release behavior of poly (vinyl alcohol)/sodium alginate hydrogels. Mater Werkst 2020;51:850–5.

[111] Jahanban-Esfahlan R, Derakhshankhah H, Haghshenas B, Massoumi B, Abbasian M, Jaymand M. A bio-inspired magnetic natural hydrogel containing gelatin and alginate as a drug delivery system for cancer chemotherapy. Int J Biol Macromol 2020.

[112] Rasool A, Ata S, Islam A, Rizwan M, Azeem MK, Mehmood A, Khan RU, Mahmood HA. Kinetics and controlled release of lidocaine from novel carrageenan and alginate-based blend hydrogels. Int J Biol Macromol 2020;47:67–78.

[113] Afshar M, Dini G, Vaezifar S, Mehdikhani M, Movahedi B. Preparation and characterization of sodium alginate/polyvinyl alcohol hydrogel containing drug-loaded chitosan nanoparticles as a drug delivery system. J Drug Deliv Sci Technol 2020;56:101530.

[114] Singh B, Kumar A. Synthesis and characterization of alginate and sterculia gum based hydrogel for brain drug delivery applications. Int J Biol Macromol 2020;148:248–57.

[115] Patrick CW, Mikos AG, McIntire LV. Prospectus of tissue engineering. In: Frontiers in tissue engineering. 1st ed. Oxford, UK: Pergamon; 1998. p. 3–11.

[116] Drury JL, David JM. Hydrogels for tissue engineering: scaffold design variables and applications. Biomaterials 2003;24:4337–51.

[117] Nishi C, Nakajima N, Ikada Y. In vitro evaluation of cytotoxicity of diepoxy compounds used for biomaterial modification. J Biomed Mater Res 1995;29(7):829–34.

[118] Lee KY, Jon AR, Petra E, Erick MM, Kamal HB, David JM. Controlling mechanical and swelling properties of alginate hydrogels independently by cross-linker type and cross-linking density. Macromolecules 2000;33(11):4291–4.

[119] Anselme K. Osteoblast adhesion on biomaterials. Biomaterials 2000;21:667–81.

[120] Hill E, Boontheekul T, Mooney DJ. Designing scaffolds to enhance transplanted myoblast survival and migration. Tissue Eng 2006;12(5):1295–304.

[121] Lee KY, Alsberg E, Hsiong S, Comisar W, Linderman J, Ziff R, Mooney D. Nanoscale adhesion ligand organization regulates osteoblast proliferation and differentiation. Nano Lett 2004;4(8):1501–6.

[122] Rowley JA, Mooney DJ. Alginate type and RGD density control myoblast phenotype. J Biomed Mater Res 2002;60(2):217–23.

[123] Park H, Lee KY. Facile control of RGD-alginate/hyaluronate hydrogelformation for cartilage regeneration. Carbohydr Polym 2011;86(3):1107–12.

[124] Yan S, Wang W, Li X, Ren J, Yun W, Zhang K, Yin J. Preparation of mussel-inspired injectable hydrogels based on dual-functionalized alginate with improved adhesive, self-healing, and mechanical properties. J Mater Chem B 2018;6(40):6377–90.

[125] Díaz-Rodríguez P, Garcia-Triñanes P, López ME, Santoveña A, Landin M. Mineralized alginate hydrogels using marine carbonates for bone tissue engineering applications. Carbohydr Polym 2018;195:235–42.

[126] Tam SK, Dusseault J, Bilodeau S, Langlois G, Halle JP, Yahia L. Factors influencing alginate gel biocompatibility. J Biomed Mater Res 2011;98(1):40–52.

[127] Jaikumar D, Sajesh KM, Soumya S, Nimal TR, Chennazhi KP, Shantikumar V, Jayakumar R. Injectable alginate-O-carboxymethyl chitosan/nano fibrin composite hydrogels for adipose tissue engineering. Int J Biol Macromol 2015;74:3318–26.

[128] Sarker JR, Raquel S, Nadine L, Rainer D, Joachim K, Ben F, Aldo RB. Alginate-based hydrogels with improved adhesive properties for cell encapsulation. Int J Biol Macromol 2015;78:72–8.

[129] Chaudhuri O, Gu L, Klumpers D, Darnell M, Bencherif SA, Weaver JC, Huebsch N, Lee H, Lippens E, Duda GN, Mooney DJ. Hydrogels with tunable stress relaxation regulate stem cell fate and activity. Nat Mater 2015;15:326–34.

[130] Nam S, Ryan S, Junzhe L, Yan X, Ovijit C. Varying PEG density to control stress relaxation in alginate-PEG hydrogels for 3D cell culture studies. Biomaterials 2019;200:15–24.

[131] Suneetha M, Rao KM, Han SS. Mechanically improved porous hydrogels with polysaccharides via polyelectrolyte complexation for bone tissue engineering. Int J Biol Macromol 2020;144:160–9.

[132] Gaharwar AK, Nicholas AP, Ali K. Nanocomposite hydrogels for biomedical applications. Biotechnol Bioprocess Eng 2014;111(3):441–53.

[133] Kumar A, Rao KM, Han SS. Synthesis of mechanically stiff and bioactive hybrid hydrogels for bone tissue engineering applications. Chem Eng J 2017;317:119–31.

[134] Al-Sabah A, Stephanie EAB, Irina NS, Zita J, Nafiseh B, Emma B, Iain SW. Structural and mechanical characterization of crosslinked and sterilised nanocellulose-based hydrogels for cartilage tissue engineering. Carbohydr Polym 2019;212:242–51.

[135] Huang Y, Yao M, Zheng X, Liang X, Su X, Zhang Y, Zhang L. Effects of chitin whiskers on physical properties and osteoblast culture of alginate based nanocomposite hydrogels. Biomacromolecules 2015;16(11):3499–507.

[136] Marrella A, Lagazzo A, Barberis F, Catelani T, Quarto R, Scaglione S. Enhanced mechanical performances and bioactivity of cell laden-graphene oxide/alginate hydrogels open new scenario for articular tissue engineering applications. Carbon 2017;115:608–16.

[137] Joddar B, Garcia E, Casas A, Stewart CM. Development of functionalized multi-walled carbon-nanotube-based alginate hydrogels for enabling biomimetic technologies. Sci Rep 2016;6(1):1–12.

[138] Homaeigohar S, Ting-Yu T, Tai-Hong Y, Hsin Ju Y, You-Ren J. An electroactive alginate hydrogel nanocomposite reinforced by functionalized graphite nanofilaments for neural tissue engineering. Carbohydr Polym 2019;224:115112.

[139] Jeon O, Bouhadir KH, Mansour JM, Alsberg E. Photocrosslinked alginate hydrogels with tunable biodegradation rates and mechanical properties. Biomaterials 2009;30(14):2724–34.

[140] Lewandowska ŁJ, Katarzyna M, Mignon A, Sandra Van V, Anna Ł, Maria N. Alginate- and gelatin-based bioactive photocross-linkable hybrid materials for bone tissue engineering. Carbohydr Polym 2017;157:1714–22.

[141] Lee JW, An H, Lee KY. Introduction of N-cadherin-binding motif to alginate hydrogels for controlled stem cell differentiation. Colloids Surf B: Biointerfaces 2017;155:229–37.

[142] Park H, Lee HJ, An H, Lee KY. Alginate hydrogels modified with low molecular weight hyaluronate for cartilage regeneration. Carbohydr Polym 2017;162:100–7.

[143] Ghosh M, Halperin SM, Grinberg I, Adler AL. Injectable alginate-peptide composite hydrogel as a scaffold for bone tissue regeneration. Nanomaterials 2019;9(4):497.

[144] Lee C, Shin J, Lee JS, Byun E, Ryu JH, Um SH, Cho SW. Bioinspired, calcium-free alginate hydrogels with tunable physical and mechanical properties and improved biocompatibility. Biomacromolecules 2013;14(6):2004–13.

[145] Bai Z, Dan W, Yu G, Wang Y, Chen Y, Huang Y, Dan N. Tough and tissue-adhesive polyacrylamide/collagen hydrogel with dopamine-grafted oxidized sodium alginate as crosslinker for cutaneous wound healing. RSC Adv 2019;8(73):42123–32.

[146] Suneetha M, Rao KM, Han SS. Mussel-inspired cell/tissue-adhesive, hemostatic hydrogels for tissue engineering applications. ACS Omega 2019;4(7):12647–56.

[147] Jammalamadaka U, Tappa K. Recent advances in biomaterials for 3D printing and tissue engineering. J Funct Biomater 2018;9(1):22.

[148] Faramarzi N, Yazdi IK, Nabavinia M, Gemma A, Fanelli A, Caizzone A, Ptaszek LM, Sinha I, Khademhosseini A, Ruskin JN, Tamayol A. Patient-specific bioinks for 3D bioprinting of tissue engineering scaffolds. Adv Healthc Mater 2018;7(11):1701347.

[149] Pan T, Wenjing S, Xiaodong C, Yingjun W. 3D bioplotting of gelatin/alginate scaffolds for tissue engineering: influence of crosslinking degree and pore architecture on physicochemical properties. J Mater Sci Technol 2016;32(9):889–900.

[150] Lorenzo M, De Wijn JR, Van Blitterswijk CA. 3D fiber-deposited scaffolds for tissue engineering: influence of pores geometry and architecture on dynamic mechanical properties. Biomaterials 2006;27(7):74–985.

[151] Xiao L, Ding M, Saadoon O, Vess E, Fernandez A, Zhao P, et al. A novel culture platform for fast proliferation of human annulus fibrosus cells. Cell Tissue Res 2017;367:339–50.

[152] Yang X, Lu Z, Wu H, Li W, Zheng LZJ. Collagen-alginate as bioink for three-dimensional (3D) cell printing based cartilage tissue engineering. Mater Sci Eng 2018;83:195–201.

12

Alginate-based nanocomposite hydrogels

G. Karthigadevi[a], Carlin Geor Malar[b],
Nibedita Dey[c], K. Sathish Kumar[d],
Maria Sarah Roseline[c], and V. Subalakshmi[c]

[a]Department of Biotechnology, Sri Venkateswara College of Engineering, Sriperumbudur, Tamilnadu, India, [b]Department of Biotechnology, Rajalakshmi Engineering College, Chennai, Tamilnadu, India, [c]Department of Biotechnology, Saveetha School of Engineering, Saveetha Institute of Medical and Technical Sciences (SIMATS), Chennai, Tamilnadu, India, [d]Department of Chemical Engineering, Sri Sivasubramaniya Nadar College of Engineering, Chennai, Tamilnadu, India

12.1 Introduction

Hydrogels are the cross-linked network of hydrophilic polymers that are capable of forming three-dimensional (3D) structures by the absorption of water. In general, nanocomposite hydrogels are produced by the interaction of nanomaterials with the polymer matrix, provided at least one phase is in the nanoscale dimension. Based on the type of the nanomaterial incorporated in the synthesis of nanocomposite hydrogel, the significant improvement in the optical, thermal, catalytic, and mechanical properties, as well as some novel properties, can be unveiled [1]. At present, various types of nanomaterials are established for this purpose such as carbonaceous nanomaterials, including graphene and graphene oxide (GO), and metal oxide nanoparticles such as magnetite, gold, and silver oxide nanoparticles for enhancing the properties [2]. In addition, the nanomaterials experience ease of processing when combined with the biopolymers [3].

The metal-based nanocomposite hydrogels are widely used in clinical applications, such as in the treatment of burns and wounds, and as antimicrobial agents due to the comprehensive properties of higher surface area and potential activity of the metal oxides. One of the drawbacks of using the metal oxide nanoparticles is the agglomeration due to the dipole-dipole interactions and high surface energy, which are found to be greater in the presence of electrolytes and by the in situ synthesis. To mitigate such agglomerations, the addition of surface ligands to cross-link with the polymeric matrix is highly suggested. It is prevalent to include such cross-links with the polymers because there is increment in the strength of the nanocomposite [4] because of the retention of smaller-sized particles.

Alginate, a class of natural anionic polysaccharide, is an encouraging biomaterial that is known to possess remarkable hydrophilicity, biodegradability, nontoxicity, and biocompatibility [5]. It also consists of interpenetrating hydrophilic polymer chains that accumulate huge water or the biological fluids, leading the materials to swell. This swelling ability empowers them to be used as an effective carrier [6, 7] because they can be administered in a minimally invasive manner. The biocompatibility, low cost, swelling property, and loading capacity qualify alginate as a perfect choice for wound dressings, tissue engineering, and drug delivery [8–10]. Apart from being used as a drug delivery carrier, alginate can also be used in immobilization as an encapsulation matrix through chemical modification [11].

This chapter discusses on the alginate nanocomposite hydrogels with a brief description on their properties and various types of preparation. The applications of alginate nanocomposite hydrogels in drug delivery, such as oral, transdermal, ocular, and nasal, and tissue engineering, such as bone, cartilage, neural, skin, and liver, are detailed. Various challenges and prospects for the effective utilization of alginate nanocomposite hydrogels are also discussed.

12.1.1 Overview on alginate nanocomposite hydrogels

Alginate, one of the most widely used polymers, is known to be obtained from seaweed. The cross-linking property of alginates enables them to be used as an effective gelling agent. The presence of various divalent cations, such as Ca^{2+} and Mg^{2+}, supports the ionic binding through the carboxylate groups of the gluconate groups. The physical properties of the alginate hydrogels can be optimized by the covalent attachment and the oxidization. Fig. 12.1 shows the various types of alginate nanocomposite hydrogel.

12.1.1.1 Structure of alginate nanocomposite hydrogels

Chemically, alginate is known to be composed of α-D-mannuronic acid and β-L-guluronic acid, as shown in Fig. 12.2. It is an effective natural linear polysaccharide and is highly soluble in water. In structure, it is the homogenous or the alternating heterogeneous arrangement of its monomeric units. Based on the number of guluronic acid residues present and

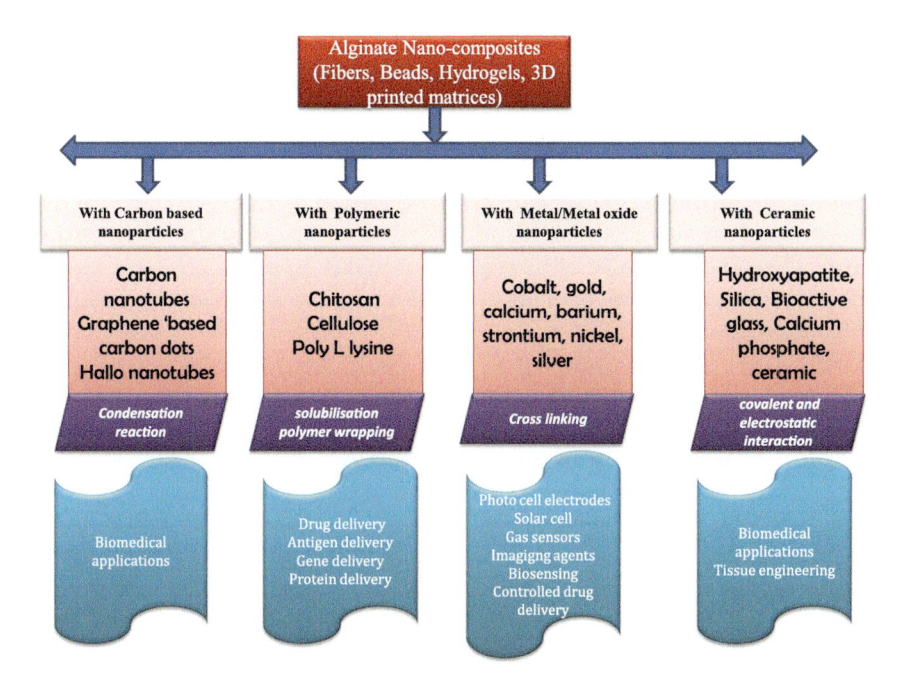

FIG. 12.1 Classification of alginate nanocomposites.

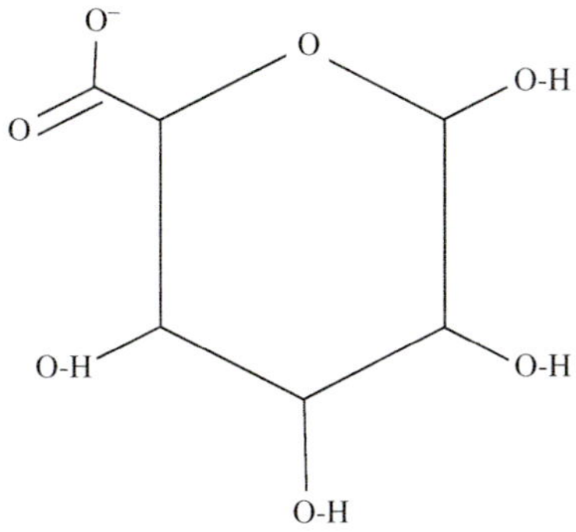

FIG. 12.2 Structure of alginate.

the molecular weight of the alginate, gelation process can result in either stronger or weaker gels. Greater hydrophilicity and solubility to form stable solution can be evidenced in the alginate salts than the alginic acids. At the same time, alginate precipitates out at much lower pH (less than 3).

Ionic cross-linking or covalent cross-linking of the polymer chains can be involved in the formation of hydrogels of alginate [12]. In the presence of divalent metal ions, alginate undergoes a rapid gelation.

The alginate nanocomposite hydrogels are formed by mixing the nanoparticles onto the preformed alginate gels [13, 14] as well as by the in situ reduction of the metallic precursors preloaded into the gel [15, 16]. The structure of the alginate nanocomposite hydrogels is extremely based on the type of the nanomaterials used as well the reaction conditions of the synthesis process. The structure can also vary by the presence of the surface ligands tailored for the improvement of the properties [17]. The structure of binding of divalent calcium ions by alginate through oxygen atoms on L-guluronate chains and interchain junction formation could be described by the egg-box model [18].

12.1.2 Properties of alginate nanocomposite hydrogels

Hydrogels are known to possess various properties that can be influenced and modified by many factors. The method of synthesis is one of the most important influencing factors and is highly responsible in determining the nanoparticle size and its interactions. Table 12.1 summarizes the influence of various properties of the alginate nanocomposite hydrogel.

12.1.2.1 Swelling property

Hydrogels acquire the swelling property by the ability of alginate to absorb water. In addition, the swelling behavior of the nanocomposite hydrogel in water relapses the toughness of the gel mechanically at a considerable level. The uncontrollable swelling of the hydrogel can cause deformation when the imbalance is caused between elastic and osmotic energies in the network [21]. The ratio of the nanoparticle to the alginate is very crucial in determining the degree of swelling, hysteresis of swelling, maintenance of the shape, and in retaining the mechanical property. Lower swelling ratio would provide better and stable mechanical properties. In addition, the swelling nature of the hydrogel is extensively pH dependent, and the swelling ratio would vary under both acidic and alkaline conditions. It is shown that the nanocomposite hydrogels with high swelling ratio at higher pH have better pH tolerance. The overswelling of

TABLE 12.1 Nanomaterials and its properties for tissue engineering applications.

Nanomaterial	Property	Impact	References
Graphene oxide	Swelling ability	Decreased	[19]
Graphene oxide	Mechanical property	Increased	[19]
Graphene oxide	Adsorption capacity	Increased	[19]
Silver nanoparticles	Rheological property	Increased	[18]
Dendrimers	Reactivity	Increased	[20]

the hydrogel can increase the sinking rate in the liquid. A well-known fact is the limited stability of the alginate-based materials and their ability to swell in the monovalent solutions [22].

Recently, the swelling behavior of the alginate hydrogel was shown to be suppressed when it was made to interact with the nanoparticles due to the formation of double networks and increased cross-linkages during the formation [19]. Hydrogen bonds can also be responsible in increasing the swelling resistance by restriction of the mobility of alginate [23].

12.1.2.2 Mechanical properties

To estimate the mechanical properties of the hydrogel, the stress-strain profiles and the Young's modulus should be studied at various concentrations of the nanomaterials. Increased nanomaterial concentration would exhibit higher Young's modulus that would directly relate the enhanced mechanical properties [4, 24]. Improved mechanical strength of the hydrogel is not only characterized by the concentrations of nanomaterials but also by the amount of cross-linker added to tailor the surface design of the gel. Therefore rigid hydrogels with better mechanical properties can be achieved by the addition of any cross-linking agents. The surface functionalization properties of nanomaterials would exploit the nature of material and its interaction with drugs will lead to alteration in their mechanical properties of the wholesome hydrogel.

12.1.2.3 Biocompatibility

It is very important to have insight knowledge on the toxic behavior of the nanocomposite hydrogel when it is used as a drug delivery carrier. The toxic behavior can be discharged either by the nanoparticles tethered to the hydrogel or by the changing environmental conditions in the release system. However, the conjugation of the nanoparticles to the hydrogel is ought to reduce the toxicity as well as improve the drug release [25]. At times, hydrogels exhibit immunoresponse that can be purely attributed to the impurities in alginates.

12.1.2.4 Adsorption properties

Higher concentrations of nanomaterials are shown to express greater adsorption capacities, enabling the application of hydrogels to be used as an efficient adsorbent of heavy metals. Among other similar adsorbents such as alginate beads [26], alginate clay [27], collagen/cellulose beads [28], activated carbon [29], and magnetite alginate beads, the alginate nanocomposite hydrogels possess relatively higher adsorption ability. The adsorption rate of the hydrogel is based on the temperature because temperature influences its electrostatic attraction, which is lower for anions and higher for cations of the heavy metals.

12.2 Preparation methods of alginate nanocomposite hydrogel

During the past decades, alginate nanocomposites have gained considerable attention in drug delivery research because of its improved mechanical and thermal properties. Nanocomposites are prepared by incorporation of various types of nanoparticles (clays, metallic nanoparticles, and CNTs) into any kind of matrix such as polymer, metal, and ceramics materials that resulted in the formation of 3D hydrogels (Table 12.2). Several methods have been reported in the literature for the formulation

TABLE 12.2   Various methods for the formulation of alginate nanocomposites.

Sl. no.	Alginate composites	Type of synthesis	Drug delivery applications	References
1	GO/PAM/sodium alginate ternary composite hydrogel	Microfluidic method	Artificial muscles	[45]
2	Sodium alginate composite hydrogel with bioactive hardystonite	**Dual ion cross-linking**	**Wound healing**	[46]
	Alginate/CaCO₃ nanocomposite	Microfluidic technology	**Wound healing**	[47]
3	Gelatin/alginate-blended nanogel	Freeze-drying	Bone marrow regeneration	[48]
4.	Silver-incorporated alginate nanocomposite	In situ gelling	Antibacterial applications	[49]
5	Alginate/carboxymethyl chitosan/ZnO-based nanocomposite	Direct precipitation method	Gastrointestinal disorders	[50]
6	Alginate hydrogel/chitosan micelle composite	Cross-linking method	Stimulant for digestion	[51]
7	Zinc oxide-incorporated alginate nanocomposites	Encapsulation	Antimicrobial and wound healing	[52]
8	Gold nanowire-incorporated alginate hydrogels	Cross-linking and lyophilization	Myocardial regeneration	[53]
9	ZnO-loaded sodium alginate-gum acacia nanohydrogels	Chemical cross-linking	Wound healing	[54]
10	Alginate/hydroxyapatite (SA/HA) nanocomposite beads	In situ generation and sol-gel method	Painkiller drug delivery	[55]
11	PEI—alginate nanocomposite	Ionotrophic gelation	Gene delivery	[56]

of nanocomposite hydrogels using physical and chemical methodologies [30]. Earlier, the nanocomposite synthesis has been performed by self-assembly of interactive polymers or through covalent cross-linking methods. Currently, nanocomposite structures have been fabricated using various techniques for drug delivery applications. The properties of the materials have been improved by modulation mechanisms that eliminate the risks that occur in the conventional strategies. Alginate-based polymeric hydrogels have been integrated with different nanostructures to tailor their properties for various applications. Normally, these hydrogels are hydrophilic, and the incorporation of nanomaterials resulted in unique structures with improved functionalities.

12.2.1 Ionic gelation methods

The reaction of polyelectrolytes to interact in presence of counter-ions to form the nanoparticles is the basic mechanism behind the ionic gelation process [31], as shown in Fig. 12.3. From the research reports, it is observed that alginates have shown better degradation profiles with a high clearance rate from the system when it is used in low molecular weight for

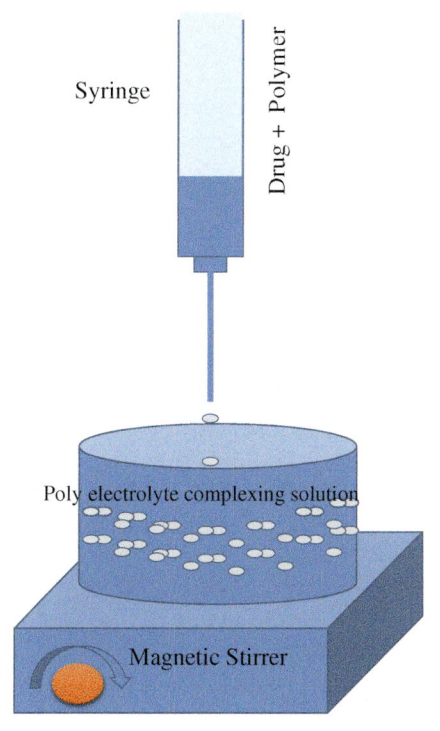

FIG. 12.3   Alginate nanocomposite synthesis using ionic gelation method.

the synthesis [32]. Ionic cross-linking methods are normally used for the preparation of alginate hydrogels, but they have limitations in the loading of drugs due to their poor mechanical strength. By increasing the gluronate ratio, the strength of the gels can be increased through ionic gelation method. Owing to their high biodegradability, there is a high possibility of forming scaffold-like structures, which are mainly used for tissue engineering applications [33].

12.2.2 Cross-linking methods

This is a physical/chemical method that involves the use of various cross-linking agents to create bonds between two components. Polymeric hydrogels are obtained by cross-linking between their hydrophilic and hydrophobic side chains that occur because of hydrogen bonding or electrostatic interactions. The incorporation of nanoparticles inside the polymer hydrogel matrix during the cross-linking process results in the formation of nanocomposite hydrogels with high tensile strength [33, 34]. The most commonly used cross-linking agents for the preparation of hydrogels are glutaraldehyde and epichlorohydrin. Treatment of hepatocellular carcinoma was performed with the help of alginate/chitosan/ hydroxyapatite nanocomposite hydrogel synthesized using gamma radiations as a cross-linking agent used for the oral delivery of the anticancer drug, doxorubicin, which was studied by Gamboa et al. [35]. Controlled gellification and sustained drug delivery were performed through these techniques, and the resulting nanocomposites were highly stable due to the intra-intermolecular cross-linking ability of calcium ions.

12.2.3 Spray drying

Spray drying techniques is an alternative technique to ionic gelation mainly used to stiffen the partially cross-linked hydrogels that are applied to deliver the thermosensitive compounds [36]. Recently, electrodynamic methods such as electrospinning and electrospraying techniques were used to fabricate fibrous scaffolds that exhibited good potential in the proliferation of cells. Alginate–chitosan fibers incorporated with nanoparticles resulted in the formation of multifunctional nanocomposites that help in the proliferation of preosteoblast cells [36, 37]. Silk fibroin has been mixed with the alginate for the preparation of nanofibrous scaffolds using thermally induced phase separation techniques that are used for a variety of tissue engineering applications [38]. This technology uses multicomponent systems for the preparation of size-controlled ultrafine powders, as depicted in Fig. 12.4. But the cost of scale-up is high, which is the major drawback of this technology. The blending of alginate with chitosan improves the mechanical

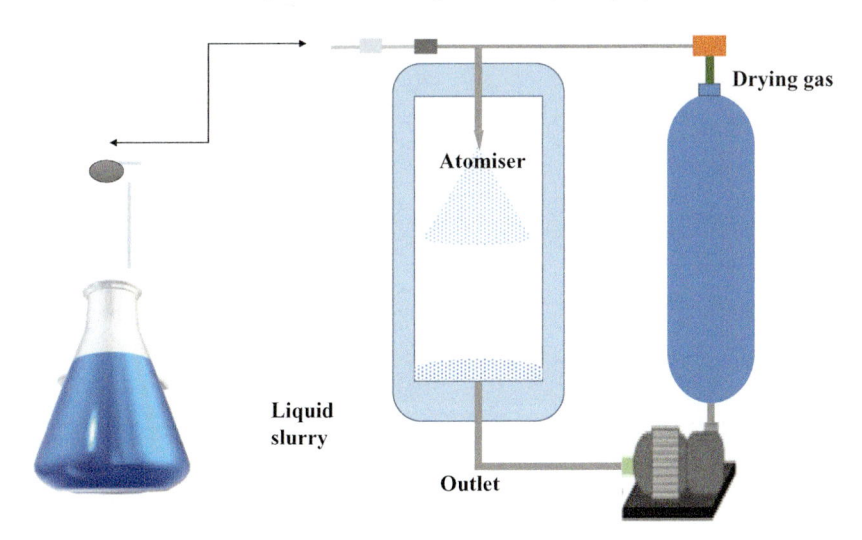

FIG. 12.4 Alginate nanocomposite synthesis using spray drying.

properties of nanocomposites, which are conducted using spray drying procedures, showed higher encapsulation capacity of prednisolone [39]. This technique works in conjunction with freeze-drying results in the formation of nanocomposite hydrogels with high mechanical strength but with minimal swelling capacity. Nanocomposite scaffold with controlled swelling ability prepared with chitosan, alginate, and silica using freeze-drying method has been successfully used for bone tissue engineering applications [40].

12.2.4 Microfluidic-aided polyelectrolyte complexation

Microfluidic technologies offer the advantage of controlling the size and polydispersity of nanoparticles by optimizing the physical and chemical parameters. In a recent study, the alginate hydrogels to respond to the external magnetic field by incorporating the magnetic nanoparticles was understood using the microfluidic device (Fig. 12.5). This technology helps to control the size of the nanoparticles, which aims to avoid the hydrogel deformation during the diffusion and delivery of drugs [41]. Single- and double-layer hydrogel fibers prepared using alginate-methacrylated gelatin composites were used to encapsulate various types of cells within the fibers, and the medium was pumped through microfluidic chips. Cell-laden microfibers promoted the proliferation of cells within the fibers showed good adhesion and proliferation. Microfluidic spinning technology used to synthesize alginate nanofibers that are used as scaffolds for the regeneration of various

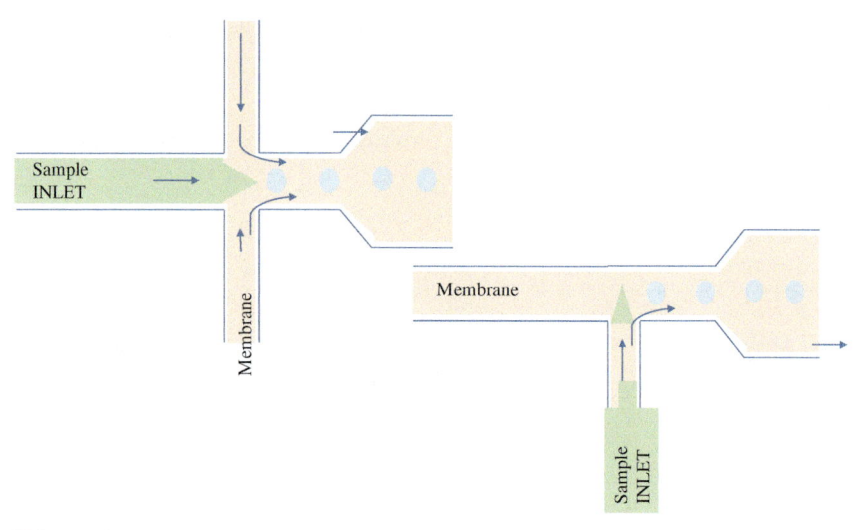

FIG. 12.5   Alginate nanocomposite synthesis using microfluidic technologies.

types of cells includes nerve cells, muscle cells, and fibroblastic cells [42]. Microfluidics, along with MEMS, enables the synthesis of alginate nanohydrogels of various morphologies with controlled size, which act as relevant platforms for 3D cell cultures [43].

12.2.5 Molecular imprinting

Polymeric nanocomposites prepared by using molecular imprinting technologies act as excellent drug delivery agents because of their unique characteristic features such as high stability, excellent drug loading capacity, and resistance to harsh conditions. This involves the reaction of the analyte with specific binding sites complementary to the template molecule in presence of a cross-linking agent. Molecularly imprinted alginate polymers are used as drug delivery carriers for vancomycin antibiotics in the treatment of wounds [44].

12.3 Application of alginate nanocomposite hydrogel in drug delivery

The main objective of the drug delivery method is to maintain the therapeutic levels of the drug in the blood circulation throughout the treatment period. Several researchers focused on various mechanisms to improve the patterns of drug delivery as well as to reduce the undesirable side effects. This involves the use of certain strategies to modify the formulation methods so that the release rate can be designed either sustained or site specific according to the type of disorders, with the advantages of biocompatibility and biodegradability. The design of the fabrication method is an essential step to achieve an efficient drug delivery system. Owing to its anionic nature, it can be able to interact with cationic molecules, so it is used for designing cationic drug delivery systems [57]. Various reports on synthesis procedures have incredibly increased in the recent decade with the improvement of physical, chemical, and biological parameters of alginate nanogels.

12.3.1 Oral drug delivery

The oral administration of drugs is the most convenient method for the treatment of various diseases. But the oral dosages faces difficulties in absorption due to the enzymatic attacks in the human system resulted in poor bioavailability. Modification strategies increase the surface area of alginate so that the intercalation of drugs deep inside the structures. When medication is administered directly, there are many hindrances because the blood supply to these regions is very limited. The degradation is also rapid, and the required dosage is also larger. Apart from these factors, there are immunological and inflammatory responses that might damage and irritate nearby nontarget cells. Controlled delivery has been opted for these regions only through specialized technologies called nanotechnology.

Nanoformulations would provide the required carriers for optimal dosage and better mechanical stability and stealth effect from the immune responses. Some very special modifiers have been used in tissue engineering as mechanical stimulations and functional system for biomolecules under the name BDS. These render great help in the regeneration process. The whole environment around the tissue to be repaired consists of numerous molecules that generate signals with an intention to initiate repair. These signals are considered while designing scaffolds in tissue engineering. The use of nanocarriers for targeted and controlled release is found to be very meritorious in overcoming delivery problems in bone and cartilage tissues [58].

These BDS have the main topic of research in the recent years because scientists all around the world focus on improvizing the hydrogel materials in combination with mesenchymal stem cells to use as a dual scaffold cum drug delivery carrier. When hydrogel is placed at target site, the drug would release under controlled circumstances. Once released, these drugs or compounds would guide the tissues toward ideal chondrogenic morphology and achieve required traits and properties. Hence BDS is a specialized platform of the hydrogel smart material community that not only can withstand external tension but also helps in regeneration of cartilage tissues by delivering many essential biomolecules and active agents. Compared with conventional methods, BDS appear to have an additional feature of providing the required stimuli and support needed by the cartilage tissue to rejuvenate [59]. They imprint the active biomolecules with great efficiency. When made up of natural polymers, these hydrogels have shown many noteworthy results. Montmorillonite-alginate nanocomposite incorporated with carboplatin, an antineoplastic drug inside, showed excellent dissolution of drugs with lower dose levels [60].

Encapsulation of protein drug inside the chitosan-alginate nanocomposites is designed as oral vaccines for the treatment of schistosomiasis, a neglected parasitic disease. Such encapsulation strategies keep nanocomposite structures remain unaltered; furthermore, they minimize the rapid release of drugs and slow their degradation in the intestinal fluids [61]. The release mechanisms can be controlled by optimizing the concentrations of alginate, chitosan, and calcium chloride using regression analysis methods. The prepared alginate nanocomposite is effectively used for the sustained release of metronidazole drug for a prolonged period [62].

12.3.2 Nasal drug delivery

Recently, stimuli-responsive hydrogels have been developed as a nasal drug delivery system, which is effective in the delivery of drugs from nose to brain without crossing the systemic circulation. Normally, the nanoparticle-mediated drug delivery is interrupted by mucociliary clearance, alginate nanocomposites effectively delivered the venlafaxine drug to the brain either intracellularly or using extracellularly. There are some limitations in following this drug delivery technique due to the chances of drug absorption in the nasal regions [63]. Mucoadhesive hydrogels act as an attractive alternative that possesses higher residence time with efficient drug absorption over days. Nasal administration of nanocomposite hydrogels was highly effective when compared with the intraperitoneal route that was observed in mice when treated with recombinant NcPDI. The intranasal application was found to protect the mice for a higher period against the infections of *Neospora cannium* tachyzoites [64].

Chitosan nanocomposites coated with alginate have been used for the intranasal delivery of hepatitis B surface antigen (HBsAg). The alginate coatings enhance the release of antigen from the chitosan, and they also protect the antigen from enzymatic degradation [65]. Alginate lipid nanogels have been accepted as potential system for the release of corticosteroid through nasal route. The studies indicated that these nanogels prolong the action of drug on the polyps beyond the nasal valve, with optimum permeation at higher residence time [66].

12.3.3 Parenteral delivery

This type of drug delivery suitable for the targeted drug delivery approaches even with lower doses of drugs. The patients who are unable to uptake medicines orally can be given through subcutaneous, intramuscular, intravenous, and intraarterial routes to the specific organs of the body. Alginate nanopowders are efficiently used as inhaling formulations for the treatment of respiratory infections with higher aerosolization efficiencies [67].

12.3.4 Ocular drug delivery

Alginate nanohydrogel systems were designed as carriers of vaccine formulations against the scorpion venoms. This study was conducted using rabbit models, and it was found that the drug encapsulated inside nanohydrogels showed high immunoprotection against scorpion envenomation [68]. Ocular delivery of daptomycin drug against bacterial endophthalmitis was studied using alginate nanocomposites. The mucoadhesive properties of the nanohydrogel systems showed enhanced permeability of the drug release, which was confirmed using epithelial cell models [69].

12.4 Application of alginate nanocomposite hydrogel in tissue engineering

The use of interdisciplinary studies in all fields is of great demand nowadays. The use of these variety of courses in the field of life sciences have brought into light many unique and remarkable features of rejuvenating tissues and body organs [70]. Hydrogels, as we see in this chapter, have many traits of smart materials of tissue engineering. They have been used in biomedical and health-care industry to compensate the functionality for real tissues. They have similar resemblance to live cells and provide support for the nearby cells to thrive well and proliferate. The tunability of these hydrogels gives the scientists to tailor the functional features of this smart material into any desired parameter of choice.

Some specific areas of the body are highly compatible to hydrogel association. These sections are the bone, vascular, dermal area, cornea of the eye, meniscus area, tendon, and various other soft tissues of the body. If an area of the body has instances of lost tissue function, hydrogel has been reported to be an ideal choice for providing support as a scaffold for the nearby cells [71]. Owing to their hydrated matrix, they can control the cellular function and development in their polymer networks. This is the fundamental behind the use of hydrogel for tissue engineering. Synthetic form of hydrogels is found to be biologically degradable, biocompatible, and similar to the natural tissue environment. Therefore they are used in tissue engineering as advanced constructs to be used as a template for target cell adhesion, binding, proliferation, and differentiation. The traditionally synthesized alginate hydrogels harbor some drawbacks in their overall structure and function. When a traditional alginate hydrogel is compared with the nanocomposite form of the same, there is a massive difference in the properties of the finished scaffold (Fig. 12.6).

The mechanical features are enhanced as the bonding is increased. Hence nanocomposites of alginate hydrogels are more preferred for tissue engineering than their former counterpart [72]. The traditional alginate hydrogels have weaker interactions compared with the nanoparticle conjugated ones; hence the hydrogel easily loosens up under different environmental and body conditions. The change in pH, concentration of the ions, and temperature have a major role on the structural integrity of the hydrogel [73].

When cross-linked alginate hydrogels are fabricated, their bonds are permanent, but the strength of the scaffold is seen to be not up to the mark. They scum easily to bends, stretches, and compresses. This might be because of shorter and irregular cross-links in the native hydrogel [74]. When unreacted cross-links from the ordinary alginate hydrogel are not conjugated with suitable conjugants, not only the features and trait of the final product go down but also the compatibility of the body becomes an issue, so the alginate nanocomposites are used for the improvement of physicochemical and biological requirements to develop native 3D biomaterials to achieve proper cell diffusion and tissue formation. In the case of tissue engineering, conventional autografting techniques are used in tissue and organ culture based on the availability of tissue donors.

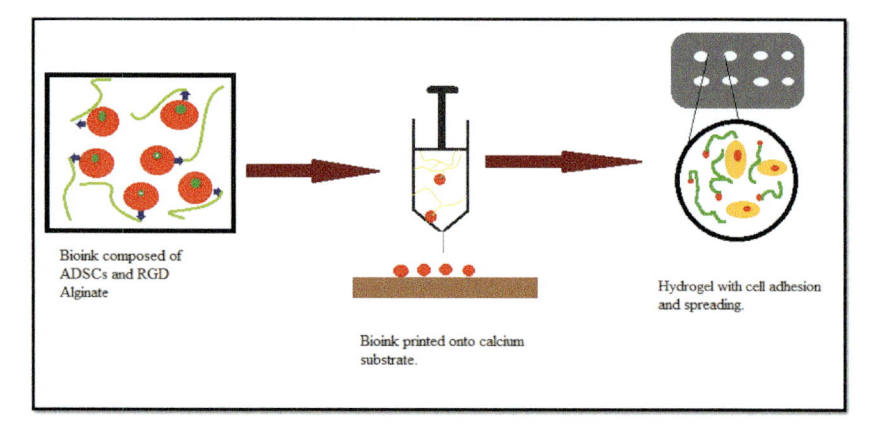

FIG. 12.6　Alginate nanohydrogels as injectable scaffolds.

It has faced complications with the morbidity of the donors, which created risks to the patients. It has been overcome by the onset of regenerative medicine principles that act as a promising alternative to organ transplant techniques.

12.4.1 Bone tissue engineering

A typical hydrogel material would have many special molecules such as growth factors and supporting cell bodies. They have an affinity for osteogenic growth and angiogenic proliferation. Hence they are found to be the go-to material to researchers associated with long bone deformities. As bone by itself is a self-healing tissue that is vascular in nature, when used along with hydrogel as scaffold, they work wonders. The support provided by this material will aid the cell to grow better in dimension and feature. This is the essential requirement for any bone healing procedure. Cartilages also have been cultured and grown well in laboratories using this material. The high water retention quality of hydrogel scaffolds has made this growth of cartilages possible in many laboratories. Compared with bone, cartilage has restricted self-healing ability. When used along with hydrogels, the repairing mechanism was escalated in these tissues.

The positive traits that make hydrogel so suitable for cartilage engineering is the support it provides mechanically, the swelling ability due to water retention, and the smooth lubricating activity. All these properties are similar to the native articular cartilage and its extracellular matrix (ECM). So the repairing action is favored well for the scaffolded cells. When opted in association with stem cells, the differentiation of the cells is increased. The essential proteins and growth factors present in them are responsible for the proper encapsulation and growth of the stem cells. Many forms of hydrogels have been tested as scaffolds for tissue engineering till date, but the most favored form among all the researchers is the injectable form of the same. They have shown great potential in 3D scaffolding techniques. Their porous back bone with high aqua retention and resemblance to the native extra cellular matrix make the bone and cartilage tissues to transplant and proliferate well without any significant invasion into the nearby cells [75].

They also have an additional ability to rectify and form of irregular deformities in the bone and cartilage tissues.

When it comes to skeletal engineering, nanocomposites form of hydrogel have been used for fabricating scaffolds for tissue engineering many bone, cartilage, and muscle cells. In the section of artificial bone development, nanoconjugate alginate hydrogel has been of great aid in addressing issues such as trauma caused by congenital defects, infections, and local damage [76, 77]. Combinations of nano-based alginate hydrogels have been promising materials that have elastic modulus similar to that of natural bone. Most the specifications for the mechanical property of novel alginate nanocomposites is kept around 0.5–1 GPa for Young's modulus (callus form) and 12–18 GPa for bone in compact form and compressive strength around 4–12 MPa. This is very essential for thriving of the repairing cells on the scaffold. Any scaffold or support that is used for engineering bone tissues should be biocompatible, avoid inflammatory responses, and the size of the pores should be apt to the damaged area supporting optimal repair mechanism.

The pore sizes in alginate nanocomposites can be tailored to various dimensions based on the application and the type of cell that would be harbored on it for repair. For the regeneration of osteogenic cells, a macrosize of greater than 100 μm is preferred because it favors effective transportation of ions and better assisting cells [78]. When the pore sizes in the hydrogel are manipulated to be less than 20 μm, this could help in growth of the bone by allowing osteoblast cells to align, position, and easily provide mounting surface for adsorption of required proteins. When the pores are increased into the alginate nanocomposite matrix, the distribution of the cells is increased for providing good efficiency in repairing of the damaged tissues [79]. The final trait of every alginate nanocomposite is the ability to deposit minerals and allow bone restoration. They are found to be osteoconductive and osteoinductive. The degradability of the scaffold should be proportional to the regeneration ability of the bone. These numerous merits of the nanocomposites of alginate hydrogels have bagged them a fame as suitable materials for bone reconstruction and engineering [80].

Nanoparticles of hydroxyapatite is mostly associated with many hydrogels for bone healing applications. It has a unique mechanical property that bears load and provides sites for nucleation of bone cells [81]. The proteins in the extracellular matrix are also activated by these nanoparticles that help in tissue formation. To name a few, these special molecules found in these scaffolds are fibronectin, osteocalcin, etc. [82]. A very famous combination for the formation of bones is alginate/nanohydroxyapatite, also written as HAP.

Generally, a simple reaction between a mineral solution such as calcium chloride and along with a basic salt such as sodium phosphate can yield a good amount of alginate/nanohydroxyapatite. The nanodimensions can be altered and tailored as per need by adding additional polymers and reagents. These special compounds have the tendency to express the alkaline phosphatase enzyme in an escalated manner. This tends to increase the inductivity of the bone [83]. When nanoform of HAP is used in combination with polymer-based hydrogel materials, the flexibility of the finished product is seen to be quite outstanding [84]. These reports in the past have stirred the curiosity of many scientists to design several high-end alginate/nanohydroxyapatite nanocombinations for bone tissue applications [85]. A novel form of nanocomposite form of hydrogel was attempted by Zuo and team. This was a unique combination of methacrylate gelatin and alginate/nanohydroxyapatite.

The pure form of alginate/nanohydroxyapatite hydrogel was compared with the experimented nanocomposite form to observe the change in properties of the latter. The newly synthesized alginate/nanohydroxyapatite hydrogel had better mechanical and biological properties. Methacrylate gelatin has functional biological markers in them that express bone growth and angiogenic features. Preosteoblast have been successfully encapsulated in the methacrylate gelatin and alginate/nanohydroxyapatite hydrogel composite along with endothelial cells in an organized and structural fashion of concentric rings. When alginate/nanohydroxyapatite hydrogel formulation is opted, the network of the matrix in the alginate gets changed.

The native physical and chemical functional features of simple alginate hydrogel get altered because of the presence of nanoparticles. When the concentration of alginate/nanohydroxyapatite is around 30% by weight in the hydrogel, the most significant feature of this material would be its osteogenic properties. The proliferation of cells is seen to be higher in this combination of hydrogel. As the concentration of alginate/nanohydroxyapatite is raised, the resulting hydrogels exhibit decrease in osteogenic functional responses [86]. If an additional 30% of alginate/nanohydroxyapatite is elevated in the hydrogel, the matrix gets mineralized and supports collagen deposition and trabecular formation of bone. The main drawback of using alginate/nanohydroxyapatite would be its inability to degrade and decompose well inside the body. Hence an alternative in the form of tricalcium phosphate has been often used by scientists instead of alginate/nanohydroxyapatite.

This material is very much biodegradable and used to man potential material combinations for tissue engineering of bone [87]. Sodium alginate cross-linked with α-tricalcium phosphate has also been used and experimented as biomaterial for scaffolds [88]. The linking is mostly found to be ionic in nature. The α-tricalcium phosphate nanoparticles are seen to be distributed uniformly in a continuous fashion on the surface of the hydrogel. A few are also found to be embedded well into the porous gel matrix. This helps in attachment of the bone tissues in the surface of the scaffold (Fig. 12.7). The hydrogels property can also be altered based on the nanoparticle and the content of the nanoparticle doped into it. Sodium alginate and tricalcium phosphate nanocomposite hydrogel manifested biocompatibility and lack of toxicity toward MC3T3 cell lines.

12.4.2 Cartilage tissue engineering

Tissue engineering enables repair of the damaged tissues either by reconstruction or regeneration using the biodegradable scaffolds that mimic the naïve tissues. Mainly for the engineering of cartilage tissues, the scaffold should be a porous one with the ability to transport the growth factors to the site of damage as well as promote the cell differentiation until

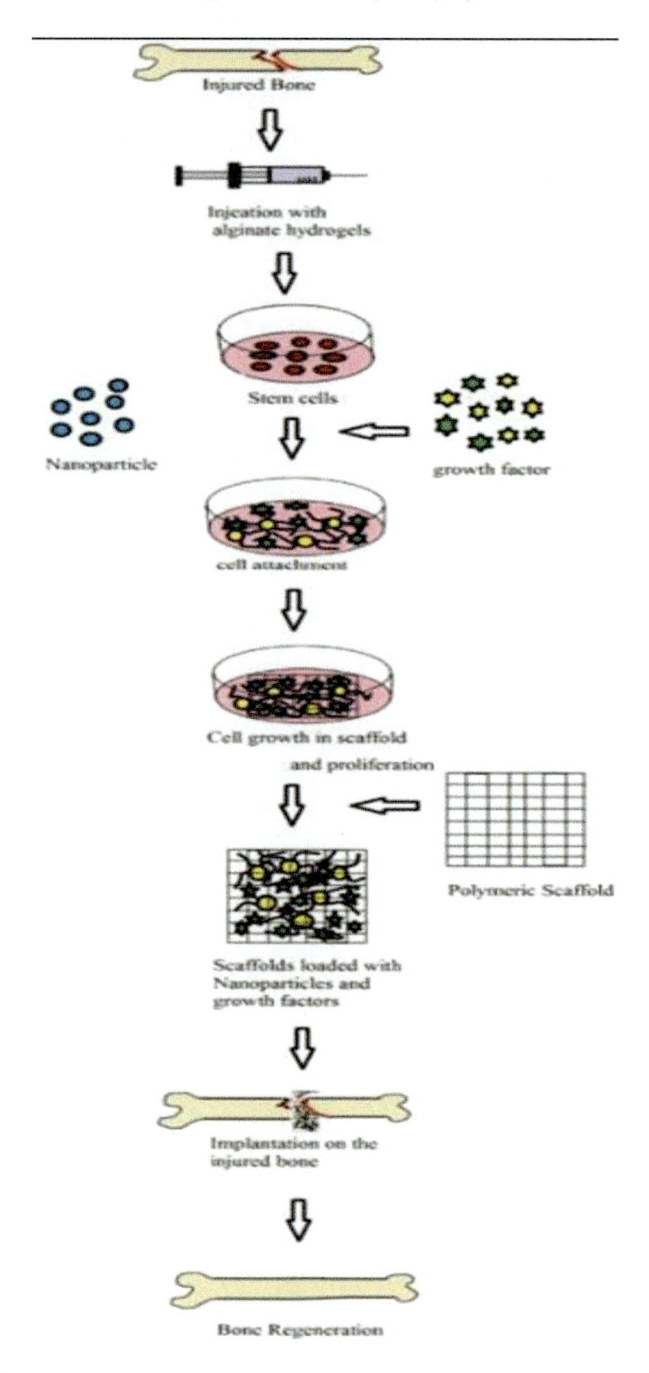

FIG. 12.7   Alginate nanohydrogels in bone regeneration.

the new tissue formation occurs [89]. In addition, alginate hydrogels possess rapid gelling with minimal inflammatory responses. Chondrogenic stem cells are incorporated into the alginate hydrogels were studied for their differentiation of cells [90]. The molecular mechanisms behind chondrogenesis were studied using mesenchymal stem cells (injectable hydrogels are used promising scaffolds for the engineering of cartilage tissues) [91], but they face limitations in maintaining their mechanical stability. This will be solved by improving their stability by blending of the alginate polysaccharide with other polymers [92, 93].

Few cartilages of our body are specialized to bear loads for the smooth functioning of the joints. The chondrocytes are found to be the building blocks of these load-bearing structures in an organized fashion. Chondrocytes are very sensitive cells that are thriving only in healthy cartilages. They aid in production and turnover of the abundant extracellular matrix of the cartilage. The supply of blood is very restricted to the articular cartilages, and their healing mechanisms are very limited. Treatment of the same externally through medications is also very tedious and difficult. Therefore many researchers have found hydrogels to be a good measure to deliver apt medications to these areas and tissues of the body. The synergistic effect of collaborating hydrogel scaffolds and mesenchymal stem cells has revolutionized regeneration of cartilages. But the mechanical property of this combination is low. Along with the stem cells and scaffolds, an additional dosage of medication is also required for regeneration of cartilage.

Starch crystals in nanoforms can also be used as an option in alginate hydrogels because they have been successfully experimented in gelatin matrix to form hydrogels [94]. Starch crystals could increase the mechanical properties of the scaffold to a great extent. Even the progenitor cells for cartilage regeneration, such as ATDC5, have good viability in the presence of starch nanocrystals. Therefore cartilage engineering researchers can always opt for starch nanocrystals as a promising scaffold for their research. For a similar function relating to cartilage regeneration, chitosan or collagen polymers are incorporated with alginate/nanohydroxyapatite nanoparticles and hydrogels are formed [95]. The structure of the matrix is porous; hence water is retained into it to a great extent. The proliferation and differentiation of the cells are readily supported by this hydrogel combination.

The Young's modulus of these nanocomposites are eight times more than its ordinary hydrogel forms and very close to natural articular cartilage's Young's modulus. In a similar study, dopamine was used to modify the alginate hydrogel and form new form of hydrogel nanocomposite. When further doping of dopamine was attempted into the same dopamine-modified alginate hydrogel, calcium ions were used to strengthen the cross-linking [96]. Polydopamine-modified alginate hydrogel nanocomposite has excellent compressive modulus for just 4% by weight content of dopamine-modified alginate hydrogel particles. This gives an optimal environment for the alginate/nanohydroxyapatite nanoparticles to mineralize and accelerate the process of cartilage repair.

12.4.3 Neural tissue engineering

Many researchers have confirmed that application of electrical signals can evoke many cells, especially those special types that need electrical excitability to function. These tissues are cardiac tissues, nerve tissues, and skeletal tissues [97]. The scaffolds associated with these cells should also be multifunctional to support the survival of these cells. Hydrogels with combination of nanoparticles have been attempted for preparation of scaffolds that are electrically stimulant and conductive as well as harbor all the pending mechanical and biological properties of an ideal hydrogel nanocomposite [98]. The nervous system is a very specialized system of the body that controls the vital features of the human system. [99]. To regenerate a damaged nerve, techniques such as neurorrhaphy and grafts are opted, but the prognosis is not very satisfactory. The recovery rate is hardly 50% from these techniques; hence tissue engineering is preferred when it comes to reviving damaged nerve cells [100]. The aim is to have ideal replacements for nerve injuries and get good functional alternatives with longer life span. Apart from mechanical support, good electrically conducive environment is needed to stimulate the elongation and maturation of axons [101].

The regeneration of nerves is also essential in many cases of trauma and damage. To revive damages, nerves scaffolds are used to nurture them with optimal growth factors and support. These hydrogels need to be biodegradable and electroactive in nature to favor the proliferation and growth of nerve cells. Graphene filaments functionalized by citric acid loaded in alginate have been designed exclusively for nerve regeneration and growth. It's a green eco-friendly approach synthesized in vitro by mesenchymal stem cells. The mechanical property is attributed to the graphene filaments present in the hydrogel. The electrical conductivity is also rendered by the graphene filaments and causes the signaling between the cells, thus stimulating the nerve cells to function well. PC12 cells were very much viable on this hydrogel formulation and spread very evidently on the surface of the scaffold. It did not trigger any immunological responses too [102].

12.4.4 Cardiac tissue engineering

When it comes to heart diseases, myocardial infraction is a predominant disorder. It has affected a lot of people all around the world. The blood flow obstruction due to plaque causes the heart tissues to be devoid of oxygen, hence leading to heart failure [103]. The regeneration of heart tissue is a herculean task; therefore heart transplant is mostly preferred as an alternative technique to deal with heart patients [104]. The drawback of transplantation is the expense associated with it and the immunological complications in the patient. Tissue engineering can easily provide repaired and revived heart tissues for effective healing of damaged tissues [105]. The scaffolds specific for cardiac engineering should be capable of mimicking the extracellular matrix of the heart region [106].

12.5 Conclusion

Alginate has been used successfully in the biomedical applications because of its biodegradability nature and feasible interaction with biological system. Although it has been effectively used as drug delivery matrix, it still faces challenges because of its poor mechanical properties. Many researchers concentrate on various designing methods to overcome the limitations. Alginate hydrogel with improved properties was formulated by incorporating carbon materials, polysaccharides, metal/metal oxide particles, and ceramic materials. There are some significant existing challenges that exist for the development of alginate nanocomposite hydrogel with high swelling ratio, poor degradation profile, and comparatively high compressive strength than other natural polymers, and elastic module showed undoubtedly holds enormous promise for the treatment of various types of diseases. By devising new design strategies and optimizing the process parameters, alginate nanocomposites have been designed with stimuli-responsive properties, cell adhesion properties, and improved mechanical properties. Based on the reviews, it is observed that alginate nanohydrogel matrices and their interaction with ECM will make them as the best possible option for tissue regeneration applications in the future.

References

[1] Karak N. Fundamentals of nanomaterials and polymer nanocomposites. Amsterdam, The Netherlands: Elsevier Inc.; 2019.

[2] Vilcinskas K, Jansen KMB, Mulder FM, Picken SJ, Koper GJM. Composition dependent properties of graphene (oxide)-alginate biopolymer nanocomposites. Polym Compos 2018;39:E236–49.

[3] Reina G, Gonzalez-Domínguez JM, Criado A, Vazquez E, Bianco A, Prato M. Promises, facts and challenges for graphene in biomedical applications. Chem Soc Rev 2017;46:4400–16.

[4] Prasher P, Sharma M, Mudila H, Gupta G, Sharma AK, Kumar D, Dua K. Emerging trends in clinical implications of bio-conjugated silver nanoparticles in drug delivery. Colloids Interfac Sci Commun 2020;35:100244. https://doi.org/10.1016/j.colcom.2020.100244.

[5] Ratner BD, Hoffman AS, Schoen FJ, Lemons JE. Biomaterials science: an introduction to materials in medicine. Toronto, ON, Canada: Academic Press; 2012.

[6] Gustafson CT, Boakye-Agyeman F, Brinkman CL, Reid JM, Patel R, Bajzer Z, Yaszemski MJ. Controlled delivery of vancomycin via charged hydrogels. PLoS ONE 2016;11, E0146401.

[7] Lu Z, Zhang J, Yu Z, Liu Q, Liu K, Li M, Wang D. Hydrogel degradation triggered by pH for the smart release of antibiotics to combat bacterial infection. New J Chem 2017;41:432–6.

[8] Li Y, Rodrigues J, Tomas H. Injectable and biodegradable hydrogels: gelation, biodegradation and biomedical applications. Chem Soc Rev 2012;41:2193–221.

[9] Matricardi P, Di Meo C, Coviello T, Hennink WE, Alhaique F. Interpenetrating polymer networks polysaccharide hydrogels for drug delivery and tissue engineering. Adv Drug Delivery Rev 2013;65:1172–87.

[10] Nguyen MK, Alsberg E. Bioactive factor delivery strategies from engineered polymer hydrogels for therapeutic medicine. Progress Polym Sci 2014;38:1236–65.

[11] Zamboni F, Collins MN. Cell based therapeutics in type 1 diabetes mellitus. Int J Pharm 2017;521:346–56.

[12] Sikorski P, Mo F, Skjak-Braek J, Stokke BT. Evidence for egg-box-compatible interactions in calcium—alginate gels from fiber x-ray diffraction. Biomacromolecules 2007;8:2098–103.

[13] Rescignano N, Hernandez R, Lopez LD, Calvillo I, Kenny JM, Mijangos C. Preparation of alginate hydrogels containing silver nanoparticles: a facile approach for antibacterial applications. Polym Inter 2016;65:921–6.

[14] Zhang F, Wu J, Kang D, Zhang H. Development of a complex hydrogel of hyaluronan and PVA embedded with silver nanoparticles and its facile studies on *Escherichia coli*. J Biomater Sci, Polymer Ed 2013;24:1410–25.

[15] Deen G, Chua V. Synthesis and properties of new "stimuli" responsive nanocomposite hydrogels containing silver nanoparticles. Gels 2015;1:117–34.

[16] Zhao X, Xia Y, Li Q, Ma X, Quan F, Geng C, Han Z. Microwave-assisted synthesis of silver nanoparticles using sodium alginate and their antibacterial activity. Coll Surf A: Physicochem Eng Asp 2014;444:180–8.

[17] Ortelli S, Costa AL. Nanoencapsulation techniques as a "safer by (molecular) design" tool. Nano-Struct Nano-Obj 2018;13:155–62.

[18] Porter GC, Schwass DR, Tompkins GR, Bobbala SKR, Medlicott NJ, Meledandri CJ. AgNP/alginate nanocomposite hydrogel for antimicrobial and antibiofilm applications. Carbohydr Polym 2021;251:117017.

[19] Zhuang Y, Yu F, Chen H, Zheng J, Ma J, Chen J. Alginate/graphene double-network nanocomposite hydrogel beads with low-swelling, enhanced mechanical properties, and enhanced adsorption capacity. J Mater Chem A 2016;4:10885–92.

[20] Malar CG, Bavanilathamuthiah. Evaluation of biocompatibity of capsaicin loaded dendrimers on zebrafish embryos. Int J Drug Delivery Technol 2015;5:54–8.

[21] Huang Z, Liu S, Zhang B, Wu Q. Preparation and swelling behavior of a novel self-assembled β-cyclodextrin/acrylic acid/sodium alginate hydrogel. Carbohydr Polym 2014;113:430–7.

[22] Cao K, Jiang Z, Zhao J, Zhao C, Gao C, Pan F, Wang B, Cao X, Yang J. Enhanced water permeation through sodium alginate membranes by incorporating graphene oxides. J Membr Sci 2014;469:272–83.

[23] He Y, Zhang N, Gong Q, Qiu H, Wang W, Liu Y, Gao J. Alginate/graphene oxide fibers with enhanced mechanical strength prepared by wet spinning. Carbohydr Polym 2012;88:1100–8.

[24] Fan J, Shi Z, Lian M, Li H, Yin J. Mechanically strong graphene oxide/sodium alginate/polyacrylamide nanocomposite hydrogel with improved dye adsorption capacity. J Mater Chem A 2013;1:7433.

[25] Deze EG, Papageorgiou SK, Favvas EP, Katsaros FK. Porous alginate aerogel beads for effective and rapid heavy metal sorption from aqueous solutions: effect of porosity in Cu^{2+} and Cd^{2+} ionsorption. Chem Eng J 2012;209:537–46.

[26] Tan WS, Ting AS. Alginate-immobilized bentonite clay: adsorption efficacy and reusability for Cu (II) removal from aqueous solution. Bioresour Technol 2014;160:115–8.

[27] Wang J, Wei L, Ma Y, Li K, Li M, Yu Y, Wang L, Qiu H. Collagen/cellulose hydrogel beads reconstituted from ionic liquid solution for Cu(II) adsorption. Carbohydr Polym 2013;98:736–43.

[28] Park HG, Kim TW, Chae MY, Yoo IK. Activated carbon-containing alginate adsorbent for the simultaneous removal of heavy metals and toxic organics. Process Biochem 2007;42:1371–7.

[29] Malar CG, Seenuvasan M, Kumar KS. Adsorption of nickel ions by surface modified magnetite nanoparticles: kinetics study. J Environ Biol 2019;40:748–52.

[30] Giri TK, Choudhary C, Ajazuddin, Alexander A, Badwaik H, Tripathi DK. Prospects of pharmaceuticals and biopharmaceuticals loaded microparticles prepared by double emulsion technique for controlled delivery. Saudi Pharm J 2013;21:125–41.

[31] Abasalizadeh F, Moghaddam SV, Alizadeh E. Alginate-based hydrogels as drug delivery vehicles in cancer treatment and their applications in wound dressing and 3D bioprinting. J Biol Eng 2020;14:8.

[32] Hernández-González AC, Téllez-Jurado L, Rodríguez-Lorenzo LM. Alginate polymer which is highly biodegradable with a high possibility of forming scaffold-like structures for tissue engineering applications. Carbohydr Polym 2020;115514.

[33] Thoniyot P, Tan MJ, Karim AA, Young DJ, Loh XJ. Nanoparticle-hydrogel composites: concept, design, and applications of these promising, multi-functional materials. Adv Sci 2015;2:1–2.

[34] Manal F, Taleb A, Alkahtani A, Mohamed SK. Radiation synthesis and characterization of sodium alginate/chitosan/hydroxyapatite nanocomposite hydrogels: a drug delivery system for liver cancer. Polym Bull 2015;72:725–42.

[35] Gamboa A, Araujo V, Caro N, Gotteland M, Abugoch L, Tapia C. Spray freeze-drying as an alternative to the ionic gelation method to produce chitosan and alginate Nanoparticles targeted to the colon. J Pharm Sci 2015;104(12):4373–85.

[36] Jeong SI, Krebs MD, Bonino CA, Samorezov JE, Khan SA, Alsberg E. Electrospun chitosan–alginate nanofibers with in situ polyelectrolyte complexation for use as tissue engineering scaffolds. Tissue Eng Part A 2010;17:59–70.4.

[37] Zhang H, Liu X, Yang M, Zhu L. Silk fibroin/sodium alginate composite nano-fibrous scaffold prepared through thermally induced phase-separation (TIPS) method for biomedical applications. Korean J Couns Psychother 2015;55:8–13.

[38] Sowjanya JA, Singh J, Mohita T, Sarvanan S, Moorthi A, Srinivasan N, et al. Biocomposite scaffolds containing chitosan/alginate/nano-silica for bone tissue engineering. Colloids Surf B 2013;109:294–300.

[39] Turnbull G, Clarke J, Picard F, Riches P, Jia L, Han F, Li B. 3D bioactive composite scaffolds for bone tissue engineering. Bioact Mater 2018;3(3):278–314.

[40] Wang Y, Shang S, Li C. Aligned biomimetic scaffolds as a new tendency in tissue engineering. Curr Stem Cell Res Ther 2016;11:3–18.

[41] Sun T, Li X, Shi Q, Wang H, Huang Q, Fukuda T. Microfluidic spun alginate hydrogel microfibers and their application in tissue engineering. Gels 2018;4(2):38.

[42] Sharifi F, Wrede AH, Kimlinger DF, Thomas DG, Vander Wiel JB, Chen Y, Montazami R, Hashemi NN. Microfibers as physiologically relevant platforms for creation of 3d cell cultures. Macromol Biosci 2017;17(12).

[43] Kurczewska J, Cegłowski M, Pecyna P, Ratajczak M, Gajęcka M, Schroeder G. Molecularly imprinted polymer as drug delivery carrier in alginate dressing. Mater Lett 2017;46–9.

[44] Peng L, Liu Y, Huang J, Li J, Gong J, Ma J. Microfluidic fabrication of highly stretchable and fast electro-responsive graphene oxide/polyacrylamide/alginate hydrogel fibers. Eur Polym J 2018;103:335–41.

[45] Li Y, Han Y, Wang X, Peng J, Xu Y, Chang J. Multifunctional hydrogels prepared by dual ion cross-linking for chronic wound healing. ACS Appl Mater Interfaces 2017;9(19):16054–62.

[46] Shi M, Zhang H, Song T, Liu X, Gao Y, Zhou J, et al. Sustainable dual release of antibiotic and growth factor from pH-responsive uniform alginate composite microparticles to enhance wound healing. ACS Appl Mater Interfaces 2019;11(25):22730–44.

[47] Sarker B, Li W, Zheng K, Detsch R, Boccaccini AR. Designing porous bone tissue engineering scaffolds with enhanced mechanical properties from composite hydrogels composed of modified alginate, gelatin, and bioactive glass. ACS Biomater Sci Eng 2016;2(12):2240–54.

[48] Shin JU, Gwon J, Lee S-Y, Yoo HS. Silver-incorporated nanocellulose fibers for antibacterial hydrogels. ACS Omega 2018;3(11):16150–7.

[49] Niu B, Jia J, Wang H, Chen S, Cao W, Yan J, et al. In vitro and in vivo release of diclofenac sodium-loaded sodium alginate/carboxymethyl chitosan-ZnO hydrogel beads. Int J Biol Macromol 2019;141:1191–8.

[50] Cong Z, Shi Y, Wang Y, Wang Y, Niu J, Chen N, Xue H. A novel controlled drug delivery system based on alginate hydrogel/chitosan micelle composites. Int J Biol Macromol 2018;855–64.

[51] Alavi M, Nokhodchi A. An overview on antimicrobial and wound healing properties of ZnO nanobiofilms, hydrogels, and bionanocomposites based on cellulose, chitosan, and alginate polymers. Carbohydr Polym 2020;227:115349.

[52] Dvir T, Timko BP, Brigham MD, Naik SR, Karajanagi SS, Levy O, Jin H, Parker KK, Langer R, Kohane DS. Nanowired three-dimensional cardiac patches. Nat Nanotechnol 2011;6:720–5.

[53] Raguvaran R, Manuja BK, Chopra M, Thakur R, Anand T, Kalia A, Manuja A. Sodium alginate and gum acacia hydrogels of ZnO nanoparticles show wound healing effect on fibroblast cells. Int J Biol Macromol 2017;96:185–91.

[54] Zhang J, Wang Q, Wang A. In situ generation of sodium alginate/hydroxyapatite nanocomposite beads as drug-controlled release matrices. Acta Biomater 2010;6(2):445–54.

[55] Patnaik S, Aggarwal A, Nimesh S, et al. PEI-alginate nanocomposites as efficient in vitro gene transfection agents. J. Control Release: Off J Control Release Soc 2006;114(3):398–409.

[56] Hariyadi DM, Islam N. Current status of alginate in drug delivery. Adv Pharmacol Pharm Sci 2020;2020:8886095.

[57] Lee G-S, Park J-H, Shin US, Kim H-W. Direct deposited porous scaffolds of calcium phosphate cement with alginate for drug delivery and bone tissue engineering. Acta Biomater 2011;3178–86.

[58] Iliescu R, Andronescu E, Ghiţulică C, Berger D, Ficai A. Montmorillonite-alginate nanocomposite beads as drug carrier for oral administration of carboplatin-preparation and characterization. UPB Sci Bull Ser B: Chem Mater Sci 2011;73(3).

[59] Oliveira CR, Rezende CM, Silva MR, Pêgo AP, Borges O, Goes AM. A new strategy based on SmRho protein loaded chitosan nanoparticles as a candidate oral vaccine against schistosomiasis. PLoS Negl Trop Dis 2012;6(11).

[60] Sabbagh HAK, Hussein-Al-Ali SH, Hussein MZ, Abudayeh Z, Ayoub R, Abudoleh SM. A statistical study on the development of metronidazole-chitosan-alginate nanocomposite formulation using the full factorial design. Polymers 2020;12:772.

[61] Haque S, Md S, Sahni JK, Ali J, Baboota S. Development and evaluation of brain targeted intranasal alginate nanoparticles for treatment of depression. J Psychiatr Res 2014;48:1–12.

[62] Debache K, Kropf C, Schütz C, Harwood L, Käuper P, Monney T, Rossi N, Laue C, McCullough KC, Hemphill A. Vaccination of mice with chitosan nanogel-associated recombinant NcPDI against challenge infection with *Neospora caninum* tachyzoites. Parasite Immunol 2011;33:81–94.

[63] Borges O, Cordeiro-da-Silva A, Tavares J, Santarém N, de Sousa A, Borchard G, Junginger HE. Immune response by nasal delivery of hepatitis B surface antigen and codelivery of a CpG ODN in alginate coated chitosan nanoparticles. Eur J Pharm Biopharm 2008;69:405–16.

[64] Dukovski BJ, Plantić I, Čunčić I, et al. Lipid/alginate nanoparticle loaded in situ gelling system tailored for dexamethasone nasal delivery. Int J Pharm 2017;533(2):480–7.

[65] Zhou QT, Leung SS, Tang P, Parumasivam T, Loh ZH, Chan HK. Inhaled formulations and pulmonary drug delivery systems for respiratory infections. Adv Drug Deliv Rev 2015;85:83–99.

[66] Nait Mohamed FA, Laraba-Djebari F. Development and characterization of a new carrier for vaccine delivery based on calciumalginate nanoparticles: safe immunoprotective approach against scorpion envenoming. Vaccine 2016;34(24):2692–9.

[67] Costa JR, Silva NC, Sarmento B, Pintado M. Potential chitosancoated alginate nanoparticles for ocular delivery of daptomycin. Eur J Clin Microbiol Infect Dis 2015;34(6):1255–62.

[68] Khandan A, Jazayeri H, Fahmy MD, Razavi M. Hydrogels: types, structure, properties, and applications. In: Frontiers in biomaterials. Sharjah, UAE: Bentham Science; 2017. p. 143–69. Chapter 4.

[69] Kopecek J. Hydrogel biomaterials: a smart future? Biomaterials 2007;28:5185–92.

[70] Carrow JK, Gaharwar AK. Bioinspired polymeric nanocomposites for regenerative medicine. Macromol Chem Phys 2015;216:248–64.

[71] Schexnailder P, Schmidt G. Nanocomposite polymer hydrogels. Colloid Polym Sci 2009;287:1–11.

[72] Haraguchi K. Stimuli-responsive nanocomposite gels. Colloid Polym Sci 2011;289:455–73.

[73] Liu M, Zeng X, Ma C, Yi H, Ali Z, Mou X, He N, Li S, Deng Y. Injectable hydrogels for cartilage and bone tissue engineering. Bone Res 2017;5:17014.

[74] Seliktar D. Designing cell-compatible hydrogels for biomedical applications. Science 2012;336:1124–8.

[75] Zhang LM, Xia K, Lu ZX, Li GP, Chen J, Deng Y, Li S, Zhou FM, He NY. Efficient and facile synthesis of gold nanorods with finely tunable plasmonic peaks from visible to near-IR range. Chem Mater 2014;26:1794–8.

[76] Bignon A, Chouteau J, Chevalier J, Fantozzi G, Carret J-P, Chavassieux P, Boivin G, Melin M, Hartmann D. Effect of micro- and macroporosity of bone substitutes on their mechanical properties and cellular response. J Mater Sci-Mater M 2003;14:1089–97.

[77] Liu X, Ma PX. Polymeric scaffolds for bone tissue engineering. Ann Biomed Eng 2004;32:477–86.

[78] Mehrali M, Thakur A, Pennisi CP, Talebian S, Arpanaei A, Nikkhah M, Dolatshahi-Pirouz A. Nanoreinforced hydrogels for tissue engineering: biomaterials that are compatible with load-bearing and electroactive tissues. Adv Mater 2017;29:1603612.

[79] Nair AK, Gautieri A, Chang SW, Buehler MJ. Molecular mechanics of mineralized collagen fibrils in bone. Nat Commun 2013;4:1724.

[80] Jensen T, Jakobsen T, Baas J, Nygaard JV, Dolatshahi-Pirouz A, Hovgaard MB, Foss M, Bunger C, Besenbacher F, Soballe K. Hydroxyapatite nanoparticles in poly-D,L-lactic acid coatings on porous titanium implants conducts bone formation. J Biomed Mater Res A 2010;95:665–72.

[81] Sadat-Shojai M, Khorasani M-T, Jamshidi A. 3-dimensional cell-laden nano-hydroxyapatite/protein hydrogels for bone regeneration applications. Mater Sci Eng C-Mater 2015;49:835–43.

[82] Cui CY, Wu TL, Gao F, Fan CC, Xu ZY, Wang HB, Liu B, Liu WG. Fabrication of strong hydrogen-bonding induced coacervate adhesive hydrogels with antibacterial and hemostatic activities. Adv Funct Mater 2018;28:1804925.

[83] Jiang YY, Zhu YJ, Li H, Zhang YG, Shen YQ, Sun TW, Chen F. Preparation and enhanced mechanical properties of hybrid hydrogels comprising ultralong hydroxyapatite nanowires and sodium alginate. J Colloid Interf Sci 2017;497:266–75.

[84] Barros J, Ferraz MP, Azeredo J, Fernandes MH, Gomes PS, Monteiro FJ. Alginate-nanohydroxyapatite hydrogel system: optimizing the formulation for enhanced bone regeneration. Mat Sci Eng C-Mater 2019;105:109985.

[85] Makvandi P, Ali GW, Sala FD, Fattah WA, Borzacchiello A. Hyaluronic acid/corn silk extract based injectable nanocomposite: a biomimetic antibacterial scaffold for bone tissue regeneration. Mat Sci Eng C-Mater 2020;107:110195.

[86] Das D, Bang S, Zhang SM, Noh I. Bioactive molecules release and cellular responses of alginate-tricalcium phosphate particles hybrid gel. Nanomaterials 2017;7:389.

[87] Wang G, Jia L, Han F, et al. Microfluidics-based fabrication of cell-laden hydrogel microfibers for potential applications in tissue engineering. Molecules 2019;24(8):1633. https://doi.org/10.3390/molecules24081633.

[88] Awad HA, Wickham MQ, Leddy HA, Gimble JM, Guilak F. Chondrogenic differentiation of adipose-derived adult stem cells in agarose, alginate, and gelatin scaffolds. Biomaterials 2004;25(16):3211–2.

[89] Balakrishnan B, Joshi N, Jayakrishnan A, et al. Self-crosslinked oxidized alginate/gelatin hydrogel as injectable, adhesive biomimetic scaffolds for cartilage regeneration. Acta Biomater 2014;10:3650–63.

[90] Park H, Lee KY. Cartilage regeneration using biodegradable oxidized alginate/hyaluronate hydrogels. J Biomed Mater Res A 2014;102:4519–25.

[91] Jaikumar D, Sajesh KM, Soumya S, et al. Injectable alginate-O-carboxymethyl chitosan/nano fibrin composite hydrogels for adipose tissue engineering. Int J Biol Macromol 2015;74:318–26.

[92] Piluso S, Labet M, Zhou C, Seo JW, Thielemans W, Patterson J. Engineered three-dimensional microenvironments with starch nanocrystals as cell-instructive materials. Biomacromolecules 2019;20:3819–30.

[93] Kaviani A, Zebarjad SM, Javadpour S, Ayatollahi M, Lair RB. Int J Polym Anal Ch 2019;24:191–203.

[94] Shen JL, Shi DJ, Dong LL, Zhang ZY, Li XJ, Chen MQ. Fabrication of polydopamine nanoparticles knotted alginate scaffolds and their properties. J Biomed Mater Res A 2018;106:3255–66.

[95] Park H, Bhalla R, Saigal R, Radisic M, Watson N, Langer R, Vunjak-Novakovic G. Effects of electrical stimulation in C2C12 muscle constructs. J Tissue Eng Regen M 2008;2:279–87.

[96] Lee JH, Lee J-Y, Yang SH, Lee E-J, Kim H-W. Carbon nanotube-collagen three-dimensional culture of mesenchymal stem cells promotes expression of neural phenotypes and secretion of neurotrophic factors. Acta Biomater 2014;10:4425–36.

[97] Bedir T, Ulag S, Ustundag CB, Gunduz O. 3D bioprinting applications in neural tissue engineering for spinal cord injury repair. Mat Sci Eng C-Mater 2020;110:110741.

[98] Lee SK, Wolfe SW. Peripheral nerve injury and repair. J Am Acad Orthop Sur 2000;8:243–52.

[99] Schmidt CE, Leach JB. Neural tissue engineering: strategies for repair and regeneration. Annu Rev Biomed Eng 2003;5:293–347.

[100] Homaeigohar S, Tsai T-Y, Young T-H, Yang HJ, Ji Y-R. An electroactive alginate hydrogel nanocomposite reinforced by functionalized graphite nanofilaments for neural tissue engineering. Carbohydr Polym 2019;224:115112.

[101] Muniyandi P, Palaninathan V, Veeranarayanan S, Ukai T, Maekawa T, Hanajiri T, Mohamed MS. ECM mimetic electrospun porous poly (L-lactic acid) (PLLA) scaffolds as potential substrates for cardiac tissue engineering. Polymers 2020;12:451.

[102] Adadi N, Yadid M, Gal I, Asulin M, Feiner R, Edri R, Dvir T. Electrospun fibrous PVDF-TrFe scaffolds for cardiac tissue engineering, differentiation, and maturation. Adv Mater Technol 2020;5:1900820.

[103] Nazari H, Heirani-Tabasi A, Hajiabbas M, Khalili M, Alavijeh MS, Hatamie S, Gorabi AM, Esmaeili E, Tafti SHA. Chitosan surface modified hydrogel as a therapeutic contact lens. Polym Adv Technol 2020;31:248–59.

[104] Shin SR, Jung SM, Zalabany M, Kim K, Zorlutuna P, Kim SB, Nikkhah M, Khabiry M, Azize M, Kong J, Wan K-T, Palacios T, Dokmeci MR, Bae H, Tang XW, Khademhosseini A. Carbon-nanotube-embedded hydrogel sheets for engineering cardiac constructs and bioactuators. ACS Nano 2013;7:2369–80.

[105] Dvir-Ginzberg M, Elkayam T, Cohen S. Induced differentiation and maturation of newborn liver cells into functional hepatic tissue in macroporous alginate scaffolds. FASEB J 2008;22:1440–9.

[106] Shteyer E, Ben Ya'acov A, Zolotaryova L, Sinai A, Lichtenstein Y, Pappo O, Kryukov O, Elkayam T, Cohen S, Ilan Y. Reduced liver cell death using an alginate scaffold bandage: a novel approach for liver reconstruction after extended partial hepatectomy. Acta Biomater 2014;10:3209–16.

13

Cellulose-based stimuli-responsive hydrogels

Manuel Palencia[a], Arturo Espinosa-Duque[a], Andrés Otálora[b], and Angélica García-Quintero[b]

[a]Research Group in Science with Technological Applications (GI-CAT), Department of Chemistry, Faculty of Natural and Exact Sciences, Universidad del Valle, Cali, Colombia, [b]Mindtech Research Group (Mindtech-RG), Mindtech s.a.s., Cali, Colombia

13.1 Introduction

The current necessity of contributing to environmental pollution problems by nondegradable materials, to promote a sustainable economy, has increased the use of easily-accessible and renewable resources for the construction of novel and new materials; cellulose is one of the most important natural raw materials for this purpose because it is the most abundant biopolymer on our planet. Cellulose can be defined as a biopolymeric material characterized by high hydrophilicity, biocompatibility, and biodegradability with multiple applications; among those that stand out is its use for making three-dimensional (3D) polymer networks with the capacity to absorb and retain large amounts of water, also called hydrogels [1–4].

Cellulose-based hydrogels (CBHGs) are characterized by their flexibility, softness, biodegradability, and biocompatibility. These properties allow its application in the development of biocompatible materials that can be used for drug-controlled release and making of medical devices, but it can also be used as scaffolding to help and promote the cultivation of different cell lines into regeneration of different tissues [3, 5–7]. On the other hand, the diversity of polymeric structures that can be designed and obtained from CBHGs has opened the possibility to obtain systems capable of undergoing a change in response to external stimuli, such as pH, ionic strength, temperature, redox processes, and electromagnetic fields, among others [8–10].

With the objective of deepening this fast-growing research field, this chapter focuses on three parts; the first is directed toward the description of structural aspects of hydrogels and their connection with physical and chemical properties, mainly those with stimuli-responsive properties. In the second part, the response and applications of stimulus-responsive hydrogels based on cellulose are described and discussed, depending on the method of obtaining them, and briefly, different methods of characterization of structural and functional properties are exposed. Finally, advances resulting from the use of cellulose-based stimulus-responsive hydrogels for drug-controlled delivery systems, growth of cell culture, and regenerative medicine and tissue engineering are shown and discussed.

13.2 Physical and chemical properties of cellulose and cellulose by-products

Cellulose is a biopolymer whose molecular structure is constituted by multiple units of β-D-glucose forming D-glucopyranose structures with the chemical formula $(C_6H_{10}O_5)_n$, where its degree of polymerization (n) is directly related to the origin of the cellulosic material; however, it has been widely established that, generally, these materials are formed between 10,000 and 15,000 β-D-glucose monomers [11, 12]. Cellulose is the most abundant polysaccharide on the planet and therefore the main source of organic carbon in nature [4]. Since the earliest times of humanity's development, and with a complete ignorance of its polymeric chemical structure, cellulose has been widely used as a fundamental raw material by ancient civilizations in the oldest constructions and in the production of energy [13]. Throughout history, cellulose has been recognized as one of the main components of ships, bridges, furniture such as chairs, boxes, and basic containers such as glasses and plates. However, its greatest historical importance is in the production of textile materials such as thread, cotton, and linen [14].

Since the beginning of the 19th century, cellulose was recognized as a compound thanks to the work of French chemist Anselme Payen who identified that, when plant samples were treated with ammonia and acid, a fibrous-consistency solidlike waste is obtained. By elementary analysis, it was determined that this solid had a molecular formula of $C_6H_{10}O_5$. However, its molecular structure was determined a century later, specifically in 1920, when German chemist Hermann Staudinger discovered that these D-glucose units are linked by covalent bonds; therefore, these were small structural units forming a more complex macromolecular structure [14, 15]. Today, cellulose continues to be a compound of interest because of its natural and renewable origin, abundance, and properties that make it a material with a wide range of relevant applications.

Cellulose, as mentioned earlier, is the biopolymer found in a major proportion in nature, mainly in plants, being the main constituent of its chemical structure and the most important substance of their cell walls [4]. It is found with lignin and hemicellulose, so the simplest method to obtain it consists of elimination of the components that are not of interest by alkaline hydrolysis with NaOH [16]. The content of cellulose in wood varies from 40% to 50%, in jute from 60% to 70%, and linen about 80%, whereas cotton consists of 95% [17]. Due to its presence in plants, it is part of the main diet of numerous animals capable of biodegrading this polymer with enzymes called cellulases, which are secreted to convert this macromolecule in free D-glucose units; whereas other species, such as ruminants, digest cellulose via microbial symbiosis between animals and microorganisms that live in their intestine. On the other hand, humans cannot synthesize and degrade cellulose because of the lack of enzymes and microorganisms that enable the metabolic pathways required for this [13].

Because cellulose is a biopolymer whose monomers correspond to glucose units, it is an excellent source of fermentable sugar, and consequently it is used for the production of acetic acid, ethanol, and ethers [13]. From an industrial point of view, the importance of cellulose is reflected in the total annual biomass production, i.e., about 1.5×10^{12} tons, which is directly associated with the large-scale production of daily use materials such as paper and cardboard, and specific materials such as regenerated cellulose films, sorption media, optical sheets, and additives for food and pharmaceutical products [16]. In addition, various more specialized processes have been developed under different conditions to manufacture other materials such as nanocellulose, rayon, and cellophane [13, 15].

Chemically speaking, cellulose can be used as a precursor of other materials by chemical reaction through its functional groups. Cellulose has in its structure β-D-glucose monomers containing three hydroxyl groups with repetitive units linked by carbons C-1 and C-4 from β-1,4 ether bonds (see Fig. 13.1) in such a way that a molecule rotates 180 degrees with respect to the adjacent unit [3]. Once the building blocks of this biopolymer are linked together, one anhydroglucose unit is formed, and two units of this form the β-D-glucopyranoside, or 1,6-Anhydro-b-D-cellobiose, which is the repetitive unit of the cellulose (see Fig. 13.1) [16, 18]. These units can be thermally fragmented at temperatures above 300°C, generating by-products for the food industry, fuel precursor compounds, and even contamination when forest fires occur [16, 19].

In cellulose, oxygen atoms of ether bond and hydroxyl groups participate in intramolecular hydrogen bonds that stabilize the β-glycosidic bond; therefore, cellulose has a linear, chiral, hydrophilic structure. It is found in

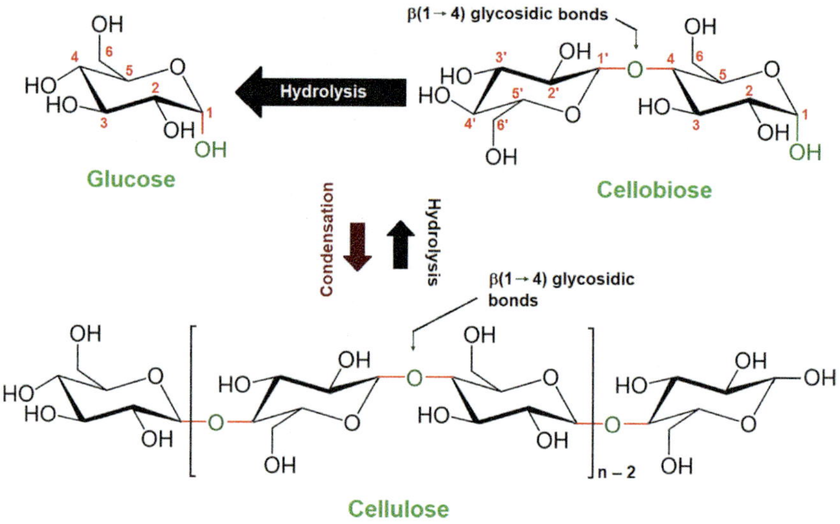

FIG. 13.1   Molecular structure of glucose, cellobiose, and cellulose.

nature forming fibrils and microfibrils (with a diameter that varies from 5 to 50 nm) due to the parallel stacking of the cellulose chains caused during its biosynthesis, providing high axial resistance, which explains the rigidity found in plants, trees, and algae [11, 13, 15]. In addition, cellulose has a hydrophobic region around carbon atoms converting it into a water-insoluble supramolecular substance, even in organic solvents. The modifications that cellulose can show in its structure are mainly due to oxidation or hydrolysis reactions that occur on the surface of amorphous areas or fibrils and the typical reactions of functionalization of the hydroxyl groups by esterification, etherification, urethanization, and sulfonation, among others [12, 20–22]. More specifically, the hydroxyl groups of cellulose polymers can react with hydroxylated methyl and ethyl units to produce water-soluble cellulose derivatives (see Fig. 13.2) such as hydroxypropyl cellulose, hydroxypropyl methylcellulose, hydroxyethyl methylcellulose, carboxymethyl cellulose, sodium carboxymethyl cellulose, methylcellulose, and ethyl cellulose [23]. The ester derivatives, on the other hand, are obtained by acid-catalyzed esterification of the cellulosic hydroxyl group using organic acids. In industry, these esters are generally obtained for the production of plastic sheets and medical applications [17, 24].

In addition to plants, another source of cellulose are bacteria such as *Acetobacter xylinum*, *Gluconacetobacter*, and *Komagataeibacter*; when cellulose is produced by bacteria, it is known as bacterial cellulose, which is chemically identical to plant cellulose. Therefore, bacterial cellulose have intramolecular hydrogen bonds, and their glucose units are linked by β-glycosidic bonds that generate a high viscosity when it is in solution (apart from the characteristic stiffness of this polymer) and high tendency

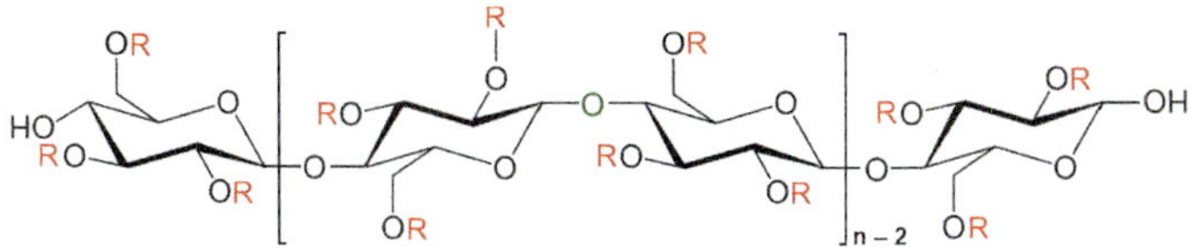

R = H	Cellulose
R = CH$_3$	Methylcellulose
R = CH$_2$CH$_3$	Ethylcellulose
R = CH$_2$CH(OH)CH$_3$	Hydroxypropylcellulose
R = CH$_3$ or CH$_2$CH(OH)CH$_3$	Hydoxypropyl methylcellulose
R = CH$_2$COOH	Carboxymethyl cellulose
R = CH$_2$COONa	Sodium carboxymethyl cellulose
R = OOCCH$_3$	Cellulose acetate

For all cases R = H depending on degree of substitution

FIG. 13.2   Chemical structure of cellulose derivatives.

to crystallize or—as mentioned before for plant cellulose—a capacity to form fibrils. Also, its structure can be highly ordered (crystalline) with the same probability of being disorderly (amorphous); the degree of crystallinity of cellulose is around of 40%–70% and depends on the isolation method and source. In this ambit, several crystalline cellulose polymorphs have been reported: (i) cellulose I, which is obtained from trees, plants, algae, and bacteria, and has metastable structures (Iα and Iβ); (ii) cellulose II, which is produced with the solubilization and subsequent recrystallization of cellulose I and has a monoclinic structure that are produced materials such as cellophane and Tencel; and finally; and (iii) cellulose III, which is obtained from cellulose I or cellulose II by treating with liquid ammonia [10, 11, 13, 16, 24, 25]. The ability that allows cellulose to absorb water and swell due to its hydrophilic nature without dissolving in the medium is one of the most relevant properties of this polymer. The hydroxyl groups primarily responsible for this particular behavior can link numerous polymers through hydrogen bonds, producing a hydrogel, a property that will be discussed in the next section [1, 26].

13.3 Cellulose-based hydrogels (CBHG)

13.3.1 Hydrogels: Concept and properties

Although hydrogels and hydrophilic materials are present in nature with low swelling ability, synthetic hydrogels were first reported in 1960 by chemists Otto Wichterle and Drahoslav Lím. They developed the first synthetic hydrogel from ethylene dimethacrylate and 2-hydroxyethyl methacrylate, which was patented for use in contact lenses [6, 16, 18]. Hydrogels can be defined in multiple ways; however, the brief and concise description recognizes that hydrogels are hydrophilic polymers that swell when in contact with water without dissolving [5, 27, 28].

The ability of hydrogels to increase their volume by absorption of water is a consequence of the osmotic, capillary, and hydration forces of the polymer chain. Thus, hydrogel swells in an aqueous medium until the thermodynamic force that causes the increase of volume is compensated by the elastic and retraction force produced by physical or chemical cross-links [1, 10]. Characteristic hydrophilicity of hydrogels is due to functional groups on the side chains or backbone of the polymer; these groups are usually $-OH$, $-COOH$, $-NH_2$, or $-SO_3H$, among others [29]. Some researchers have determined that water should be at least 10% of the mass of the swollen material to be classified as a hydrogel to achieve an adequate distinction of other cross-linked polymers usually named as resins [5, 6, 16]. Thus, both hydrogels and resins can be hydrophilic cross-linked polymers, however, hydrophilic resins are expected to show low-swelling ability in water, and consequently these can be described in many cases as rigid materials.

On the other hand, hydrogels are classified to be physical or chemical gels according to their formation mechanism (see Fig. 13.3). The first case corresponds to hydrogels whose cross-linking is formed by hydrogen bonds and/or electrostatic interactions resulting from polar groups in their molecular structure [7, 30]. This type of hydrogel is referred to as reversible because the links between polymer chains can be weakened or enhanced depending on the chemical environment to which they are exposed. In general, the linking strength is weakened by the presence of

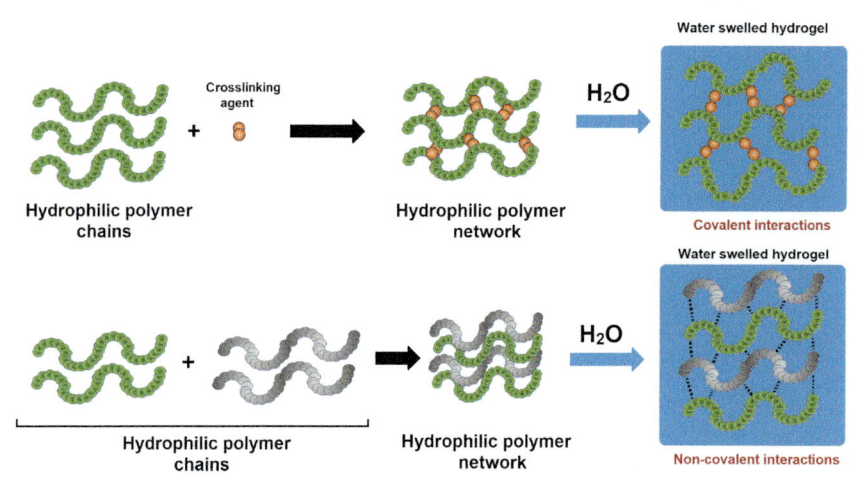

FIG. 13.3   Illustration of formation mechanism of hydrogels.

external electrostatic fields produced by the presence of ions in the medium; thus, a hydrogel formed only by electrostatic interactions will be unstable at high ionic forces. A similar effect is observed at extreme acidity or alkalinity values, for example, at very low pH, the concentration of hydrogen ions is very high and promotes the weakening of interactions between different interacting groups [6–8]. On the other hand, chemical gels are made from chemical reactions directed toward the formation of new covalent bonds between functional groups on different chains. In an analogy with physical gels, these are referred to as permanent or covalent-bonding gels, and their ability to swell is affected by the number of hydrophilic groups defining the hydrophilic domains of the network and by the degree of cross-linking resulting in interchain covalent bonds [7].

Another way in which hydrogels are classified is based on the origin of the polymer; thus, hydrogels can be referred to as natural or synthetic polymers. Although the latter have the advantage of having major water absorption capacity and a strength structure as a result of the synthetic design, natural hydrogels are better raw materials environmentally and sustainably speaking because they are usually biodegradable and biocompatible materials, in many cases with biomimetic characteristics and null or low toxicity [8, 9, 27, 31]. Because hydrogels show transitions from a swollen state in excess water to a no-swollen state in the absence of water, besides the swelling controlled by external factors such as humidity, temperature, pH, ionic strength, among others, their applications are diverse but at the same time limited when adequate mechanical properties are required. In this way, hydrogels are adequate for the development of biomedical devices, contact lenses, bioactive gels, water reservoirs, artificial muscles, food additives, humidity sensors, and drug-controlled delivery systems, among others. However, they are a very bad alternative for the retaining phase of ions in column packing systems, porous membranes, or coating of exterior surfaces [9, 10].

13.3.2 Cellulose as a raw material for hydrogel development

As mentioned before, hydrogels have multiple applications depending on their degree of biodegradability and biocompatibility, and since these features are enhanced and practically ensured when hydrogels are obtained from natural polymers, the natural polymers are an excellent candidate for making this kind of hydrogel. Natural polymers usually used are cellulose, chitosan, collagen, and starch, among others. In the specific case of CBHGs, these are generally prepared from water-soluble ethers derived from cellulose by a physical cross-linking of polymer chains like methyl-, ethyl-, propyl-, carboxymethyl-, hydroxypropyl methyl-, and hydroxyethyl methylcellulose, and also polyelectrolytes like sodium carboxymethyl cellulose, which has high sensitivity to the ionic strength or pH and therefore is commonly called a smart polymer. Hydrogels that are manufactured from sodium carboxymethyl cellulose have a major capacity to swell when polymer chains are characterized by a high molecular weight and high charge density since electrostatic repulsion occurring between particles of the same charge promotes that polymer chain to expand [10].

CBHGs can be obtained by physical stabilization or chemical reaction of synthetic or natural polymers, a mixture of them, or from their derivatives [8, 9]. Cross-linking reactions can be carried out using water or organic solvents with the subsequent elimination of solvent by some adequate method, but these can also be synthesized in the absence of solvent. Several cross-linking methods can be found in the literature, but two main processes are frequently used: (i) direct cross-linking of water-soluble polymer chains, and (ii) reticulation or bonded-covalently network formation of hydrophilic polymer chains using a cross-linking agent. The function of a cross-linking agent is to react with functional groups of hydrophilic polymers to form new bonds. Typical reactions are esterification between hydroxyl and carboxylic acid groups (e.g., R_1 $-OH + R_2-COOH \rightarrow R_1-COO-R_2 + H_2O$), formation of amide-type linking (e.g., $R_1-NH_2 + R_2-COOH \rightarrow R_2-CONH-R_1 + H_2O$ or $R_1-NH_2 + R_2-COX \rightarrow R_2-CONH-R_1 + HX$ with X = halogen), formation of urethane-type linking (e.g., $R_1-OH + R_2-NCO \rightarrow R_2-HNCOO-R_1$), and formation of imine-type linking (e.g., $R_1-NH_2 + R_2-COH \rightarrow R_2-CHN-R_1 + H_2O$), among others. For cellulose, the cross-linking agents commonly used are reagents based on aldehydes, epichlorohydrin, urea derivatives, and multifunctional carboxylic acids, among others, which should be used to direct chemical reactions with hydroxyl groups on cellulose. In addition, these can be classified into two groups: etherifying agents (e.g., epoxides, vinyl compounds, and organochlorines) and esterifying agents (e.g., anhydrides and carboxylic acids) [9, 16].

Also, it is possible to produce the cross-linking of cellulose chains by sequential reactions without the use of etherifying or esterifying agents. For that, it is necessary to first carry out a chemical reaction between hydroxyl groups of cellulose and a molecule with at least one functional group and a reactive double bond, e.g., $NCO-R_2-CH=CH_2$; thus, in a first stage that can be called an *"activation stage"*, cellulose or another polyhydroxylated polymer can react to produce the partial modification of a number of hydroxyl groups on the polymer structure. Thus, cellulose-OH $+ NCO-R_2-CH=CH_2 \rightarrow$ cellulose-ONHCO-R_2-CH=CH$_2$. Note that in this stage, easily polymerizable double bonds are inserted on the side chains of cellulose or derivatives of cellulose; as a consequence, in a second stage, *"by-polymerization cross-linking stage"*, linear hydrophilic polymers can be used as cross-linking agents by their in situ polymerization. The advantage of this procedure is that hydrophilicity of cellulose can be significantly increased depending on the nature of the monomer used for the forming of the polymeric cross-linking agent and by control of polymer chain length, which is controlled by the amount of radical initiator (e.g., ammonium peroxodisulfate, potassium persulfate, 2,2-azo-isobutyronitrile, benzoyl peroxide, or UV-radiation, among others) [9, 16].

13.3.2.1 Chemical CBHGs

The production of chemical hydrogels can be carried out by the use of high energy radiation or chemical agents to obtain stable cross-linked chains. In general terms, the cross-linking degree influences the mechanical properties, the ability of water absorption, the volume increase resulting from swelling, the facility of degradation, and its biodegradability [10]. For example, when esterifying agents such as citric acid, fumaric acid, or 1-ethyl-3-(3-dimethylaminopropyl)carbodiimide are employed, high temperatures for the generation of the cross-linked network are required. Esterification occurs between the hydroxyl groups of the cellulose or its derivatives with the functional groups from the cross-linking agent. With respect to 1-ethyl-3-(3-dimethylaminopropyl)carbodiimide, its use generates efficient and environmentally friendly cross-linking of carboxyl and hydroxyl group with nontoxic urea derivatives; in addition, products of reaction are easily separable. When etherifying agents are used, such as epoxides, an alkaline medium (at pH 11) and a slightly high temperature of 60°C are required [16].

Chemical hydrogels also can be obtained from cellulose by esterifying with succinic anhydride and 1,2,3,4-butanetetracarboxylic dianhydride or by etherifying using epichlorohydrin [1]. The absorption capacity of CBHGs produced via catalytic esterification with succinic anhydride depends on the amount of agent employed, the solvent, and the reaction temperature. Generally, syntheses of these hydrogels are developed in the presence of 4-dimethylaminopyridine and a mixture of LiCl/N-methyl-2-pyrrolidone. On the other hand, 1,2,3,4-butanetetracarboxylic dianhydride has two acidic anhydrous groups available for reacting with cellulose; therefore, two carboxylate groups are formed while the cross-linking with the polymer chains occurs. If more cross-linking agent is added to the reaction system, then more water molecules will be absorbed. On the other hand, epichlorohydrin is a cross-linking agent commonly used for polysaccharides during the etherification reaction catalyzed by bases between the hydroxyl groups of cellulose [1]. A good example of the use of this cross-linking agent is the work performed by Peng et al., who synthesized a superabsorbent hydrogel from a chemical cross-linking process with epichlorohydrin using cellulose modified with quaternary ammonium groups in aqueous NaOH/urea solution, reaching desirable properties for hydrogels such as high mechanical resistance, biocompatibility, and antibacterial activity against *Saccharomyces cerevisiae* [27, 32].

13.3.2.2 Physical CBHGs

Physical hydrogels can be obtained from cellulose derivatives like methyl-, hydroxypropyl-, hydroxypropyl methyl-, and sodium carboxymethyl cellulose because strongly interacting polymer chains permit the physical reticulation and consequent hydrogel formation. These materials are physically gelled due to two factors; the first is the noncovalent interaction between polymer chains, and the second is the physical impediment that restricts the mobility of the chains because they are entangled between them. Nevertheless, if the tangle of chains increases, then the hydrogel decreases its hydration ability as a result of the restriction in the mobility of the chains, which is associated with less swelling. The temperature at which this transition occurs depends on the type and degree of substitution presented by the cellulose-derived polymer, since this degree is directly associated with changes in the hydrophobic character of the polymer network and, consequently, with the hydrophobic character that is inversely related to the temperature required for the formation of hydrogel. Thus, freezing and subsequent defrosting process generate microcrystals forming the polymer network, being an optimal method for the improvement of the mechanical properties by easy control of temperature or time. To obtain products for biomedical applications, a variant of the previous process has been developed and is based on the addition of salts to the polymer solution for the decreasing of the hydration level. However, this type of physical hydrogel can be easily and excessively degraded under certain conditions, so they should be evaluated previous to their use in vivo, even when a cross-linking reaction is seen to be favored by the physiological environment [10, 16].

CBHGs have the advantage that their abundant hydroxyl groups cause numerous inter- and intramolecular hydrogen bonds between the polymer chains; as a result of these interactions, the insolubility in water is achieved, as well as a limited solubility in ethanol and methanol that are solvents easing the physical cross-linking. Thus, dispersive molecular interactions such as Van der Waals forces, London dispersion forces, and hydrogen bonds promote the physical entanglements. CBHGs can be obtained from chemical dissolution with ionic liquids, urea, 4-methylmorpholine 4-oxide, bacterial cellulose, and LiCl/dimethylacetamide to break the hydroxyl at position C-6 with the subsequent formation of hydrogen bonds. In this way, Cl$^-$ ions interact with hydroxyl groups through ion-dipole forces with free dimethylacetamide molecules. On the other hand, when dissolution is performed using 4-methylmorpholine 4-oxide, it is imperative to control the water amount, because at 100°C, the 4-methylmorpholine 4-oxide molecules replace the water molecules trapped by cellulose, whereas at 150°C, the crystalline structure is destroyed and a homogeneous dissolution is obtained [8, 16].

When bacterial cellulose is used as a material to develop the hydrogel, notable improvements in its purity, resistance, thermostability, and high biocompatibility are obtained [1]. In addition, it has been described that bacterial CBHGs properties can be improved by mixing cellulosic material with other biopolymers such as chitosan, gelatin, or starch, among others [16]. Chunshom et al. published the synthesis of blends based on bacterial lyophilized CBHGs and poly(vinyl alcohol) and suggested that it is a promissory material for application in pharmaceutical products. According to researchers, hydrogen bonds were formed in the cross-linked network of the biopolymeric mixture, being thermostable up to a temperature of 200°C and presenting an optimal swelling capacity [33].

Physical CBHGs can also be achieved from cellulose derivatives like hydroxypropyl cellulose and methylcellulose in a mixture of NaOH/thiourea. In particular, methylcellulose is an optimal cellulose derivative when the hydrogel is desired to respond to variations in temperature [1]. Hydrogels based on carboxymethyl cellulose are obtained from physical cross-linking by hydrogen bonds between the polymer chains. In 2015, Zheng et al. described the synthesis of physical hydrogels from sodium carboxymethyl cellulose pastes by immersion during a certain period of time in citric acid; see Fig. 13.4A. These hydrogels were transparent with optimal mechanical properties and good stretching capacity as illustrated in Fig. 13.4B [34, 35].

13.4 Stimuli-responsive CBHGs

In nature, there are numerous phenomena occurring due to the need to maintain an optimal functioning of an organism, or system, in response to environmental stimulus [16]. Investigations in the last few years, mainly for biomedical applications, have had as an object of analysis the study and development of hydrogels with the ability to change their properties, such as their swelling and porosity power, when external physical factors such as light, ultrasonic waves, electric and magnetic fields, or chemical factors such as pH, ionic strength, humidity, and concentration of specific species are varied. Due to the great versatility and properties of cellulose polymers and their derivatives, stimuli-responsive CBHGs have been obtained and studied to determine the influence of cellulose in physical, chemical, and functional properties of these smart systems [16, 28, 36].

13.4.1 CBHGs with physical stimulus response

Thermosensitive CBHGs, as their name suggests, are those whose properties are altered when the temperature of the external environment varies. The effect of temperature can be directed to produce changes of

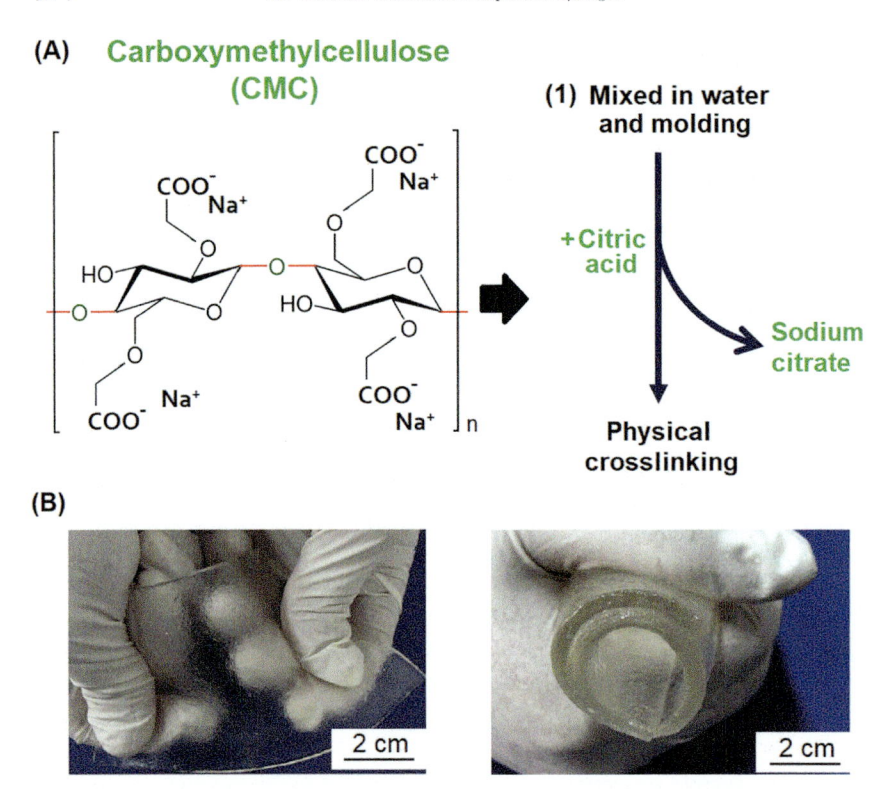

FIG. 13.4   Physical hydrogel based on carboxymethyl cellulose. (A) Two steps to obtain the hydrogel. The first consists of preparation of the carboxymethyl cellulose paste from respective powder with water and subsequent acidification in citric acid. (B) Transparent physical hydrogel with good stretching capacity and optimal mechanical properties. *Reprinted from Zheng WJ, Gao J, Wei Z, Zhou J, Chen YM, Facile fabrication of self-healing carboxymethyl cellulose hydrogels. Eur Polym J 2015;75: 514–22. Copyright (2015) with permission from Elsevier.*

some physical or chemical property like size or solubility, respectively; but also, the change can be reversible or irreversible. Thermosensitive CBHGs are classified as negative thermosensitive hydrogels when they are obtained in a higher temperature of low critical solution temperature (LCST) (since, at a lower temperature, all components are soluble with each other), where the polymer undergoes phase separation, which gives rise to the hydrogel. On the contrary, hydrogels that collapse at temperatures below the upper critical solution temperature (UCST) are called positive thermosensitive hydrogels. Thermosensitive CBHGs are characterized by hydrophobic groups that also affect UCST and LCST when they vary [36, 37].

Natural polymers that form the basis of cross-linked networks in thermosensitive hydrogels must have a thermal response, such as starch, chitosan, gelatin/collagen, and of course, cellulose [37]. When the LCST is reached, water-water and polymer-polymer interactions predominate over polymer-water interactions. This generates a hydrophobic structure due to dehydration in the transition, lowering the sol-gel transition temperature [27]. These hydrogels have been applied on oral- and transdermal-drug development and cancer drug therapies [36]. Cellulose and its derivatives are not used frequently because they have high LCST (for example, methylcellulose's LSCT is 60°C-80°C) [38]; however, one of the first and most famous thermosensitive CBHGs was synthesized by Liu et al. (2004) [39]. In this work, hydrogels based on methylcellulose and poly(N-isopropylacrylamide) were synthesized by free radical polymerization using N,N,N',N'-tetramethyl ethylenediamine and ammonium persulfate as activator and initiator, respectively. This hydrogel presented a thermosensitive behavior depending on contents of methylcellulose; in this way, it was observed that, if methylcellulose content was low, then the LCST was decreased. The transition time was about 1 min and very close to body temperature, being therefore a suitable material for biomedical applications [39].

On the other hand, electrical-field-sensitive hydrogels are characterized by undergoing changes of size and/or shape after swelling and deflation when they are exposed to electric fields; usually for this behavior to be evidenced it is necessary to introduce the hydrogel in an electrolyte solution, thus, when the system solution-hydrogel is subjected to an electric field, an organized and directional movement of the ions generates opposite potential and electrophoretic interactions causing the contraction of the hydrogel. In addition, this produces an imbalance in charges, causing a difference in osmotic pressure, therefore, the hydrogel will absorb water by electroosmotic movement; thus, by this mechanism, the cross-linked network swells when the osmotic pressure increases, and decreases its volume when the pressure decrease [40]. Also, the electrically sensitive property can be associated with ionic strength, pH, field strength, and the time in which the hydrogel is exposed to the stimulus [37]. Polymers such as chitosan, poly(acrylamide), poly(2-hydroxyethyl methacrylate), poly(acrylic acid), and poly(2-(acrylamide)-2-methylpropanesulfonic acid) have been reported as constituent chains of hydrogel networks with responses to electric fields [41]. With respect to electrically sensitive CBHGs, Shi et al. published the synthesis of a hydrogel composed of nanofibers from bacterial cellulose with an anionic polysaccharide such as sodium alginate, which is also pH sensitive, and its behavior in drug release such as ibuprofen was evaluated. The variations of electric field intensity from 0.0 to 0.5 V caused a greater water absorption by the hydrogel, increasing its size up to 14 times the initial one. These hydrogels were a novelty and are a promising material for drug delivery [40].

When a magnetic field is applied, only hydrogels with magnetic additives such as cobalt or magnetite nanoparticles respond to that stimulus. Hydrogels sensitive to magnetic fields generally are developed with magnetite due to their superparamagnetic properties, as well as being friendly to the environment. These additives cause hydrogels to act in synchrony with the direction of a magnetic field applied wirelessly, so they are employed when accuracy is relevant as in the design of drug delivery systems and artificial muscles [40]. Liu et al. proved that, when magnetite is coated with chitosan-CBHG and dispersed in ionic liquids, it can be considered to be an optimal material for heavy metal adsorption; see Fig. 13.5. These hydrogels showed affinity with ions such as Zn^{2+}, Mn^{2+}, and Ni^{2+} [42].

A light-responsive hydrogel must also contain additives known as photoactivators. Hydrogels with light response have modifications in their physicochemical properties, and the speed at which this phenomenon occurs will depend on the intensity absorbed and the quantum efficiency. The latter depends on the wavelength, the depth at which the light penetrates, and mainly on reagents concentrations, since it is only valid at high concentrations. As the absorbed intensity and quantum efficiency are greater, the observed response will be faster, and the change in the hydrogel's physicochemical properties will be effective [16]. The response manifested by this type of hydrogel will depend on the polymer chain nature constituting the network and can be based on processes such as photoisomerization, photodimerization, photoconjugation, and photocleavage [37]. In photoisomerization, for example, a *cis-trans* change occurs, which influences polarity and, consequently, its hydrophobicity, such as azobenzene compound hydrogels, which produce a response when irradiated with wavelength light inside of the 360 nm range (*trans*-to-*cis*) and 440 nm (*cis*-to-*trans*) [16, 27]. Information about light-sensitive CBHGs is scarce; however, these can become promising materials for engineering or biomedical applications.

13.4.2 CBHGs with chemical stimulus response

The pH-sensitive hydrogels are polymer networks absorbing water in function of pH of the medium, being obviously a property directly connected with the functional groups on polymer chains since these should accept or donate protons as the pH is perturbed [28, 41]. In general, monomers constituting the hydrogel are characterized by having amino or carboxylic acid groups on their structure. However, it is important to indicate that any hydrogel can respond to variations of pH when some ionic group is incorporated into its structure [37]. The mechanism by which these hydrogels act is related to the functional groups on the side chains in the polymer backbone; thus, functional groups are ionized by the effect of pH producing a redistribution of the charges to guarantee

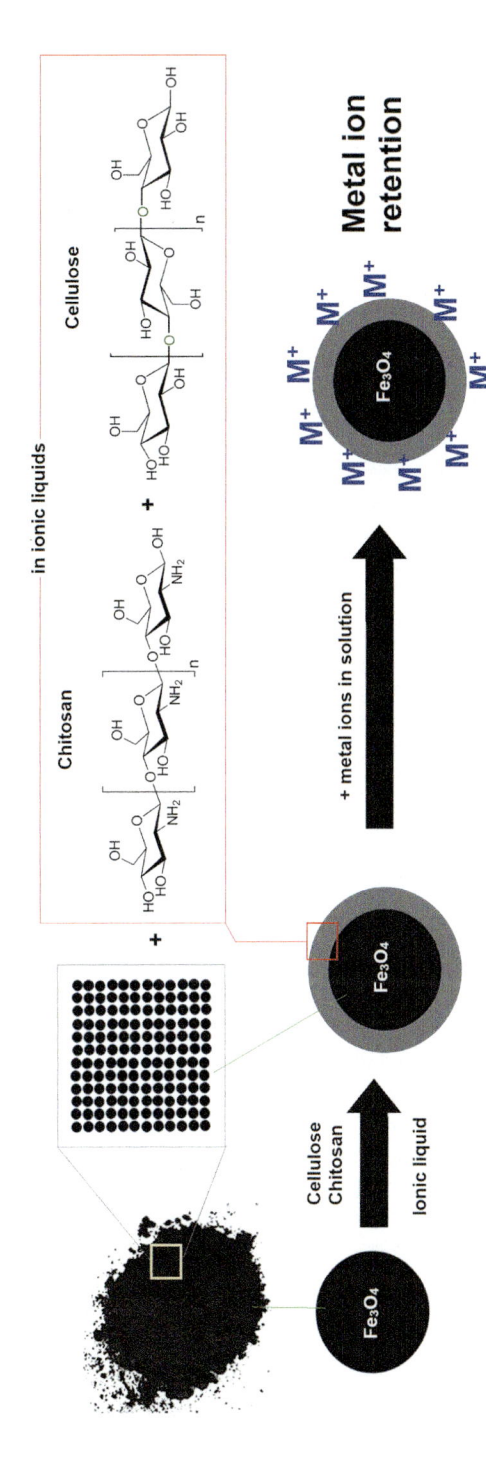

FIG. 13.5 Illustration of cellulose and chitosan hydrogel with response to magnetic field for heavy metal adsorption.

electroneutrality. The appearance of charges produces electrostatic repulsion between them, and because these are found fixed on the polymer chains, these are expanded to decrease the electrostatic repulsion generated. As a consequence, water absorption is favored, and hydrodynamic volume of the hydrogel is increased. pH-sensitive hydrogels are classified as anionic and cationic, and the magnitude of the effect on the hydrogel will depend mainly on the dissociation of their functional groups and their corresponding apparent pKa. When functional groups are anionic, pH must be larger than pKa to generate negatively charged groups, while for cationic groups the inverse behavior is expected [41, 43].

Biopolymers such as alginate, gelatin, chitosan, and albumin have been used to obtain hydrogels that respond to pH variations [41]. Conversely, cellulose cannot be directly used to obtain pH-sensitive hydrogels, since its multiple hydroxyl groups are unable to respond to acidity variations. As a consequence, the route for obtaining `pH-sensitive CBHGs is usually based on the functionalization of cellulose chains with carboxylic acid groups, amines, or any other ionizable group (see Fig. 13.6) [27]. pH-sensitive CBHGs are promissory materials for biomedical applications in vivo since these could control the release of a certain drug due to changes of acidity in the application zone by the effect of pathological conditions or by inherent condition (e.g., pH acid of the stomach) [27, 36].

Another way in which hydrogels respond to changes in their environment is when they undergo some modification resulting from the presence

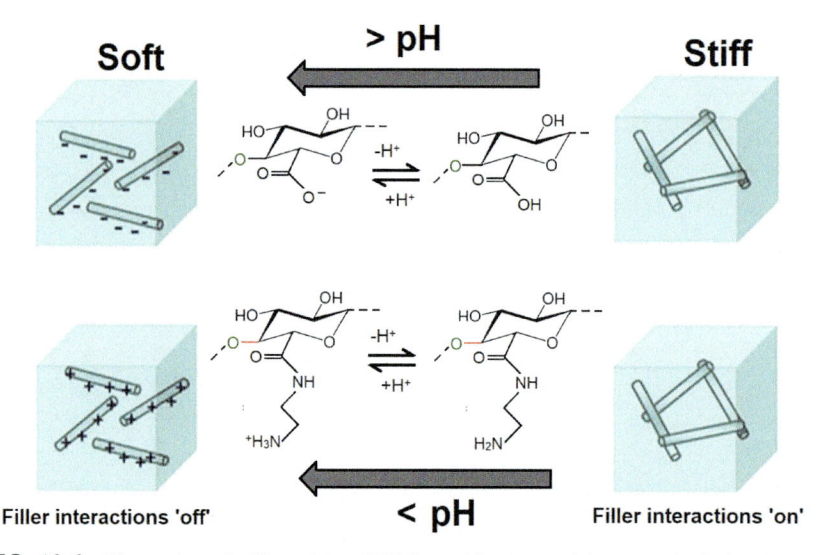

FIG. 13.6   Illustration of pH-sensitive CBHG resulting in modification of cellulose by insertion of carboxylic acid groups (upper) and amine groups (lower). *Reprinted from Chen Y. Hydrogels based on natural polymers; 2020, p. 175. Copyright (2020) with permission from Elsevier.*

of salts or counterions. The main reason why salt-responsive hydrogels exhibit this behavior is due to the changes of osmotic pressure, which is directed toward the conservation of the balance between among ionic concentrations inside and outside of the hydrogel. Thus, if the internal ionic concentration is increased, then hydrogel swells, whereas it deflates when the external ionic concentration is increased [43]. Polyelectrolytes based on sodium carboxymethyl cellulose are expected to be effective for the development of salt-responsive hydrogels [44]. Hydrogels based on sodium carboxymethyl cellulose cross-linked with fumaric acid were shown to have high water absorption capacity, which depended on the charge of the metal ions in the medium. Those that were in the presence of Na^+ had greater swelling than hydrogels in an Al^{3+} solution. On the other hand, Chang et al. published the development of salt-sensitive CBHGs from carboxymethyl cellulose and quaternized cellulose with epichlorohydrin in the presence of NaOH that exhibited a smart behavior in aqueous solutions of NaCl, $FeCl_3$, and $CaCl_2$, where quaternized cellulose was added to produce the charge regulation [45].

Also, hydrogels can respond to redox systems by incorporating redox centers into their structure to use reversible oxidation-reduction cycles to produce changes of hydrogel properties [46]. Redox-responsive hydrogels are of interest in biomedical research because, in organisms, the regulation and redox balance are relevant for optimal cellular functioning; a redox imbalance has been associated with diseases such as cancer, diabetes, fibrosis, and neurodegenerative diseases. In the area of controlled drug release, the synthesis of these hydrogels is of interest since they can release drugs in places with high redox potential [47]. For example, Li et al. reported the synthesis of a redox-responsive CBHG with thiol-disulfide groups from carboxymethyl cellulose nanocrystals that were functionalized with L-cysteine through amide bonds. According to the researchers, the resulting hydrogel responded correctly to redox changes. It is expected that this material will serve in the adsorption of organic dyes; however, it can be extended to drug release and tissue engineering applications [48].

13.4.3 Obtention methods

Fig. 13.7 shows the design and obtention of stimuli-responsive CBHGs. It can be seen that the strategies are focused in two ways: (i) the inclusion of natural or physically modified cellulose (dimensions and physical presentation, for example, nanoparticles or fibrils) within of a matrix, together with polymers and/or chemical species that have a response to a certain stimulus, for example, synthetic polymers, peptides, nanoparticles, ligands, among others [42, 49–52], and (ii) chemical modification of cellulose through redox, radical, or condensation reactions to obtain derivatives, such as methylcellulose, carboxymethyl cellulose, hydroxypropyl

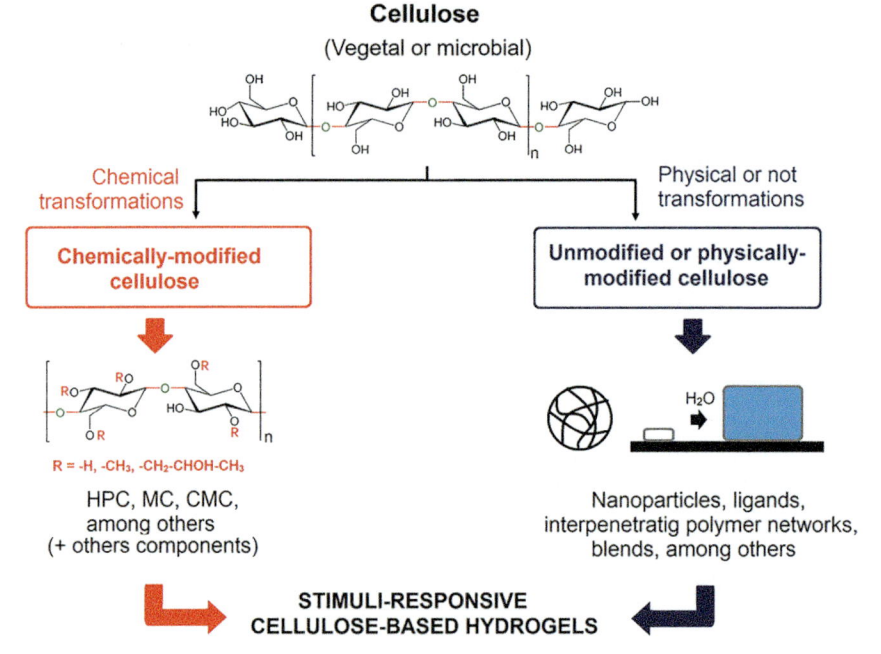

FIG. 13.7 Schematic representation of the general methodologies for obtaining stimuli-responsive CBHGs.

methylcellulose, or any other functionalized cellulosic material with the addition (or not) of other components to obtain hydrogels with stimulus responses [34, 45, 48, 53].

Cellulose can be used as a filler material of hydrogel to obtain composite and nanocomposite materials. By this approach, mechanical and physical properties of hydrogels can be improved. Commonly improved properties include pore size and structure, swelling degree, viscoelasticity, and self-healing properties, among others [54, 55]. When cellulose is used as a filler, physical interactions between the hydrogel components are promoted such as hydrogen bonds, and Van der Waals and dispersion forces. For example, recently obtaining CBHG from celery cellulose by a slow gelation process was described [56]. Initially, cellulose was dissolved in a solution of LiCl/dimethylacetamide. Subsequently, the resulting solution was subjected to an ethanol atmosphere producing the gelation of the cellulose gradually over a time of 24 h (see Fig. 13.8). The resulting CBHG showed ultrasound sensitivity and was successfully applied in controlled release of short chain fatty acids [56].

On the other hand, the dispersion of cellulosic material within a monomer solution and its subsequent chemical polymerization has allowed the obtaining of stimuli-responsive CBHGs. Thus, Sun et al. developed

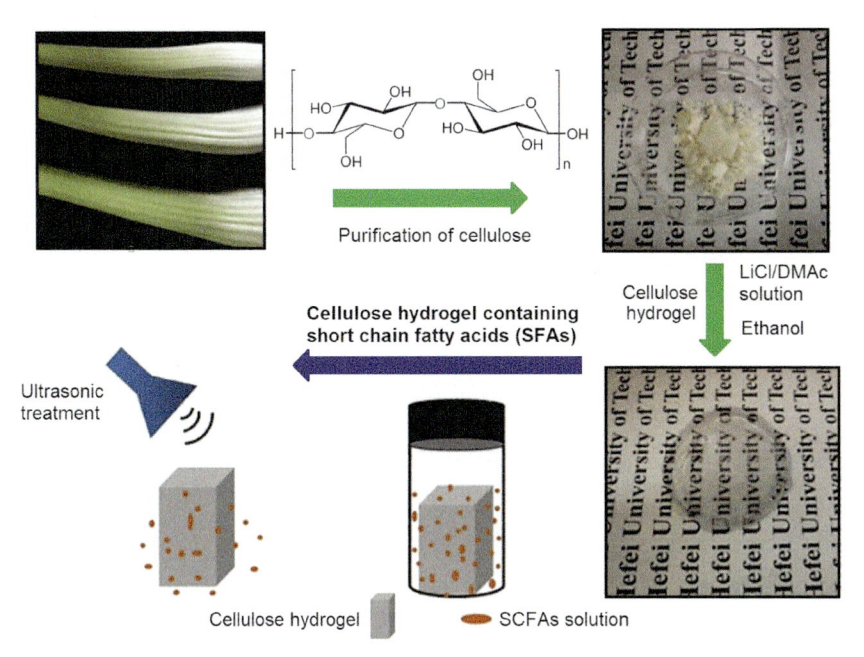

FIG. 13.8 Schematic representation of the synthesis of a celery cellulose hydrogel for fatty-acids delivery assisted by ultrasound. *Reprinted from Yan L, Wang L, Gao S, Liu C, Zhang Z, Ma A, Zheng L. Celery cellulose hydrogel as carriers for controlled release of short-chain fatty acid by ultrasound. Food Chem, 2020;309:125717. Copyright (2020) with permission from Elsevier.*

a composite-type hydrogel based on cellulose nanocrystals and poly(*N*-isopropylacrylamide); for that, *N*-isopropylacrylamide was polymerized by free radical polymerization in the presence of cellulose nanocrystals using isopropanol as solvent; in addition, polymerization was initiated using ultraviolet-visible light. The hydrogel showed a thermoresponse; but also, optical and mechanical properties were controlled by the number of cellulose nanocrystals added in the obtaining process. Similarly, thermosensitive hydrogels have been developed using cellulose microfibers and poly(*N*-isopropylacrylamide) [55, 57].

The physical coating of cellulosic material with some type of functional polymer has been another strategy for the development of stimuli-responsive CBHGs. Wang et al. developed pH-sensitive CBHGs from microcrystalline cellulose, Konjac glucomannan, and poly(dopamine). Initially, microcrystalline cellulose was coated with poly(dopamine) by oxidative polymerization of dopamine with the microcellulosic material in aqueous solution. Subsequently, the inclusion of poly(dopamine)-coated microcrystalline cellulose in a solution with Konjac glucomannan allowed the obtaining of hydrogels with physical cross-linking by hydrogen bonds through a process of heating and subsequent cooling, as shown in Fig. 13.9. The hydrogels showed a pH-dependent release of ofloxacin, associated with the formation of a hydrogen-bonded network at low pH, while this network was ruptured at neutral pH [58].

When cellulose is chemically modified, it provides its functionality for the developed hydrogels in terms of producing a response to one or several stimuli; also modification can be directed toward the improvement of mechanical and physical properties of a hydrogel [27]. In this way, it has been possible to obtain "multiresponsive" or polyfunctional smart hydrogel [59]. This is of utmost importance because, due to the versatility of structures, polymers and other types of functional species that can be obtained through chemical modification included within CBHGs allows open countless applications for these types of materials. In this way, Karzar and Mahkam prepared CBHGs from carboxymethyl cellulose nanocrystals, sodium alginate, chitosan, and magnetite nanoparticles (Fe_3O_4) (see Fig. 13.10A) [60]. Initially, carboxymethyl cellulose crystals were obtained by two steps: (i) the acid hydrolysis of alpha-cellulose and (ii) the carboxymethylation of the nanocrystals using monochloroacetic acid. Subsequently, nanoparticles of Fe_3O_4 were synthesized in a dispersion of carboxymethyl cellulose crystals using a chemical reduction in a basic ammonia solution, obtaining "magnetized" carboxymethyl cellulose crystals. Dispersion of magnetized crystals/sodium alginate were added drop by drop to a solution of $CaCl_2$ allowing the obtaining of physically cross-linked hydrogels by electrostatic interactions. Finally, the hydrogels were physically coated with chitosan (see Fig. 13.10B). It was observed that the hydrogels showed a release of dexamethasone phosphate controlled by pH changes; this behavior was explained by the presence of two types of functional groups on the polymeric structure (amino and carboxylic acid groups). But also, a characteristic property of these materials was their response to the presence of a magnetic field (see Fig. 13.10C).

Dutta et al. developed CBHGs based on carboxymethyl cellulose and poly(N-isopropylacrylamide) using chemical pathways [59, 60]. The methodology was based on radical polymerization with two different approaches: (i) the formation of a polymer network by copolymerization of methacrylate carboxymethyl cellulose, N,N'-methylene-bis-acrylamide or N,N'-bis-(acryloyl)cysteamine, and N-isopropylacrylamide; and (ii) the formation of semi-interpenetrating polymer networks by polymerization of N,N'-methylene-bis-acrylamide and N-isopropylacrylamide in a carboxymethyl cellulose solution. It was determined that the greater the amount of carboxymethyl cellulose incorporated into the hydrogel structure, the faster the swelling kinetics were observed due to the increase of polymer hydrophilicity. In addition, it was observed that the formation of hydrogels via semi-interpenetrating polymer networks from N,N'-bis-(acryloyl)cysteamine, nonmethacrylate carboxymethyl cellulose,

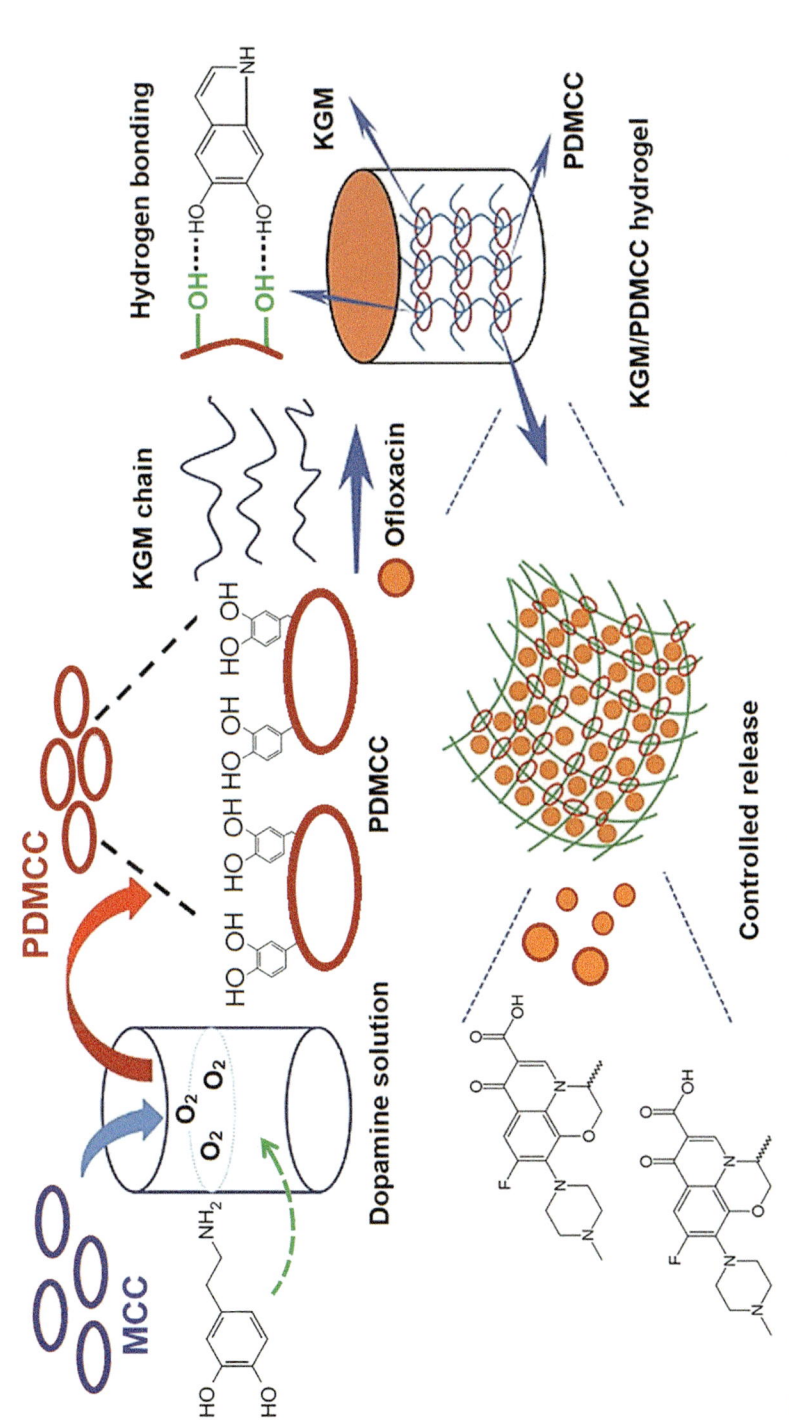

FIG. 13.9 Schematic representation of obtaining hydrogels from Konjac glucomannan and poly(dopamine)-coated microcrystalline cellulose through a physical process. Reprinted from Wang L, Du Y, Yuan Y, Mu RJ, Gong J, Ni Y, Wu C. Mussel-inspired fabrication of konjac glucomannan/microcrystalline cellulose intelligent hydrogel with pH-responsive sustained release behavior. Int J Biol Macromol, 2018;113:285–293. Copyright (2018) with permission from Elsevier.

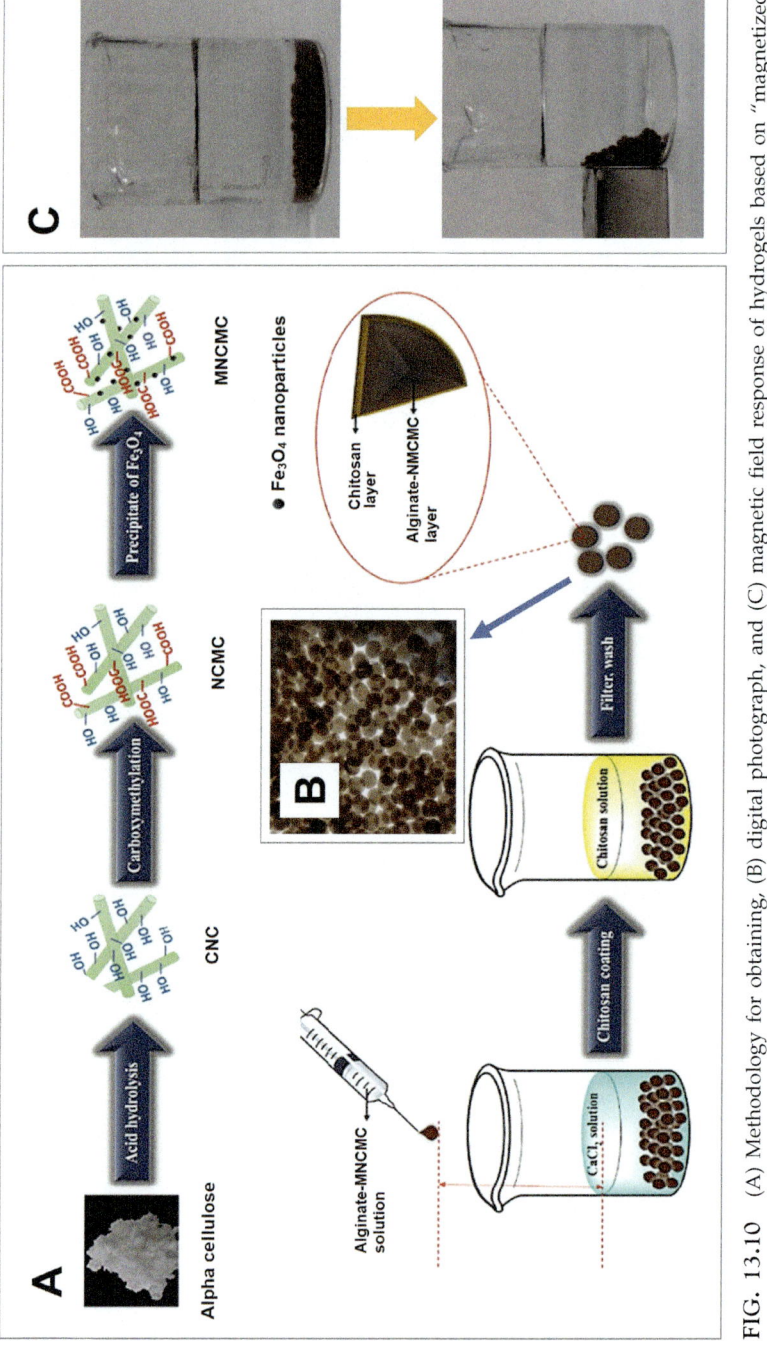

FIG. 13.10 (A) Methodology for obtaining, (B) digital photograph, and (C) magnetic field response of hydrogels based on "magnetized" carboxymethyl cellulose nanocrystals, sodium alginate, and chitosan. *Adapted from Karzar M, Malikam M. Magnetic nano carboxymethyl cellulose-alginate/chitosan hydrogel beads as biodegradable devices for controlled drug delivery. Int J Biol Macromol 2019;135:829–38. Copyright (2019) with permission from Elsevier.*

and poly(N-isopropylacrylamide) allows the obtaining of polyfunctional smart hydrogels with response to pH, temperature, and redox processes. Multiresponsiveness was explained by the presence of carboxylic acid and thiol groups on the structure of the hydrogel. Other types of chemical modification have been used to obtain stimuli-responsive CBHGs, such as oxidation of cellulosic material to generate aldehyde groups in their structure and cross-linking by imine bonds, functionalization with quaternary ammonium groups through substitution reactions, inclusion of disulfide bonds by chemical cross-linking with molecules of that nature, and chemical functionalization with chelating groups for cross-linking by coordination bonds, among others [34, 53, 61–63].

13.4.4 Characterization methods

Similar to the characterization of other types of hydrogels, characterization methods of stimuli-responsive CBHGs can be classified as: (i) structural or chemical characterization, (ii) mechanical or physical characterization, and (iii) functional characterization. However, it is important to indicate that this classification is only in a practical sense, and therefore other classifications could be defined depending on the desired objective. In our case, it is important for one stimuli-responsive CBHG to describe its chemical structure and nature, its reactivity or chemical affinity, the study of physicochemical properties, the determination of mechanical resistance, its thermal stability, and those characteristics associated directly with its application [64–66].

13.4.4.1 Structural characterization

Structural characterization aims to obtain information about the chemical structure of polymers or about any other component, constituting the hydrogel to confirm that it was correctly incorporated in the polymeric matrix and its content. This characterization focuses on the qualitative and quantitative description of the hydrogel. A wide number of techniques and methods can be employed, including spectroscopic techniques such as Raman spectroscopy, Fourier transform infrared spectroscopy (FTIR), and nuclear magnetic resonance (NMR) in solid-state.

FTIR and Raman spectroscopy have similar approaches, since they allow determined characteristic bonds in the hydrogel structure by absorption of radiation associated with vibrational transitions. Both techniques turn out to be complementary, since FTIR appreciates spectral bands associated with vibrational modes that lead to changes in the total dipole moment, to identify bonds like O–H, C–H, C=O, and C–O. Conversely, Raman spectroscopy appreciates spectral bands associated with vibration modes that lead to changes in the molecule polarizability to identify bonds like S–S, C–C, and C–H [66–69]. Many vibrational transitions absorb infrared radiation in only one of the two techniques, making them complementary. Generally, in these techniques, the spectral comparison of the final material with the starting reagents is used to verify the adequate formation of the hydrogel [53, 62]. For example, Liu et al. carried out a successful structural characterization of a pH- and redox-sensitive hydrogel by FTIR and Raman spectroscopy (see Fig. 13.11A and B) [70]. The hydrogel was based on cellulose acetoacetate with chemical cross-linking using cysteamine hydrochloride. It was possible to identify bands associated with stretching vibrations of O–H, C=O, and C–H bonds present in the cellulose acetoacetate structure. In addition, it was corroborated by the presence of disulfide and enamine bonds by the identification of new spectral bands after cysteamine hydrochloride cross-linking. Its relevant mention, in most cases of multicomponent materials such as hydrogels composed by cellulose and their derivatives, is expected that the infrared and/or Raman spectra present overlapped signals; this can be solved by employing derivative spectroscopy. A relatively new tool is the functionally enhancement derivative spectroscopy (FEDS), a simple algorithm that permits the deconvolution of spectra to obtain the signals of overlapped bands. This tool have been demonstrated effective in the deconvolution of the spectra of a complex matrix such as a mixture of humified substances of soils, a mixture of substance with similar regions of infrared absorption, and multicomponent polyurea-base hydrogels [71, 72].

On the other hand, the CBHG's insolubility in different types of organic solvents due to their high degree of cross-linking has directed attention toward the use of solid-state NMR, mostly carbon-13 (^{13}C NMR) to obtain information about different carbons atoms associated with cellulose and other components of the polymer structure [73]. For example, Dai et al. reported the successful characterization through solid-state ^{13}C NMR of stimuli-responsive CBHGs (see Fig. 13.11C) based on carboxymethyl cellulose obtained from pineapple peel, acrylic acid, acrylamide, and graphene oxide. Signals associated with carbons in the hydrogel structure were identified but also signals from methylene carbons ($-CH_2-$) associated with the acrylic acid and acrylamide polymer chains, allowing corroboration of their correct insertion in the structure of the hydrogel [74].

The description of solid structure and morphology of CBHGs have been extensively carried out by transmission electron microscopy (TEM) and scanning electron microscopy (SEM). Both techniques employ the interaction of the sample with an electron beam to construct an image of its structure. Through SEM, the information about the polymer surface is obtained, while internal structure information is obtained by TEM, as exemplified in Fig. 13.11D [75]. Lu et al. characterized the morphological structure of a hydrogel based on TEMPO-oxidized cellulose nanofibrils,

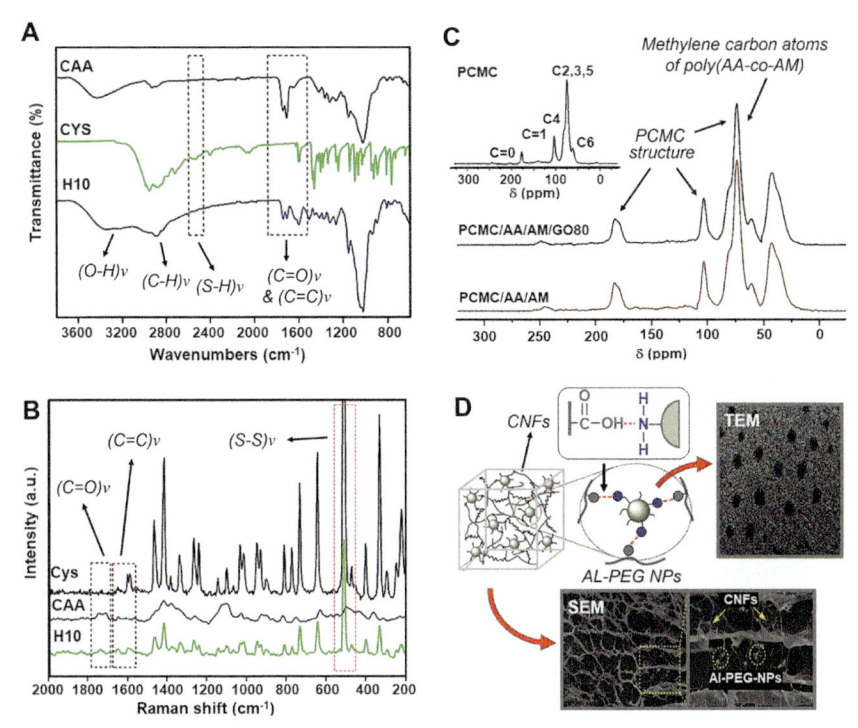

FIG. 13.11 Examples of chemical and morphological characterization of some CBHGs. (A) FTIR and (B) Raman comparative spectra of cysteamine hydrochloride, cellulose acetoacetate, and obtained hydrogel by chemical cross-linking with cysteamine hydrochloride designated as H10. (C) Comparative spectra of solid state ^{13}C NMR for a hydrogel synthetized from carboxymethyl cellulose obtained from pineapple peel, acrylic acid, acrylamide, and graphene oxide, and (D) TEM/SEM characterization of hydrogels obtained by cellulose nanofibrils and lignin/amine-terminated polyethylene glycol nanoparticles (*v: stretching vibration; δ: chemical displacement). *Adapted from Lu J, Zhu W, Dai L, Si C, Ni Y. Fabrication of thermo- and pH-sensitive cellulose nanofibrils-reinforced hydrogel with biomass nanoparticles. Carbohydr Polym 2019;215:289–95. Copyright (2019) with permission from Elsevier; Liu H, Rong L, Wang B, Xie R, Sui X, Xu H, Zhang L, Zhong Y, Mao Z. Facile fabrication of redox/pH dual stimuli responsive cellulose hydrogel. Carbohydr Polym 2017;176:299–306. Copyright (2017) with permission from Elsevier; and Dai H, Zhang H, Ma L, Zhou H, Yu Y, Guo T, Zhang Y, Huang H. Green pH/ magnetic sensitive hydrogels based on pineapple peel cellulose and polyvinyl alcohol: synthesis, characterization and naringin prolonged release. Carbohydr Polym 2019;209:51–61. Copyright (2019) with permission from Elsevier.*

poly(N-isopropylacrylamide), and lignin/amine-terminated polyethylene glycol nanoparticles by means of SEM/TEM. Thus, it was possible to appreciate the dependence of nanoparticle diameters in the function of pH of the medium using TEM micrographs. Besides a mesh structure for the hydrogel, the "bridge" function of the lignin/amine-terminated polyethylene glycol nanoparticles were satisfactorily determined by SEM [76].

In addition to these, atomic force microscopy (AFM) and X-ray diffraction (XRD) are also employed in the structural characterization of CBHGs [77]. Through XRD, information on the crystallinity of the sample can be obtained, which has a direct influence on sample mechanical properties [78]. AFM allows study of the morphology of a hydrogel in its swollen state and to obtain 3D images of its surface contrary to TEM and SEM, which require a complete drying of the hydrogel and only 2D images can be obtained [66].

13.4.4.2 Mechanical characterization

The mechanical characterization of stimuli-responsive CBHGs aims to obtain information about the resistance of the material to external forces with stress-strain tests and dynamic mechanical analysis as the most used methodologies [79]. Both tests are carried out using rheometers. With stress-strain tests, the main measured property is the stiffness of the CBHG through Young's module, such that hydrogels with a greater Young's modulus are characterized by greater rigidity or greater resistance to deformation. Whereas through dynamic mechanical analysis, viscoelastic properties of the CBHG are quantified through three parameters: (i) shear storage module, (ii) shear loss modulus, and (iii) loss factor [66]. Thus, the study of rheological properties of CBHGs has allowed researchers to determine direct relationships between the mechanical behavior of hydrogels and its type of structure; for example, CBHGs with ionic, covalent, and hydrogen bond links have been evidenced that mechanical properties are controlled by a change in type and quantity of each component in the polymeric matrix [27, 80–82].

13.4.4.3 Functional characterization

Functional properties can be defined as those properties of CBHGs associated directly with their use. For example, if a hydrogel, or any material, is going to be used for regenerative medicine of tissue, then biocompatibility is an important property associated with that specific application (functional property), and consequently, the methods used to evaluate or measure the biocompatibility can be defined to be functional characterization methods. As it can be easily concluded, there are many methods, strategies, and approaches to evaluate a functional property, but it is extremely complex to achieve a complete description of them all. However, the main functional characterization for hydrogel is described here as well as the swelling degree and also an approximation of functional properties in the biomedical.

The more important functional properties of hydrogels are: (i) swelling degree, which is directly associated with their water absorption capacity, and (ii) hydrolytic stability. However, other important properties in more specific areas of application are directed to determine the influence of certain stimulus on hydrogel functional behavior (e.g., pH, temperature, presence of salts, etc.) [59]. Also, depending on the potential application for which the system was designed, the capacity of encapsulation release of drugs, cell encapsulation, antibacterial activity, cell culture, and/or biocompatibility assays, such as cell viability and hemocompatibility test, among others, can be defined as functional properties in the biomedical engineering field [74, 77].

First, swelling degree and water retention capacity are terms commonly used to quantitatively describe the hydrogel's ability for absorbing water. However, while "swelling capacity" is a concept that describes a change in the dimension of the hydrogel, "water retention capacity" is a term related to the affinity of the hydrogel for water and its ability to store it inside. Since the swelling capacity depends on the water retention capacity, both parameters can be used to describe the intrinsic nature of hydrogels, and therefore it is common for these terms to be used interchangeably. However, for some specialized studies, differentiation is required. For example, for experiments with a mixture of solvents, the water retention capacity cannot be directly related to the swelling capacity. A simple method for determining the water retention capacity is the gravimetric method, which is also often called the "tea bag method." The gravimetric method is based on the determination of the changes of mass between the swollen hydrogel and the dry hydrogel. Although it is a simple method, it is important to reduce the sources of error to obtain reproducible results. Common mistakes are incorporation into surface water results as a result of improper drainage, very short contact times, measurements not made at maximum swelling capacity, and a small number of replicates without having considered the heterogeneity of the sample. This is common when the highly heterogeneous sample is mechanically crushed and sieved [2, 64]. Also, the swelling degree can be monitored over time (in days, generally) to obtain information of structure hydrolytic stability by variations in system components and environment conditions [53, 83].

On the other hand, studies of encapsulation release of drugs or model drugs are carried out through spectroscopic techniques due to the high sensitivity of these methods. For drug-loading experiments, a known amount of hydrogel is added to a solution containing a known concentration of the target drug. Later, hydrogel is usually removed and the drug contents remaining are quantified. Note that, for many applications, it is very important to warrant the amount of drug inside the hydrogel; as a consequence, before drug-loading experiments, it is recommended to measure the water absorption capacity at working conditions. Moreover, the amount of drug incorporated in the hydrogel can be affected by properties of the hydrogel and also by properties associated with the experimental design. For example, when the dried hydrogel is added to the drug dissolution, initially, the drug entering the hydrogel is mainly promoted by the flux of water. Thus, it is equivalent to take a fraction of the dissolution and incorporate it into the interior of the hydrogel; as a consequence, the change of drug concentration inside the hydrogel and in the dissolution is zero. However, in a second stage, it is possible that the diffusion mechanism promotes the entering or exiting of drugs from the hydrogel to dissolution or from dissolution to the hydrogel, respectively. The direction of drug flux in this second stage is determined by chemical potentials of the drug. Otherwise, if the amount of solution is established to be lower than the maximum water absorption capacity, then all drug dissolution is expected to be absorbed by a single mechanism (water flux). this case, the drug load in a specific amount of hydrogel is easily quantified. But also, a third design can be easily identified; note that hydrogel can be swelled previous to the addition of the drug solution. In this case, only diffusion mechanism is possible, and information obtained could be used to determine when water flux and diffusion mechanisms are consecutively acting [53, 74–77, 83–86].

On the other hand, drug-release experiments are performed by addition of loaded hydrogel in a dissolution or medium with a composition describing the best possible action site, or the working environment where the hydrogel will be applied. Note that, for these experiments, several experimental designs can also be carried out. For example, the drug-loaded hydrogel in its swelled state can be added to the target medium, dissolution as a simple example. In this case, the release is expected to occur by one or more mechanisms depending on the nature of the hydrogel and possible interactions between the hydrogel and the medium. Possible mechanisms are diffusion; chemical erodibility of the hydrogel structure by external factors, for example, pH; biochemical degradation by enzymatic activity; and water flux when hydrogel is added to a medium with a hydric potential lower than that contained in the hydrogel; among others. But another possibility is the addition of dried drug-loaded hydrogel, and as a consequence, when hydrogel is introduced to the target medium, it will absorb water, and therefore, only after hydration will the diffusion of the drug occur [53, 74–77, 83–86]. In addition, it is clear that the variation of environment properties and a certain stimulus allows us to determine its influence on the controlled drug release, and also it was concluded that researchers should carefully analyze what is the best design for the description of the functionality of hydrogel.

In the case of CBHGs developed for their application on tissue engineering, the determinations of encapsulation capacity and cell viability are carried out by subjecting the material to a suspension of target cells with the respective supplements for their growth. The hydrogel can encapsulate or support the cells by adhesion. Subsequently, the growth and cell morphology are monitored over time to determine its viability and system influence on its morphology [85, 86]. Additionally, it could be relevant to determine the biocompatibility of the hydrogel with biological fluids, such as blood components. In this sense, the hemocompatibility test consists of placing a determined amount of the material in contact with a blood solution, then the system is incubated and centrifuged. Later Drabkin's reagent is added to the supernatant, and the hemoglobin is oxidized to methemoglobin and complexed to cyanmethemoglobin, which absorbs in the visible region at 540 nm. Because of this, the substance can be quantified to determine the amount of red blood cells that suffer hemolysis [87]. There are other assays of interest when the material is obtained for medical applications; one of the most common is antibacterial activity that consists of determining bacterial growth in a strain in contact with the material. This can be performed by setting the inhibition halo in disk diffusion method or by the determining the optical density of a bacterial suspension by the McFarland's scale [3, 28, 72].

Other methods of functional characterization can be based on the monitoring of some properties that permit inferring the behavior of the hydrogel. These methods can be denominated to be semiempirical methods as they are based on models requiring input data for the computation and obtention of the results. For example, if it were in our interest to determine the potential interaction of hydrogel with biological fluids, one alternative is using a semiempirical approach. It could be the determination of the superficial energy of the hydrogel by Van Oss-Chaudhury-Good theory in conjunction with measures of contact angle, as these parameters have demonstrated a direct correlation with the prediction of the physisorption of biological substances, such as blood proteins. Finally, there are also several optic methods based on the use of an image and the digital analysis of them, usually by the use of specific algorithms. By this approach, it is possible to evaluate parameters such as particle size and shape distribution, surface anisotropy, porosity, and changes associated with fouling or biofouling, among others [12, 87].

13.5 Stimuli-responsive CBHGs for drug-controlled release

Since the beginning of the last decade, numerous stimuli-responsive CBHGs with potential applications as drug delivery systems have been developed, using a variety of functional and structural components of cellulose and its derivatives (see Table 13.1). Likewise, different types of model drugs with anticancer, anti-inflammatory, and antibacterial properties, among others, have been evaluated on the release process assisted by hydrogels and modulated by the exploitation of their sensitivity to a certain stimulus. Some drugs evaluated under this approach are insulin,

TABLE 13.1 Some works on cellulose-based stimuli-responsive hydrogels applied to drug delivery: pH, temperature (T), redox, ultrasound (US), and magnetic field (mf), among others.

Raw materials	Response to	Drug model	Administration route	Ref.
Bacterial cellulose, poly(acrylic acid)	pH	Insulin	Oral	[88]
Carboxymethyl cellulose, chitosan and cysteamine	Redox	5-Fluorouracil and tetracycline hydrochloride	Not established	[53]
Celery cellulose	US	Short-chain fatty acids	Not established	[56]
Konjac glucomannan, microcrystalline cellulose, poly(dopamine)	pH	Ofloxacin	Oral	[58]
"Methacrylated" carboxymethyl cellulose, poly(N-isopropylacrylamide)	pH, T, redox	Lysozyme	Not established	[59]
Carboxymethyl cellulose nanocrystals, magnetite, sodium alginate, chitosan	pH, mf	Dexamethasone	Oral	[60]
Cellulose acetoacetate, cysteamine	pH, redox	Rhodamine B	Not established	[70]
Nanocellulose, carboxymethyl cellulose, polyvinyl alcohol, magnetite	pH, mf	Naringin	Not established	[74]
Modified cellulose nanofibrils	pH	Doxorubicin	Not established	[80]
Cellulose nanofibrils, poly(dopamine)	pH, IR light	Tetracycline hydrochloride	Transdermal	[86]
Xanthan gum, methyl cellulose	T	Doxorubicin	Not established	[82]
Poly(acrylamidoglycolic acid), cellulose nanocrystals	pH	Sodium diclofenac	Oral	[83]
Chitosan, functionalized graphene, modified cellulose nanocrystals	pH	Doxorubicin and curcumin	Subcutaneous	[84]
Carboxymethyl cellulose, tobramycin, β-cyclodextrin	pH	Tobramycin and borneol	Transdermal	[89]
Ethyl cellulose, poly(N-isopropylacrylamide)	T	Rhodamine B and vitamin B12	Not established	[90]
Hydroxypropyl methylcellulose, cyclodextrin	T	Insulin	Subcutaneous	[91]
Carboxymethyl cellulose, 2-hydroxyethyl acrylate	pH	Naringenin	Transdermal	[92]
Cellulose, poly(4-vinylboronic acid)	pH, glucose	Insulin	Not established	[93]

doxorubicin, diclofenac, curcumin, vitamin B12, and short-chain fatty acids, among others. For this, the use of CBHGs can be considered to be "a versatile alternative" for drug-controlled release [34, 80, 83, 84, 89, 90]. Some works carried out on CBHGs with applications in smart drug delivery have been based on the chemical degradation of a hydrogel or in the transport controlled by some type of potential, usually, chemical potential; however, both the degradative processes as the transport can be modulated using some type of external stimulus [6, 91, 94]. For example, pH is a characteristic stimulus producing reversible and irreversible changes in the structure of CBHGs. Usually it is used for drug-controlled oral release by taking advantage of pH changes throughout the digestive system and in different body tissues resulting in some type of disease, while the temperature can be useful both for oral and transdermal release due to the gelation processes at body temperatures. Other stimuli frequently studied are the application of a magnetic field, an electric field, and some redox processes [27, 53, 58, 84, 91, 92, 94–96].

Stimuli-responsive CBHGs with an ability to respond to two or more stimuli is another important approach for drug-controlled release systems because of higher control of the release rate and processes, which are a result of a combination of various types of stimuli (both chemical and physical) for a single objective [59]. This strategy has been considered for increasing the site specificity and effectiveness of the drug in the treatment of disease; in addition, it has the advantage to allow different administration routes for the same hydrogel. Thus, stimuli-responsive CBHGs with physical and chemical responses are usually designed for two or three stimuli, e.g., pH/magnetic field and pH/infrared light (physical and chemical stimuli); pH/redox reactions (two chemical stimuli); and pH/temperature/redox processes (three stimuli, one physical stimulus and two chemical stimuli) [59, 62, 74, 86].

13.5.1 Stimuli-responsive CBHGs for oral delivery

Oral drug delivery is one of the most widely used methodologies for drug administration to humans and animals. The importance of this delivery route is the result of the availability of different sites for drug absorption including mouth, esophagus, stomach, small intestine, and large intestine, but also it is a simple, fast, and not painful administration route. The drug-controlled release using stimuli-responsive CBHGs has been based on the use of changes of properties along this path, mainly enzymatic activity and pH changes. In both cases, enzymes and pH are external factors that promote the degradation of the drug carrier (i.e., release mechanisms by erosion of the polymer matrix), which in this case is the hydrogel. However, if the drug reaches the small intestine, the hydrogel must not only act as a drug transporter but must also protect the active component from enzyme activity and heartburn. Therefore, it is clear that there is no single method for the manufacture of stimuli-responsive CBHGs, since the purpose of the active ingredient (drug) and the characteristics of the disease to be treated influence the characteristics that must be borne in mind when the hydrogel is designed [97, 98]. In this way, the drug administration assisted by stimuli-responsive CBHGs makes it possible to protect the drug and release it in the intestinal tract, which presents less severe biological conditions since it is characterized by a neutral to basic pH and low enzymatic activity. Likewise, the intestinal tract has a long surface area of specialized cells for the absorption of nutrients, called M cells, which can easily absorb the drug [99].

The frequent stimulus used for drug administration via oral is pH; as a consequence, stimuli-responsive CBHGs are mainly designed to respond to changes of pH, not only as a result of stomach acidity (the determining factor of this tendency) but also the effect of pH on chemical and physical properties of the hydrogel. For example, Ahmad et al. (2016) reported the design of microparticulate hydrogels based on bacterial cellulose and polyacrylic acid for improving the availability of insulin when it is orally administered. The polymerization was carried out through electron beam irradiation. The obtained polymer was characterized for absorbing large amounts of water, being highly pH-sensitive, and its ability to store and release insulin in a controlled way. In spite of the protonation of the carboxylic acid groups of the hydrogel, it was possible to protect the insulin of enzymatic degradation and also degradation resulting from strongly acidic environments. On the other hand, ex vivo tests appreciated the good cytocompatibility of the hydrogel and their mucoadhesion to intestinal tissues; this fact is associated with the presence of cellulose in their structure. In addition, in vivo studies on diabetic rats appreciated that the administration of insulin assisted by CBHG improved the bioavailability of the drug and its hypoglycemic effects [88].

In this way, stimuli-responsive CBHGs were developed from poly(dopamine)-coated microcrystalline cellulose in a solution with Konjac glucomannan [58]. This hydrogel showed an ability to control the release of ofloxacin as a function of pH by in vitro experiments. It was observed that the release rate of the antibiotic was less at low pH than at neutral pH, and this fact was associated with the formation of a network with a high amount of hydrogen bonds at low pH, thus avoiding the release of the drug. At neutral pH, this physical cross-linking was ruptured, allowing the consequent release of ofloxacin. Accordingly, the obtained materials were postulated as potential drug-release systems for oral administration. Likewise, other works have been carried out to obtain stimuli-responsive CBHGs for oral drug administration [60, 83]. Despite the importance of the oral delivery as a drug administration route, there are still some limitations in this methodology, such as low penetration through the mucosa, biodegradation of the released drug (presystemic metabolism), low biocompatibility of the delivery systems, and even the construction of delivery systems at commercial scale [98]. In part, stimuli-responsive CBHGs have been developed for drug release by other routes, e.g., transdermal and subcutaneous routes.

13.5.2 Stimuli-responsive CBHGs for transdermal delivery

Transdermal drug delivery is another alternative approach to the design of stimuli-responsive CBHGs. Transdermal drug delivery is frequently used in treatment of wounds and skin conditions, since it facilitates efficient therapy with a low dosage, suppresses potential side effects of the drug in the body, allows obtaining constant plasma levels of the drug, and avoids hepatic presystemic metabolism [100]. It is important to indicate that this route requires an efficient passage of the drug through the stratum corneum of the epidermis with $10-20\,\mu m$ in thickness and minimizes any effect on the skin properties; for this, adequate contact between the surface (skin) and the drug-transporting vehicle (hydrogel) is very important. In this sense, to promote hydrogel-skin contact, it is important that the hydrogel possess suitable adhesive properties to avoid losses during its application; in addition, it should not irritate the skin and minimize the losses of the active component, which must be efficiently dispersed in the polymer matrix. At the same time, the hydrogel must be correctly distributed on the surface. Drugs that have been administered or researched through this route are insulin, naringenin, tobramycin, sodium fluoride, progesterone, and theophylline [97, 101].

Some stimuli-responsive CBHGs have been designed to be patches covering the wound and releasing the drug [86, 87, 89, 90, 101, 102]. For example, Park et al. synthesized a CBHG from carboxymethyl cellulose and 2-hydroxyethyl acrylate with low cytotoxicity, adequate rheological properties, and high permeation of the drug through the skin, for the controlled transdermal release of naringenin, a flavonoid with potential therapeutic effects on atopic dermatitis [92]. The presence of carboxylic acid groups in the hydrogel structure provided the system with sensitivity to pH, such that the release rate was lower at pH 5.5 (normal skin pH) compared with the release at pH 7.5 (acne skin pH) and 8.5 (atopic skin pH). Therefore, it was demonstrated that it is possible to modulate the release of the drug by the CBHG depending on skin condition. Similar work was carried out by Fan et al. [89]; in this case, they synthesized CBHGs from carboxymethylcellulose, β-cyclodextrin, and tobramycin, a broad-spectrum antibiotic, using chemical cross-linking by imine bonds. In this case, the antibiotic was part of the covalent polymer network, while β-cyclodextrin was used to encapsulate borneol, which has therapeutic effects on skin wounds. The resulting polymeric system exhibited pH sensitivity, promoting the controlled release of tobramycin and borneol at the wound site by breaking of imine bonds. Thus, the obtained materials promoted wound healing in in vivo models, which was the result of the therapeutic action of borneol and the antimicrobial activity of tobramycin. For this reason, they were classified as potential transdermal drug delivery systems in wound healing [89].

13.5.3 Stimuli-responsive CBHGs for subcutaneous delivery

Stimuli-responsive CBHGs have been designed with the possibility of being injected subcutaneously [84, 91]. Through this administration route, the drug is deposited in the interstitial region of the subcutis to promote the absorption by the cardiovascular system. This type of absorption tends to be faster than noninvasive administration routes; however, its use depends on the type of drug. Additionally, ideal subcutaneous drug delivery systems should present a high biocompatibility and potential biodegradability [91, 97, 103]. In the case of hydrogels, these are generated in situ through rapid and effective intermolecular interactions or ultrafast chemical reactions [84].

Injectable hydrogels based on cellulose nanocrystals, amino-functionalized graphene oxide, and chitosan for the controlled release of doxorubicin and curcumin, which have anticancer activity have been recently reported [84]. The formation of the stimuli-responsive CBHGs was carried out in situ through chemical cross-linking by a synthetic di-aldehyde with a polymerization time of 3 min. Hydrogels showed pH response due to the presence of imine groups resulting in chemical reaction between dialdehyde molecule and chitosan, and dialdehyde molecule and amino groups on graphene oxide, high biocompatibility due to the nature of their raw materials (cellulose nanocrystals and chitosan), injectability defined by the fluency of reactive components, and sensitivity to aldehyde or amino compounds, such as cysteine or benzaldehyde, as a result of "free" or unreacted groups on chitosan and the cross-linking agent. The applicability of these systems for the controlled release of drugs subcutaneously was adequate.

On the other hand, Okubo et al. reported the fabrication of stimuli-responsive CBHGs based on hydroxypropyl methylcellulose and cyclodextrin through physical interactions. Initially, the inclusion of the modified cellulose side chains in the cyclodextrin-facilitated host-guest interactions, which were altered by temperature changes [91]. The hydrogel was formed at body temperatures ($\sim$ 37°C) by promoting hydrophobic interactions between the hydrophobic side chains and disfavoring host-guest interactions between cellulose and cyclodextrin. However, at lower temperature, the rupture of the network is induced. These stimuli-responsive CBHGs showed successful results in the subcutaneous release of insulin in experiments with mice, promoting a prolonged hypoglycemic effect of the drug.

On the other hand, it is important to indicate that, so far, stimuli-responsive CBHGs have not been reported for controlled drug delivery by other routes than those discussed here; however, it is a research field in continuous development. However, various works associated with the design and obtaining of stimuli-responsive CBHGs have allowed us to appreciate how their important properties, such as biocompatibility, multifunctionality, structural diversity, and stimuli response, may facilitate the approach of other release pathways, e.g., ocular, rectal, pulmonary, or nasal delivery [16, 21, 97]. A clear example of this is the numerous applications of pharmaceutical formulations and CBHGs for the treatment of ocular, nasal, and rectal conditions [10, 15]. Furthermore, it is widely accepted that the design of multisensitive systems based on cellulose would allow its application as a delivery system through different routes with high site-specificity and a precise release methodology [59, 60].

13.6 Stimuli-responsive CBHGs focused on tissue engineering

Tissue engineering and regenerative medicine are two areas of current technology that aim to combine different disciplines to create tissues for medical purposes, either through ex situ production for subsequent implantation in patients who require it or through the construction of artificial cell growth supports that allow the in situ construction of a new functional tissue. In particular, at present, tissue engineering in conjunction with the material engineering are focused on the design of materials, biocompatible and/or biodegradable, that fulfill the function of an extracellular matrix to support some type of cell, guarantee its adequate growth, and regulate the release of factors that promote it. In particular, it is more or less widely accepted that biopolymer-based stimuli-responsive hydrogels are promising candidates for this function. This type of material satisfies the characteristics previously mentioned, but they also have the advantage of offering the possibility of controlling the release of substances with ability to enhance cell growth and express various genes in tissue. Also hydrogels can be designed with structural reversibility properties, which facilitates the release of cells once tissue is formed or recovered [104, 105]. In this way, various types of stimuli-responsive CBHGs with potential functionality as "scaffold" have been developed, and several examples are summarized in Table 13.2.

The strategies for obtaining stimuli-responsive CBHGs have mainly focused on two approaches; the first one is based on the use of chemically modified cellulosic material through oxidation processes, chemical

TABLE 13.2 Stimuli-responsive CBHGs with potential application in tissue engineering.

Precursors	Response to	Application	Ref.
Cellulose nanocrystals and poly(N-isopropylacrylamide)	Temperature	Cancer spheroid culture	[91]
Carboxymethylcellulose functionalized with chelating agents	ClO^-/SCN^-	Cancer spheroid culture	[106]
Cellulose acetoacetate and EDTA	Ca^{2+}/Mg^{2+}	Culture of mesenchymal cells from adipose tissue	[107]
Carboxyethyl cellulose functionalized with hydrazide dipropionate and dibenzaldehyde-terminated polyethylene glycol	pH, redox	Encapsulation and culture of L929 cells	[108]
TEMPO-oxidized cellulose nanofibrils	Shear, sonication, pH, Ca^{2+}/Fe^{3+}	Capsules for human breast cancer cells and mouse embryonic stem cells	[109]
Carboxymethylcellulose functionalized with norbornene groups and thiolate agents	Temperature	Human mesenchymal stem cell culture	[110]
Cellulose nanocrystals and poly(N-isopropylacrylamide-co-N,N'-dimethyl aminoethyl methacrylate)	Temperature	Capsules and culture media of fibroblasts and T-cells	[111]
Hydroxypropyl cellulose functionalized with allyl isocyanate	Temperature	Cytocompatibility with several cell lines	[112]

functionalization, polymer insertion, etc., while the second one is based on insertions in a controlled way of interactions promoting the reticulation, generally corresponding to hydrogen bonding, ionic interactions, and, more recently, coordination interactions [91, 93, 104–106]. The stimuli-responsive CBHGs developed by these methods have the ability to imitate the cartilage, bone structure, and neuronal tissue, among others, due to their wet nature, porous morphology, and soft structure, reasons that make them promissory materials for applications in the tissue engineering [113]. A brief description of outstanding applications in relation to regeneration of bone tissue, regeneration of cartilage tissues, regeneration of neural tissues, wound dressing, and cell culture will be exposed in the following sections.

13.6.1 Bone tissue regeneration

Bones are rigid organs that form the endoskeleton of some animals and humans; they are made up of cells (2%) and a highly resistant, flexible, and low-density extracellular matrix (98%), consisting of hydroxyapatite (~ 70%), collagen and other components of an organic nature (30%). They form a solid structure of varied architecture depending on their location. They have an interface in direct contact with the muscles, blood, and bone marrow. Therefore, a synthetic structure with suitable mechanical properties and biocompatibility is an excellent candidate as a bone substitute; however, these two properties alone are not sufficient for the functional biomimetic of the bones. Bone fractures, osteoporosis, and diseases caused by aging are common in athletes, high-risk workpeople, people with congenital chronic pathologies, and in people over 50 years old because their bones lose the ability to self-repair [114–116].

One of the great challenges in the engineering of bone tissue is the development of biocompatible porous materials with high mechanical resistance that satisfy, from a biomechanical point of view, the same requirements that bones have for their correct functioning [117]. Rusu et al. established that, although CBHGs are biocompatible materials, they do not possess important properties for the regeneration of bone tissue such as biomineralization and osseointegration; therefore, for correct functionality, these must be accompanied by inorganic compounds like hydroxyapatite, which is the most important and abundant mineral in the bones, to allow hydrogels to acquire good mechanical properties to carry out biomineralization and osteoconductivity processes [105, 118]. Thermoresponsive injectable CBHGs based on methylcellulose, gelatin, and citric acid, in conjunction with bioceramic components of hydroxyapatite, tetracalcium phosphate, dehydrated calcium sulfate, and dehydrated dicalcium phosphate have been obtained; these have been characterized by a low degradation rate and optimal viscoelastic and mechanical properties [119].

Despite the novelties and advantages of these CBHGs, currently there are no in vivo studies of these cellulosic materials, and as a consequence, properties associated with their activity, effectiveness, and compatibility with the body of the hydrogel host are still unidentified. However, it cannot be ignored that they are a promising material for bone recovery due to the properties of composites based on cellulose and biominerals.

13.6.2 Cartilage tissues regeneration

Cartilage is part of the connective tissue, and in a broad sense it is an elastic material that does not have any blood supply, made up of a highly complex extracellular matrix of a biopolymeric nature consisting mainly of collagen of various types, hyaluronan, and proteoglycan. When weakening, damage, or alterations in the cartilage is evidenced in a patient, there is a clinical challenge from the orthopedic point of view, in particular, the cartilages are tissues that lack blood vessels and are distant from the progenitor cells; therefore, they are tissues incapable of self-repair when they present an affectation [120, 121]. It is important to indicate that, at the present, there is no effective solution available for the clinical treatment of cartilage tissue damage [105, 121].

The complexity of the clinical problem, and of the science of materials, lies in the fact that the scaffolding for cartilage remediation must promote the proliferation of tissue cells called chondrocytes, which are present in greater proportion. Furthermore, an ideal material should be stable and flexible to adequately mimic real cartilage [105]. However, although it is a complex task involving not only the biocompatibility but also the stimulation of cell growth, some research has shown notable progress in this direction. In this way, Vinatier et al. developed pH-sensitive CBHGs based on hydroxypropyl methylcellulose and silanol, in which they successfully cultivated chondrocytes for their subsequent proliferation. However, although the researchers demonstrated in vitro that this material was biocompatible and functionally viable, its efficacy in vivo has not yet been evaluated due to the difficulty of determining the pH in the damaged cartilage, which is why the tissue response to CBHGs can be aggressive [122, 123]. Other researchers have described CBHGs with magnetic response from cellulose and dextran; sensitivity to magnetic stimuli was achieved by grafting superparamagnetic iron oxide, while the objective behind the design of this material was to allow its monitoring by magnetic resonance. These researchers integrated kartogenin into hydrogels, which is a nonprotein compound that allows differentiation of host cells into chondrocytes for cartilage repair. In a very positive way, in vivo studies showed that the regenerated cartilage was similar to natural tissue, signifying an enormous advance for the development of novel treatment alternatives [124].

Evidently, tissue engineering is a multidisciplinary field of application with promising results in the field of materials, particularly those based on CBHGs; however, multiple evaluations must be satisfied before a fully functional system can be established, for example, setting long-term effects. Therefore, it is a constantly advancing research area.

13.6.3 Neural tissues regeneration

The nervous system is responsible for vital functions of the body, so any damage between nerve links and the brain or other parts can cause paralysis, sensory loss, or serious malfunctions both consciously and unconsciously. These injuries cause permanent disability, reduce the quality of life, and represent economic, social, and individual problems [125, 126].

In this sense, CBHGs emerge as a remediation strategy due to their versatility and properties. First, it has been investigated that thermosensitive CBHGs can be used as "scaffolds" because they are noninvasive. It has been described, from studies in rats, that temperature-sensitive methylcellulose-based hydrogels have optimal stability and biocompatibility with tissues of the nervous system [127]. But in addition, laminin-1-bound methylcellulose hydrogels have been shown to be suitable for cell viability in rats [128]. However, the application of methylcellulose has been limited by its low adsorption of proteins that can promote the repair of neuronal tissues [129]. On the other hand, the complexity of the nervous tissues complicates the decision of an appropriate material for the regeneration of these tissues. Although stimuli-responsive CBHGs have multiple properties mentioned throughout this chapter, research on neuronal repair is scarce and highly specialized, and its evaluation in this area should be explored for its potential usefulness and efficacy.

13.6.4 Wound dressing

Tissue injuries can be severely aggravated because they can be colonized by opportunistic microorganisms, causing infections that, in the worst case, lead to amputation and even death. It is important that wounds are kept moist, as this is the optimal conditions for tissue regeneration and pain relief. Temperature-sensitive physical CBHGs are attractive materials such as wound gauze. Its function is essential because, in addition to maintaining a humid environment, they also absorb excess tissue fluid generated by the wound (hydrogel-assisted in-situ water drainage). Furthermore, hydroxyl groups allow the adhesion of this material from epithelial tissues [16, 130]. Zubik et al. developed temperature-sensitive physical hydrogels based on cellulose nanocrystals and poly(N-isopropylacrylamide), which exhibited optimal mechanical strength and high temperature sensitivity, making them an attractive material for wound dressings [131].

CBHGs sensitive to pH are also used, since an acidic environment prevents the colonization of bacterial species in wounds [16]. Among the most common strategies is the use of the antibacterial activity carried out for the quaternary ammonium groups; therefore, the insertion of these in a suitable matrix will give the material bacterial asepsis and also a significant degree of hydrophilicity [132]. However, the applications of CBHGs go beyond contact protection of wounds, sometimes being, through appropriate stimulation, excellent platforms for the monitoring of the evolution of wounds; for example, Kassal et al. synthesized CBHGs with pH indicator dyes so that, when changes in wound acidity occur, hydrogels change color and consequently allow constant monitoring of the wound [133].

13.6.5 Cell culture

In tissue engineering, regardless of the area to be repaired, it is important that biomaterials can encapsulate cells with regenerative properties, and under the right conditions, allow and promote cell growth. Research has shown that CBHGs are attractive candidates for this purpose by allowing the construction of porous three-dimensional structures from the hydrogel, and that they can be used as scaffolds for cell growth. The construction of this type of system may involve specific methodological processes, such as emulsification, lyophilization, porogen leaching, 3D printing, and photolithography, among others [91, 93, 102].

One of the best-known examples is the development of a CBHG from TEMPO-oxidized cellulose nanofibrils with thixotropic properties and response to stimuli such as shear stress, ultrasound, pH, and presence of Ca^{2+} and Fe^{3+} ions, for encapsulation of breast cancer and mouse embryonic stem cells by simple homogenization of these in the polymer matrix. The hydrogel showed an adequate preservation of cells for about 7 days with a maximum cell loss of 30%. Likewise, the structure decreased its storage module G' (loss of its elastic behavior) by being subjected to constant stress, ultrasound, and pH increases, due to a breakdown of physical interactions between polymer chains, thus able to be "broken" with the consequent release of the cells [106].

Another example is the work developed by Dadoo et al. [110], who photolithographed hydrogels from carboxymethylcellulose functionalized with norbornene groups and chemically cross-linked with dithiolated molecules for encapsulation and culture of human mesenchymal stem cells. These showed a response to changes of temperature with a narrowing of the 3D grid structure due to an increase in temperature (above 32°C). In addition, the high cell viability was demonstrated with the use (or not) of cell adhesion by peptides [110].

Other types of CBHGs were developed from the functionalization of cellulosic material with high hydrophobic molecules and polymers, for example, allyl isocyanate, poly(N-isopropylacrylamide) and poly(N-isopropylacrylamide-co-N,N'-dimethylaminoethyl methacrylate) to generate thermoresponsive CBHGs for encapsulation and cell culture [91, 108, 109]. It was even opted for the design of CBHGs with stimuli response that does not compromise the cell viability (as some stimulus can generate changes in temperature, for example). Thus, Hai et al. developed CBHGs sensitive to anionic species such as ClO^- and SCN^- from functionalized carboxymethylcellulose with chelating groups of Eu(III) ions to generate cross-linking by coordination bonds. The hydrogels were successfully employed for the cultivation of cancer spheroids, and they showed a rupture of the polymeric structure due to ClO^- presence and its formation by subsequent addition of SCN^- ions [93].

According to this, it can be seen that the application of CBHGs in the development of scaffolds and extracellular matrices for encapsulation and cell culture is growing. Thus, this allows us to appreciate the versatility of this type of hydrogel and the importance of using cellulose as a material for obtaining polymeric networks with high hydrophilicity (water absorption capacity), good cytocompatibility, adequate mechanical properties, and multifunctionality. This fact allows us to think about the potential applications and benefits generated by the continuous development and application of CBHGs in the biomedical field.

13.7 Conclusions and perspectives

Throughout history, cellulose has been used for many important applications, from instruments and structures used in everyday life to reaching devices used in the biomedical field. The properties of this polymeric material, such as its high hydrophobicity, biocompatibility, and biodegradability, in addition to its high availability as a resource, as the most abundant natural polymer, have allowed us to direct attention to the construction of useful materials and systems from cellulose. Among these materials, there are hydrogels, which have been studied and developed successfully from cellulose and applied in various areas, primordially, in the medical field.

As discussed, the diversity of functional polymer structures that can be obtained from natural cellulose or its derivatives provides greater importance to this type of renewable resource in the development of intelligent systems, even reaching to be developed from the beginning of the last decade, CBHGs sensitive to different stimuli or CBHGs, whether of a physical type (temperature, light, electromagnetic fields, among others) or a chemical type (pH, redox processes, among others). The methodological alternatives for obtaining CBHGs have focused on two ways: the use of natural or physically modified cellulose and the use of modified cellulose through chemical processes. Both types of methodologies have been used successfully for the construction of CBHGs with response to different types of stimuli, even presenting a "multiresponse."

Controlled drug release and tissue engineering have been fields of research in current growth for which various types of CBHGs have been designed and evaluated for the controlled release of substances, from anti-inflammatory to anticancer drugs, through different stimuli; some of the most studied are pH, temperature, and redox processes. Likewise, CBHGs have been developed to fulfill the function of extracellular matrix for the encapsulation and promotion of the growth of various cell lines—a fact that opens a wide window of functions for the consideration of this type of cellulose-based systems in future biomedical applications and, possibly, daily life.

References

[1] Popa V, Volf I. Biomass as renewable raw material to obtain bioproducts of high-tech value. Amsterdam: Elsevier; 2018.

[2] Palencia M, Lerma T, Combatt E. Hydrogels based in cassava starch with antibacterial activity for controlled release of cysteamine-silver nanostructured agents. Curr Chem Biol 2017;11:28–35.

[3] Kumar T, Ghosh B. Polysaccharide-based nano-biocarrier in drug delivery. Boca Raton, FL: CRC Press; 2019.

[4] Rudin A, Choi P. The elements of polymer science & engineering. Boston, MA: Academic Press; 2013.

[5] Ahmed EM. Hydrogel: preparation, characterization, and applications: a review. J Adv Res 2015;6(2):105–21.

[6] Biswas S. Emerging concepts in analysis and applications of hydrogels. London: InTechOpen; 2016.

[7] Caló E, Khutoryanskiy VV. Biomedical applications of hydrogels: a review of patents and commercial products. Eur Polym J 2015;65:252–67.

[8] Kabir SMF, Sikdar PP, Haque B, Bhuiyan MAR, Ali A, Islam MN. Cellulose-based hydrogel materials: chemistry, properties and their prospective applications. Prog Biomater 2018;7(3):153–74.

[9] Palantöken S, Bethke K, Zivanovic V, Kalinka G, Kneipp J, Rademann K. Cellulose hydrogels physically crosslinked by glycine: synthesis, characterization, thermal and mechanical properties. J Appl Polym Sci 2020;137(7):48380.

[10] Sannino A, Demitri C, Madaghiele M. Biodegradable cellulose-based hydrogels: design and applications. Materials 2009;2(2):353–73.

[11] Bajpai P. Pulp and paper industry. Amsterdam: Elsevier; 2017.

[12] Palencia M, Mora MA, Palencia SL. Biodegradable polymer hydrogels based in sorbitol and citric acid for controlled release of bioactive substances from plants (polyphenols). Curr Chem Biol 2017;11(1):36–42.

[13] Rodríguez A, Eugenio ME. Cellulose. London: IntechOpen; 2019.

[14] Kamide K. Cellulose and cellulose derivatives. Amsterdam: Elsevier; 2005.

[15] Klemm D, Heublein B, Fink H, Bohn A. Cellulose: fascinating biopolymer and sustainable raw material. Angew Chem 2005;44(22):3358–93.

[16] Mondal IH. Cellulose-based superabsorbent hydrogels. Cham: Springer; 2018.

[17] Ebnesajjad S. Handbook of biopolymers and biodegradable plastics. Boston, MA: William Andrew Publishing; 2013.

[18] Suhas GVK, Carrot PJM, Singh R, Chaudhary M, Kushwaha S. Cellulose: a review as natural, modified and activated carbon adsorbent. Bioresour Technol 2016;216:1066–76.

[19] Krumm C, Pfaendtner J, Dauenhauer PJ. Millisecond pulsed films unify the mechanisms of cellulose fragmentation. Chem Mater 2016;28(9):3108–14.

[20] Arbeláez N, Lerma T, Córdoba A. Modification of membranes by insertion of short-chain alcohols on reactive porous substrates: effect of chain length on the surface free energy. J Sci Technol Appl 2017;2:75–83.

[21] Lerma TA, Benítez E, Córdoba A. Making of porous ionic surfaces by sequential polymerization: polyurethanes + grafting of polyelectrolytes. J Sci Technol Appl 2017;2:44–53.

[22] Palencia M, Córdoba A, Lerma T. Polyurethanes with boron retention properties for the development of agricultural fertilization smart systems. J Sci Tech Appl 2016;1:39–52.

[23] Sadasivuni KK, Ponnamma D, Kim J, Cabibihan JJ, AlMaadeed MA. Biopolymer composites in electronics. Amsterdam: Elsevier; 2017.

[24] Rojas OJ. Cellulose chemistry and properties: fibers, nanocelluloses and advanced materials. Cham: Springer; 2016.

[25] Van De Ven TGM. Cellulose—fundamental aspects. London: IntechOpen; 2013.

[26] Ficai D, Grumezescu AM. Nanostructures for novel therapy. Amsterdam: Elsevier; 2017.

[27] Chen Y. Hydrogels based on natural polymers. Amsterdam: Elsevier; 2020.

[28] Palencia M, Otálora A, Lerma TA. Synthesis and characterization of polyurea-base hydrogels by multicomponent polycondensation of 1,6-hexamethylene diisocyanate, sorbitol and cysteine. J Sci Tech Appl 2020;7:5–19.

[29] Palencia M, Garcés V. Development of bacterial inoculums based on biodegradable hydrogels for agricultural applications. J Sci Technol Appl 2017;2:13–23.

[30] Malmonge SM. Reference module in materials science and materials engineering. Amsterdam: Elsevier; 2018.

[31] Rivas B, Urbano BF, Palencia M, Palacio DA. Preparation of alkylated chitosan-based polyelectrolyte hydrogels: the effect of monomer charge on polymerization. Eur Polym J 2019;118:551–60.

[32] Peng N, Wang Y, Ye Q, Liang L, An Y, Li Q, Chang C. Biocompatible cellulose-based superabsorbent hydrogels with antimicrobial activity. Carbohydr Polym 2016;37:59–64.

[33] Chunshom N, Chuysinuan P, Techasakul S, Ummartyotin S. Dried-state bacterial cellulose (*Acetobacter xylinum*) and polyvinyl-alcohol-based hydrogel: an approach to a personal care material. J Sci Adv Mater Devices 2018;3(3):296–302.

[34] Tang J, Javaid MU, Pan C, Yu G, Berry RM, Tam KC. Self-healing stimuli-responsive cellulose nanocrystal hydrogels. Carbohydr Polym 2020;229:115486.

[35] Zheng WJ, Gao J, Wei Z, Zhou J, Chen YM. Facile fabrication of self-healing carboxymethyl cellulose hydrogels. Eur Polym J 2015;72:514–22.

[36] Popa L, Violeta M, Dinu-Pîrvu. Hydrogels—smart materials for biomedical applications. London: IntechOpen; 2019.

[37] Mohamed MA, Fallahi A, El-Sokkary AMA, Salehi S, Akl MA, Jafari A, Tamayol A, Fenniri H, Khademhosseini A, Andreadis ST. Stimuli-responsive hydrogels for manipulation of cell microenvironment: from chemistry to biofabrication technology. Prog Polym Sci 2019;98:101147.

[38] Huang H, Qi X, Chen Y, Wu Z. Thermo-sensitive hydrogels for delivering biotherapeutic molecules: a review. Saudi Pharm J 2019;27(7):990–9.

[39] Liu W, Zhang B, Lu WW, Li X, Zhu D, De Yao K, Wang Q, Zhao C, Wang C. A rapid temperature-responsive sol–gel reversible poly(N-isopropylacrylamide)-g-methylcellulose copolymer hydrogel. Biomaterials 2004;25(15):3005–12.

[40] Shi X, Zheng Y, Wang G, Lin Q, Fan J. pH- and electro-response characteristics of bacterial cellulose nanofiber/sodium alginate hybrid hydrogels for dual controlled drug delivery. RSC Adv 2014;4(87):47056–65.

[41] Koetting MC, Peters JT, Steichen SD, Peppas NA. Stimulus-responsive hydrogels: theory, modern advances, and applications. Mater Sci Eng R 2015;93:1–49.

[42] Liu Z, Wang H, Liu C, Jiang Y, Yu G, Mu X, Wang X. Magnetic cellulose–chitosan hydrogels prepared from ionic liquids as reusable adsorbent for removal of heavy metal ions. Chem Commun 2012;48(59):7350–2.

[43] Shi Q, Liu H, Tang D, Li Y, Li X, Xu F. Bioactuators based on stimulus-responsive hydrogels and their emerging biomedical applications. NPG Asia Mater 2019;11(1):1–21.

[44] Akar E, Altınışık A, Seki Y. Preparation of pH- and ionic-strength responsive biodegradable fumaric acid crosslinked carboxymethyl cellulose. Carbohydr Polym 2012;90(4):1634–41.

[45] Chang C, He M, Zhou J, Zhang L. Swelling behaviors of pH- and salt-responsive cellulose-based hydrogels. Macromolecules 2011;44(6):1642–8.

[46] Amiri S. Amiri S. Properties and Industrial Applications. John Wiley & Sons, Hoboken: Cyclodextrins; 2017.

[47] Jana S, Maiti S. Biopolymer-based composites. Singapore: Woodhead Publishing; 2017.

[48] Li Y, Hou X, Pan Y, Wang L, Xiao H. Redox-responsive carboxymethyl cellulose hydrogel for adsorption and controlled release of dye. Eur Polym J 2020;123:109447.

[49] Lu Q, Zhang S, Xiong M, Lin F, Tang L, Huang B, Chen Y. One-pot construction of cellulose-gelatin supramolecular hydrogels with high strength and pH-responsive properties. Carbohydr Polym 2018;196:225–32.

[50] Spagnol C, Rodrigues FHA, Pereira AGB, Fajardo AR, Rubira AF, Muniz EC. Superabsorbent hydrogel composite made of cellulose nanofibrils and chitosan-graft-poly(acrylic acid). Carbohydr Polym 2012;87(3):2038–45.

[51] Yang X, Liu G, Peng L, Guo J, Tao L, Yuan J, Chang C, Wei Y, Zhang L. Highly efficient self-healable and dual responsive cellulose-based hydrogels for controlled release and 3D cell culture. Adv Funct Mater 2017;27(40):1703174.

[52] Li N, Chen W, Chen G, Tian J. Rapid shape memory TEMPO-oxidized cellulose nanofibers/polyacrylamide/gelatin hydrogels with enhanced mechanical strength. Carbohydr Polym 2017;171:77–84.

[53] Wang F, Zhang Q, Huang K, Li J, Wang K, Zhang K, Tang X. Preparation and characterization of carboxymethyl cellulose containing quaternized chitosan for potential drug carrier. Int J Biol Macromol 2020;154:1392–9.

[54] Ge W, Cao S, Shen F, Wang Y, Ren J, Wang X. Rapid self-healing, stretchable, moldable, antioxidant and antibacterial tannic acid-cellulose nanofibril composite hydrogels. Carbohydr Polym 2019;224:115147.

[55] Halake KS, Lee J. Superporous thermo-responsive hydrogels by combination of cellulose fibers and aligned micropores. Carbohydr Polym 2014;105(1):184–92.

[56] Yan L, Wang L, Gao S, Liu C, Zhang Z, Ma A, Zheng L. Celery cellulose hydrogel as carriers for controlled release of short-chain fatty acid by ultrasound. Food Chem 2020;309:125717.

[57] Sun X, Tyagi P, Agate S, Lucia L, McCord M, Pal L. Unique thermo-responsivity and tunable optical performance of poly(N-isopropylacrylamide)-cellulose nanocrystal hydrogel films. Carbohydr Polym 2019;208:495–503.

[58] Wang L, Du Y, Yuan Y, Mu RJ, Gong J, Ni Y, Pang J, Wu C. Mussel-inspired fabrication of konjac glucomannan/microcrystalline cellulose intelligent hydrogel with pH-responsive sustained release behavior. Int J Biol Macromol 2018;113:285–93.

[59] Dutta S, Samanta P, Dhara D. Temperature, pH and redox responsive cellulose based hydrogels for protein delivery. Int J Biol Macromol 2016;87:92–100.

[60] Karzar M, Mahkam M. Magnetic nano carboxymethyl cellulose-alginate/chitosan hydrogel beads as biodegradable devices for controlled drug delivery. Int J Biol Macromol 2019;135:829–38.

[61] Jeong D, Joo SW, Hu Y, Shinde VS, Cho E, Jung S. Carboxymethyl cellulose-based superabsorbent hydrogels containing carboxymehtyl β-cyclodextrin for enhanced mechanical strength and effective drug delivery. Eur Polym J 2018;105:17–25.

[62] Wang F, Zhang Q, Li X, Huang K, Shao W, Yao D, Huang C. Redox-responsive blend hydrogel films based on carboxymethyl cellulose/chitosan microspheres as dual delivery carrier. Int J Biol Macromol 2019;134:413–21.

[63] Zhang T, Cheng Q, Ye D, Chang C. Tunicate cellulose nanocrystals reinforced nanocomposite hydrogels comprised by hybrid cross-linked networks. Carbohydr Polym 2017;169:139–48.

[64] Carpi A. Progress in molecular and environmental bioengineering. IntechOpen; 2011.

[65] Mohd-Amin M, Ahmad N, Halib N, Ahmad I. Synthesis and characterization of thermo- and pH-responsive bacterial cellulose/acrylic acid hydrogels for drug delivery. Carbohydr Polym 2012;88(2):465–73.

[66] Raghuwanshi V, Garnier G. Characterization of hydrogels: linking the nano to the microscale. Adv Colloid Interface 2019;274:102044.

[67] Biswas N, Waring AJ, Walther FJ, Dluhy RA. Structure and conformation of the disulfide bond in dimeric lung surfactant peptides SP-B1–25 and SP-B8–25. BBA-Biomembranes 2007;1768(5):1070–82.

[68] Xue J, Shi Y, Li C, Xu X, Xu S, Cao M. Methylcellulose and polyacrylate binary hydrogels used as rectal suppository to prevent type I diabetes. Colloid Surface B 2018;172:37–42.

[69] Yu H, Xiao C. Synthesis and properties of novel hydrogels from oxidized konjac glucomannan crosslinked gelatin for in vitro drug delivery. Carbohydr Polym 2008;72:479–89.

[70] Liu H, Rong L, Wang B, Xie R, Sui X, Xu H, Zhang L, Zhong Y, Mao Z. Facile fabrication of redox/pH dual stimuli responsive cellulose hydrogel. Carbohydr Polym 2017;176:299–306.

[71] Palencia M. Functional transformation of Fourier-transform mid-infrared spectrum for improving spectral specificity by simple algorithm based on wavelet-like-functions. J Adv Res 2018;14:53–62.

[72] Otalora A, Palencia M. Application of functionally-enhanced derivative spectroscopy (FEDS) to the problem of the overlap of spectral signals in binary mixtures: triethylamine-acetone. J Sci Technol Appl 2019;6:96–107.

[73] Kobe R, Iwamoto S, Endo T, Yoshitani K, Teremoto Y. Stretchable composite hydrogels incorporating modified cellulose nanofiber with dispersibility and polymerizability: mechanical property control and nanofiber orientation. Polymer 2016;97:480–6.

[74] Dai H, Zhang H, Ma L, Zhou H, Yu Y, Guo T, Zhang Y, Huang H. Green pH/magnetic sensitive hydrogels based on pineapple peel cellulose and polyvinyl alcohol: synthesis, characterization and naringin prolonged release. Carbohydr Polym 2019;209:51–61.

[75] Rodriguez YA, Castro RI, Arenas FA, López-Cabaña ZE, Carreño G, Carrasco-Sánchez V, Marican A, Villaseñor J, Vargas E, Santos LS, Durán-Lara EF. Preparation of hydrogel/silver nanohybrids mediated by tunable-size silver nanoparticles for potential antibacterial applications. Polymers 2019;11(4):716.

[76] Lu J, Zhu W, Dai L, Si C, Ni Y. Fabrication of thermo- and pH-sensitive cellulose nanofibrils-reinforced hydrogel with biomass nanoparticles. Carbohydr Polym 2019;215:289–95.

[77] Li Y, Khuu N, Gevorkian A, Sarjinsky S, Therien-Aubin H, Wang Y, Cho S, Kumacheva E. Supramolecular nanofibrillar thermoreversible hydrogel for growth and release of cancer spheroids. Angew Chem Int Ed Eng 2017;56(22):6083–7.

[78] Du W, Deng A, Guo J, Chen J, Li H, Gao Y. An injectable self-healing hydrogel-cellulose nanocrystal conjugate with excellent mechanical strength and good biocompatibility. Carbohydr Polym 2019;223:115084.

[79] De Vicente J. Rheology. IntechOpen; 2012.

[80] Hujaya SD, Lorite GS, Vainio SJ, Liimatainen H. Polyion complex hydrogels from chemically modified cellulose nanofibrils: structure-function relationship and potential for controlled and pH-responsive release of doxorubicin. Acta Biomater 2018;75:346–57.

[81] Liu Y, Sui Y, Liu C, Liu C, Wu M, Li B, Li Y. A physically crosslinked polydopamine/nanocellulose hydrogel as potential versatile vehicles for drug delivery and wound healing. Carbohydr Polym 2018;188:27–36.

[82] Liu Z, Yao P. Injectable thermo-responsive hydrogel composed of xanthan gum and methylcellulose double networks with shear-thinning property. Carbohydr Polym 2015;132:490–8.

[83] Rao KM, Kumar A, Han SS. Poly(acrylamidoglycolic acid) nanocomposite hydrogels reinforced with cellulose nanocrystals for pH-sensitive controlled release of diclofenac sodium. Polym Test 2017;64:175–82.

[84] Omidi S, Pirhayati M, Kakanejadifard A. Co-delivery of doxorubicin and curcumin by a pH-sensitive, injectable, and in situ hydrogel composed of chitosan, graphene, and cellulose nanowhisker. Carbohydr Polym 2020;231:115745.

[85] Chang C, Zhang L. Cellulose-based hydrogels: present status and applications prospects. Carbohydr Polym 2011;84:40–53.

[86] Thérien-Aubin H, Wang Y, Nothdurft K, Prince E, Cho S, Kumacheva E. Temperature-responsive nanofibrillar hydrogels for cell encapsulation. Biomacromolecules 2016;17(10):3244–51.

[87] Palencia M. Surface free energy of solid by contact angle measurements. J Sci Technol Appl 2017;2:84–93.

[88] Ahmad N, Amin M, Ismail I, Buang F. Enhancement of oral insulin bioavailability: in vitro and in vivo assessment of nanoporous stimuli-responsive hydrogel microparticles. Expert Opin Drug Delivery 2016;13(5):621–32.

[89] Fan X, Yang L, Wang T, Sun T, Lu S. pH-responsive cellulose-based dual drug-loaded hydrogel for wound dressing. Eur Polym J 2019;121:109290.

[90] Yu YL, Zhang MJ, Xie R, Ju XJ, Wang JY, Pi SW, Chu LY. Thermo-responsive monodisperse core–shell microspheres with PNIPAM core and biocompatible porous ethyl cellulose shell embedded with PNIPAM gates. J Colloid Interface Sci 2012;376(1):97–106.

[91] Okubo M, Iohara D, Anraku M, Higashi T, Uekama K, Hirayama F. A thermoresponsive hydrophobically modified hydroxypropylmethylcellulose/cyclodextrin injectable hydrogel for the sustained release of drugs. Int J Pharm 2020;575:118845.

[92] Park SH, Shin HS, Park SN. A novel pH-responsive hydrogel based on carboxymethyl cellulose/2-hydroxyethyl acrylate for transdermal delivery of naringenin. Carbohydr Polym 2018;200:341–52.

[93] Peng H, Ning X, Wei G, Wang S, Dai G, Ju A. The preparations of novel cellulose/phenylboronic acid composite intelligent bio-hydrogel and its glucose, pH-responsive behaviors. Carbohydr Polym 2018;195:349–55.

[94] Zhou H, Zhu H, Yang X, Zhang Y, Zhang X, Cui K, Shao L, Yao J. Temperature/pH sensitive cellulose-based hydrogel: synthesis, characterization, loading, and release of model drugs for potential oral drug delivery. Bioresources 2015;10(1):760–71.

[95] Chen N, Wang H, Ling C, Vermerris W, Wang B, Tong Z. Cellulose-based injectable hydrogel composite for pH-responsive and controllable drug delivery. Carbohydr Polym 2019;225:115207.

[96] Yue Z, Wen F, Gao S, Ang MY, Pallathadka PK, Liu L, Yu H. Preparation of three-dimensional interconnected macroporous cellulosic hydrogels for soft tissue engineering. Biomaterials 2010;31:8141–52.

[97] Sosnik A, Seremeta KP. Polymeric hydrogels as technology platform for drug delivery applications. Gels 2017;3(3):25.

[98] Homayun B, Lin X, Choi HJ. Challenges and recent progress in oral drug delivery systems for biopharmaceuticals. Pharmaceutics 2019;11(3):129.

[99] Sharpe LA, Daily AM, Horava SD, Peppas NA. Therapeutic applications of hydrogels in oral drug delivery. Expert Opin Drug Delivery 2014;11(6):901–15.

[100] Boddé HE, Van Aalten AC, Junginger HE. Hydrogel patches for transdermal drug delivery; in-vivo water exchange and skin compatibility. J Pharm Pharmacol 1989;41(3):152–5.

[101] Ahsan A, Tian WX, Farooq MA, Khan DH. An overview of hydrogels and their role in transdermal drug delivery. Int J Polym Mater 2020;70(8):574.

[102] An YH, Lee J, Son DU, Kang DH, Park J, Cho KW, Kim S, Kim SH, Ko J, Jang MH. Facilitated transdermal drug delivery using nanocarriers-embedded electroconductive hydrogel coupled with reverse electrodialysis-driven iontophoresis. ACS Nano 2020;14(4):4523–35.

[103] Jones GB, Collins DS, Harrison MW, Thyagarajapuram NR, Wright JM. Subcutaneous drug delivery: an evolving enterprise. Sci Transl Med 2017;9(405):eaaf9166.

[104] Mantha S, Pillai S, Khayambashi P, Upadhyay A, Zhang Y, Tao O, Pham HM, Tran SD. Smart hydrogels in tissue engineering and regenerative medicine. Materials 2019;12(20):3323.

[105] Rusu D, Ciolacu D, Simionescu BC. Cellulose-based hydrogels in tissue engineering applications. Cellul Chem Technol 2019;53(9-10):907–23.

[106] Hai J, Zeng X, Zhu Y, Wang B. Anions reversibly responsive luminescent nanocellulose hydrogels for cancer spheroids culture and release. Biomaterials 2019;194:161–70.

[107] Melero A, Senna A, Domingues J, Motta A, Haussen M, Junior AR, Duek E, Botaro V. Chelating effect of cellulose acetate hydrogel crosslinked with EDTA dianhydride used as a platform for cell growth. Adv Mater Sci Eng 2019;8684753.

[108] Sultana T, Gwon J, Lee B. Thermal stimuli-responsive hyaluronic acid loaded cellulose based physical hydrogel for post-surgical de novo peritoneal adhesion prevention. Mater Sci Eng C 2020;110661.

[109] Sanandiya ND, Vasudevan J, Das R, Lim CT, Fernandez JG. Stimuli-responsive injectable cellulose thixogel for cell encapsulation. Int J Biol Macromol 2019;130:1009–17.

[110] Dadoo N, Landry S, Bomar J, Gramlich W. Synthesis and spatiotemporal modification of biocompatible and stimuli-responsive carboxymethyl cellulose hydrogels using thiol-norbornene chemistry. Macromol Biosci 2017;17(9):1700107.

[111] Treesuppharata W, Rojanapanthu P, Siangsanoh C, Manuspiya H, Ummartyotin S. Synthesis and characterization of bacterial cellulose and gelatin-based hydrogel composites for drug-delivery systems. Biotechnol Rep 2017;15:84–91.

[112] Way AE, Hsu L, Shanmuganathan K, Weder C, Rowan SJ. pH-responsive cellulose nanocrystal gels and nanocomposites. ACS Macro Lett 2012;1(8):1001–6.

[113] Fu LH, Qi C, Ma MG, Wan P. Multifunctional cellulose-based hydrogels for biomedical applications. J Mater Chem B 2019;7:1541–62.

[114] Mills LA, Aitken SA, Simpson AHRW. The risk of non-union per fracture: current myths and revised figures from a population of over 4 million adults. Acta Orthop 2017;88(4):434–9.

[115] Qu H, Fu H, Han Z, Sun Y. Biomaterials for bone tissue engineering scaffolds: a review. RSC Adv 2019;9(45):26252–62.

[116] Ren B, Betz VM, Thirion C. Osteoinduction within BMP-2 transduced muscle tissue fragments with and without a fascia layer: implications for bone tissue engineering. Gene Ther 2019;26:16–28.

[117] Orciani M, Fini M, Di Primio R, Mattioli-Belmonte M. Biofabrication and bone tissue regeneration: cell source, approaches, and challenges. Front Bioeng Biotechnol 2017;5(17):1–15.

[118] Liu Z, Liu J, Cui X, Wang X, Zhang L, Tang P. Recent advances on magnetic sensitive hydrogels in tissue engineering. Front Chem 2020;8(24):1–17.

[119] Demir Oğuz Ö, Ege D. Rheological and mechanical properties of thermoresponsive methylcellulose/calcium phosphate-based injectable bone substitutes. Materials 2018;11(4):604.

[120] Li H, Hu C, Yu H, Chen C. Chitosan composite scaffolds for articular cartilage defect repair: a review. RSC Adv 2018;8(7):3736–49.

[121] Zhang Y, Yu JK, Ren K, Zuo J, Ding J, Chen X. Thermosensitive hydrogels as scaffolds for cartilage tissue engineering. Biomacromolecules 2019;20(4):1478–92.

[122] Vinatier C, Magne D, Weiss P. A silanized hydroxypropyl methylcellulose hydrogel for the three-dimensional culture of chondrocytes. Biomaterials 2005;26(33):6643–51.

[123] Balakrishnan B, Banerjee R. Biopolymer-based hydrogels for cartilage tissue engineering. Chem Rev 2011;111(8):4453–74.

[124] Yang W, Zhu P, Huang H, Zheng Y, Liu J, Feng L, Guo H, Tang S, Guo R. Functionalization of novel theranostic hydrogels with kartogenin grafted USPIO nanoparticles to enhance cartilage regeneration. ACS Appl Mater Interfaces 2019;11(38):34744–54.

[125] Bedir T, Ulag S, Ustundag CB, Gunduz O. 3D bioprinting applications in neural tissue engineering for spinal cord injury repair. Mater Sci Eng C 2020;110:110741.

[126] Patel BB, Sharifi F, Stroud DP, Montazami R, Hashemi NN, Sakaguchi DS. 3D microfibrous scaffolds selectively promotes proliferation and glial differentiation of adult neural stem cells: a platform to tune cellular behavior in neural tissue engineering. Macromol Biosci 2019;19(2), e1800236.

[127] Tate MC, Shear DA, Hoffman SW, Stein DG, LaPlaca MC. Biocompatibility of methylcellulose-based constructs designed for intracerebral gelation following experimental traumatic brain injury. Biomaterials 2001;22(10):1113–23.

[128] Stabenfeldt SE, García AJ, LaPlaca MC. Thermoreversible laminin-functionalized hydrogel for neural tissue engineering. J Biomed Mater Res A 2006;77(4):718–25.

[129] Wang Q. Smart materials for tissue engineering: applications. London: RSC Smart Materials Series; 2017.

[130] Boateng J, Catanzano O. Advanced therapeutic dressings for effective wound healing—a review. J Pharm Sci 2015;104(11):3653–80.

[131] Zubik K, Singhsa P, Wang Y, Manuspiya H, Narain R. Thermo-responsive poly(N-isopropylacrylamide)-cellulose nanocrystals hybrid hydrogels for wound dressing. Polymers 2017;9(12):119.

[132] Wang Y, Wang Z, Wu K, Wu J, Meng G, Liu Z, Guo X. Synthesis of cellulose-based double-network hydrogels demonstrating high strength, self-healing, and antibacterial properties. Carbohydr Polym 2017;168:112–20.

[133] Kassal P, Zubak M, Scheipl G, Mohr GJ, Steinberg MD, Murković SI. Smart bandage with wireless connectivity for optical monitoring of pH. Sensor Actuat B-Chem 2017;246:455–60.

14

Hydrogels based on cellulose nanocomposites

Neslihan Kayra[a], Yaprak Petek Koraltan[b], and Ali Özhan Aytekin[a]

[a]Genetics and Bioengineering Department, Engineering Faculty, Yeditepe University, Istanbul, Turkey, [b]Biotechnology Graduate Program, Graduate School of Natural and Applied Sciences, Yeditepe University, Istanbul, Turkey

14.1 Introduction

Nanocomposite materials are multiphase structures; at least one of its components are nanosized. Hydrogels, including nanomaterials as filler or reinforcement agents, are also defined as nanocomposites. When nanomaterials are considered as a biomaterial, it is essential to have some criteria. For example, being biocompatible, biodegradable, renewable, and eco-friendly are considered properties when deciding on nanomaterial sources. Various natural polymers can be used for this purpose, for example, chitin, chitosan, alginate, and cellulose. Among these sources, cellulose is most favored due to its impressive properties such as abundance in nature, capability of various surface modifications, and being environmentally friendly. In comparison to bulk cellulose, nanosized cellulose (cellulose nanocrystal [CNC] and cellulose nanofibril [CNF]) exhibits straightforward surface modification, biocompatibility, bioavailability, high surface area characteristics, and tunable surface properties that make it suitable for biomedicine applications.

This chapter mainly involves knowledge regarding plant-originated nanocelluloses and a summary of plant nanobased hydrogels in drug delivery and tissue engineering studies explicitly reported in the last 3 years. The chapter gives information about cellulose types and characteristics of plant-based nanocellulose (CNC and CNF), preparation techniques

Plant and Algal Hydrogels for Drug Delivery and Regenerative Medicine
https://doi.org/10.1016/B978-0-12-821649-1.00013-1

of nanocellulose, and a brief explanation of nanocomposites and hydrogels. Then nanocellulose-based hydrogels and their functionality in biomedicine, specifically in drug delivery and tissue engineering fields, are explained by giving examples from the latest research. As a result, this chapter summarizes nanocomposite hydrogels produced from plant-originated CNC and CNF that are favorable materials with broad applications in drug delivery and tissue engineering.

14.2 Structure and types of cellulose

Cellulose is the most abundant polymer in nature. It can be either a structural part of plants or the product of fungi, algae, or bacteria [1]. Plant-based cellulose does not occur as an isolated structure; it is found in lignocellulosic biomass with other plant structures [1, 2]. Lignocellulose consists of three main polymers: hemicellulose, lignin, and cellulose polymers; in addition to these polymers, acetyl groups, minerals, and phenolic compounds can be found in small quantities [2]. These polymers are grouped as nonuniformly and three-dimensionally in the structure with different composition and degree according to the type of lignocellulosic biomass [2]. Although the distribution of these polymers in the cell wall is not uniform [2] and can be changeable according to species, tissues, and maturity of the cell wall [2], among these polymers, the major part of the lignocellulosic biomass is made up from cellulose [3]. Cellulose is responsible for the mechanical strength of plants [1]. Cellulose is a linear-chain homopolysaccharide, and its structure is composed of repeating D-glucopyranose (glucose) units that link together via β-(1–4)-glycosidic linkages as shown in Fig. 14.1 [1, 4]. After the linkage, anhydroglucose is formed, and two anhydroglucose units form anyhydrocellobiose (β-D-glucopyranose), which is a repeating part.

Each anhydroglucose unit is composed of six carbon atoms and three hydroxyl groups located at C2, C3, and C6 atoms. These hydroxyl groups on the monomer are essential for forming hydrogen bonds and plays a

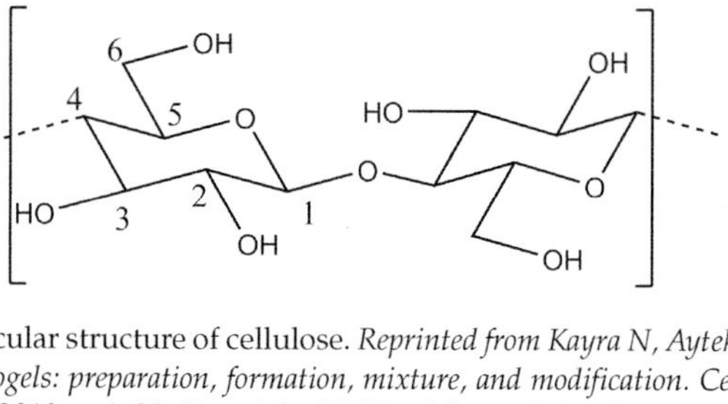

FIG. 14.1   Molecular structure of cellulose. *Reprinted from Kayra N, Aytekin AÖ. Synthesis of cellulose-based hydrogels: preparation, formation, mixture, and modification. Cellulose-based superabsorbent hydrogels 2018; p. 1–28. Copyright (2018), with permission from Springer.*

role in the cellulose's crystalline structure [4]. The cellobiose units are bonded via covalent bonds through acetal functions between the equatorial OH groups of C4 and C1 atoms [1]. The difference of cellulose from other glucan polymers is that the repeating unit is disaccharide cellobiose, not glucose [2], and it consists of β-(1–4) glycosidic bonds instead of α-(1–4) bonds as found in other polysaccharides [1]. Cellobiose structure includes extended intramolecular and intermolecular hydrogen bonds to tightly bind glucose units [2].

Cellulose is generally located in the secondary wall of the plant structure. A cell wall composed of nanosized cellulose microfibrils is embedded in the lignin matrix and forms a continuous and dynamic network through the whole plant [4, 5]. These microfibrils consist of crystalline and amorphous regions [6], and supramolecular cellulose structure is composed of networks of nanocellulose fibers that are fixed irreversibly [5] (Fig. 14.2). Jute, kenaf, cotton, flax, and all-natural fiber are examples of cellulose [6].

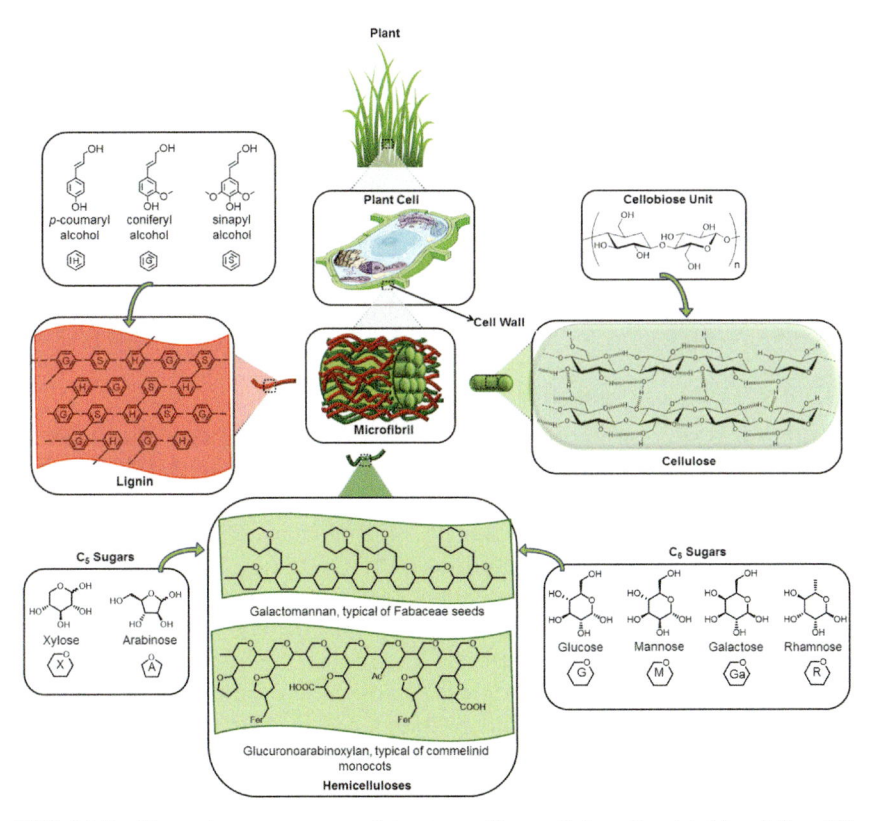

FIG. 14.2 The main components and structure of lignocellulose. *Reprinted from Isikgor FH, Becer CR. Lignocellulosic biomass: a sustainable platform for the production of bio-based chemicals and polymers. Polym Chem 2015;6:4497–559. https://doi.org/10.1039/c5py00263j. Copyright (2015), published by The Royal Society of Chemistry.*

Recently, most industrial areas considered sustaining their productions from renewable, biodegradable, environmentally friendly components. Although cellulose meets these properties, it also presents some specific features such as hydrophilicity, chirality, chain stiffness, and chemical modifying capacity because of extensive hydroxyl groups and semicrystalline structure, hydrolysis, and oxidation of chain-forming acetal groups that make it favorable and distinctive among other polymers [5, 7]. The extraction of cellulose from plant sources can be achieved by removing impurities via mechanical and chemical methods such as sodium hydroxide [1]. In the case of sodium hydroxide treatment, acid concentration and process time are crucial factors affecting polymerization [8]. In addition to this, pretreatment with ammonia, microwaves, and ultrasonication methods have been applied in the literature [1].

14.2.1 Types of plant-based nanocellulose

It is possible to obtain cellulose in small-dimension scales with additional degradation processes after isolating from a plant source. This leads to the classification of cellulose according to its shape and dimensions. "Nanocellulose" means the cellulose has at least one dimension in the nanometric scale [4]. Nanocellulose can be extracted from various sources such as jute, sisal, flax wood, cotton, eucalyptus, etc. [6]. The features of nanocellulose that make it attractive are low thermal expansion [4]; high aspect ratio, defined as the ratio of the length to diameter [4, 9]; nanoporosity and transparency in their dispersion; its composite forms a large surface area; the chance for surface chemical modifications [10]; and its solubility in water.

14.2.1.1 Cellulose nanofibrils (CNF)

There are several synonym nomenclatures of this size cellulose in the literature, such as CNF, nanofibrillated cellulose (NFC), microfibrils, microfibrilated cellulose (due to its length) [11], nanofibrillar cellulose, and cellulose nanofiber [4]. In this chapter, it is named CNF. CNF is flexible fiberlike [3] cellulose with a length in micrometer scale, whereas its width is in a nanometer scale [12]. Generally, CNF has a diameter in the 5–50 nm dimension and length of a few micrometers [10]. CNF includes both amorphous and crystalline regions, and due to the amorphous part, it is more flexible compared with CNC [9, 12] and has a lower degree of crystallinity than CNC [1] (Fig. 14.3). which has near-perfect crystallinity (ca. 90%) [13]. CNF can form physically entangled networks and structures when dispersed in aqueous media, even at low concentrations [9, 12]. Highly viscous aqueous suspensions can be produced due to the entanglement of relatively low concentration (below 1 wt%) of CNF [13].

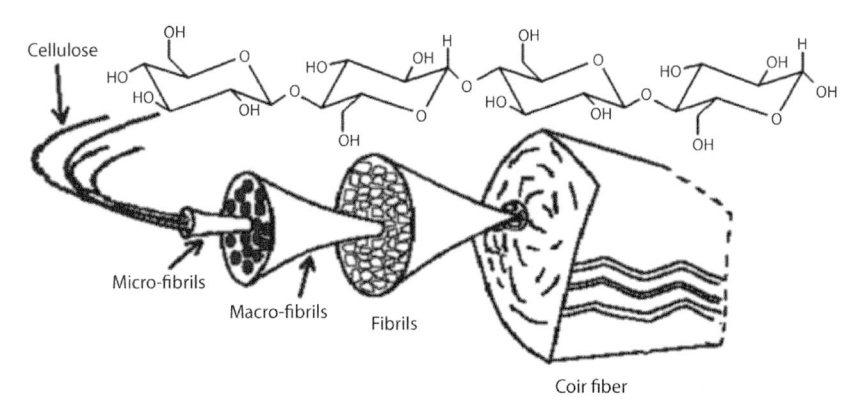

Micro-fibrils

Macro-fibrils

Fibrils

Coir fiber

FIG. 14.3 The structure of cellulose nanofibrils (CNF). *Reprinted from Raji M, Essabir H, Bouhfid R, El Kacem Qaiss A. Impact of chemical treatment and the manufacturing process on mechanical, thermal, and rheological properties of natural fibers-based composites. Handb Compos from Renew Mater 2017;1–8:225–252. https://doi.org/10.1002/9781119441632.ch71. Copyright (2017), with permission from John Wiley and Sons.*

CNF is obtained by its release from fundamental fiber matrix and microfiber bundles [12] via several treatments. Generally, mechanical forces such as high-pressure homogenization, high-intensity sonication, grinding cryocrushing, microfluidization, and milling [6, 13] are used to extract CNF from cellulosic fibers. However, these techniques might require high energy demand depending on the scale of the process. Therefore, to decrease energy consumption, chemical pretreatments (alkaline-acid treatment), chemical treatments (TEMPO oxidation) [9, 13], biological treatments (enzymes), and a combination of chemical and mechanical treatments [6, 13] are other techniques to achieve CNF extraction. A brief description of these techniques can be seen in Fig. 14.4.

The features of CNF like high aspect area (length to diameter: L/d) and properties related to its weight present an opportunity to use nanofillers in nanocomposites and bionanocomposites productions in different industrial [6] and research areas.

14.2.1.2 Cellulose nanocrystals (CNC)

CNC, also called nanocrystalline cellulose (NCC) or cellulose nanowhiskers (CNW), is a rigid rodlike-, nanorod-, or nanowhisker-shaped particle in a 10–30 nm diameter and several 100 nm in length [3]. The CNC's length and diameter can vary depending on cellulose source and extraction conditions [14]. The length dimension of CNC is not higher than CNF [1], and CNC has a lower aspect ratio when compared with CNF [12]. Additionally, because of the lack of amorphous regions, CNC shows limited flexibility compared with CNF [4]. CNC is extracted from cellulose fibers through the acid hydrolysis process. Amorphous regions

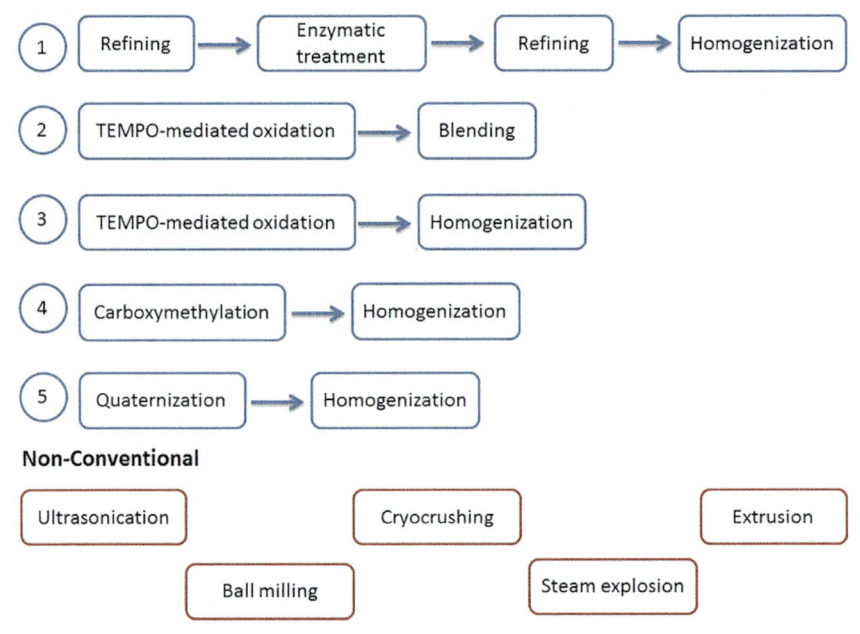

FIG. 14.4   Conventional and nonconventional methods for cellulose nanofibril extraction. *Reprinted from Kayra N, Aytekin AÖ. Synthesis of cellulose-based hydrogels: preparation, formation, mixture, and modification. Cellulose-based superabsorbent hydrogels 2018; p. 1–28. Copyright (2018), with permission from Springer.*

are degraded during the acid hydrolysis process, and highly crystalline cellulose nanoparticles occur [12]. After the hydrolysis process, obtained particles are pure cellulose with 54% and 88% crystalline zones [15]. The hydrolysis method and cellulosic material are determinative factors of the degree of crystallinity, dimensional diversity, and CNC morphology [4]. The degree of crystallinity, cellulose source, hydrolysis reaction conditions such as process time, temperature, and acid concentration are crucial parameters that influence nanocrystals' dimensions [11]. CNC hydrolysis treatments can be achieved using sulfuric acid, hydrochloric acid, phosphoric acid, hydrobromic acid, or a combination of inorganic and organic acids [14]. During the hydrolysis process, polysaccharide bounds that are found on the surface of fibrils are first eliminated, then amorphous regions are broken up to reveal crystalline rodlike cellulose [11]. After the optimum level of glucose chain depolymerization centrifugation and dialysis, processes are applied to remove acid and residual impurities. An additional mechanical method is applied to obtain uniform nanocrystals [11]. The types of acid used in the hydrolysis process can contribute to surface functionalization. For example, at the end of the sulfuric acid treatment, the nanoparticles' surface is grafted with negatively charged sulfate-ester groups. This functionalization prevents aggregation because of electrostatic repulsion between particles [13]. In addition to sulfuric acid, HCl treatment leads to weakly negative charges on CNC but less than sulfuric acid [11].

CNC exhibits good mechanical properties, and rare optical and self-assembly properties [13, 16]. These unique features of CNC provide optically transparent and lightweight materials such as nanocomposites for different purposes [16].

14.3 Fundamental modification reaction of cellulose

Cellulose is an excellent polymer with attractive features. Although advantageous because of the hydrophilic nature of nanocellulose and hydrophobic nature of the polymeric matrix (thermoset and thermoplastics), desired interfacial adhesion with the polymeric matrix cannot occur during the manufacturing of nanocomposites [6]. This weak adhesion directly affects nanocomposites' mechanical and structural properties as it leads to poor resistance to moisture absorption, low tensile strength, and formation of agglomerates [6]. Therefore, adding specific functional groups on cellulose can improve its reactivity, solubility, mechanical properties [13], and dispersion in hydrophobic media or polymer matrices [17]. With the chemical treatments, high dense hydrogen bonds are formed between nanocellulose and polymer matrix [6]. The advantageous features of the nanocellulose, mainly surface hydroxyl groups and large specific surface areas, contribute to extensive active sites for modification [13]. Oxidation, esterification, etherification, polymer grafting (grafting from or onto), silylation, Diels-Alder, thiol-one, and Huisgen cycloaddition are some modification reactions used to introduce functional groups or help for further modification [13, 14].

Because of exciting mechanical and optical properties, CNC is more preferred for modification than CNF [13]. Additionally, extensive reactive hydroxyl groups on the surface of CNC provide the potential of various modification ways to introduce functional groups to its surface [18]. Surface hydrophobization by silylation or acylation, carboxylation, esterification, fluorescein isothiocyanate (FITC) labeling, polymer grafting, and cationic surface functionalization are some examples of modification that have been applied for the modification of CNC [11]. The critical point that must be considered before modification of CNC is selecting the correct reagent and reaction medium that will not dissolve CNC and introduce undesired bulk changes [11]. The hydrophobization contributes to the improvement of compatibility because the hydroxyl groups of CNC cause low dispersion of CNC nonpolar solvents and polymer matrices [13]. For this purpose, alkyl groups, fluorine, alkenyl, alkynyl, thiol groups, and pyridine moieties were used [13]. Besides hydrophobization, polymer grafting can improve adhesion between the polymer matrix and CNC, enabling stress transfer to enhance the produced nanocomposite material [13].

14.4 Nanocomposite

14.4.1 Preparation method of nanocomposite

The term "nanomaterial" is used for particles with at least one dimension smaller than 100 nm [19]. This small-scale dimension allows some unique chemical and physical characteristics compared with bulk forms such as a particular surface area and impressive electrical, optical, mechanical, magnetic, and thermal features [19]. Because of these features, nanomaterials are mostly preferred in various fields such as environment, optics, electronics, medicine, etc.

Nanocomposites are new generation multiphase materials containing more than one component, and at least one component is in the nanosized dimension [4, 6, 20]. They are considered an alternative to conventional composites thanks to good compatibility between matrix and nanomaterials and the desired dispersibility of the nanomaterial in the polymer matrix [20]. Several factors affect nanocomposites' properties: the polymer matrix's nature, the interaction between polymer and nanoparticles, and the conformation of large interphase elements [4]. Compared with microsized reinforcement agents, including composites, nanocomposites possess large surface areas and low deficiency in the reinforcing part [4]. Among nanomaterials used in the construction of nanocomposites, natural fibers have been favored in various fields because of its mechanical features, thermal stability, biodegradability, cheapness, abundance, and being environmentally friendly [4, 16, 21].

In addition to these impressive characteristics, using natural fibers as reinforcement agents increases the chance of producing green nanocomposite materials [4]. Fiber size, aspect ratio, volume fraction and orientation, fiber-matrix adhesion, and stress transfer through the interface are some parameters that might be effective on nanocomposites characterization reinforced by fiber [4]. Like all other nanomaterials, nanocellulose has significant properties due to nanometric sizes such as high mechanical strength, high aspect ratio, and being lightweight. Thanks to these properties, it is an excellent filler or reinforcement agent for nanocomposite production, mainly in the medicine, electronic, and energy fields [6, 16].

Among the nanocelluloses, CNF is favored as a reinforcement agent because of its large surface area, transparency, water retention, high strength and stiffness, low weight, and homogenous dispersibility in polymer matrixlike properties [16]. However, the primary purpose of using CNF in nanocomposites is to develop the final product's mechanical properties [6].

When using hydrophilic cellulose in a polymer matrix, some difficulties can appear. For example, desired adhesion in nonpolar polymer matrices cannot be enabled, which causes weak interfacial bonding between the polymer and cellulosic components [12]. Additionally, the entanglements due to nanofibers' length might cause aggregation problems during the dispersion of nanofibers in the polymer matrix [11]. There have been some techniques to produce a nanocomposite. Dispersing dried cellulose into a hydrophobic matrix, dispersing cellulose and polymer matrix in a common solvent, and using aqueous nanocellulose dispersion are the main production methods of nanocellulose [12]. Among these methodologies, aqueous nanocellulose dispersion is not suitable for nonpolar polymers because of insufficient mixing and adhesion [12].

14.4.2 Hydrogel

Hydrogels are 3D, physically or chemically cross-linked mono- or co-polymer chains of natural or synthetic materials that have embedded water. The hydrophilic groups of hydrogel-forming polymers like $-OH$, $-CONH-$, $-CONH_2-$, and $-SO_3H$ are mainly responsible for hydrogels' water absorption ability [22]. Hydrogels can be formed via chemical or physical methods. In chemically formed hydrogels, covalent interactions exist between functional groups of the polymer chains [23]. The mainly used covalent coupling reactions are Michael addition, click reaction, Schiff's base formation, photocross-linking, and enzyme-mediated cross-linking [23]. In chemically cross-linked hydrogels, cross-linking agents are used to construct covalent interactions between polymer chains [22]. Particular functional groups of polymers readily available or obtained by several chemical modifications are the primary needs for cross-linking chemistry [23].

On the other hand, physically formed hydrogels utilize physical interactions like Van der Waals forces, hydrogen bonding, chain entanglements, and hydrophobic forces to cross-link polymer chains [22, 23]. Instead of the chemical cross-linking method, the physical method can be chosen to produce safe, environmentally friendly hydrogels. Especially tailorable mechanical, chemical, and physical properties of hydrogels make them advantageous in biomedicine applications. Its high water content and solidlike properties make it preferable for biomedical applications, especially for tissue engineering, wound healing, and drug delivery [18]. Hydrogels used for that purpose have self-healing, injectable, and stimuli-responsive properties compared with chemical hydrogels [18].

14.4.3 Preparation of nanocomposite hydrogel

Nanocellulose-based hydrogels have attracted attention for biomedical applications because of their low toxicity, biodegradability, biocompatibility, and mechanical properties [3], especially because the contribution of nanocellulose to hydrogel is for the modification of its mechanical properties. By incorporation of CNC and CNF into synthetic polymers like poly(vinyl alcohol) (PVA), polyacrylamides (PAM), poly(ethylene glycol) (PEG), or natural polymers like alginate, gelatin, chitosan, it is possible to obtain mechanically improved hydrogels [3]. Hydrogels produced completely from biopolymers and reinforced with nanocellulose can be recognized as "green" nanocomposites because their structures are renewable, biodegradable, and eco-friendly [14]. The main difference between nanocomposite hydrogels from conventional ones is higher elasticity and strength. Because of nanocomposite hydrogel's elasticity, during stretching of the polymer network, the filler polymer is switched off and contributes to swelling of the hydrogel several times its mass [14].

Nanocomposite hydrogel formation can typically succeed in chemical and physical manners. Ionic interactions, hydrogen bonds, freeze–thaw method, supramolecular assembly, and chemically cross-linking are examples of the 3D network formation method. The physical network formation was ensured by electrostatic and ionic interactions, hydrogen bonding, and chain entanglements. Chemical hydrogel formation is enhanced by covalent bonds due to radical polymerization, enzymatic reaction, irradiation, chemical reactions, and various cross-linking agents [24]. In the case of nanocomposite hydrogel formation, modification or functionalization surface of nanocellulose can facilitate network formation. For example, surface modification of CNCs contributed to the formation of carboxyl or aldehyde groups that served as covalent cross-linking sites or surface groups that can be screened with salt addition thus ionic cross-linking is ensured [9]. And surface modification of CNCs can enhance gel formation due to colloidal instability by reducing electrostatic interactions between particles [9]. During hydrogel formation, some critical parameters should be taken into account that affects hydrogels' characteristics and functionality. For example, porosity can be arranged by controlling cross-linking density [24]. It is crucial to transmit various compounds such as drugs, nutrients, or waste mainly in drug absorption and release studies. Also, swelling ratio, shear modulus, and mechanical features are influenced by interconnected chains [24]. The next section (Table 14.1) comprises some recent nanocomposite hydrogels formation applications by chemical, physical, and both.

TABLE 14.1 Nanocomposite hydrogel preparation methods.

Nanocellulose type	Nanocellulose role	Method type	Method name	References
		Chemically	Radical polymerization	[25]
TEMPO-oxidized cellulose nanofibrils	Main material	Chemically and physically	ECH/Fe^{3+}	[26]
Cellulose nanocrystals	Supporting material	Chemically	Genipin	[27]
Cellulose nanocrystals	Supporting material	Chemically	Radical polymerization	[28]
Cellulose nanocrystal TEMPO-oxidized cellulose nanofibers Bacterial cellulose fibers	Supporting material	Chemically	Ca^{2+}, MBA	[29]
Cellulose nanocrystals	Supporting material	Chemically		[30]
P4VP-cellulose nanocrystals	Supporting material	Chemically	Free radical polymerization	[31]
β-Cyclodextrin modified tunicate cellulose nanocrystals	Supporting material	Physically	Cellulose nanocrystals/Fe^{3+}	[32]
Lignin-containing cellulose nanocrystals	Supporting material	Physically	Freeze–thaw	[33]
TEMPO-oxidized cellulose nanofibrils	Main material	Physically	Ionic cross-linking (Zn^{2+})	[34]
Methylcellulose/cellulose nanocrystals	Main material	Physically	Electrostatic interactions	[35]

14.4.3.1 Chemically cross-linked nanocomposite hydrogels

A hydrogel nanocomposite was formed from acrylic acid and cellulose nanofibers, including urea, as a functional reactant by radical polymerization method [25]. The process was achieved using N-N'-methylene–bisacrylamide (MBA) as a cross-linker at 0.2 wt% and potassium persulfate (KPS) as an initiator at 0.04 wt% concentrations at 70 °C. The polymerization mechanism was summarized so that KPS produces sulfate anion radicals. These radicals contribute to the formation of alkoxy radicals on cellulose by subtracting hydrogen atoms of hydroxyl groups of hemicellulose [25]. Then cellulose radicals are recognized by neutralized acrylic acid monomers, and these monomers behave as free radical donors for other close molecules. In this way, polymerization is completed [25]. The study's characterization results indicated that polymerization was achieved, and the presence of the urea led to high cross-linking density by acting as cross-linking agents besides MBA, as suggested. Another chemically cross-linked hydrogel nanocomposite example was a genipin cross-linked chitosan hydrogel reinforced with CNCs [27]. The cross-linking reaction of chitosan with genipin continued for 7 days, and blue-colored hydrogel was formed. It was seen that, by increasing CNCs concentration, hydrogel mechanical strength was improved; therefore, CNCs might be useful for hydrogel formation at low genipin concentrations. An interpenetrating polymer network (IPN)-structured hydrogel was formed from polyacrylamide used for the flexible part. The polyelectrolyte sodium alginate was used for the rigid part in three types of nanocellulose: bacterial cellulose fibers, CNCs, and TEMPO-oxidized cellulose nanofibers (TOCN) [29]. Hydrogel formation between sodium alginate and polyacrylamide was ensured by chemical cross-linking with Ca^{2+} and MBA. Analysis of the hydrogels' structures revealed that all three types of nanocellulose behaved as multifunctional cross-linking agents. CNCs extracted from grape pomace by deep eutectic solvent were used to prepare guar gum-based self-healing hydrogel by facilitating borax as a cross-linking agent and Fe^{3+} as the cross-linking site [30]. It was proven that the addition of the CNCs at higher amounts enriched the number of cross-linking density and hydrogen bonds and improved the mechanical strength of the hydrogel. A self-healing nanocomposite hydrogel was produced from acrylic acid and surface-modified CNCs, which served as reinforcement agents by in situ free radical polymerization in KPS (Fig. 14.5) [31].

Surface modification of CNCs was carried by metal-free photoinduced electron transfer atom transfer radical polymerization (PET-ATRP). The surface initiation of produced PET-ATRP was conducted in a functional monomer, photocatalyst, light source, 4-vinyl pyridine (4VP), 10-phenylphenothiazine (pH-PTZ), and ultraviolet light at 365 nm, respectively. Surface-modified CNCs-reinforced hydrogels exhibited 85.9% self-healing and 6.6 MPa mechanical strength characteristics.

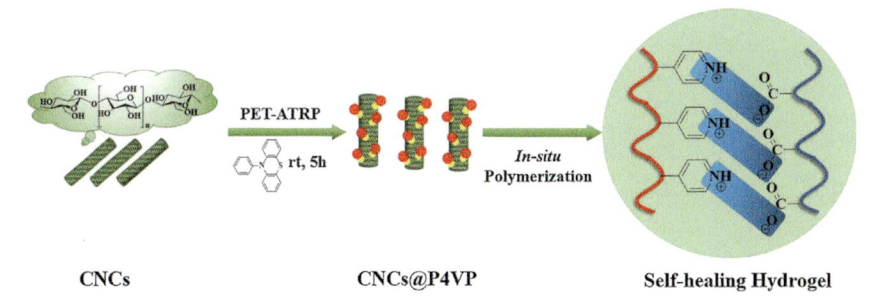

FIG. 14.5 Self-healing hydrogel-based P4VP-cellulose nanocrystals. *Reprinted from Bai L, Jiang X, Sun Z, Pei Z, Ma A, Wang W, et al. Self-healing nanocomposite hydrogels based on modified cellulose nanocrystals by surface-initiated photoinduced electron transfer ATRP. Cellulose 2019;26:5305–19. https://doi.org/10.1007/s10570-019-02449-2. Copyright (2019), with permission from Springer.*

14.4.3.2 Physically cross-linked nanocomposite hydrogels

In addition to chemical cross-linking, physical cross-linking can be applied to form nanocomposite hydrogels. A current study synthesized a nanocomposite hydrogel from tunicate CNCs by doubly physical cross-linking [32]. First, cross-linking was succeeded between β-cyclodextrin-modified tunicate CNCs and monomers of acrylic acid, acrylamide, and adamantane acrylamide by the aid of APS and TEMED at 60°C. After the first cross-linking, stretching was applied to hydrogels to align CNCs inside the hydrogel network. Then prestretched hydrogel doubly cross-linked with the aid of Fe^{3+}. It was explained that tunicated CNCs acted as both cross-linker agents, particularly at the first stage, and filler. By ion cross-linking, hydrogel mechanical strength was improved to ~ 56 MPa. The freeze–thaw method was used to synthesize physical cross-linked nanocomposite hydrogel from polyvinyl alcohol (PVA) reinforced with lignin-containing CNCs (Fig. 14.6) [33].

Homogenized PVA and CNCs suspensions (at different contents of 0.1, 0.25, 0.5, and 1.0 wt%) were treated twice at $-20°C$ for 8 h and then thawed at room temperature for 3 h. The researchers concluded that lignin-containing CNCs contributed to hydrogel formation by only two freeze–thaw cycles with high G'max (max storage modulus) (5176 Pa). These results were more reasonable than found in the literature. TEMPO-mediated oxidized cellulose possesses negative carboxylate groups that allow easy screening by counterions such as Ca^{2+} and Fe^{3+}, and this ionic cross-linking enhances network formation to produce hydrogel. A recent study was facilitated in this manner of hydrogel formation from bagasse-based TEMPO-oxidized nanocellulose fibers in the presence of Zn^{2+} and self-assembled nanocomposite hydrogel loaded with pH-responsive colors for the monitoring of chicken freshness [34]. Methylcellulose and CNCs-based nanocomposite hydrogels were

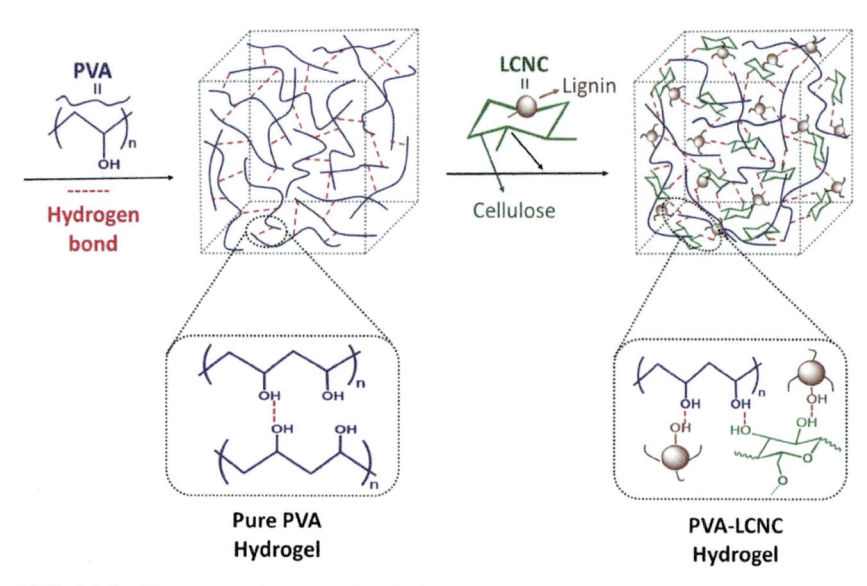

FIG. 14.6　Illustration of pristine PVA hydrogel and lignin-containing cellulose nanocrystals reinforced PVA hydrogel-formation mechanism. *Reprinted from Wang Y, Liu S, Wang Q, Fu X, Fatehi P. Performance of polyvinyl alcohol hydrogel reinforced with lignin-containing cellulose nanocrystals. Cellulose 2020;27:8725–8743. https://doi.org/10.1007/s10570-020-03396-z. Copyright (2020), with permission from Springer.*

produced to obtain nanocomposite fibers by the continuous spinning procedure [35]. Two cellulose components were mixed for hydrogel formation, and methylcellulose content was kept constant (1 wt%), whereas CNC concentration varied between 0 and 3 wt%. Hydrogel formation was assessed due to electrostatic interactions.

A recent study was used sequentially to form doubly cross-linked nanocellulose hydrogel with improved mechanical features [26]. Chemical cross-linking of the TEMPO-oxidized nanocellulose was performed in the presence of epichlorohydrin (ECH) as a cross-linker, and then physical cross-linking was achieved by the addition of multivalent metals (Fe^{3+}, Ca^{2+}) in salt form (Fig. 14.7).

The doubly cross-linked nanocellulose hydrogel's compressive strength was increased to 450 kPa compared with only physically (Fe^{3+}) and chemically formed hydrogels' compressive strength of 117 and 17 kPa, respectively.

Beyond the formation process, the structuring of produced nanocomposite hydrogels is crucial for versatile purposes. The 3D printed, injectable, 2.5 D-structured hydrogels are the most preferred structured techniques by current studies, especially in the biomedicine field, to appropriately target tissue or deliver drugs to targeted tissue or organs. For example, a 2.5D-structured nanocomposite hydrogel manufactured from

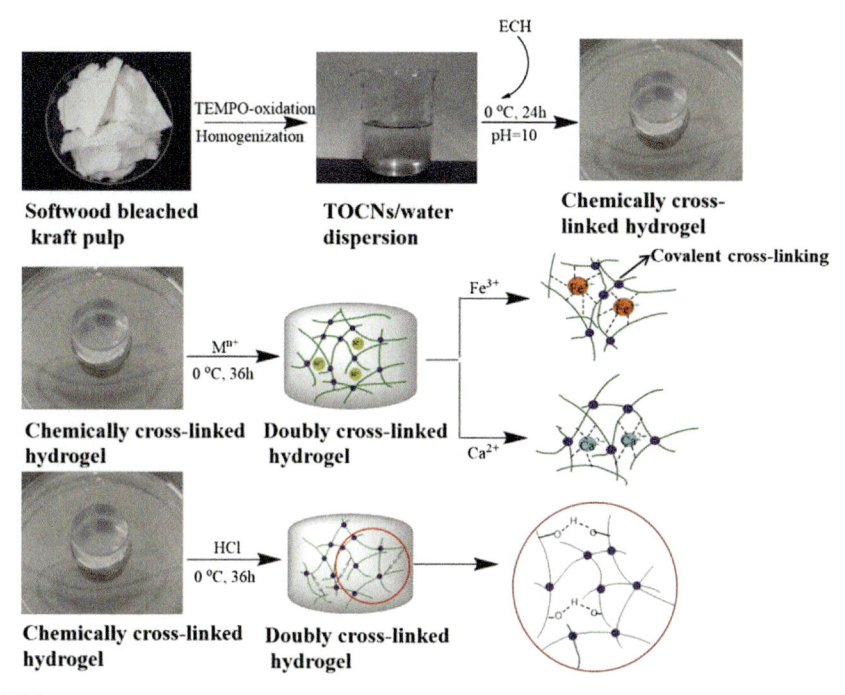

FIG. 14.7 Doubly cross-linked process of nanocellulose hydrogel. *Reprinted from Xu H, Liu Y, Xie Y, Zhu E, Shi Z, Yang Q, et al. Doubly cross-linked nanocellulose hydrogels with excellent mechanical properties. Cellulose 2019;26:8645–8654. https://doi.org/10.1007/s10570-019-02689-2. Copyright (2019), with permission from Springer.*

CNCs, aldehyde, and hydrazide-functionalized poly(oligo ethylene glycol methacrylate) (POEGMA) by spin-coating procedure was structured by the thermal shrinking method [36]. The injectability of the hydrogels can be arranged by checking the viscoelasticity of the hydrogel during the process. 3D printing is mostly defined as additive manufacturing or rapid prototyping [37]. First of all, a hydrogel is formed according to the specific intended use, and the produced hydrogel is used as ink for 3D structuring. For example, CNCs were used at 0.5–25 wt% concentrations to prepare hydrogels and then evaluate its 3D printability [38]. 3D printed hydrogels' analysis demonstrated that hydrogels produced at 20 wt% CNCs possessed optimal print resolution and a great orientation degree (72%–73%).

Hydrogels are evaluated by way of different parameters. Generally, composition analysis is done by Fourier transform infrared spectrophotometry (FTIR). Pore size and morphology are examined by scanning electron microscope (SEM). Mechanical characterization is done to measure tensile strength, compression, physical features like viscoelasticity, and rheological measurements examine storage modulus. In addition, the morphology of the filling agents can be characterized by a transmission electron microscope (TEM). Besides hydrogel characterization analyses, in vitro and in vivo studies must be done considering the interested hydrogel composition and application biomedicine area. For example, biocompatibility tests like cytotoxicity must be done to understand the interaction between the hydrogel and related sites by looking at cell attachment, cell proliferation, and viability results.

14.5 Nanocellulose-based hydrogel applications in drug delivery and tissue engineering

There is increased popularity in hydrogel studies based on drug delivery and tissue engineering fields. The important points that should be considered are hydrogel's ability to deliver and release drugs without side effects with no damage to healthy tissue and organs. The feature that makes hydrogels attractive is that they can be prepared from biodegradable, biocompatible, and nontoxic materials. Therefore, cellulose, one of the most abundant polymers on Earth and its derivatives, is excellent for hydrogel formation. Besides its chemical form, indifferent physical forms such as nanocrystal or nanofiber forms increase its application numbers.

14.5.1 Drug delivery applications

The inherent nature of hydrogel makes it a promising environment for drugs having aqueous insolubility. Loading of hydrogels with therapeutics can enable their sustained or control release, protect sensitive drugs from extreme conditions such as pH before reaching the target site, improve the solubility of hydrophobic drugs, and protect from side effects of the drug via targeting to the particular site. Drug delivery-based hydrogel studies have been mostly based on the medium characteristics of the drug's following pathway before the target site. For example, researchers have produced nanocarboxymethylcellulose (NCMC) by acid hydrolysis and carboxymethylation processes and then magnetized by Fe_3O_4 nanoparticles [39]. NCMC has been produced from CNC by alkalization and etherification processes. Magnetized NCMC has been used in alginate spherical hydrogel production. They have suggested that beads with well-ordered size and shape are suitable for drug delivery studies because of high surface area and the opportunity to encapsulate various drugs. After the formulation of hydrogel beads, coating with chitosan has been applied to prevent solubility in tested mediums.

The formulated magnetic hydrogel beads were tested for the delivery of dexamethasone in simulated gastric (pH 1.2), intestinal (pH 7.4), and cancer cell (pH 5.8) fluids. In vitro, drug release studies have shown that NCMCs presented promising results in drug loading, swelling, and drug release. Also, pH-sensitive results have been obtained for a pH of 5.8 rather than other mediums. In further study, CNCs produced by acid hydrolysis of microcrystalline cellulose (MCC) were used as a nanoreinforcement agent. Starch-based click hydrogel was produced by the Diels-Alder click cross-linking reaction of furan-functionalized starch derivative and water-soluble tetrafunctional maleimide compound [40]. While the starch-based hydrogel has been tested for the delivery of chloramphenicol, CNC's effect has been evaluated in terms of swelling, rheological, and morphological aspects. The CNC effect has been assessed at 2.5 and 5 wt% concentrations, and results have revealed that the CNC content has positively contributed to stiffness.

On the other hand, the incorporation of CNC to the hydrogel has prevented hydrogel's mobility and led to a lower swelling ratio value. Also, as the CNC content increased, the porosity of the hydrogel increased. The drug loading amount has been similar for the CNC-filled hydrogel and unfilled hydrogels.

Drug release from hydrogels was investigated for various drugs such as antibiotic agents or cancer therapy agents. Besides the sustained release or target site-reaching advantages, another reason for using hydrogels is their inherent hydrophilic nature. The insolubility of lipophilic drugs in an aqueous environment limits their use; therefore, hydrogels can be an excellent material to reduce this problem. Researchers have suggested that clofazimine (CFZ) solubility, which is a lipophilic antibiotic in water, could be improved by preparing the hydrogel ionotropic gelation technique of TEMPO-oxidized cellulose in the presence of Tween 20 as a nonionic surfactant agent [41]. Hydrogels have been prepared at different CFZ concentrations and constant CFZ but varying Tween 20 concentrations. Releasing studies of CFZ have been conducted both in water and in ethanol, and the effect of cations from cross-linker agents has been examined. The study results have revealed that, although NC hydrogels loaded with dry CFZ had a reasonable release, the addition of Tween 20 led to an improvement in the solubility of CFZ in water. Similarly, nanocellulose-filled chitosan hydrogel was prepared for the delivery of lipophilic curcumin extract [42]. Because the group's previous outputs have stated that nanocellulose had a positive impact on the mechanical and swelling properties of chitosan hydrogel, a recent study group focused on only the curcumiñs solubility extract. To increase the curcumin extract's solubility, Tween 20, a nonionic surfactant, was added. In addition to the surfactant's effect on solubility, hydrogel formation under atmospheric and CO_2 gas was evaluated. The drug entrapment efficiency of new hydrogel decreased from $92.09 \pm 0.15\%$ to $77.92 \pm 0.70\%$ and $70.21 \pm 0.26\%$ by the addition of 5 and 30 (w/v)% Tween 20, respectively. The effect of hydrogel produced under gas foaming and atmospheric conditions on drug delivery revealed that entrapment efficiency was better atmospherically produced. This situation was associated with large-size pore formation during the gas foaming process, therefore less entrapment of the drug. Hydrogel beads were prepared by incorporating magnetic CNCs and alginate to deliver ibuprofen as a modal drug [22]. First, CNCs were modified with Fe^{2+} and Fe^{3+} ions by the coprecipitation method and then incorporated into the hydrogel. The utilization of magnetic CNCs aimed to improve the mechanical properties of the hydrogel and drug release manner. Consequently, although magnetic CNCs improved mechanical strength, hydrogel beads showed a decreasing drug release rate. A pH stimuli-responsive delivery of doxorubicin was performed via a hydrogel of anionic CNFs and cationic CNFs [43]. Chemical modification of CNFs ensured carboxylic acid groups and quaternary ammonium groups to anionic and cationic CNFs. The hydrogel was formed via self-standing of oppositely charged CNFs at acidic pH. The pH-dependent release of the doxorubicin was evaluated at pH 7.4 and pH 4. For pH 7.4, at the first 6 h, 35% entrapped doxorubicin was released at burst phase, but then release was not observed. On the other hand, drug release at pH 4 displayed fast release for the first 8.5 h then continued slowly until the end of 5 days. Biocompatibility tests of the polyion hydrogel indicated no cytotoxicity effect on NIH3T3 cells up to 900 μg/mL CNF concentration. TEMPO-oxidized and ultrasonicated (TOUS) cellulose nanofibers were used to form a hydrogel cross-linked by calcium ions for ibuprofen's control release [44]. The cross-linking of fibers was established due to the interaction between cations and carboxylic groups. Rheological analysis of the hydrogels indicated that 2% TOUS nanofibers and 10 mM $CaCl_2$ formed hydrogel with higher dynamic viscosity and pseudoplastic properties. After hydrogel formation, drug loading was done with the addition of β-cyclodextrins, which are mostly used to stabilize and aid the solubility of the drugs. The research proved that hydrogel's physiochemical properties could be tailored to TOUS nanofibers and cross-linking agent concentration. It is also possible to regulate drug release only by the addition of carriers like β-CD. In addition, biocompatibility analysis of the TOUS nanofibers injectable gel on the L929 murine fibroblast cell line revealed that cell viability was higher than 70% for 1, 3, and 7 day cultures. Similarly, self-assembly cellulose hydrogel was produced from CNCs cross-linked by NaCl [45]. The hydrogel was designed to inject bovine serum albumin (BSA), a low soluble drug (tetracycline), and a readily soluble drug (doxorubicin). Besides shear rheology, which is commonly used for analysis injectability of hydrogel, capillary rheology was performed to get reliable results. Measurements showed that CNCs hydrogels had plug flow, and they were injectable by saving structure and mechanical strength. While tetracycline exhibited burst release profile, protein and doxorubicin had sustained release that continued for 2 weeks. Additionally, whereas 80% of tetracycline and protein were released, doxorubicin completely released loaded drugs. These results were attributed to CNC's concentration, solubility, molecular size, and interactions between drug and cellulose as more important aspects of the release profile. Additionally, CNC hydrogel had no cytotoxic effect on HeLa cells. CNCs-incorporated hydrogel was synthesized from carboxymethyl cellulose and hydroxypropyl β-cyclodextrin by cross-linking with citric acid to release neohesperidin–copper (II) (NH-Cu(II)) [46]. The contribution of CNCs to swelling, drug loading, and controlled release profile was investigated. The CNC amount up to 4wt% led to improved tensile strength and elastic modulus; however, greater than this amount caused it to decrease. This amount improved loading and release capacity by 753.75mg/g and 85.08%, respectively. The drug release profile of hydrogels was burst release at an initial 30min, then diffusion control release. Self-assembly hydrogel formation of nanocellulose fibers modified by periodate-chlorite oxidation was studied to release piroxicam (PRX), a nonsteroidal anti-inflammatory drug [47]. Gel formation was assisted by vacuum filtration. Unlike the common surface-modification method of TEMPO-mediated oxidation, sequential periodate-chlorite oxidation was preferred to tune the surface charge of nanocellulose with a higher number of carboxyl moieties. As a result, surface modification of nanocellulose succeeded with 0.74–2.00mmol/g carboxylate group amount. The increasing amount of surface charge contributed to 30–60mg/g drug loading, which was ensured in less duration than release. It was suggested that anisotropic nanocellulose gel membrane might be used as a patch for transdermal drug delivery. 3D printed poly(lactic acid) capsules were filled with cellulose nanofiber hydrogel for release performance of metoprolol and nadolol as model drugs [48]. The study's aim was underlined as controlling drug release by arranging the capsules' inner geometry. PLA capsules were formed in three different shapes: small and large capsule, and tube design composed of an inner reservoir cavity and single release channel. The hydrogel part was prepared as a monolith dispersion of cellulose nanofiber, and 19G needles ensured nadolol and metoprolol injection of dispersion into the capsules. At the beginning of the release study, all designs demonstrated a brief profile but then continuously released linearly for 3 weeks. For both drugs, tube design showed higher cumulative release and small capsule showed less release. The study results represented that, by regulation of the capsules' inner geometry, sustained release can be achieved. The later addition of the drugs' printing capsules is a way of protecting drugs from side effects of processing conditions like heat. A hydrogel system was made up of chitosan, which is a digestible polymer, and CNCs used as a reinforcing agent for delayed and spatially controlled delivery of macromolecules [49]. The digestion of cellulose chitosan hydrogel and release of protein at the same time was investigated in the intestinal tract. It was revealed that new cellulose hydrogels were not degraded by lysozyme. However, cellulose chitosan hydrogel cylinders were exposed to degradation due to the presence of chitosan as requested. Protein release was sustained as slow, and in the sigmoidal profile and delivery path, it was associated with a hydrogel-formation process such as molding. Besides delivering one type of drug, codelivery of curcumin and doxorubicin was observed from chitosan, graphene, and CNW-based hydrogel under pH-, aldehyde-, and amine compound-stimulated response [50]. The hydrogel was manufactured from chitosan, aminated nanowhisker, and aminated via Schiff base reaction, including synthetic dialdehyde (2P). The released amount of both drugs increased at low pH, and at an initial 12 h, 56.1% and 63% of the curcumin and doxorubicin released at pH 5.4, respectively. At higher pH (7.4), both drugs' released amounts declined to 26% and 35% for curcumin and doxorubicin, respectively. Also, the drugs' codelivery demonstrated that, again, low pH was better for the release of both drugs, but curcumin release was lower than doxorubicin at low pH (5.4) and high pH (7.4). Research showed that chitosan/graphene/CNW-based hydrogel might be useful for delivery of curcumin, doxorubicin, and their combination form under pH stimuli. Periodate-oxidized CNCs were used to attain dialdehyde nanocellulose, and this modified nanocellulose served as a cross-linking agent and matrix for hydrogel formation from chitosan and CNCs (Fig. 14.8) [51]. Manufactured hydrogel was designed for delivery of theophylline as a model drug. The higher drug encapsulation (92.31%) was achieved at high chitosan concentration. Similarly, drug release profile showed an increasing trend with a rise in chitosan content. Chitosan- and nanocellulose-based hydrogel represented 85% and 23% cumulative drug release at pH 1.5 and 7.4, which are properties of gastric and intestinal fluids, respectively.

Stimuli-responsive hydrogels give well-timed reactions to alterations in the environment, such as pH, temperature, light, magnetic or electric field, ultrasound, and so on [41, 52]. Stimuli-responsive hydrogels are useful mainly for gastrointestinal drug delivery systems because of the changeable pH environment.

A pH-responsive hydrogel has been produced from surface-modified CNC and studied for the targeted release of paclitaxel (PTX), used in cancer therapy [53]. Surface modification has been achieved by oxidation with acetic anhydride to obtain CNC with carboxyl groups (O-CNC). Hydrogel from O-CNC was formed in the presence of hexadecyl amine (HAD). The drug release has been examined under different pH conditions (pH 5.5, 6.8, 7.4). The in vitro PTX release results revealed that, under acidic conditions (pH 5.5), while hydrogel lost its formation, the release of the PTX was better than in the gel form compared with its free form, but it kept its stability at pH 7.4. Besides release studies, research has searched for the inhibition effect of PTX-loaded O-CNC hydrogel, which has been tested on human HCC cell (HepG2) and adenocarcinoma human alveolar basal epithelial cell (A549) lines by in vitro cytotoxicity (MTT assay). The physicochemical

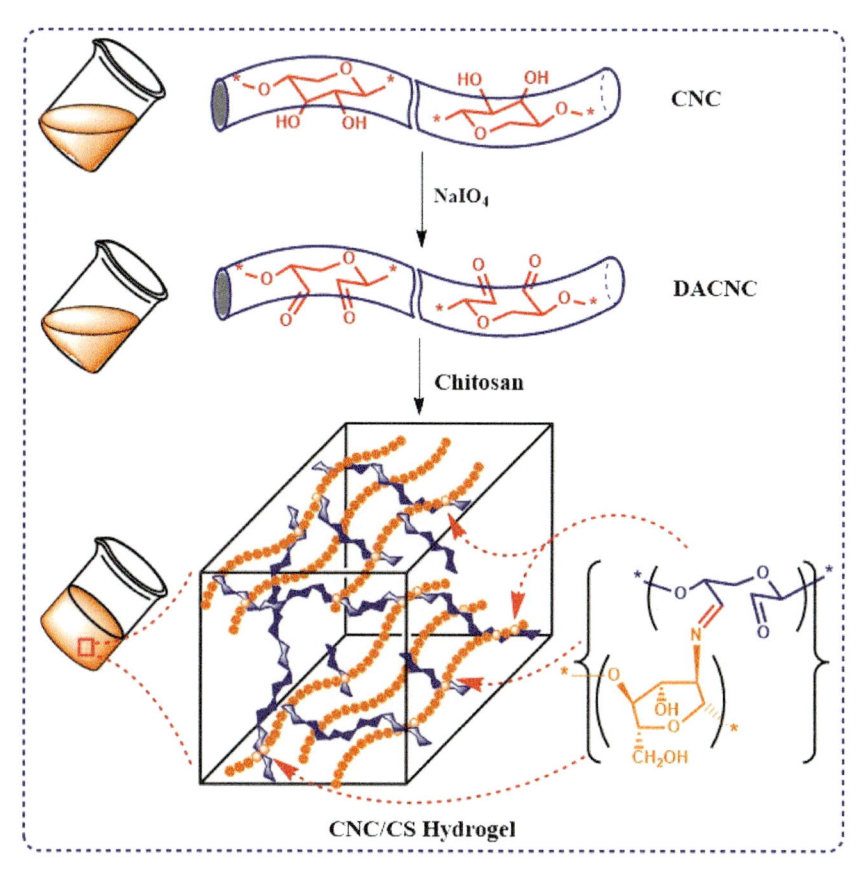

FIG. 14.8 Hydrogel formation from dialdehyde cellulose nanocrystals and chitosan. *Reprinted from Xu Q, Ji Y, Sun Q, Fu Y, Xu Y, Jin L. Fabrication of cellulose nanocrystal/chitosan hydrogel for controlled drug release. Nanomaterials 2019;9. https://doi.org/10.3390/nano9020253. Copyright (2019), with permission from Multidisciplinary Digital Publishing Institute.*

analyses and in vitro studies of the PTX-loaded O-CNC hydrogel indicated that surface-modified CNC hydrogel was a promising pH-sensitive vehicle for targeting drug delivery of PTX. In a similar study, pH and near-infrared (NR) responsive hydrogel was produced by physical cross-linking of CNFs (TOCNFs) produced by 2,2,6,6,-tetramethylpiperidine-1-oxyl (TEMPO)-mediated oxidation and polydopamine (PDA) in the presence of calcium ions [52]. It was aimed at loading the PDA, a photothermal agent with an antibiotic agent (tetracycline hydrochloride (TH)), and releasing it under NR and low pH-featured environments. Besides drug-releasing and wound-healing results, it was shown that, from characterization analysis, the PDA's addition to the TOCNF hydrogels enhanced hydrogel in terms of deformation and compression modulus.

14.5.2 Tissue engineering applications

Tissue engineering relies on engineering and life science knowledge to construct scaffolds instead of biological ones to repair, regenerate, and restore tissues at the lesion site [23]. Blood vessels, bone, cartilage, skin, and heart valves are some examples of tissue-engineered scaffolds. Besides general properties like biodegradability, noncytotoxicity, and mechanical and physical characteristics, viscosity and cellular response such as attachment, viability, and proliferation are featured properties that should be considered during the designing of scaffolds for tissue engineering [54]. Structural and compositional similarities between the scaffolds and extracellular matrix (ECM) of the relevant tissues represent tissue engineering's success [23]. There are some crucial parameters of hydrogels produced for tissue engineering applications that must be analyzed. For example, mechanical strength is essential for bone and disc applications. It must not restrict movement and be biocompatible to allow cell attachment, viability, and related tissue proliferation. Another important parameter is viscosity that must be considered particularly for injectable 3D printable hydrogels.

Besides drug delivery studies, tissue engineering is another popular area of hydrogels. There might be skin loss due to several reasons such as surgeries, burns, accidents, and decreased wound-healing time. A suitable wound cover that accelerates healing and protects the wound is required [55]. As in drug delivery studies, tissue engineering-based hydrogels can be loaded with therapeutic agents such as synthetic drugs or natural composites have healing properties. For example, curcumin incorporation into the PVA hydrogel has been studied due to its antioxidant property, collagen synthesis, and cellular proliferation-like effects of curcumin (Fig. 14.9) [55].

PVA hydrogel has been formed physically by the freeze–thaw method, and porosity enhancement has been achieved by TOCN. Hydrogel formation between TOCN and PVA occurred thanks to hydrogen bonds between carboxyl (–COOH) and hydroxyl (–OH) groups of TOCN and –OH groups of PVA. Apart from direct contact of hydrogels with the skin, there are injectable applications in tissue engineering studies. For example, pectin and chitosan-based injectable hydrogel have been produced in CNCs [56]. The CNC has been used to increase the biomaterials' mechanical strength and enhance cell migration, proliferation, and differentiation of the focused organs. Besides the reinforcement performance of CNC, aldehyde-modified CNC has been produced to improve mechanical properties and Schiff's structural performance of base reaction-based injectable hydrogels. The study results have noticed that high CNC content has affected hydrogels by contributing stiffness, lower equilibrium swelling ratio, and protecting against degradation. Another nanocellulose composed of injectable hydrogel has been formulated to prevent postsurgical

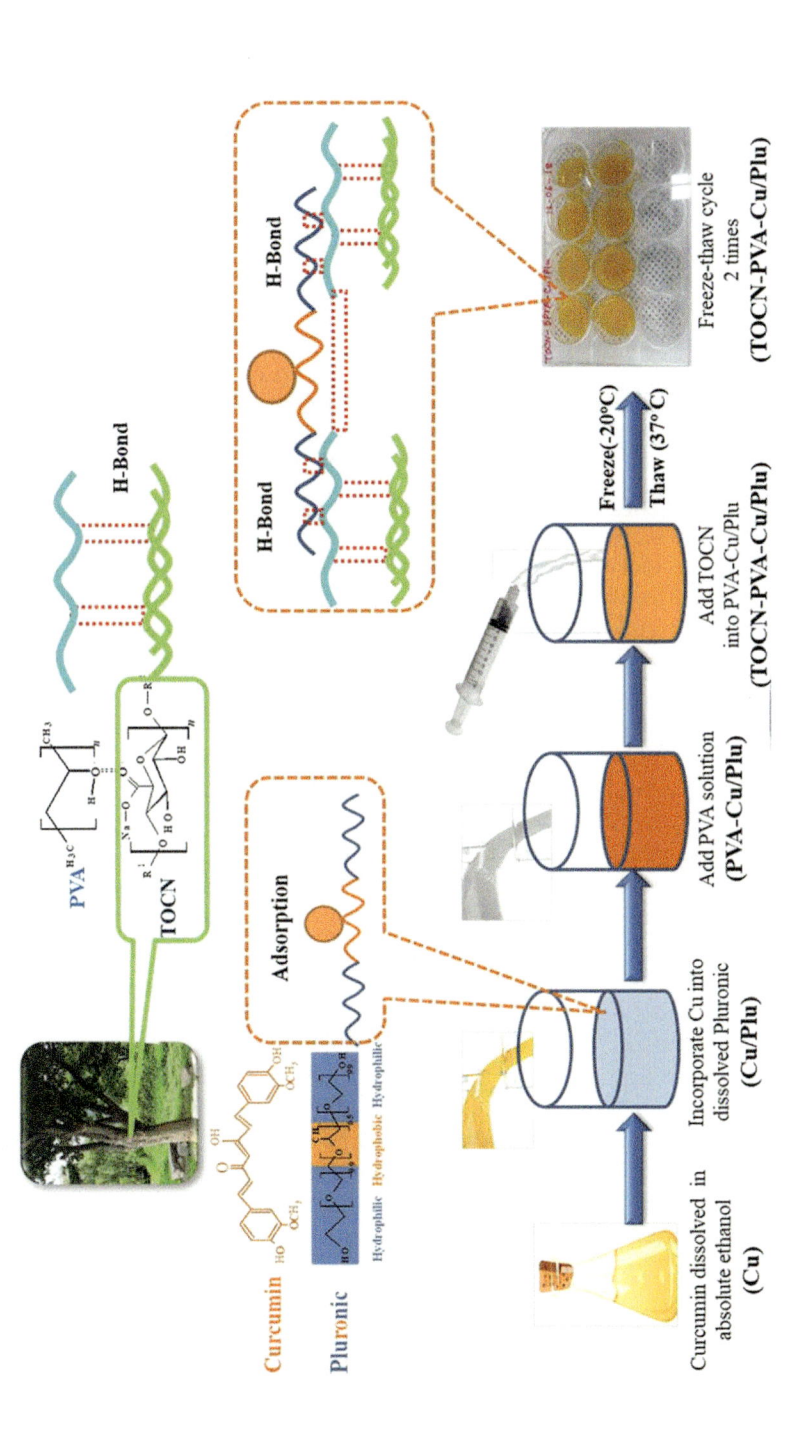

PVA=Polyvinyl Alcohol; TOCN=TEMPO(2,2,6,6-Tetramethylpiperidin-1-yl)oxyl)-oxidized cellulose nanofiber

FIG. 14.9 Schematic illustration process of oxidized cellulose nanofiber-polyvinyl alcohol hydrogel system. *Reprinted from Shefa AA, Sultana T, Park MK, Lee SY, Gwon JG, Lee BT. Curcumin incorporation into an oxidized cellulose nanofiber-polyvinyl alcohol hydrogel system promotes wound healing. Mater Des 2020;186:108313. https://doi.org/10.1016/j.matdes.2019.108313. Copyright (2020), with permission from Elsevier.*

adhesion [57]. For this purpose, a thermosensitive, antiadhesion, injectable hydrogel has been produced from TOCN, methylcellulose, and carboxymethyl cellulose, polyethylene glycol (PEG). The TOCN effect has been evaluated at 0.2, 0.5, 0.8, and $1\,w/v\%$ concentrations. TOCN content at $0.2\,w/v\%$ produced stable hydrogel without an additional chemical cross-linker and showed short gelation time. This concentrations in vitro studies revealed that it had no cytotoxicity effect against rat bone marrow mesenchymal stem cells (RBMSCs) and L929 fibroblast cells. The injectable hydrogel with a $0.2\,w/v\%$ TOCN concentration reduced peritoneal adhesion in the rat. An injectable hydrogel was produced from NC with biodegradable, biofunctionalized, and thixotropic properties to enhance cell infiltration and promote in vivo tissue remodeling [58]. Biodegradability of the NC was gained in the sodium periodate by cleaving C2-C3 bonds of glucose units (DAC), and then biofunctionality was accomplished by sulfonation (sNC). Then sNC/G gel matrix was formed by Schiff base formation. The thixotropic hydrogel was produced to overcome complex injection procedures faced in chemically cross-linked injectable hydrogels and improve cell infiltration and biochemically upregulation cellular activity by single syringe injection. Biofunctionality of the sNC was tested on mouse fibroblast cells (L929), and the results displayed that sulfonation enhanced bonding of proteins to sNC/G, and sNC/G served as scaffolds for fibroblast cells. The cell infiltration, vascularization, and macrophage polarization of the sNC were examined in in vivo tissue remodeling via subcutaneous implantation in rats. Results showed that biofunctionalized, thixotropic, cell-infiltrative hydrogel could be used as a single syringe injectable hydrogel to promote in vivo tissue remodeling.

Artificial bone is an essential topic of tissue engineering. Studies are conducted to produce bones with properties nearest to the real ones to overcome side effects and drawbacks of current medical applications. For this purpose in regenerative therapy, biomimetic scaffolds are produced and implanted to form new bone tissue via adhering, spreading, and proliferating cells [59]. Hydroxyapatite (HAP) is the main mineral composition of bone and gives it its mechanical strength. Additionally, HAP is essential for improving bone cell proliferation and activity, and preventing cell apoptosis and collagen formation during the regeneration process [59]. An artificial porous bone scaffold was produced from in situ HAP-coated CNC cross-linked with poly(methyl vinyl ether-alt-maleic acid) (PMVEMA) and PEG by esterification reaction [59]. For HAP coating, CNCs were dispersed in simulated body fluid (SBF), and then HAP coating was achieved by ionic and hydrogen bonding. As mentioned previously, HAP is important for the regeneration of bone tissue, and it was stated that HAP content increase was directly proportional to CNC content. The maximum 40.1% HAP content was obtained, but it was lower than the predicted value (62%). Porous (91.0%), lightweight (60–$70\,mg/cm^3$)

CNCs/HAP scaffold displayed mechanical strength that increased with HAP content but decreased with excess HAP content. Biocompatibility of the CNCs/HAP scaffold was tested with BSA protein, and results exhibited that, with increasing HAP content, protein denaturation was replaced with protein stabilization.

Consequently, the study indicated that a biocompatible, lightweight, mechanically strong CNCs/HAP composite is a candidate for bone regeneration therapy. Similar tissue-engineered bone scaffolds were produced from 3D printed alginate/TEMPO-oxidized CNFs hydrogel cross-linked by calcium ions [60]. The study was the first that used alginate/TEMPO-oxidized CNFs hydrogel for 3D printing. The TEMPO-oxidized CNFs were used to enhance the shape formation because pure alginate has insufficient rheological characteristics. Also, carboxylate groups of TEMPO-oxidized CNFs affect the biomimetic mineralization process. A two-step cross-linking procedure was applied. Its first goal, partially cross-linking, was to prepare printable hydrogel by ensuring the shape and fidelity, and inhibiting filament collapse. Subsequent cross-linking was immediately applied to give mechanical strength to the printed hydrogel that was produced. Then the created hydrogel was mineralized by using HAP in SBF. Outputs of the study indicated that 3D printable, thixotropic, HAP-coated (20.1%) scaffold could be manufactured from alginate/TEMPO-oxidized CNFs with fidelity and improved mechanical properties for bone tissue engineering applications. A methacrylate gellan gum (GGMA) hydrogel reinforced with CNCs was produced by ionic cross-linking for the regeneration of annulus fibrosus (AF) tissue [61]. The effect of the CNC addition to GGMA responded positively to matrix entanglements at even low GGMA concentration rather than the requirement of high GGMA concentration, cell spreading, cytoskeleton rearrangement, and stiffness. Reported results of the research demonstrated that CNC-reinforced GGMA hydrogel with noncytotoxic, native human AF with likely mechanical properties and suitability for AF cell spreading features might be used as an injectable, self-gelling composite for regeneration of AF.

An injectable, in situ-gelling, cellulose nanofiber-reinforced, viscous chitosan solution was prepared with the purpose of repair and regeneration of intervertebral disc [62]. The report proposed that cellulose nanofibers' role in the composite is as a reinforcement agent as collagen fibrils do naturally in discs. It was shown that cellulose nanofibers contribute to chitosan solution increasing elastic modulus. Also, the effect of the cellulose nanofibers' addition in chitosan solution was evaluated by using human fibroblast cells. It was shown that cellulose nanofiber had no negative impact on the biocompatibility of chitosan. Unlike most of the research that used one type of nanocellulose, a recent study first used different nanocellulose types: bacterial nanocellulose, cellulose nanofibers, and CNCs to reinforce biomimetic, 3D printable, photochemically cross-linked, regenerated silk fibroin (RSF) hydrogel [54]. In addition to mechanical strength effects, hydrogels were evaluated in cell attachment, viability, and proliferation using L929 fibroblast cell lines. The research indicated that the addition of nanocellulose to hydrogels leads to a decrease in optical size, diameter, and water uptake capacity to bacterial cellulose, cellulose nanofibers, and CNCs. Moreover, the incorporation of nanocellulose to RSF hydrogel reduced pore size from ~ 9.2 µm, and CNCs were the most effective. It was suggested that cellulose nanofiber and bacterial nanocellulose-added hydrogels exhibited a more appropriate environment for the proliferation of fibroblast cells than CNCs. This was attributed to low swelling capacity, and a small pore size of CNC-included RSF hydrogel. Consequently, it was understood that bacterial nanocellulose, cellulose nanofibers, and CNCs contributed to RSF hydrogel in different aspects like mechanical strength, biocompatibility, and printability. Aforementioned studies were related to the utilization of various types of nanocellulose, mainly as reinforced agents in other polymers-based hydrogels. In a recent study, instead of nanocellulose, emulsion was used as a filler in cellulose nanofiber-based hydrogel as an alternative to commonly manufactured hydrogels for tissue engineering applications [63]. An emulsion of clove essential oil was prepared via high-intensity ultrasound (HIUS) technique. First, cellulose nanofibers hydrogel (continuous phase) was achieved via the HIUS method, and then clove essential oil (dispersed phase) emulsion, at 0.1, 0.5, and 1.0 wt% concentrations, filled the hydrogel again by performing the HIUS method. The best-entrapped oil concentration was chosen as 0.5 wt%, and the rise of the oil concentration of hydrogels caused a decreasing trend in water retention and swelling capacity. Cytocompatibility evaluation of hydrogels for human gingival fibroblast cells displayed up to the essential oil concentration of 0.5 wt% with no cytotoxic effect (cell viability was 74%–101%), but 1 wt% concentration showed the cytotoxic effect. It was suggested that clove essential oil emulsion-filled cellulose nanofiber hydrogel might be an alternative scaffold, especially for periodontal tissue engineering studies. CNCs-filled gelatin (GA)-hyaluronic acid (HA) hydrogel was produced as wound dressings for the treatment of skin defects [64]. CNCs were added to GA-HA hydrogel produced via the freeze-drying method. Hydrogel morphology indicated that addition of CNCs improved pore size. Incorporation of CNCs to the GA-HA hydrogel increased swelling ratio and viability of NIH-3T3 cells. A wound dressing hydrogel system was produced to examine the combined effect of antibiotics and steroids, which were neomycin and diosgenin, respectively, for skin defects [65]. Diosgenin conjugated carboxylated nanocellulose was cross-linked with gelatin by a natural extract, which was genipin. After hydrogel formation, the antibiotic drug was included in hydrogel by the swelling diffusion method. Besides characterization studies, the hydrogel was tested for in vitro cytotoxicity assay against human dermal fibroblast (HDF) and for antibacterial activity against human pathogenic Gram (−) and Gram (+) bacteria, which were *E. coli* and *S. aureus*, respectively. Results displayed that hydrogel could be a candidate for wound-healing therapy with 50%–88% antibacterial activity and higher than 80% cell viability properties. TEMPO-mediated oxidized CNFs hydrogel was formed by cross-linking with Ca^{2+} as wound dressings [66]. Hydrogels were loaded with BSA, lysozyme, and fibrinogen proteins, which possess distinct isoelectric point and size. The importance of interactions between CNFs and protein on the loading manner was pointed out. Loaded amounts were 0.78%, 0.86%, and 4.12%; isoelectric points were 4.7, 5.1–6.3, and 11.1 for BSA, fibrinogen, and lysozyme, respectively. It was suggested that the incorporation of proteins before cross-linking might be an alternative manner for loading. Simultaneously, the release profile of proteins depends on the effect of their size and net charge. For example, negatively charged BSA and fibrinogen released 97.1% and 98% of loaded content, respectively, whereas positively charged lysozyme released 61.3% loaded amount. Hydrogels had no negative effect on stability of proteins; therefore, it was suggested that surface properties of ion cross-linked CNFs hydrogels can be tailored for wound dressing applications loaded with therapeutic agents. CNCs-based hydrogel patches were synthesized by cation-induced gelation technique by using various mono- and divalent cations like Na^+, Ca^+, and Mg^{2+} [67]. Because hydrogel membrane was produced with the purpose of melanoma phototherapy, toxicity evaluation was conducted particularly on melanoma cell lines (A375 and M14) and human fibroblasts. When gelation is mediated by addition of Na^+ or Mg^{2+}, biocompatible hydrogel membranes were produced, and also Mg^{2+}-including hydrogels presented long-term stability. Wood-based NFC was used to prepare ion cross-linked hydrogel for treatment of wound infections caused especially from pathogenic bacteria [68]. Hydrogels were formed with the addition of Ca^{2+} and Cu^{2+}, and antibacterial assessment was done on *Staphylococcus epidermis* and *Pseudomonas aeruginosa* as tested bacteria. Experiment results of the *S. epidermis* indicated that both Ca^{2+} and Cu^{2+} led to a decline in growth of the bacteria in comparison to control groups. For *Pseudomonas aeruginosa*, Ca^{2+} acted as protective agent against biofilm formation, and Cu^{2+} represents bacteriostatic behavior. Consequently, it was proposed that Ca^{2+} and Cu^+ cross-linked NFC hydrogel might be an advantageous medical material for wound healing. An anisotropic wood hydrogel was produced from wood nanofibers to benefit from its stiffness and polyacrylamide hydrogel to take advantage of its flexibility as a simulation of muscle structure (Fig. 14.10) [69]. The wood hydrogel's mechanical strength reached to 36 MPa for tensile strength through L direction and ionic conductivity was 5×10^{-4} S/cm because of cellulose nanofibers. It was stated that the muscle-inspired wood cellulose hydrogel was suitable for application of soft tissues, sensor devices, and (Table 14.2) nanofluidic.

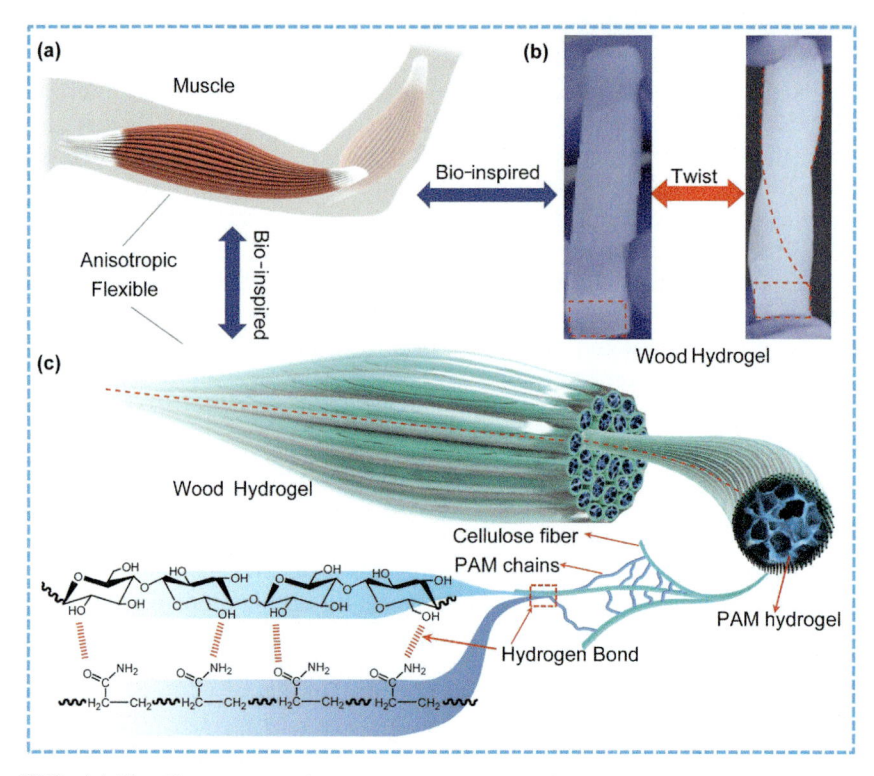

FIG. 14.10 Illustration and microscopic structure of wood hydrogel. *Reprinted from Kong W, Wang C, Jia C, Kuang Y, Pastel G, Chen C, et al. Muscle-inspired highly anisotropic, strong, ion-conductive hydrogels. Adv Mater 2018;30:1–7. https://doi.org/10.1002/adma.201801934. Copyright (2018), with permission from John Wiley and Sons.*

14.6 Conclusion

Nanocellulose has excellent properties like tunable surface chemistry, biocompatibility, nontoxicity, mechanical stability and strength properties, and high surface-to-volume ratio. It makes them favorable materials for nanocomposite hydrogel applications in versatile fields, particularly biomedicine. In this chapter, recent advancements in nanocomposite hydrogels based on plant nanocellulose in drug delivery and tissue engineering research were summarized. In light of the latest studies, it was proven that nanocellulose, especially CNCs and cellulose fibers, are promising and multifunctional materials that can be used both as reinforcement materials and the main matrix in hydrogel formulations because of the aforementioned outstanding properties. Additionally, it is a fact that the utilization of nanocellulose and its derivatives, instead of chemical compounds for the same function, ends up with hydrogel formation with upgraded properties

TABLE 14.2 Summary of recent nanocellulose-based hydrogel studies based on type and role of nanocellulose and application field.

Nanocellulose type	Role in hydrogel	Intended application	References
Nano carboxymethyl cellulose	Supporting material	Drug delivery	[39]
Cellulose nanocrystals	Supporting material	Drug delivery	[40]
TEMPO-oxidized nanocellulose	Matrix	Drug delivery	[41]
Cellulose nanocrystals	Supporting material	Drug delivery	[42]
Charged cellulose nanofibrils	Matrix	Drug delivery	[43]
TEMPO-oxidized cellulose nanofibers	Matrix	Drug delivery	[44]
Cellulose nanocrystals	Matrix	Drug delivery	[45]
Cellulose nanocrystals	Supporting material	Drug delivery	[46]
Cellulose nanofibers	Matrix	Drug delivery	[47]
Cellulose nanofibers	Matrix	Drug delivery	[48]
Cellulose nanocrystals	Supporting material	Drug delivery	[49]
Cellulose nanowhisker	Supporting material	Drug delivery	[50]
Cellulose nanocrystals	Matrix/Supporting material	Drug delivery	[51]
TEMPO-oxidized cellulose nanofibers	Matrix	Drug delivery/ Wound healing	[52]
Oxidized Cellulose nanocrystals	Matrix	Drug delivery	[53]
Cellulose nanofiber/cellulose nanocrystals/bacterial nanocellulose	Supporting material	Tissue engineering	[54]
TEMPO-oxidized cellulose nanofibers	Supporting material	Tissue engineering	[55]

Continued

TABLE 14.2 Summary of recent nanocellulose-based hydrogel studies based on type and role of nanocellulose and application field—cont'd

Nanocellulose type	Role in hydrogel	Intended application	References
Cellulose nanocrystals	Supporting material	Tissue engineering	[56]
TEMPO-oxidized cellulose nanofibers	Supporting material	Tissue engineering	[57]
Nanocellulose	Matrix	Tissue engineering	[58]
Cellulose nanocrystals	Supporting material	Tissue engineering	[59]
TEMPO-oxidized cellulose nanofibrils	Supporting material	Tissue engineering	[60]
Cellulose nanocrystals	Supporting material	Tissue engineering	[61]
Cellulose nanofiber	Supporting material	Tissue engineering	[62]
Cellulose nanofiber	Matrix	Tissue engineering	[63]
Cellulose nanocrystals	Supporting material	Tissue engineering–Wound dressing	[64]
Diosgenin modified nanocellulose	Supporting material	Tissue engineering–Wound healing	[65]
Nanofibrilated cellulose	Matrix	Tissue engineering–Wound dressing	[66]
Cellulose nanocrystals	Matrix	Tissue engineering	[67]
Cellulose nanofibrils	Matrix	Tissue engineering–Wound dressing	[68]
Cellulose nanofibers	Supporting material	Tissue engineering	[69]

and protection from both environment and targeted biological sites from side effects of chemical compounds. Consequently, nanocellulose and its derivatives are favorable materials with their multifunctional properties for nanocomposite hydrogel applications of release studies of therapeutic agents and tissue-engineered supporting materials.

References

[1] Kayra N, Aytekin AÖ. Synthesis of cellulose-based hydrogels: preparation, formation, mixture, and modification. In: Cellulose-based superabsorbent hydrogels; 2018. p. 1–28. https://doi.org/10.1007/978-3-319-76573-0_16-1.

[2] Isikgor FH, Becer CR. Lignocellulosic biomass: a sustainable platform for the production of bio-based chemicals and polymers. Polym Chem 2015;6:4497–559. https://doi.org/10.1039/c5py00263j.

[3] Du H, Liu W, Zhang M, Si C, Zhang X, Li B. Cellulose nanocrystals and cellulose nanofibrils based hydrogels for biomedical applications. Carbohydr Polym 2019;209:130–44. https://doi.org/10.1016/j.carbpol.2019.01.020.

[4] Abdul Khalil HPS, Davoudpour Y, Islam MN, Mustapha A, Sudesh K, Dungani R, et al. Production and modification of nanofibrillated cellulose using various mechanical processes: a review. Carbohydr Polym 2014;99:649–65. https://doi.org/10.1016/j.carbpol.2013.08.069.

[5] Klemm D, Schumann D, Kramer F, Hebler N, Koth D, Sultanova B. Nanocellulose materials—different cellulose, different functionality. Macromol Symp 2009;280:60–71. https://doi.org/10.1002/masy.200950608.

[6] Abdellaoui H, Raji M, Essabir H, Bouhfid R, El Kacem Qaiss A. Nanofibrillated cellulose-based nanocomposites. Bio-Based Polym Nanocompos Prep Process Prop Perform 2019;67–86. https://doi.org/10.1007/978-3-030-05825-8_4.

[7] Klemm D, Heublein B, Fink HP, Bohn A. Cellulose: fascinating biopolymer and sustainable raw material. Angew Chemie Int Ed 2005;44:3358–93. https://doi.org/10.1002/anie.200460587.

[8] Hivechi A, Bahrami SH. A new cellulose purification approach for higher degree of polymerization: modeling, optimization and characterization. Carbohydr Polym 2016;152:280–6. https://doi.org/10.1016/j.carbpol.2016.07.001.

[9] De France KJ, Hoare T, Cranston ED. Review of hydrogels and aerogels containing nanocellulose. Chem Mater 2017;29:4609–31. https://doi.org/10.1021/acs.chemmater.7b00531.

[10] Nechyporchuk O, Belgacem MN, Bras J. Production of cellulose nanofibrils: a review of recent advances. Ind Crop Prod 2016;93:2–25. https://doi.org/10.1016/j.indcrop.2016.02.016.

[11] Klemm D, Kramer F, Moritz S, Lindström T, Ankerfors M, Gray D, et al. Nanocelluloses: a new family of nature-based materials. Angew Chemie Int Ed 2011;50:5438–66. https://doi.org/10.1002/anie.201001273.

[12] Salas C, Nypelö T, Rodriguez-Abreu C, Carrillo C, Rojas OJ. Nanocellulose properties and applications in colloids and interfaces. Curr Opin Colloid Interface Sci 2014;19:383–96. https://doi.org/10.1016/j.cocis.2014.10.003.

[13] Abitbol T, Rivkin A, Cao Y, Nevo Y, Abraham E, Ben-Shalom T, et al. Nanocellulose, a tiny fiber with huge applications. Curr Opin Biotechnol 2016;39:76–88. https://doi.org/10.1016/j.copbio.2016.01.002.

[14] Nascimento DM, Nunes YL, Figueirêdo MCB, De Azeredo HMC, Aouada FA, Feitosa JPA, et al. Nanocellulose nanocomposite hydrogels: technological and environmental issues. Green Chem 2018;20:2428–48. https://doi.org/10.1039/c8gc00205c.

[15] Moon RJ, Martini A, Nairn J, Simonsen J, Youngblood J. Cellulose nanomaterials review: structure, properties and nanocomposites. Chem Soc Rev 2011;40:3941–94. https://doi.org/10.1039/c0cs00108b.

[16] Erbas Kiziltas E, Kiziltas A, Bollin SC, Gardner DJ. Preparation and characterization of transparent PMMA-cellulose-based nanocomposites. Carbohydr Polym 2015;127:381–9. https://doi.org/10.1016/j.carbpol.2015.03.029.

[17] Raji M, Essabir H, Bouhfid R, El Kacem Qaiss A. Impact of chemical treatment and the manufacturing process on mechanical, thermal, and rheological properties of natural fibers-based composites. Handb Compos Renew Mater 2017;1–8:225–52. https://doi.org/10.1002/9781119441632.ch71.

[18] Du WB, Deng A, Guo J, Chen J, Li H, Gao Y. An injectable self-healing hydrogel-cellulose nanocrystals conjugate with excellent mechanical strength and good biocompatibility. Carbohydr Polym 2019;223:115084. https://doi.org/10.1016/j.carbpol.2019.115084.

[19] Azizi A. Green synthesis of Fe3O4 nanoparticles and its application in preparation of Fe3O4/cellulose magnetic nanocomposite: a suitable proposal for drug delivery systems. J Inorg Organomet Polym Mater 2020;30(9):3552–61. https://doi.org/10.1007/s10904-020-01500-1.

[20] Gibril ME, Lekha P, Andrew J, Sithole B, Ramjugernath D, Khosla A. Fabrication, physical and optical properties of functionalized cellulose based polymethylmethacrylate nanocomposites. Microsyst Technol 2019;8. https://doi.org/10.1007/s00542-019-04686-8.

[21] Thomas MG, Abraham E, Jyotishkumar P, Maria HJ, Pothen LA, Thomas S. Nanocelluloses from jute fibers and their nanocomposites with natural rubber: preparation and characterization. Int J Biol Macromol 2015;81:768–77. https://doi.org/10.1016/j.ijbiomac.2015.08.053.

[22] Supramaniam J, Adnan R, Mohd Kaus NH, Bushra R. Magnetic nanocellulose alginate hydrogel beads as potential drug delivery system. Int J Biol Macromol 2018;118:640–8. https://doi.org/10.1016/j.ijbiomac.2018.06.043.

[23] Radhakrishnan J, Subramanian A, Krishnan UM, Sethuraman S. Injectable and 3D bioprinted polysaccharide hydrogels: from cartilage to osteochondral tissue engineering. Biomacromolecules 2017;18:1–26. https://doi.org/10.1021/acs.biomac.6b01619.

[24] Curvello R, Raghuwanshi VS, Garnier G. Engineering nanocellulose hydrogels for biomedical applications. Adv Colloid Interface Sci 2019;267:47–61. https://doi.org/10.1016/j.cis.2019.03.002.

[25] Shahzamani M, Taheri S, Roghanizad A, Naseri N, Dinari M. Preparation and characterization of hydrogel nanocomposite based on nanocellulose and acrylic acid in the presence of urea. Int J Biol Macromol 2020;147:187–93. https://doi.org/10.1016/j.ijbiomac.2020.01.038.

[26] Xu H, Liu Y, Xie Y, Zhu E, Shi Z, Yang Q, et al. Doubly cross-linked nanocellulose hydrogels with excellent mechanical properties. Cellul 2019;26:8645–54. https://doi.org/10.1007/s10570-019-02689-2.

[27] Pomari AAdN, Montanheiro TLdA, de Siqueira CP, Silva RS, Tada DB, Lemes AP. Chitosan hydrogels crosslinked by genipin and reinforced with cellulose nanocrystals: production and characterization. J Compos Sci 2019;3:84. https://doi.org/10.3390/jcs3030084.

[28] Wu R, Liu K, Ren J, Yu Z, Zhang Y, Bai L, et al. Cellulose nanocrystals extracted from grape pomace with deep eutectic solvents and application for self-healing nanocomposite hydrogels. Macromol Mater Eng 2020;305:1–11. https://doi.org/10.1002/mame.201900673.

[29] Yue Y, Wang X, Han J, Yu L, Chen J, Wu Q, et al. Effects of nanocellulose on sodium alginate/polyacrylamide hydrogel: mechanical properties and adsorption-desorption capacities. Carbohydr Polym 2019;206:289–301. https://doi.org/10.1016/j.carbpol.2018.10.105.

[30] Fan Q, Jiang C, Wang W, Bai L, Chen H, Yang H, et al. Eco-friendly extraction of cellulose nanocrystals from grape pomace and construction of self-healing nanocomposite hydrogels. Cellul 2020;27:2541–53. https://doi.org/10.1007/s10570-020-02977-2.

[31] Bai L, Jiang X, Sun Z, Pei Z, Ma A, Wang W, et al. Self-healing nanocomposite hydrogels based on modified cellulose nanocrystals by surface-initiated photoinduced electron transfer ATRP. Cellul 2019;26:5305–19. https://doi.org/10.1007/s10570-019-02449-2.

[32] Hu D, Cui Y, Mo K, Wang J, Huang Y, Miao X, et al. Ultrahigh strength nanocomposite hydrogels designed by locking oriented tunicate cellulose nanocrystals in polymeric networks. Compos Part B Eng 2020;197:108118. https://doi.org/10.1016/j.compositesb.2020.108118.

[33] Wang Y, Liu S, Wang Q, Fu X, Fatehi P. Performance of polyvinyl alcohol hydrogel reinforced with lignin-containing cellulose nanocrystals. Cellul 2020;27:8725–43. https://doi.org/10.1007/s10570-020-03396-z.

[34] Lu P, Yang Y, Liu R, Liu X, Ma J, Wu M, et al. Preparation of sugarcane bagasse nanocellulose hydrogel as a colourimetric freshness indicator for intelligent food packaging. Carbohydr Polym 2020;249:116831. https://doi.org/10.1016/j.carbpol.2020.116831.

[35] Hynninen V, Mohammadi P, Wagermaier W, Hietala S, Linder MB, Ikkala O, et al. Methyl cellulose/cellulose nanocrystal nanocomposite fibers with high ductility. Eur Polym J 2019;112:334–45. https://doi.org/10.1016/j.eurpolymj.2018.12.035.

[36] De France KJ, Babi M, Vapaavuori J, Hoare T, Moran-Mirabal J, Cranston ED. 2.5D hierarchical structuring of nanocomposite hydrogel films containing cellulose nanocrystals. ACS Appl Mater Interfaces 2019. https://doi.org/10.1021/acsami.8b16232.

[37] Athukoralalage SS, Balu R, Dutta NK, Choudhury NR. 3D bioprinted nanocellulose-based hydrogels for tissue engineering applications: a brief review. Polymers (Basel) 2019;11:1–13. https://doi.org/10.3390/polym11050898.

[38] Ma T, Lv L, Ouyang C, Hu X, Liao X, Song Y, et al. Rheological behavior and particle alignment of cellulose nanocrystal and its composite hydrogels during 3D printing. Carbohydr Polym 2020;253:117217. https://doi.org/10.1016/j.carbpol.2020.117217.

[39] Karzar Jeddi M, Mahkam M. Magnetic nano carboxymethyl cellulose-alginate/chitosan hydrogel beads as biodegradable devices for controlled drug delivery. Int J Biol Macromol 2019;135:829–38. https://doi.org/10.1016/j.ijbiomac.2019.05.210.

[40] González K, Guaresti O, Palomares T, Alonso-Varona A, Eceiza A, Gabilondo N. The role of cellulose nanocrystals in biocompatible starch-based clicked nanocomposite hydrogels. Int J Biol Macromol 2020;143:265–72. https://doi.org/10.1016/j.ijbiomac.2019.12.050.

[41] Piotto C, Bettotti P. Surfactant mediated clofazimine release from nanocellulose-hydrogels. Cellul 2019;26:4579–87. https://doi.org/10.1007/s10570-019-02407-y.

[42] Sampath Udeni Gunathilake TM, Ching YC, Chuah CH, Illias HA, Ching KY, Singh R, et al. Influence of a nonionic surfactant on curcumin delivery of nanocellulose reinforced chitosan hydrogel. Int J Biol Macromol 2018;118:1055–64. https://doi.org/10.1016/j.ijbiomac.2018.06.147.

[43] Hujaya SD, Lorite GS, Vainio SJ, Liimatainen H. Polyion complex hydrogels from chemically modified cellulose nanofibrils: structure-function relationship and potential for controlled and pH-responsive release of doxorubicin. Acta Biomater 2018;75:346–57. https://doi.org/10.1016/j.actbio.2018.06.013.

[44] Fiorati A, Negrini NC, Baschenis E, Altomare L, Faré S, Schieroni AG, et al. TEMPO-nanocellulose/Ca2+ hydrogels: ibuprofen drug diffusion and in vitro cytocompatibility. Materials (Basel) 2020;13:183. https://doi.org/10.3390/ma13010183.

[45] Bertsch P, Schneider L, Bovone G, Tibbitt MW, Fischer P, Gstöhl S. Injectable biocompatible hydrogels from cellulose nanocrystals for locally targeted sustained drug release. ACS Appl Mater Interfaces 2019;11:38578–85. https://doi.org/10.1021/acsami.9b15896.

[46] Xia N, Wan W, Zhu S, Liu Q. Preparation of crystalline nanocellulose/hydroxypropyl β cyclodextrin/carboxymethyl cellulose polyelectrolyte complexes and their controlled

release of neohesperidin-copper (II) in vitro. Int J Biol Macromol 2020;163:1518–28. https://doi.org/10.1016/j.ijbiomac.2020.07.272.

[47] Plappert SF, Liebner FW, Konnerth J, Nedelec JM. Anisotropic nanocellulose gel–membranes for drug delivery: tailoring structure and interface by sequential periodate–chlorite oxidation. Carbohydr Polym 2019;226:115306. https://doi.org/10.1016/j.carbpol.2019.115306.

[48] Auvinen VV, Virtanen J, Merivaara A, Virtanen V, Laurén P, Tuukkanen S, et al. Modulating sustained drug release from nanocellulose hydrogel by adjusting the inner geometry of implantable capsules. J Drug Deliv Sci Technol 2020;57:101625. https://doi.org/10.1016/j.jddst.2020.101625.

[49] Maestri CA, Motta A, Moschini L, Bernkop-Schnürch A, Baus RA, Lecca P, et al. Composite nanocellulose-based hydrogels with spatially oriented degradation and retarded release of macromolecules. J Biomed Mater Res Pt A 2020;108:1509–19. https://doi.org/10.1002/jbm.a.36922.

[50] Omidi S, Pirhayati M, Kakanejadifard A. Co-delivery of doxorubicin and curcumin by a pH-sensitive, injectable, and in situ hydrogel composed of chitosan, graphene, and cellulose nanowhisker. Carbohydr Polym 2020;231:115745. https://doi.org/10.1016/j.carbpol.2019.115745.

[51] Xu Q, Ji Y, Sun Q, Fu Y, Xu Y, Jin L. Fabrication of cellulose nanocrystal/chitosan hydrogel for controlled drug release. Nanomaterials 2019;9. https://doi.org/10.3390/nano9020253.

[52] Liu Y, Sui Y, Liu C, Liu C, Wu M, Li B, et al. A physically crosslinked polydopamine/nanocellulose hydrogel as potential versatile vehicles for drug delivery and wound healing. Carbohydr Polym 2018;188:27–36. https://doi.org/10.1016/j.carbpol.2018.01.093.

[53] Ning L, You C, Zhang Y, Li X, Wang F. Synthesis and biological evaluation of surface-modified nanocellulose hydrogel loaded with paclitaxel. Life Sci 2020;241:117137. https://doi.org/10.1016/j.lfs.2019.117137.

[54] Dorishetty P, Balu R, Athukoralalage SS, Greaves TL, Mata J, De Campo L, et al. Tunable biomimetic hydrogels from silk fibroin and nanocellulose. ACS Sustain Chem Eng 2020;8:2375–89. https://doi.org/10.1021/acssuschemeng.9b05317.

[55] Shefa AA, Sultana T, Park MK, Lee SY, Gwon JG, Lee BT. Curcumin incorporation into an oxidized cellulose nanofiber-polyvinyl alcohol hydrogel system promotes wound healing. Mater Des 2020;186:108313. https://doi.org/10.1016/j.matdes.2019.108313.

[56] Ghorbani M, Roshangar L, Soleimani RJ. Development of reinforced chitosan/pectin scaffold by using the cellulose nanocrystals as nanofillers: an injectable hydrogel for tissue engineering. Eur Polym J 2020;130:109697. https://doi.org/10.1016/j.eurpolymj.2020.109697.

[57] Sultana T, Van Hai H, Abueva C, Kang HJ, Lee SY, Lee BT. TEMPO oxidized nanocellulose containing thermo-responsive injectable hydrogel for post-surgical peritoneal tissue adhesion prevention. Mater Sci Eng C 2019;102:12–21. https://doi.org/10.1016/j.msec.2019.03.110.

[58] Nishiguchi A, Taguchi T. A thixotropic, cell-infiltrative nanocellulose hydrogel that promotes in vivo tissue remodeling. ACS Biomater Sci Eng 2020;6:946–58. https://doi.org/10.1021/acsbiomaterials.9b01549.

[59] Huang C, Hao N, Bhagia S, Li M, Meng X, Pu Y, et al. Porous artificial bone scaffold synthesized from a facile in situ hydroxyapatite coating and crosslinking reaction of crystalline nanocellulose. Materialia 2018;4:237–46. https://doi.org/10.1016/j.mtla.2018.09.008.

[60] Abouzeid RE, Khiari R, Beneventi D, Dufresne A. Biomimetic mineralization of three-dimensional printed alginate/TEMPO-oxidized cellulose nanofibril scaffolds for bone tissue engineering. Biomacromolecules 2018;19:4442–52. https://doi.org/10.1021/acs.biomac.8b01325.

[61] Pereira DR, Silva-Correia J, Oliveira JM, Reis RL, Pandit A, Biggs MJ. Nanocellulose reinforced gellan-gum hydrogels as potential biological substitutes for annulus fibrosus tissue regeneration. Nanomed Nanotechnol Biol Med 2018;14:897–908. https://doi.org/10.1016/j.nano.2017.11.011.

[62] Doench I, Torres-Ramos MEW, Montembault A, de Oliveira PN, Halimi C, Viguier E, et al. Injectable and gellable chitosan formulations filled with cellulose nanofibers for intervertebral disc tissue engineering. Polymers (Basel) 2018;10. https://doi.org/10.3390/polym10111202.

[63] Huerta RR, Silva EK, El-Bialy T, Saldaña MDA. Clove essential oil emulsion-filled cellulose nanofiber hydrogel produced by high-intensity ultrasound technology for tissue engineering applications. Ultrason Sonochem 2020;104845. https://doi.org/10.1016/j.ultsonch.2019.104845.

[64] Yin F, Lin L, Zhan S. Preparation and properties of cellulose nanocrystals, gelatin, hyaluronic acid composite hydrogel as wound dressing. J Biomater Sci Polym Ed 2019;30:190–201. https://doi.org/10.1080/09205063.2018.1558933.

[65] Ilkar Erdagi S, Asabuwa Ngwabebhoh F, Yildiz U. Genipin crosslinked gelatin-diosgenin-nanocellulose hydrogels for potential wound dressing and healing applications. Int J Biol Macromol 2020;149:651–63. https://doi.org/10.1016/j.ijbiomac.2020.01.279.

[66] Basu A, Strømme M, Ferraz N. Towards tunable protein-carrier wound dressings based on nanocellulose hydrogels crosslinked with calcium ions. Nanomaterials 2018;8. https://doi.org/10.3390/nano8070550.

[67] Meschini S, Pellegrini E, Maestri CA, Condello M, Bettotti P, Condello G, et al. In vitro toxicity assessment of hydrogel patches obtained by cation-induced cross-linking of rod-like cellulose nanocrystals. J Biomed Mater Res Pt B Appl Biomater 2020;108:687–97. https://doi.org/10.1002/jbm.b.34423.

[68] Basu A, Heitz K, Strømme M, Welch K, Ferraz N. Ion-crosslinked wood-derived nanocellulose hydrogels with tunable antibacterial properties: candidate materials for advanced wound care applications. Carbohydr Polym 2018;181:345–50. https://doi.org/10.1016/j.carbpol.2017.10.085.

[69] Kong W, Wang C, Jia C, Kuang Y, Pastel G, Chen C, et al. Muscle-inspired highly anisotropic, strong, ion-conductive hydrogels. Adv Mater 2018;30:1–7. https://doi.org/10.1002/adma.201801934.

15

Composite hydrogels of pectin and alginate

Laura Sánchez-González, Kamil Elkhoury, Cyril Kahn, and Elmira Arab-Tehrany

Université de Lorraine, Laboratoire Ingénierie des Biomolécules, Vandoeuvre-lès-Nancy, France

15.1 Introduction

Hydrogels are classified based on their configuration (crystalline, amorphous, or semicrystalline), their polymeric composition (homopolymeric, copolymeric, or multipolymeric), their network electrical charge (ionic, nonionic, amphoteric electrolyte, or zwitterionic), or their cross-linking method (physical or chemical) [1]. Hydrogels can be created by cross-linking synthetic or natural polymers, which present advantages and disadvantages (Table 15.1) [1, 2]. Synthetic hydrogels are mechanically strong, and their degradation rate and structure can be controlled. However, they possess a low biocompatibility and sometimes induce immunogenic responses. On the other hand, the low mechanical properties of natural hydrogels and batch-to-batch variation sometimes limit their use. However natural hydrogels are the preferred choice when it comes to choosing a tissue engineering scaffold because of their excellent biocompatibility, low cytotoxicity, and tunable biodegradability [3].

15.1.1 General information about alginate

Alginate is a linear polysaccharide quite abundant in nature and composed of ß-D-mannuronic acid (M) and α-L-guluronic acid (G) linked in $(1 \rightarrow 4)$ (Fig. 15.1A). Alginate is a polyanionic biopolymer that presents many advantages such as its nontoxicity and biodegradability. Commercial alginates are mainly extracted from brown algae (Phaeophyceae) and

Plant and Algal Hydrogels for Drug Delivery and Regenerative Medicine
https://doi.org/10.1016/B978-0-12-821649-1.00012-X

TABLE 15.1   Advantages and disadvantages of using natural or synthetic polymers for the preparation of hydrogels [1, 2].

	Synthetic hydrogels	Natural hydrogels
Advantages	• Long shelf life • Controllable degradation • Controllable microstructure • Wide varieties of raw chemical resources • Tailored functionality • Strong mechanical properties	• Promote cells proliferation • Promote cells differentiation • Promote cells ECM secretion • No inflammatory response • No immunological response • Biocompatible • Biodegradable
Disadvantages	• Risk of inflammatory response • Low biocompatibility • Risk of immunological response	• Batch variation • Low mechanical strength

telluric bacteria (acetylated alginate) and have different M and G contents. Alginate from algae generally present a high proportion of G blocks contrarily to polymer produced by *Pseudomonas aeruginosa*. The proportion and distribution of M and G blocks significantly influence physicochemical properties of alginate [4].

Gelation of this polymer results from the establishment of interactions between G residues and Ca^{2+} ions. Alginate is widely used in food industry as a stabilizer, emulsifier, and thickener.

15.1.2 General information about pectin

Pectin, a water-soluble polysaccharide, is extracted from plant cell walls. Heteropolysaccharides rich in galacturonic acid are usually consider as pectins. Pectin is an anionic biopolymer widely used in the food industry as a texturizer, emulsifier, and for thickening and gelling. From a chemical point of view, pectin mainly contains α-D-galacturonic acid residues [5]. This heteropolysaccharide is composed of at least 17 different kinds of monosaccharide with main components D-galacturonic acid, D-galactose, and L-arabinose [6]. A schematic representation of pectin structure is presented in Fig. 15.1B and C. The degree of esterification is an important parameter allowing classification of pectins in two groups with different properties: high methoxyl pectin (more than 50% degree of esterification) and low methoxyl pectin (LMP) (less than 50%). This biopolymer is generally extracted with acidified (pH range 1.5–3) hot water (60–100 °C) for several hours [7]. Different alternative methods of extraction are described in the literature to improve pectin quality [8] such as enzymatic, ultrasound-assisted extraction or a combination of subcritical water with ultrasound-assisted extraction. The degree of esterification varies with the source [9].

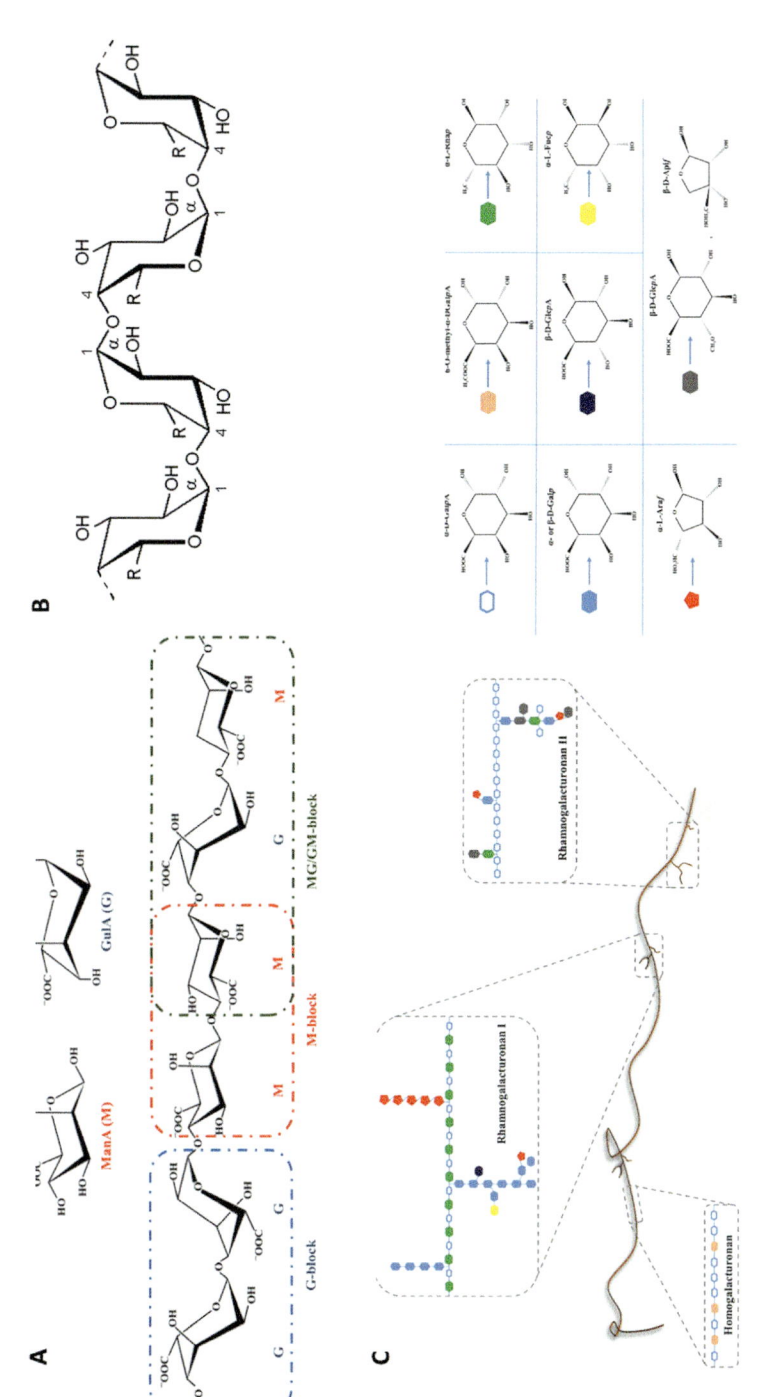

FIG. 15.1 (A) Chemical structure of alginate (ManA (M) β-D-mannuronic acid; GulA (G) α-L-guluronic acid), (B) zigzag-shaped pectin chain, and (C) schematic representation of pectin structure with monosaccharide composition and main domains. *Reprinted from Williams PA, Endress HU, editors. Renewable resources for functional polymers and biomaterials. In: Pectins: production, properties and applications. RSC Polymer Chemistry Series No. 1. Copyright (2011), with permission from RSC; adapted from Martau GA, Mihai M, Vodnar DC. The use of chitosan, alginate, and pectin in the biomedical and food sector—biocompatibility, bioadhesiveness, and biodegradability. Polymers 2019;11:1837.*

Commercial pectins are produced from citrus peels, apple pomace, and sugar beet pulp in smaller proportion. Pectins are used by the food industry basically as thickening and gelling agents. Depending on their molecular weight, different viscosities and gel strengths are observed. Pectins are nonsoluble in organic solvent and very stable under acidic conditions (pH range from 2 and 4.5).

15.1.3 Egg-box model-based gelation of alginate and pectin

Gelation of alginate and pectin depend on different intrinsic (molecular weight, Ca-binding blocks distribution, degree of methoxylation [DM]) and extrinsic factors (pH, temperature, ion strength). The rheological properties of gels are therefore modified according to these parameters.

15.1.3.1 Intrinsic factors

Alginate or pectin with higher molecular weight present longer molecular chains and a larger number of Ca-binding sites. A high number of active binding sites contribute to the structuration of gel and significantly improved their properties (increased viscosity, higher modulus of elasticity, faster gelling velocity). Concerning gel syneresis, this parameter decreased with decreasing molecular weight of alginate. For example, the degree of syneresis was reduced by 50% when the molecular weight of alginate decreases from 320 to 50 kDa [10]. Hydrogels produced by pectin with high molecular weight (generally more than 300 kDa) present compact network structures with interesting mechanical properties (strength). Pectin with low molecular weight (less than 10 kDa) do not allow the formation of gels due to a lack of Ca-binding sites [11].

The percentage of guluronic acid in alginate and galacturonic acid in pectin are essential to allow the formation of Ca-dependent gels [12]. Gels produced by alginate with a high percentage of guluronic acid present better heat stability and water holding capacity. Alginate chains are short and rigid, allowing predominant intermolecular aggregations. Conversely, the use of alginate with a low proportion of guluronic acid leads to the formation of more elastic and less strength gels [12]. This is explained by the polymer structure; alginate present long and flexible chains, and intramolecular aggregation is predominant. The percentage of guluronic acid therefore significantly modifies the interchain association of alginate.

The length and the distribution of calcium-bindings blocks—guluronic acid blocks (G blocks) and nonmethoxylated galacturonic acid blocks (GalA blocks) for alginate and pectin, respectively—are also parameters to be considered to understand the differences in terms of gels' properties (strength, elasticity, water retention capacity). According to previous studies [10, 13], alginate and pectin with respectively long G blocks or

GalA blocks produce gels with interesting mechanical properties (high strength) due to the formation of long cross-links.

In the literature, a pectin methoxylation step is often carried out before the gelation of the polymer. The DM significantly influences gel properties. Pectin with a low DM leads to the formation of gels with high viscosity and strength.

Another intrinsic parameter to take into account is the acetylation of pectin. Pectin is naturally acetylated contrarily to alginate. The acetylation of GalA in pectin reduces the number of Ca-binding sites and the gelation properties of the polymer [14].

Finally, amidation is one of the most important chemical modifications that may affect the ability of pectin to gel in the presence of calcium. Amidated pectin leads to the formation of gels with higher stability and strength, and hydrogen bonds between amide groups and amidated pectin facilitates gel formation especially when the pH is low [15]. For example, Lootens et al. reported that amidated pectin gels present higher strength than nonamidated gels at pH < 3 [16]. Moreover, amidated pectin forms pH-sensitive and thermally reversible gels.

15.1.3.2 Extrinsic factors

Several extrinsic factors such as the concentration of biopolymers and Ca^{2+}, pH, ion strength, and temperature may affect gelation of alginate and pectin. According to Farrés et al., an increase in the polymer concentration leads to a strengthening of the mechanical gel properties (hardness, strength, rupture strength) [17]. However, high concentrations of alginate may prove unfavorable to gel formation. In this case, Ca-independent gelled clusters can form, which decrease the diffusion of free Ca^{2+} and reduces the establishment of bonds between this ion and the polymer [18]. It therefore seems important to select the suitable alginate concentration to form gel with interesting properties (mechanical properties, porosity, controlled release). With regard to the second polymer, pectin, Ca-dependent gels can only be formulated within a concentration range of the polymer. At high concentrations, the dissolution of pectin is not possible, and at low concentrations, gel formation does not occur [19].

The effects of the concentration of calcium ions is equally described in the literature. An increase of the Ca^{2+} concentration accelerates the gelation rate and leads to a dense and elastic gel structure, this being due to the formation of monocomplexes and egg-box dimers [20]. Excessive calcium concentration induces gel syneresis [21]. According to Wang et al., an increase in calcium concentration leads to the formation of a dense and elastic pectin gel (increase of strength and elasticity) [22].

Ion strength and pH significantly influence alginate and pectin gelation. For example, at low ionic strength, electrostatic interactions can be established between alginate and Ca^{2+}, but in the presence of high levels of cationic ions, a phenomenon of competition is observed with Ca^{2+} leading to unstable gels [23]. The dissociation of alginate and pectin carboxylic groups and their binding with Ca^{2+} can be altered by the pH value [24, 25]. The shear modulus (G′G″) of calcium-dependent gels does not change at pH values between 3.5 and 5.0 but increases significantly for pH values lower than 3.5 [16].

Temperature is another extrinsic factor to consider. An increase in temperature may help the formation of a dense network structure through the development of linear structures between alginate chains [26].

Fig. 15.2 summarizes the similarities and differences between alginate and pectin Ca-dependent gelation from intrinsic and extrinsic factors.

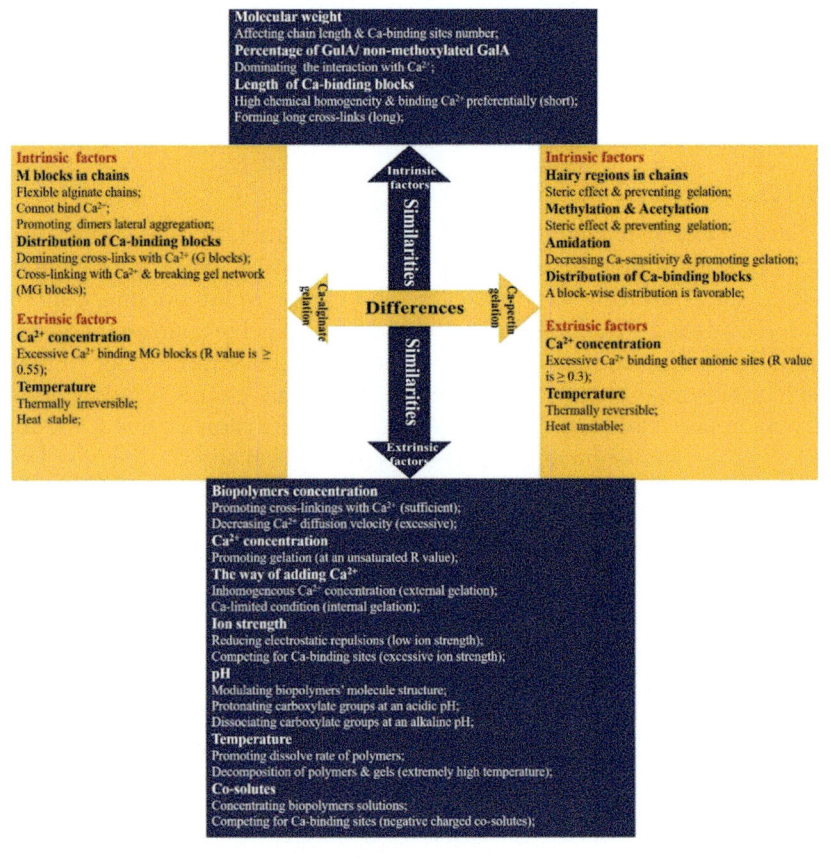

FIG. 15.2 Differences and similarities between alginate and pectin Ca-dependent gelation. (GulA, guluronic acid; GalA, galacturonic acid; G blocks, guluronic acid blocks; M blocks, mannuronic acid blocks; MG blocks, mixed guluronic acid and mannuronic acid blocks). *Reprinted from Cao L, Lu W, Mata A, Nishinari K, Fang Y. Egg-box model-based gelation of alginate and pectin: a review. Carbohydr Polym 2020;242:116389, Copyright (2020), with permission from Elsevier.*

15.1.3.3 Gelation mechanism

The first description of alginate Ca-dependent gelation mechanism as an egg-box model dates to 1973 [27] (Fig. 15.3A). Two G or MG blocks of two adjacent polymer chains may be cross-linked in the presence of a divalent cation by electrostatic interaction between carboxyl groups of the polysaccharide COO–. When two polymer strands are facing each other, the conformation of G or MG blocks form cavities that are housed the Ca^{2+} ions. This block's dimerization is named an "egg box" structure. Due to the existent symmetry conformation between alginate and pectin chains, this model can also be applied to pectin [28, 29] (Fig. 15.3B). However, egg-box models of alginate and pectin present differences in terms of structure and driving force [30–32]. Galacturonic acid and guluronic acid for pectin and alginate, respectively, present well-defined chelation sites and present high specificity for Ca^{2+} [30, 33]. To form stable cross-linking, different studies reported that 6–8 adjacent guluronic acid units and 6–20 consecutive galacturonic acid units were required in alginate and pectin, respectively [34–36].

15.2 Applications in drug delivery

15.2.1 Interest of composite hydrogels in drug delivery

Alginate hydrogels represent a type of biomaterials with a wide range of applications in many fields such as food [37], nutraceutical [38], environment, and water treatment [39]. The interest of alginate hydrogels also gave rise to the development of a wide range of biomaterials with different architectures such as plane or spherical hydrogels (beads and capsules), fibers, and anisotropic structures at milli-, micro-, and nanoscale. Pectin is equally a promising encapsulation material due to its properties (emulsion stabilizer, gelling properties, binding abilities). Pectin is biodegradable, biocompatible, and has an interesting matrix in drug delivery. This polysaccharide is widely used for the development of colon-specific drug delivery systems because this polymer is resistant to the enzymes present in the upper gastrointestinal tract but degraded by some enzymes produced by colonic microflora [40].

The association of both polymers, alginate and pectin, appears as an interesting strategy for applications in controlled release. The properties of alginate-pectin mixed gels depend on the polymer's ratio, the degree of methylesterification of pectin, and the mannuronic/guluronic acid ration of alginate [41]. The formation of a synergistic gel upon acidification of pH below polysaccharides pK_a was reported by Walkenström et al. [41]. The conditions favoring this synergistic effect are the following: alginate with high proportion of guluronate, pectin with high degree of

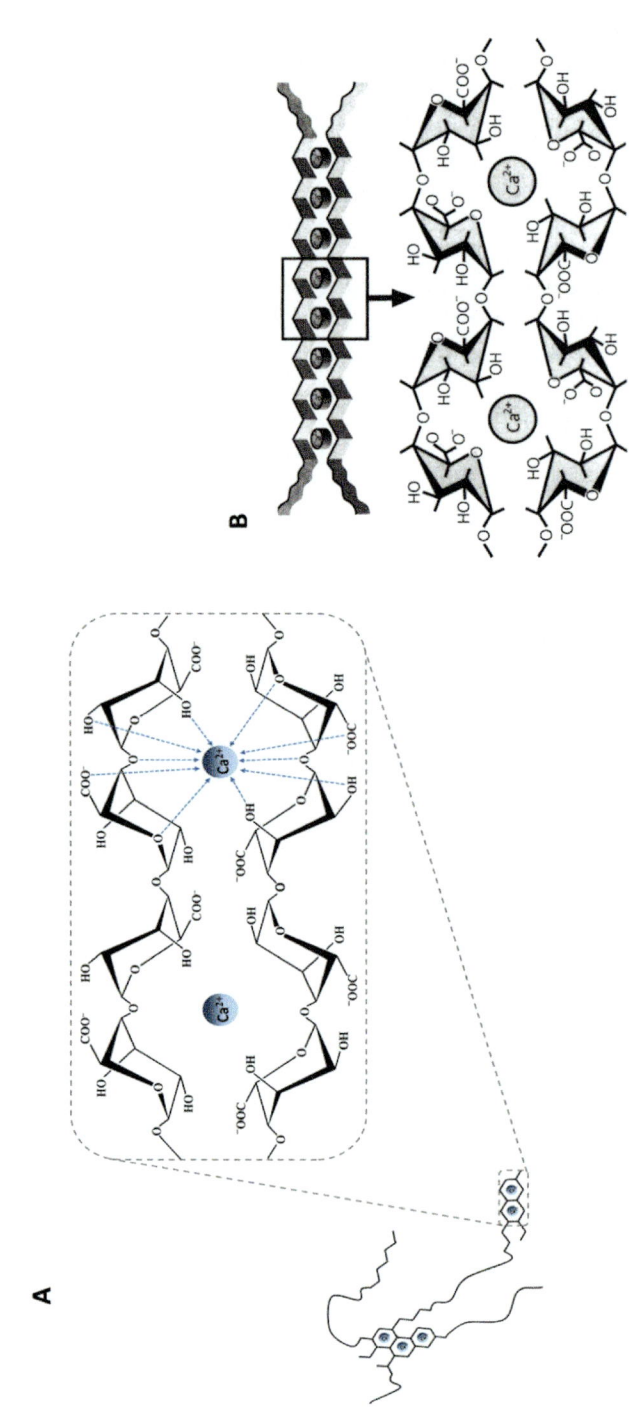

FIG. 15.3 (A) Model describing alginate ionic gel formation by the formation of interactions between G blocks and Ca^{2+} and (B) gelation of LM pectin by Ca^{2+} (egg-box model). *Reprinted from Williams PA, Endress HU, editors. Renewable resources for functional polymers and biomaterials. In: Pectins: production, properties and applications. RSC Polymer Chemistry Series No. 1, Copyright (2011), with permission from RSC; adapted from Martau GA, Mihai M, Vodnar DC. The use of chitosan, alginate, and pectin in the biomedical and food sector—biocompatibility, bioadhesiveness, and biodegradability. Polymers 2019;11:1837.*

methylesterification, and use of alginate:pectin ratio of 1:1. The structural similarity between these polymers can explain the synergistic interaction between the pectin galacturonic acid chains and the alginate guluronic acid blocks [42]. Intermolecular bindings can lead to an increased formation of coupled networks. Koo et al. reported that the alginate-pectin combination makes it possible to develop more interesting systems than pectin microcapsules [43].

15.2.2 Methods of formulation

Several encapsulation techniques using alginate and pectin were developed to obtain particles with a wide size range [44]. Indeed, the diameter of gel particles can be higher than 1000 μm (macro), from 0.2 to 1000 μm (micro), or lower than 0.2 μm (nanoparticles). Electrospinning, a relatively new encapsulation method, can also be used to produce fiberlike structures. Some examples of alginate-pectin gel particles (beads, fibers) with techniques used and bioactive compounds encapsulated are reported in Table 15.2. Bioactive compounds as essential oils, vitamin, minerals, or bacteria are encapsulated in alginate-pectin systems. Images of different alginate-pectin microbeads or fiber developed recently are shown in Fig. 15.4.

TABLE 15.2 Use of alginate-pectin gels as carrier for bioactive compounds.

Encapsulation technique	Ratio Alginate:Pectin	Bioactive compounds	Particle size	References
Extrusion (vibrating technology)	Different ratios tested but best results with 75:25	Lactic acid bacteria (*Lactococcus lactis* subsp. *lactis*)	$272 \pm 11\,\mu m$ (ratio 75:25)	[45]
Vibration technology	55:45	*Lactobacillus* spp.	160 μm	[46]
Vibration technology	Different ratios tested (100:0 to 50:50)	Antacids	300–1660 μm	[47]
Spray-drying	50:50	Carvacrol	Between 2.58 and 5.30 μm	[48]
Coextrusion	66:34	Canola oil	$367 \pm 9\,\mu m$	[49]
Electrospinning (fibers)	70:30 (+30% PEO (poly(ethylene oxide))	Folic acid		[50]

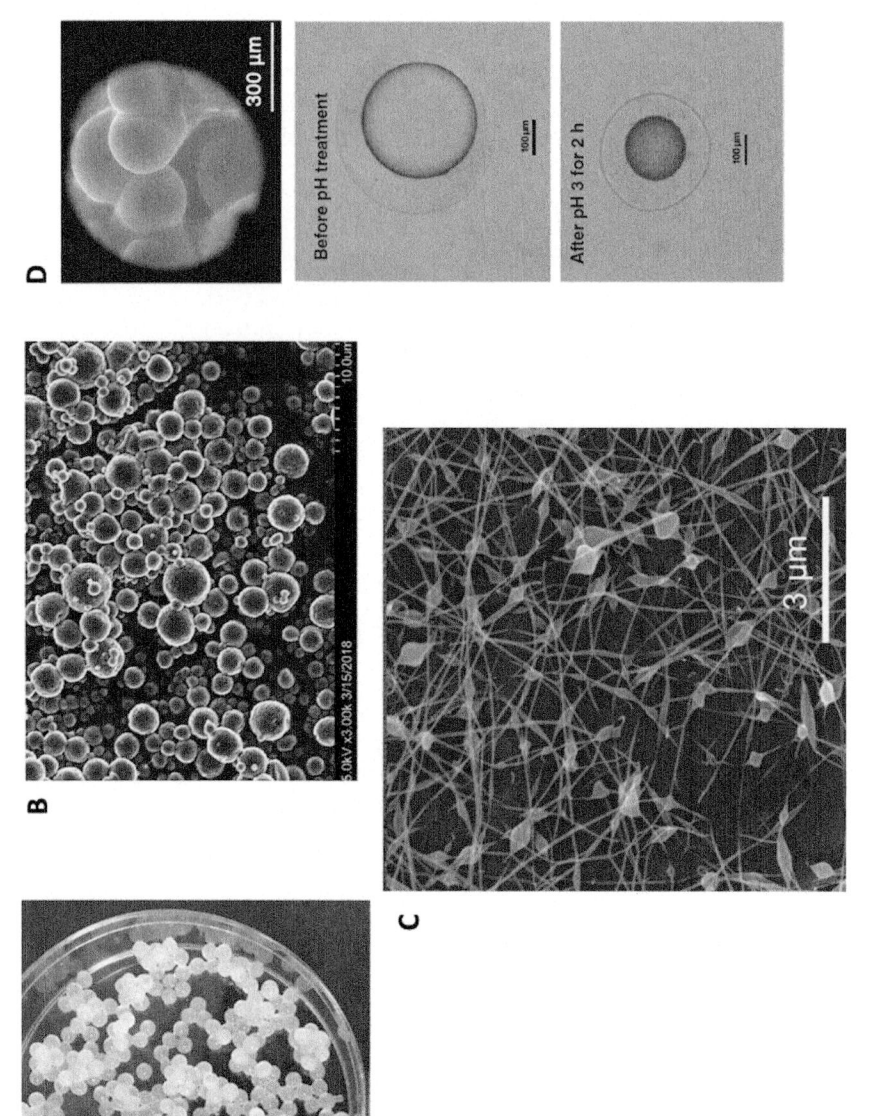

FIG. 15.4   See figure legend on opposite page.

Among alginate-pectin composite particles, liquid-core microcapsules were promising systems with interesting results in bacterial encapsulation, for example. The liquid-core capsules with an alginate hydrogel membrane can be prepared using different techniques: inverse spherification, coextrusion, and multilayer polymerization. A promising approach is the use of minifluidic or millifluidic instruments, by coextrusion or by electro-coextrusion of the core of the capsule (internal mixing) and the alginate solution (outer solution) in a bath of CaCl2 to produce alginate capsules. By changing the ratio between the flow rates of inner and outer solutions, it is possible to modulate the thickness of the membrane [51]. Concerning the inverse spherification, the CaCl2 droplets containing the molecules to be encapsulated are injected into an alginate bath, and an alginate gel membrane instantly forms when these two solutions come in contact. To complete and finalize the cross-linking process, the partially gelled capsules are then transferred into a CaCl2 solution. It is possible to control the membrane thickness of the capsules by varying the sodium alginate concentration and the contact time in the polymer solution [52]. Another technique used to prepare liquid-core microcapsules is multilayer polymerization. This method is based on the formation of alginate beads by simple extrusion of an alginate solution into a bath of CaCl2. Spherical alginate hydrogels are then coated by the addition of a layer of cationic polymer or more coating layers, alternating alginate with an opposite charged polymer such as poly-L-lysine or chitosan. The coating operation may be repeated until reaching the desired number of layers [53]. Finally, the core alginate was dissolved by incubating the capsules in a solution of chelating agent (sodium citrate, EDTA).

FIG. 15.4, CONT'D   Example of alginate-pectin gels as a carrier for bioactive compounds. (A) Alginate-pectin microgels produced using a syringe. (B) Scanning electronic microscopy images of carvacrol in pectin-alginate matrix microcapsules (3000 K). (C) SEM micrograph of electrospun fibers obtained from 3% sodium alginate-pectin/PEO (70/30). (D) SEM and microscopy images of canola oil beads prepared with shell formulation (alginate + high methoxyl pectin). *Reprinted from Wang W, Waterhouse GIN, Sun-Waterhouse D. Co-extrusion encapsulation of canola oil with alginate: effect of quercetin addition to oil core and pectin addition to alginate shell on oil stability. Food Res Int 2013;54(1):837–851, Copyright (2013), with permission from Elsevier; Alborzi S, Lim LT, Kakuda Y. Release of folic acid from sodium alginate pectin-poly(ethylene oxide) electrospun fibers under in vitro conditions. LWT Food Sci Technol 2014;59:383–388, Copyright (2014), with permission from Elsevier; Chen F, Zhang Z, Deng Z, Zhang R, Fan G, Ma D, McClements DJ, Controlled-release of antacids from biopolymer microgels under simulated gastric conditions: impact of bead dimensions, pore size, and alginate/pectin ratio. Food Res Int 2018;106:745–751, Copyright (2018), with permission from Elsevier; Sun X, Cameron RG, Bai J. Microencapsulation and antimicrobial activity of carvacrol in a pectin-alginate matrix. Food Hydrocoll 2019;92:69–73, Copyright (2019), with permission from Elsevier.*

The main limitation to the use of liquid-core capsules with sodium alginate membrane is the rapid and significant loss of their contents. The physicochemical properties (mechanical properties, porosity, membrane permeability) of these capsules may be improved by the incorporation of a second polymer such as pectin. For example, Bekhit et al. observed that the physical properties and entrapped efficiency of alginate-pectin beads are significantly affected by the polysaccharide ratio [45]. The best mechanical properties, stability, and higher release of nisin were observed for a 75:25 alginate-pectin ratio. The preparation of alginate/pectin interpenetrating network resulted in better control of physicochemical properties of composite microbeads and potentially of the hydrogel mesh size.

Another method of interest to produce alginate-pectin microparticles is spray-drying. A homogenized mixture of encapsulating agent (wall material) and encapsulated agent (core material) is converted into a powder. The encapsulating agent surrounds the core material with spraying, and high temperature is utilized to quickly volatilize the solvent [54]. Spray-drying conditions, particularly inlet air temperature, are key factors to optimize efficiency of encapsulation. Correa-Filho et al. reported that the inlet air temperature of the spray-drier can modify the physicochemical properties of the microparticles [55].

More recently, electrospinning appears as a simple and flexible fiber-forming technique with interesting applications in the encapsulation field. A basic electrospinning setup requires three essential parts: advancement pump, conductive target, and high voltage source [56]. The positive end of the voltage source is usually wired to the polymer solution/melt that is placed a set distance away from the target, which in turn is connected to the other end of the voltage source. The growing interest in polymer electrospinning stems from the capacity of the technique to produce continuous, controllable, and uniform fibers with diameters reaching the nanometer scale [57]. The geometry of fibers (high surface area-to-volume ratio) makes this encapsulation method more attractive due to an improvement of porosity and an increase of available surface for chemical modifications and interactions. Two difficulties arise when you want to produce fibers from natural polymers: solvent choice and the need for additional carrier polymers. Due to their solvent insolubility, natural polymers are often electrospun in more toxic solvent than those used for synthetic polymers. Polyethylene oxide (PEO), a linear semicrystalline polymer, is often the chosen polymer blend due to its properties (biocompatibility, fiber spinning reproducibility, and water solubility). Alborzi et al. produced sodium alginate-pectin-poly(ethylene oxide) electrospun fibers [50]. These fibers had good potential as an acid folic carrier in acidic food products (pH < 3).

15.2.3 Gels' properties

15.2.3.1 Size and morphology

Size and morphology of particles may vary depending on the nature of the polymeric matrix composition and the technique chosen for their production. Composite alginate-pectin microparticles present a more grooved surface than alginate beads [58]. Higher concentration of alginate leads to the production of microparticles with smoother surface microrelief [40]. According to Awasthi et al., the polymer nature and degree of cross-linking have a significant effect on the morphology of alginate-pectin beads [59]. An increase in the degree of cross-linking leads to the production of microparticles with a higher surface smoothness. Chen et al. observed an increase in the amount of pectin leads to microparticles slightly larger and less spherical [47]. Rheological properties of alginate-pectin gels depend on the polymer's ratio, differences in the initial viscosity, gelation time of solution, and impact shape of microparticles produced by extrusion. Concerning microparticles produced by spray-drying, Sun et al. observed by SEM that microcapsules at 100 and 130 °C were regular round spheres with fairly smooth surface [60]. The average particle sizes were significantly smaller when the temperature was 100 °C or 130 °C.

15.2.3.2 Mechanical properties

The microcapsules' functionality is closely related to their chemical and mechanical stability. In fact, microspheres are sensitive to deformations that may lead to their rupture or to undesirable early release of their contents. To evaluate the mechanical stability of the prepared systems, microbeads were compressed between two parallel plates. According to Günter et al., a significant positive correlation was observed between gel strength of composite microparticles and alginate concentration [40]. An increase in terms of alginate concentration (from 0.2% to 1.0%) leads to an increase in gel strength. In the case of mixed alginate-pectin gels, polysaccharide is a key ratio to control mechanical properties. In the case of alginate-pectin microcapsules produced by extrusion, ratios 25:75 and 75:25 showed better stability [45]. The differences of mechanical stability could be related to potential synergy between alginate and pectin [41]. This synergism is attributed to a heterogeneous association of the G blocks of alginate and the methyl ester regions of pectin [61]. On the other hand, molecular modeling showed that the G blocks and methylesterified polygalacturonic acid ribbons could pack together in parallel two-fold crystalline arrays [62].

15.2.3.3 Bioactive compounds release

Bioactive compounds release is closely related to porosity and swelling properties of gel matrix. A significant positive correlation between the swelling degree and the alginate concentration used to produce composite microparticles was reported by Günter et al. [40]. Swelling properties are equally modified by Ca^{2+} content, and microparticles with higher Ca^{2+} content and gel strength have a greater swelling degree.

The method used for production of alginate-pectin particles also influences the structuration, the properties of the gel, and the protection of encapsulated bioactive molecules. According to Sun et al., the encapsulation of carvacrol in alginate/pectin matrix by spray-drying is interesting to preserve effectiveness of the bioactive compound [60]. The drying temperature is a key factor, as the powder dried at lower temperature (100 and 130 °C) showed higher antimicrobial and antioxidant properties with lower minimum inhibitory concentration (MIC) (against *E. coli*) and higher value of DPPH assay.

It is possible not only to protect the encapsulated active biomolecules but to control their release by choosing the encapsulation technique and composition of the gelled matrix in particular.

The release behavior of folic acid from alginate-pectin/PEO electrospun fibers was studied by Alborzi et al. [50]. Results are reported in Fig. 15.5A. The highest amount of folic acid released from the electrospun fibers in aqueous solution occurred at pH 7.8, and the lowest was at pH 3. The highest release at pH 7.8 was due to swelling of fibers as evidence from the SEM images (Fig. 15.5B). The release of folic acid at pH 1.2 was likely due to the degradation of the electrospun fibers under highly acidic conditions. pH has a significant effect on the release behavior of folic acid from sodium alginate-pectin fibers.

15.3 Applications in tissue engineering

15.3.1 Interest of hydrogels in tissue engineering

The initial goal of tissue engineered constructs was to replace damaged or diseased tissues. However, these constructs have now found various new applications beyond that initial goal, as they are emerging as research tools that could improve our understanding of biological processes [63–65] and pathophysiology of diseases [66, 67]. In addition, the development of personalized medicine is expected to be facilitated by the use of patient-specific cells and biological factors [68, 69]. Combining the advances in biomaterials, biomanufacturing, drug delivery biology, and on-chip technologies can result in the production of more complex, yet functional tissues and organoids [70–75].

Despite these developments, many challenges still persist [76–80], such the formation of a proper niche that can support cellular adhesion, growth, and differentiation, and mimic the natural extracellular environment. This extracellular environment is composed of a highly defined

A

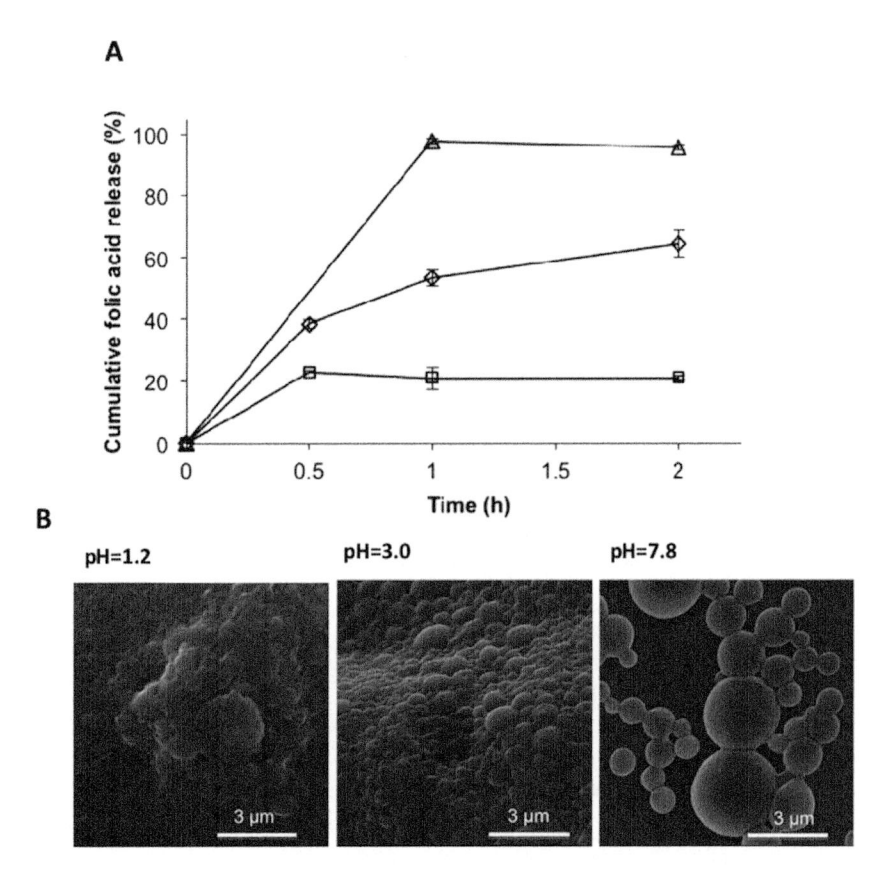

B

FIG. 15.5 Encapsulation of folic acid in sodium alginate-pectin-poly(ethylene oxide) electrospun fibers. Release of folic acid in aqueous solution. (A) Release of folic acid in aqueous solution at pH 1.2 (◊), 3.0 (□), and 7.8 (Δ) at 37°C. (B) SEM images of alginate-pectin/PEO fibers after soaking at different pH. *Reprinted from Alborzi S, Lim LT, Kakuda Y. Release of folic acid from sodium alginate pectin-poly(ethylene oxide) electrospun fibers under in vitro conditions. LWT Food Sci Technol. 2014;59:383–388, Copyright (2014), with permission from Elsevier.*

microarchitecture that defines and modulates the physical and chemical properties on the cellular and tissue level [81–83]. The development and function of different tissues and organs in the human body require proper oxygenation and nutrient transport, as well as the presence of a cocktail of factors affecting biological processes at different stages of tissue development and maturation [84, 85].

The successful engineering of advanced biomaterials with controlled biological, chemical, physical, and electrical properties can facilitate the formation of functional tissues [64, 86–89]. Hydrogels, which are composed of cross-linked three-dimensional (3D) hydrophilic polymer networks, are one type of biomaterial suitable for tissue engineering applications [85, 90], as in addition to their tunable physical and biological properties, high biocompatibility, and robustness in biofabrication, they can mimic the native extracellular matrix (ECM) [74, 91, 92]. As a result of these desirable characteristics, hydrogels are widely used for biomedical applications [93–95], such as drug delivery [96–99] and tissue engineering [91, 100–102].

Polysaccharides are one family of natural polymers that have an immense potential to be used as tissue engineering scaffolds, since they are highly biocompatible, biodegradable, and mechanically tunable, as well as they are a key component of native ECM. The most popular polysaccharide-based hydrogels used as tissue engineering scaffolds are alginate [103], pectin [104], cellulose [105], hyaluronic acid [106], and chitosan [107], although other polysaccharide-based hydrogels such as chitin, gellan gum, etc., have been also used as tissue engineering scaffolds [108, 109].

15.3.2 Alginate-based hydrogels in tissue engineering

Alginate, also known as algin or alginic acid, is a linear copolymer comprising 1,4-linked β-D-mannuronic and α-L-guluronic acid residues in different sequences and varying proportions [110–112]. This hydrophilic, biocompatible, and nonimmunogenic polysaccharide is mainly produced from brown algae but can also be biosynthesized from bacterial sources [110, 113]. Alginate hydrogels have been widely used in tissue engineering, regenerative medicine, and drug delivery [114].

Alginate can also be copolymerized or used in the formation of interpenetration network polymers to add different functionality [74, 115]. In one example, Zhao et al. prepared thermosensitive semi-interpenetrating polymer hydrogels in the presence of sodium alginate via in situ copolymerization of N-isopropylacrylamide with poly(ethylene glycol)-copoly(epsilon-caprolactone) macromer by ultraviolet irradiation technology [116]. The use of sodium alginate enhanced the cumulative release percentage of bovine serum albumin and the mechanical strength of the hydrogels. In the absence of chemical cross-linking agents, cells can be used as an alternative cross-linker, as cells have the ability to bind multiple polymer chains and form long-distance reversible networks when alginate is modified with cell adhesion ligands; this has proven to be a very useful way to make hydrogels from alginate solutions, as it is repeatable and shear reversible [117, 118]. Alginate has many biomedical applications due to its proper biological properties like small chemical drugs and protein delivery in pharmaceutical applications [119]. As a result, alginate has been utilized as the base material for engineering hydrogel scaffolds with the capability of controlled release of drugs and biological factors. In one example, alginate was used to carry platelet-rich plasma (PRP) that can release a cocktail of biological factors essential for tissue healing and growth (Fig. 15.6A and B) [68]. The utilized hydrogels could facilitate vascularization and stem cell migration.

Alginate hydrogels can be prepared by chemical or physical cross-linking of alginate chains. Ionic cross-linking is one of the most commonly used cross-linking methods and is based on replacing Na^+ ions with $2+$ ions such as Ca^{2+} or Br^{2+} to create cross-linked networks [120]. The ionic cross-linking process is very fast, and the formed networks offer tensile modulus in the range of $100–1000\,kPa$. These properties make alginate a suitable candidate for use in many microfabrication technologies including fiber-based technologies and 3D bioprinting. Furthermore, the ionic cross-linking is reversible, and upon the replacement of the $2+$ ions, the network dissociates. The attribute of reversible cross-linking makes alginate a suitable material for engineering sacrificial networks or structures (Fig.15.6C–E) [121]. The use of calcium chelators has been shown to quickly dissolve alginate networks.

Key reasons for the popularity of alginate-based hydrogels in tissue engineering applications are its stability, ease of handling, and fast cross-linking process. As a result, alginate-based hydrogels have been frequently used in fiber-based techniques including biotextiles fabrication and bioploting [121, 122]. In addition, alginate capsules formed by spraying, electrospraying, bubble-based microfluidic platforms, and gravitational droplet formation have been widely used for engineering biocompatible cell-carriers. Key challenges associated with alginate-based hydrogels are their small pore size distribution and lack of cell-binding moieties. Thus, methods for creating macropores within alginate-based hydrogels have been developed to facilitate cellular migration within the fabricated scaffold. In addition, functionalizing alginate with peptides and proteins containing RGD sequences have been developed to enhance cell-substrate interaction and adhesion. The fabrication of interpenetrating network of polymers from alginate and another hydrogel with cell-binding sequences has also been shown to significantly improve the biological activity of the hydrogel (Fig. 15.6E) [121].

15.3.3 Pectin-based hydrogels in tissue engineering

Pectin is a natural polysaccharide found in citrus and is promising for biomedical applications since it can be easily formulated into nanoparticles, microparticles, films, hydrogels, and scaffolds [123]. Pectin chemical structure is composed of (1,4)-linked α-D-galacturonic acid residues with varying degrees of methylation of carboxylic acid residues. Pectin forms a gel in an acidic medium when its degree of methylation is high, and in the presence of multivalent ions when its degree of methylation is low.

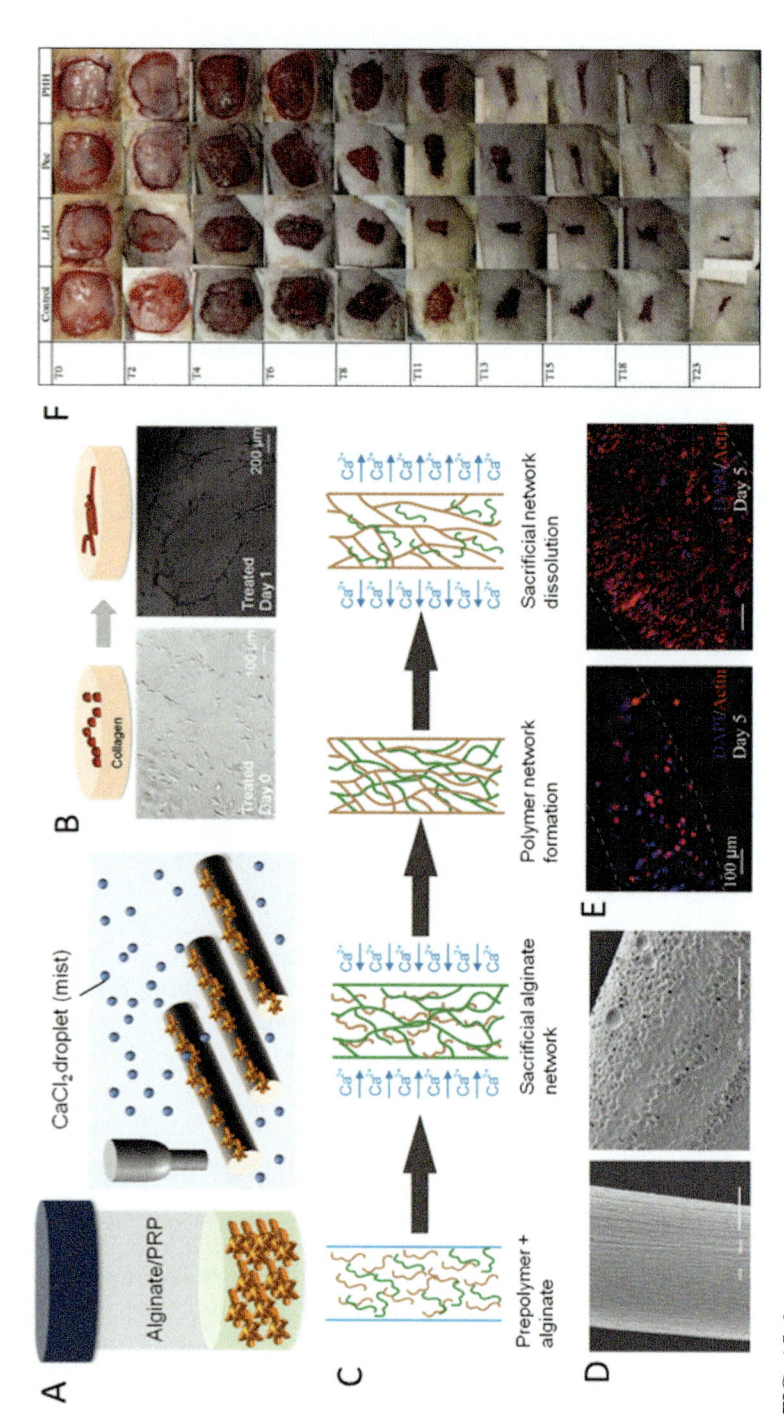

FIG. 15.6   See figure legend on opposite page.

Although pectin composes around 30% of plants' primary cell walls, only a few types of plants are used to produce commercial pectins [124]. More importantly, pectin is still mainly extracted from cider, juice, and apple waste materials via hot water extraction, enzymatic extraction, or extraction with chelating compounds [125].

Few studies investigated the use of pectin for tissue engineering, which might be due to cells' nonadhesiveness on it. Nevertheless, pectin hydrogels have found some applications for bone tissue engineering and wound healing (Fig. 15.6F). Munarin et al. proposed injectable pectin–apatite hybrid hydrogels as an alternative to alginate scaffolds for bone tissue engineering [126]. They reported that the pectin hybrid system promoted, when immersed in adequate physiological solutions, the nucleation of a mineral phase and better mimicked the bone natural architecture by the formation of biomimetic constructs. Moreover, other modified pectin microspheres, coatings, and hydrogels were studied for the 2D and 3D culture of bone cells and showed good cell viabilities and prompted metabolic activities and differentiation [126, 127].

Recently, hydrogels have found new active functions in wound healing other than their previous passive functions of maintaining a moist environment and preventing infections. Some of these novel functions are forming matrices for skin regeneration, delivering drugs or growth factors locally, and preventing harmful postsurgical adhesions. Since pectin is hydrophilic, can retain an acidic environment, and can deliver active molecules locally, it can remove exudates, act as a barrier against bacteria, and treat wounds. Because of these impressive wound healing

---

FIG. 15.6, CONT'D Alginate-based hydrogels in tissue engineering applications. (A) The use of alginate for carrying PRP as a source of biological factors in tissue engineering. The hydrogel fibers could be printed in the presence of $CaCl_2$ mist on dry substrates. (B) The effect of PRP encapsulated in alginate in releasing angiogenic factors facilitating vascularization. (C) The use of alginate for engineering IPN hydrogels with various materials or its use as a sacrificial network for creating fibers from polymers and protein-based hydrogels. (D) SEM image of IPN fibers of GelMA and alginate (*left*) and the removal of alginate from the construct to fabricate pure GelMA fibers (*right*). (E) Cellular morphology shown by F-actin staining in IPN fibers of GelMA and alginate (*left*) and GelMA fibers after the removal of alginate from the network (*right*). (F) Wound healing pictures of liquid Manuka honey (LH), pectin hydrogel (Pec), and pectin-honey hydrogel (PHH) groups on days 0, 2, 4, 6, 8, 11, 13, 15, 18, 21, and 23. *Reprinted from Tamayol A, Najafabadi AH, Aliakbarian B, Arab-Tehrany E, Akbari M, Annabi N, et al. Hydrogel templates for rapid manufacturing of bioactive fibers and 3D constructs. Adv Healthc Mater 2015;4:2146–2153, Copyright (2015), with permission from Wiley; Faramarzi N, Yazdi IK, Nabavinia M, Gemma A, Fanelli A, Caizzone A, et al. Patient-specific bioinks for 3D bioprinting of tissue engineering scaffolds. Adv Healthc Mater 2018;7:1701347, Copyright (2018), with permission from Wiley; adapted from Giusto G, Vercelli C, Comino F, Caramello V, Tursi M, Gandini M, A new, easy-to-make pectin-honey hydrogel enhances wound healing in rats. BMC Complement Altern Med 2017;17:266.*

properties, many pectin-based wound dressings have been approved for commercial use, such as CombiDERM®, DuoDERM®, Granuflex®, Hydrocoll®, GranuGel®, and CitruGel® [125]. These dressings are mainly formed from absorbent and adhesive polymers, pectin, and sodium carboxy-methylcellulose.

15.3.4 Composite hydrogels in tissue engineering

All in all, alginate and pectin have found multiple applications in the tissue engineering field because of their biocompatibility, and their biomimetic physical and mechanical properties. However, to the best of our knowledge, only one study investigated the use of an alginate-pectin hydrogel for tissue engineering. In that study, Archana et al. freeze-dried a chitosan-pectin-alginate hybrid scaffold and evaluated its mechanical properties, swelling behavior, biodegradability, antibacterial activity, and cytotoxicity [128]. They reported that the chitosan-pectin-alginate scaffold had good mechanical strength, high swelling property, moderate biodegradability, and excellent antibacterial activity, and recommended its use as a potential scaffold for tissue engineering applications.

15.4 Conclusions

Natural polymers alginate and pectin appear as promising materials for applications ranging from food processing to biomedical engineering due to their properties of nontoxicity, biodegradability, and biocompatibility. The egg-box model described the Ca-dependent gelation mechanisms of these biopolymers. Extrinsic (polysaccharides and Ca^{2+} concentration, ion strength, pH) and intrinsic (molecular weight, percentage of guluronic acid/galacturonic acid, acetylation) factors can affect polysaccharides' gelation and gels' physicochemical properties. Several encapsulation techniques (extrusion/coextrusion, spray-drying, electrospinning) using alginate and pectin were developed to obtain particles (beads, microcapsules, fibers) with a wide size range (from a millimetric to a nanometric scale). It is important to optimize the composition and structuration of the matrix, in particular by the choice of the microparticle or fiber production technique to control the release of the active biomolecule. Composite alginate-pectin gels present interesting applications in drug delivery and particularly in colon-specific drug delivery systems. Concerning applications in tissue engineering, polysaccharide association still remains little studied to this day.

References

[1] Ahmed EM. Hydrogel: preparation, characterization, and applications: a review. J Adv Res 2015;6:105–21.

[2] Zhao W, Jin X, Cong Y, Liu Y, Fu J. Degradable natural polymer hydrogels for articular cartilage tissue engineering: degradable natural polymer hydrogels for articular cartilage tissue engineering. J Chem Technol Biotechnol 2013;88:327–39. https://doi.org/10.1002/jctb.3970.

[3] Elkhoury K, Russell CS, Sanchez-Gonzalez L, Mostafavi A, Williams TJ, Kahn C, et al. Soft-nanoparticle functionalization of natural hydrogels for tissue engineering applications. Adv Healthc Mater 2019;1900506. https://doi.org/10.1002/adhm.201900506.

[4] Hecht H, Srebnik S. Structural characterization of sodium alginate and calcium alginate. Biomacromolecules 2016;17(6):2160–7.

[5] Roy MC, Alam M, Saeid A, Das BC, Mia MB, Rahman MA, et al. Extraction and characterization of pectin from pomelo peel and its impact on nutritional properties of carrot jam during storage. J Food Process Preserv 2018;42(1), e13411.

[6] Yapo BM. Pectic substances: from simple pectic polysaccharides to complex pectins. A new hypothetical model. Carbohydr Polym 2011;86:373–85.

[7] Wang W, Ma X, Jiang P, Hu L, Zhi Z, Chen J, et al. Characterization of pectin from grapefruit peel: a comparison of ultrasound-assisted and conventional heating extractions. Food Hydrocoll 2016;61:730–9.

[8] Grassino AN, Brnčić M, Vikić-Topić D, Roca S, Dent M, Brnčić SR. Ultrasound assisted extraction and characterization of pectin from tomato waste. Food Chem 2016;198:93–100.

[9] Marić M, Grassino AN, Zhu Z, Barba FJ, Brnčić M, Brnčić SR. An overview of the traditional and innovative approaches for pectin extraction from plant food wastes and by-products: ultrasound-, microwaves-, and enzyme-assisted extraction. Trends Food Sci Technol 2018;76:28–37.

[10] Draget KI, Gåserød O, Aune I, Andersen PO, Storbakken B, Stokke BT, et al. Effects of molecular weight and elastic segment flexibility on syneresis in Ca-alginate gels. Food Hydrocoll 2001;15(4):485–90.

[11] Capel F, Nicolai T, Durand D, Boulenguer P, Langendorff V. Influence of chain length and polymer concentration on the gelation of (amidated) low methoxylpectin induced by calcium. Biomacromolecules 2005;6(6):2954–60.

[12] Cao L, Lu W, Mata A, Nishinari K, Fang Y. Egg-box model-based gelation of alginate and pectin: a review. Carbohydr Polym 2020;242:116389. https://doi.org/10.1016/j.carbpol.2020.116389.

[13] Kim Y, Wicker L. Valencia PME isozymes create charge modified pectins with distinct calcium sensitivity and rheological properties. Food Hydrocoll 2009;23(3):957–63.

[14] BeMiller JN. An introduction to pectins: Structures and properties. Chemistry and Function of Pectins: Washington, DC; 1986.

[15] Vithanage CR, Grimson MJ, Wills PR, Harrison P, Smith BG. Rheological and structural properties of high-methoxyl esterified, low-methoxyl esterified and low-methoxyl amidated pectin gels. J Texture Stud 2010;41(6):899–927.

[16] Lootens D, Capel F, Durand D, Nicolai T, Boulenguer P, Langendorff V. Influence of pH, Ca concentration, temperature and amidation on the gelation of low methoxyl pectin. Food Hydrocoll 2003;17(3):237–44.

[17] Farrés IF, Douaire M, Norton IT. Rheology and tribological properties of Ca-alginate fluid gels produced by diffusion-controlled method. Food Hydrocoll 2013;32(1):115–22.

[18] Skjåk BG, Draget KI, Moe ST. Food polysaccharides and their applications. Chemical Rubber Company Press; 2006. p. 189–234.

[19] Han W, Meng Y, Hu C, Dong G, Qu Y, Deng H, et al. Mathematical model of Ca2+ concentration, pH, pectin concentration and soluble solids (sucrose) on the gelation of low methoxyl pectin. Food Hydrocoll 2017;66:37–48.

[20] Ramdhan T, Ching SH, Prakash S, Bhandari B. Time dependent gelling properties of cuboid alginate gels made by external gelation method: effects of alginate-CaCl2 solution ratios and pH. Food Hydrocoll 2019;90:232–40.

[21] Donati I, Mørch YA, Strand BL, Skjåk-Bræk G, Paoletti S. Effect of elongation of alternating sequences on swelling behavior and large deformation properties of natural alginate gels. J Phys Chem B 2009;113(39):12916–22.

[22] Wang H, Fei S, Wang Y, Zan L, Zhu J. Comparative study on the self assembly of pectin and alginate molecules regulated by calcium ions investigated by atomic force microscopy. Carbohydr Polym 2020;231:115673.

[23] Leusden PV, Hartog GJMD, Bast A, Postema M, Linden EVD, Sagis LMC. Permeation of probe molecules into alginate microbeads: effect of salt and processing. Food Hydrocoll 2017;73:255–61.

[24] Moreira HR, Munarin F, Gentilini R, Visai L, Granja PL, Tanzi MC, et al. Injectable pectin hydrogels produced by internal gelation: pH dependence of gelling and rheological properties. Carbohydr Polym 2014;103(1):339–47.

[25] Yang X, Nisar T, Liang D, Hou Y, Sun L, Guo Y. Low methoxyl pectin gelation under alkaline conditions and its rheological properties: using NaOH as a pH regulator. Food Hydrocoll 2018;79:560–71.

[26] Studart AR, Gonzenbach UT, Tervoort E, Gauckler LJ. Processing routes to macroporous ceramics: a review. J Am Ceram Soc 2006;89(6):1771–89.

[27] Grant GT, Morris ER, Rees DA, Smith PJC, Thom D. Biological interactions between polysaccharides and divalent cations: the egg-box model. Bull Fed Eur Biochem Soc Lett 1973;32(1):195–8.

[28] Morris ER, Rees DA, Thom D, Boyd J. Chiroptical and stoichiometric evidence of a specific, primary dimerisation process in alginate gelation. Carbohydr Res 1978;66(1):145–54.

[29] Powell DA, Morris ER, Gidley MJ, Rees DA. Conformations and interactions of pectins II. Influence of residue sequence on chain association in calcium pectate gels. J Mol Biol 1982;155(4):517–31.

[30] Braccini I, Pérez S. Molecular basis of Ca2+-induced gelation in alginates and pectins : the egg-box model revisited. Biomacromolecules 2001;2:1089–96.

[31] Fang Y, Al-Assaf S, Phillips GO, Nishinari K, Funami T, Williams PA, et al. Multiple steps and critical behaviors of the binding of calcium to alginate. J Phys Chem B 2007;111(10):2456–62.

[32] Ventura I, Jammal J, Bianco-Peled H. Insights into the nanostructure of lowmethoxyl pectin–calcium gels. Carbohydr Polym 2013;97(2):650–8.

[33] Kohn R. Ion binding on polyuronates-alginate and pectin. Pure Appl Chem 1975;42(3):371–97.

[34] Stokke BT, Smidsrød O, Zanetti F, Strand W, Skjåk-Bræk G. Distribution of uronate residues in alginate chains in relation to alginate gelling properties-2: enrichment of β-d-mannuronic acid and depletion of α-l-guluronic acid in sol fraction. Carbohydr Polym 1993;21(1):39–46.

[35] Fraeye I, Duvetter T, Doungla E, Loey AV, Hendrickx M. Fine-tuning the properties of pectin–calcium gels by control of pectin fine structure, gel composition and environmental conditions. Trends Food Sci Technol 2010;21(5):219–28.

[36] Bowman KA, Aarstad OA, Nakamura M, Stokke BT, Skjåk-Bræk G, Round AN. Single molecule investigation of the onset and minimum size of the calcium-mediated junction zone in alginate. Carbohydr Polym 2016;148:52–60.

[37] Farris S, Schaich KM, Liu L, Piergiovanni L, Yam KL. Development of polyion-complex hydrogels as an alternative approach for the production of bio-based polymers for food packaging applications: a review. Trends Food Sci Technol 2009;20(8):316–32.

[38] Chen L, Remondetto GE, Subirade M. Food protein-based materials as nutraceutical delivery systems. Trends Food Sci Technol 2006;17(5):272–83.

[39] Crini G. Recent developments in polysaccharide-based materials used as adsorbents in wastewater treatment. Prog Polym Sci 2005;30(1):38–70.

[40] Günter EA, Popeyko OV, Belozerov VS, Martinson EA, Litvinets SG. Physicochemical and swelling properties of composite gel microparticles based on alginate and callus cultures pectins with low and high degrees of methylesterification. Int J Biol Macromol 2020;164:863–70. https://doi.org/10.1016/j.ijbiomac.2020.07.189.

[41] Walkenström P, Kidman S, Hermansson AM, Rasmussen PB, Hoegh L. Microstructure and rheological behavior of alginate/pectin mixed gels. Food Hydrocoll 2003;17:593–603.

[42] Lara-Espinoza C, Carvajal-Millán E, Balandrán-Quintana R, López-Franco Y, Rascón-Chu A. Pectin and pectin-based composite materials: beyond food texture—a review. Molecules 2018;23:942–76.

[43] Koo SY, Cha KH, Song DG, Chung D, Pan CH. Microencapsulation of peppermint oil in an alginate–pectin matrix using a coaxial electrospray system. Int J Food Sci Technol 2014;49:733–9.

[44] Ching SH, Bansal N, Bhandari B. Alginate gel particles—a review of production techniques and physical properties. Crit Rev Food Sci Nutr 2017;57(6):1133–52.

[45] Bekhit M, Sánchez-González L, Ben Messaoud G, Desobry S. Encapsulation of Lactococcus lactis subsp. lactis on alginate/pectin composite microbeads: effect of matrix composition on bacterial survival and nisin release. J Food Eng 2016;180:1–9.

[46] Eckert C, Agnol WD, Dallé D, Serpa VG, Maciel MJ, Lehn DN, Volken de Souza CF. Development of alginate-pectin microparticles with dairy whey using vibration technology: effects of matrix composition on the protection of Lactobacillus spp. from adverse conditions. Food Res Int 2018;113:65–73.

[47] Chen F, Zhang Z, Deng Z, Zhang R, Fan G, Ma D, McClements DJ. Controlled-release of antacids from biopolymer microgels under simulated gastric conditions: impact of bead dimensions, pore size, and alginate/pectin ratio. Food Res Int 2018;106:745–51.

[48] Sun X, Cameron RG, Bai J. Microencapsulation and antimicrobial activity of carvacrol in a pectin-alginate matrix. Food Hydrocoll 2019;92:69–73.

[49] Wang W, Waterhouse GIN, Sun-Waterhouse D. Co-extrusion encapsulation of canola oil with alginate: effect of quercetin addition to oil core and pectin addition to alginate shell on oil stability. Food Res Int 2013;54:837–51.

[50] Alborzi S, Lim LT, Kakuda Y. Release of folic acid from sodium alginate pectin-poly(ethylene oxide) electrospun fibers under in vitro conditions. LWT Food Sci Technol 2014;59:383–8.

[51] Bremond N, Santanach-Carreras E, Chu LY, Bibette J. Formation of liquidcore capsules having a thin hydrogel membrane: liquid pearls. Soft Matter 2010;6(11):2484–8.

[52] Blandino A, Macías M, Cantero D. Formation of calcium alginate gel capsules: influence of sodium alginate and CaCl2 concentration on gelation kinetics. J Biosci Bioeng 1999;88(6):686–9.

[53] Breguet V, Gugerli R, Pernetti M, von Stockar U, Marison IW. Formation of microcapsules from polyelectrolyte and covalent interactions. Langmuir 2005;21(21):9764–72.

[54] Assadpour E, Jafari SM. Advances in spray-drying encapsulation of food bioactive ingredients: from microcapsules to nanocapsules. Annu Rev Food Sci Technol 2019;10:103–31.

[55] Correa-Filho LC, Lourenco MM, Moldao-Martins M, Alves VD. Microencapsulation of beta-carotene by spray drying: effect of wall material concentration and drying inlet temperature. Int J Food Sci 2019;8914852.

[56] Rockwell PL, Kiechel MA, Atchison JS, Toth LJ, Schauer CL. Various-sourced pectin and polyethylene oxide electrospun fibers. Carbohydr Polym 2014;107:110–8. https://doi.org/10.1016/j.carbpol.2014.02.026.

[57] Reneker DH, Yarin AL. Electrospinning jets and polymer nanofibers. Polymer 2008;49(10):2387–425.

[58] Belščak-Cvitanović A, Komes D, Karlović S, Djaković S, Špoljarić I, Mršić G, Ježek D. Improving the controlled delivery formulations of caffeine in alginate hydro-gel beads combined with pectin, carrageenan, chitosan and psyllium. Food Chem 2015;167:378–86.

[59] Awasthi R, Kulkarni GT, Ramana MV, de Jesus Andreoli Pinto T, Kikuchi IS, Dal Molim Ghisleni D, de Souza Braga M, De Bank P, Dua K. Dual crosslinked pectin–alginate network as sustained release hydrophilic matrix for repaglinide. Int J Biol Macromol 2017;97:721–32.

[60] Sun X, Cameron RG, Bai J. Effect of spray-drying temperature on physico-chemical, antioxidant and antimicrobial properties of pectin/sodium alginate microencapsulated carvacrol. Food Hydrocoll 2020;100:105420. https://doi.org/10.1016/j.foodhyd.2019.105420.

[61] Oakenfull D, Scott A, Chai E. The mechanism of formation of mixed gels by high methoxyl pectins and alginates. In: Phillips GO, Wedlock DJ, Williams PA, editors. Gums and Stabilisers for the Food Industry, vol. 5. London: Elsevier Applied Science Publishers; 1990. p. 243e264.

[62] Thom D, Dea IC, Morris ER, Powell DA. Interchain association of alginate and pectins. Prog Food Nutr Sci 1982;6:97–108.

[63] Khademhosseini A, Langer R, Borenstein J, Vacanti JP. Microscale technologies for tissue engineering and biology. Proc Natl Acad Sci 2006;103:2480–7. https://doi.org/10.1073/pnas.0507681102.

[64] Gaharwar AK, Peppas NA, Khademhosseini A. Nanocomposite hydrogels for biomedical applications. Biotechnol Bioeng 2014;111:441–53. https://doi.org/10.1002/bit.25160.

[65] Uto K, Tsui JH, DeForest CA, Kim D-H. Dynamically tunable cell culture platforms for tissue engineering and mechanobiology. Prog Polym Sci 2017;65:53–82. https://doi.org/10.1016/j.progpolymsci.2016.09.003.

[66] Bhatia SN, Underhill GH, Zaret KS, Fox IJ. Cell and tissue engineering for liver disease. Sci Transl Med 2014;6:245sr2. https://doi.org/10.1126/scitranslmed.3005975.

[67] Ma X, Qu X, Zhu W, Li YS, Yuan S, Zhang H, et al. Deterministically patterned biomimetic human iPSC-derived hepatic model via rapid 3D bioprinting. Proc Natl Acad Sci 2016;113:2206–11. https://doi.org/10.1073/pnas.1524510113.

[68] Faramarzi N, Yazdi IK, Nabavinia M, Gemma A, Fanelli A, Caizzone A, et al. Patient-specific bioinks for 3D bioprinting of tissue engineering scaffolds. Adv Healthc Mater 2018;7:1701347. https://doi.org/10.1002/adhm.201701347.

[69] Neves LS, Rodrigues MT, Reis RL, Gomes ME. Current approaches and future perspectives on strategies for the development of personalized tissue engineering therapies. Exp Rev Prec Med Drug Dev 2016;1:93–108.

[70] Bhatia SN, Ingber DE. Microfluidic organs-on-chips. Nat Biotechnol 2014;32:760–72. https://doi.org/10.1038/nbt.2989.

[71] Byambaa B, Annabi N, Yue K, Trujillo-de Santiago G, Alvarez MM, Jia W, et al. Bioprinted osteogenic and vasculogenic patterns for engineering 3D bone tissue. Adv Healthc Mater 2017;6:1700015. https://doi.org/10.1002/adhm.201700015.

[72] Caldorera-Moore M, Peppas NA. Micro- and nanotechnologies for intelligent and responsive biomaterial-based medical systems. Adv Drug Deliv Rev 2009;61:1391–401. https://doi.org/10.1016/j.addr.2009.09.002.

[73] Culver HR, Daily AM, Khademhosseini A, Peppas NA. Intelligent recognitive systems in nanomedicine. Curr Opin Chem Eng 2014;4:105–13. https://doi.org/10.1016/j.coche.2014.02.001.

[74] Khademhosseini A, Peppas NA. Micro- and nanoengineering of biomaterials for healthcare applications. Adv Healthc Mater 2013;2:10–2. https://doi.org/10.1002/adhm.201200444.

[75] Liechty WB, Caldorera-Moore M, Phillips MA, Schoener C, Peppas NA. Advanced molecular design of biopolymers for transmucosal and intracellular delivery of chemotherapeutic agents and biological therapeutics. J Control Release 2011;155:119–27. https://doi.org/10.1016/j.jconrel.2011.06.009.

[76] Amini AR, Laurencin CT, Nukavarapu SP. Bone tissue engineering: recent advances and challenges. Crit Rev Biomed Eng 2012;40:363–408. https://doi.org/10.1615/critrevbiomedeng.v40.i5.10.

[77] Onoe H, Takeuchi S. Cell-laden microfibers for bottom-up tissue engineering. Drug Discov Today 2015;20:236–46. https://doi.org/10.1016/j.drudis.2014.10.018.

[78] Peppas NA, Hoffman AS. Chapter I.2.5—Hydrogels. Biomaterials science. 3rd ed. Academic Press; 2013. p. 166–79. https://doi.org/10.1016/B978-0-08-087780-8.00020-6.

[79] Peppas NA, Slaughter BV, Kanzelberger MA. Hydrogels. Polymer science: a comprehensive reference. Elsevier; 2012. p. 385–95. https://doi.org/10.1016/B978-0-444-53349-4.00226-0.

[80] Vacanti JP, Vacanti CA. The history and scope of tissue engineering. In: Principles of tissue engineering. Elsevier; 2014. p. 3–8. https://doi.org/10.1016/B978-0-12-398358-9.00001-X.

[81] Hay ED. Cell biology of extracellular matrix. Springer Science & Business Media; 2013.

[82] Hynes RO. The extracellular matrix: not just pretty fibrils. Science 2009;326:1216–9. https://doi.org/10.1126/science.1176009.

[83] Yannas IV. Hesitant steps from the artificial skin to organ regeneration. Regen Biomater 2018. https://doi.org/10.1093/rb/rby012.

[84] Bae H, Puranik AS, Gauvin R, Edalat F, Carrillo-Conde B, Peppas NA, et al. Building vascular networks. Sci Transl Med 2012;4:160ps23. https://doi.org/10.1126/scitranslmed.3003688.

[85] De Witte T-M, Fratila-Apachitei LE, Zadpoor AA, Peppas NA. Bone tissue engineering via growth factor delivery: from scaffolds to complex matrices. Regen Biomater 2018;5:197–211. https://doi.org/10.1093/rb/rby013.

[86] Culver HR, Clegg JR, Peppas NA. Analyte-responsive hydrogels: intelligent materials for biosensing and drug delivery. Acc Chem Res 2017;50:170–8. https://doi.org/10.1021/acs.accounts.6b00533.

[87] Culver HR, Peppas NA. Protein-imprinted polymers: the shape of things to come? Chem Mater 2017;29:5753–61. https://doi.org/10.1021/acs.chemmater.7b01936.

[88] Wagner AM, Gran MP, Peppas NA. Designing the new generation of intelligent biocompatible carriers for protein and peptide delivery. Acta Pharmaceut Sin B 2018;8:147–64. https://doi.org/10.1016/j.apsb.2018.01.013.

[89] Wagner AM, Spencer DS, Peppas NA. Advanced architectures in the design of responsive polymers for cancer nanomedicine: REVIEW. J Appl Polym Sci 2018;135:46154. https://doi.org/10.1002/app.46154.

[90] Peppas NA, Vela Ramirez J. Molecularly and cellularly imprinted, intelligent scaffolds for tissue engineering and regenerative medicine, Beijing; 2018.

[91] Annabi N, Tamayol A, Uquillas JA, Akbari M, Bertassoni LE, Cha C, et al. 25th anniversary article: rational design and applications of hydrogels in regenerative medicine. Adv Mater 2014;26:85–124. https://doi.org/10.1002/adma.201303233.

[92] Peppas NA, Van Blarcom DS. Hydrogel-based biosensors and sensing devices for drug delivery. J Control Release 2016;240:142–50. https://doi.org/10.1016/j.jconrel.2015.11.022.

[93] Hoffman AS. Hydrogels for biomedical applications. Adv Drug Deliv Rev 2012;64:18–23. https://doi.org/10.1016/j.addr.2012.09.010.

[94] Klouda L, Mikos AG. Thermoresponsive hydrogels in biomedical applications. Eur J Pharm Biopharm 2008;68:34–45. https://doi.org/10.1016/j.ejpb.2007.02.025.

[95] Koetting MC, Peters JT, Steichen SD, Peppas NA. Stimulus-responsive hydrogels: theory, modern advances, and applications. Mater Sci Eng R Rep 2015;93:1–49. https://doi.org/10.1016/j.mser.2015.04.001.

[96] Caldorera-Moore ME, Liechty WB, Peppas NA. Responsive theranostic systems: integration of diagnostic imaging agents and responsive controlled release drug delivery carriers. Acc Chem Res 2011;44:1061–70. https://doi.org/10.1021/ar2001777.

[97] Hoare TR, Kohane DS. Hydrogels in drug delivery: progress and challenges. Polymer 2008;49:1993–2007. https://doi.org/10.1016/j.polymer.2008.01.027.

[98] Peppas NA. Hydrogels and drug delivery. Curr Opin Colloid Interface Sci 1997;2:531–7. https://doi.org/10.1016/S1359-0294(97)80103-3.

[99] Qiu Y, Park K. Environment-sensitive hydrogels for drug delivery. Adv Drug Deliv Rev 2001;53:321–39. https://doi.org/10.1016/S0169-409X(01)00203-4.

[100] Drury JL, Mooney DJ. Hydrogels for tissue engineering: scaffold design variables and applications. Biomaterials 2003;24:4337–51. https://doi.org/10.1016/S0142-9612(03)00340-5.

[101] Lee KY, Mooney DJ. Hydrogels for tissue engineering. Chem Rev 2001;101:1869–80. https://doi.org/10.1021/cr000108x.

[102] Slaughter BV, Khurshid SS, Fisher OZ, Khademhosseini A, Peppas NA. Hydrogels in regenerative medicine. Adv Mater 2009;21:3307–29. https://doi.org/10.1002/adma.200802106.

[103] Venkatesan J, Bhatnagar I, Manivasagan P, Kang KH, Kim SK. Alginate composites for bone tissue engineering: a review. Int J Biol Macromol 2015;72:269–81. https://doi.org/10.1016/j.ijbiomac.2014.07.008.

[104] Li N, Xue F, Zhang H, Sanyour HJ, Rickel AP, Uttecht A, et al. Fabrication and characterization of pectin hydrogel nanofiber scaffolds for differentiation of mesenchymal stem cells into vascular cells. ACS Biomater Sci Eng 2019;5:6511–9. https://doi.org/10.1021/acsbiomaterials.9b01178.

[105] Dugan JM, Gough JE, Eichhorn SJ. Bacterial cellulose scaffolds and cellulose nanowhiskers for tissue engineering. Nanomedicine 2013;8:287–98. https://doi.org/10.2217/nnm.12.211.

[106] Collins MN, Birkinshaw C. Hyaluronic acid based scaffolds for tissue engineering—a review. Carbohydr Polym 2013;92:1262–79. https://doi.org/10.1016/j.carbpol.2012.10.028.

[107] Madihally SV, Matthew HWT. Porous chitosan scaffolds for tissue engineering. Biomaterials 1999;20:1133–42. https://doi.org/10.1016/S0142-9612(99)00011-3.

[108] Freier T, Montenegro R, Shan Koh H, Shoichet MS. Chitin-based tubes for tissue engineering in the nervous system. Biomaterials 2005;26:4624–32. https://doi.org/10.1016/j.biomaterials.2004.11.040.

[109] Oliveira JT, Martins L, Picciochi R, Malafaya PB, Sousa RA, Neves NM, et al. Gellan gum: a new biomaterial for cartilage tissue engineering applications. J Biomed Mater Res 2009;9999A. https://doi.org/10.1002/jbm.a.32574.

[110] Bayer CL, Herrero ÉP, Peppas NA. Alginate films as macromolecular imprinted matrices. J Biomater Sci 2011;22:1523–34. Polymer Edition https://doi.org/10.1163/092050610X514115.

[111] Draget KI, Østgaard K, Smidsrød O. Homogeneous alginate gels: a technical approach. Carbohydr Polym 1990;14:159–78.

[112] Martinsen A, Skjåk-Braek G, Smidsrød O. Alginate as immobilization material: I. Correlation between chemical and physical properties of alginate gel beads. Biotechnol Bioeng 1989;33:79–89.

[113] Pawar SN, Edgar KJ. Alginate derivatization: a review of chemistry, properties and applications. Biomaterials 2012;33:3279–305. https://doi.org/10.1016/j.biomaterials.2012.01.007.

[114] Augst AD, Kong HJ, Mooney DJ. Alginate hydrogels as biomaterials. Macromol Biosci 2006;6:623–33. https://doi.org/10.1002/mabi.200600069.

[115] Knipe JM, Peters JT, Peppas NA. Theranostic agents for intracellular gene delivery with spatiotemporal imaging. Nano Today 2013;8:21–38. https://doi.org/10.1016/j.nantod.2012.12.004.

[116] Zhao S, Cao M, Li H, Li L, Xu W. Synthesis and characterization of thermo-sensitive semi-IPN hydrogels based on poly(ethylene glycol)-co-poly(ε-caprolactone) macromer, N-isopropylacrylamide, and sodium alginate. Carbohydr Res 2010;345:425–31. https://doi.org/10.1016/j.carres.2009.11.014.

[117] Lee KY, Kong HJ, Larson RG, Mooney DJ. Hydrogel formation via cell crosslinking. Adv Mater 2003;15:1828–32. https://doi.org/10.1002/adma.200305406.

[118] Drury JL, Boontheekul T, Mooney DJ. Cellular cross-linking of peptide modified hydrogels. J Biomech Eng 2005;127:220. https://doi.org/10.1115/1.1865194.

[119] Lee KY, Mooney DJ. Alginate: properties and biomedical applications. Prog Polym Sci 2012;37:106–26. https://doi.org/10.1016/j.progpolymsci.2011.06.003.

[120] Kuo CK, Ma PX. Ionically crosslinked alginate hydrogels as scaffolds for tissue engineering: part 1. Structure, gelation rate and mechanical properties. Biomaterials 2001;22:511–21. https://doi.org/10.1016/S0142-9612(00)00201-5.

[121] Tamayol A, Najafabadi AH, Aliakbarian B, Arab-Tehrany E, Akbari M, Annabi N, et al. Hydrogel templates for rapid manufacturing of bioactive fibers and 3D constructs. Adv Healthc Mater 2015;4:2146–53. https://doi.org/10.1002/adhm.201500492.

[122] Onoe H, Okitsu T, Itou A, Kato-Negishi M, Gojo R, Kiriya D, et al. Metre-long cell-laden microfibres exhibit tissue morphologies and functions. Nat Mater 2013;12:584–90. https://doi.org/10.1038/nmat3606.

[123] Mishra RK, Banthia AK, Majeed ABA. Pectin based formulations for biomedical applications: a review. Asian J Pharm Clin Res 2012;5:1–7.

[124] Hui YH, Sherkat F, editors. Handbook of Food Science, Technology, and Engineering—4 Volume Set. CRC Press; 2005. https://doi.org/10.1201/b15995.

[125] Munarin F, Tanzi MC, Petrini P. Advances in biomedical applications of pectin gels. Int J Biol Macromol 2012;51:681–9. https://doi.org/10.1016/j.ijbiomac.2012.07.002.

[126] Munarin F, Guerreiro SG, Grellier MA, Tanzi MC, Barbosa MA, Petrini P, et al. Pectin-based injectable biomaterials for bone tissue engineering. Biomacromolecules 2011;12:568–77. https://doi.org/10.1021/bm101110x.

[127] Coimbra P, Ferreira P, de Sousa HC, Batista P, Rodrigues MA, Correia IJ, et al. Preparation and chemical and biological characterization of a pectin/chitosan polyelectrolyte complex scaffold for possible bone tissue engineering applications. Int J Biol Macromol 2011;48:112–8. https://doi.org/10.1016/j.ijbiomac.2010.10.006.

[128] Archana D, Upadhyay L, Tewari RP, Dutta J, Huang YB, Dutta PK. Chitosan-pectin-alginate as a novel scaffold for tissue engineering applications. Indian J Biotechnol 2013;12:475–82.

16

Clinical applications of biopolymer-based hydrogels

Bijaya Ghosh[a] and Moumita Das Kirtania[b]

[a]Department of Pharmaceutical Technology, School of Health Sciences, NSHM Knowledge Campus, Kolkata Group of Institutions, Kolkata, West Bengal, India, [b]School of Pharmaceutical Technology, Adamas University, Kolkata, West Bengal, India

16.1 Introduction

As an entity, hydrogel is not new. The existence of the swell-gels has been known for more than 50 years. But recently, the scientific community is showing an increased interest to realize its full potential in various biomedical fields [1, 2]. Hydrogels can be classified into two distinct categories: natural and synthetic [3]. Of the two, hydrogels obtained from the natural sources have caught the fancy of the drug delivery scientists because many of them exhibit strong similarity with the human tissue and can be used as ideal excipients for drug delivery. As high water content makes it a good medium of growth for live cells, it has caught the fancy of tissue engineering scientists too [4, 5]. Presently, it is being investigated for delivery of small molecules [6–8], proteins [9, 10] live cells [11], and some difficult to deliver biomolecules such as DNA pieces [12]. It has opened the promise of repairing complex tissues and biological systems by integrating the knowledge of materials engineering, stem cell architecture, and developmental biology [13].

However, natural hydrogels suffer from two distinct disadvantages: first, their mechanical properties and gelation conditions are poorly understood; second, their composition may vary depending on the source [14]. Yet in spite of this natural constraint, it is the natural hydrogels that drew significant attention of drug delivery scientists because it is endowed with the most important property desired in a system for in vivo application. Most of the natural hydrogels are biocompatible and biodegradable [15].

Plant and Algal Hydrogels for Drug Delivery and Regenerative Medicine
https://doi.org/10.1016/B978-0-12-821649-1.00015-5

On the basis of response to external stimuli, hydrogels can be divided into two categories: conventional gels and environmentally sensitive gels. The swelling behavior of conventional hydrogels is more or less constant, whereas that of environmentally sensitive hydrogels is highly influenced by the changes external conditions. The latter type, that is, the gels whose swelling depends on pH, temperature, concentration of indigenous biomolecules, etc. is mostly used in drug delivery as sensors and controlled release switches.

Over the years, many other possibilities of the hydrogels got unveiled for various types of biomedical applications, and some of them have already been commercially exploited [16]. Hydrogels can carry huge volume of water in their structure. Because water is the main connective medium of the human body, this gives hydrogels some inherent biocompatibility. They can be processed under mild conditions, allowing the incorporation of drugs and cells of labile nature without compromising their physical or chemical stability [17]. Release of drugs in the body is largely influenced by size, shape, and tortuosity level of the dosage form. Because hydrogels can be formulated in various sizes and shapes, they can serve as convenient vehicles for development of almost every type of dosage form. Hydrogels are made of polymers. Nature provides a wide variety of polymers; however, to qualify for in vivo applications, certain requirements are to be met namely, biocompatibility/biodegradability, nontoxicity, nonimmunogenicity, and suitable mechanical strength. When a hydrogel is designed to serve as a tissue scaffold, there may be some additional requirements such as easy removability and ability to provide cues for cells [16]. Most of the biopolymers have these desired properties.

By definition, biopolymers are macromolecules produced by living organisms. There are three main classes of biopolymers: polynucleotides, polypeptides, and polysaccharides. A large number of hydrogel products are already available in the drug delivery and tissue engineering market. They are being used to deliver both inorganic and organic molecules belonging to every possible category. However, most of them are beyond the scope of this chapter.

This chapter mainly gives a glimpse of clinical applications of the biopolymer-based hydrogels derived from plant and algal sources. Some products that are on the verge of commercial application are also discussed.

16.1.1 The business prospects of hydrogel

As per a market analysis study conducted in 2016, global hydrogel market was valued at USD 10.87 billion in 2016 and was projected to reach 15.33 billion in 2022 at a compound annual growth rate of 6.04%. It showed that increased demand for the health-care sector was a major factor contributing to this growth [18]. At this moment, Johnson & Johnson (United States), Cardinal Health (United States), the 3M Company (United States), B. Braun

Melsungen (Germany), Smith & Nephew (United Kingdom), and Derma Sciences (United States) are the key players operating in the hydrogel market. Almost all the companies have wound healing topical hydrogels in their repertoire. Some of the important products are summarized in Table 16.1.

Tegaderm is an amorphous hydrogel wound filler indicated for surgical wounds as well as dermal and neuropathic ulcers. It provides a moist environment that is conducive to wound healing. It is available in single-dose tubes.

NU-GEL by Johnson and Johnson contains sodium alginate. It is a transparent hydroactive amorphous gel that causes rehydration of the wound. Sodium alginate hydrogel provides the moistness that hydrates and help in auto-debridement. This natural rehydration facilitates wound healing.

Cardinal Health too markets a group of products relevant to wound healing. In addition to the Kendall amorphous hydrogel, it also markets Hydrogel, Hydrogel + Ag (antibacterial hydrogel), Kendall hydrogel wound dressing (for prolonged wear time), and Kendall hydrogel impregnated gauze, which conforms to the contours of the wound.

Prontosan is a ready-to-use colorless gel marketed by B. Braun Melsungen, Germany. It is meant for application in hard-to-heal wound cavities. It contains betaine and polyhexanide, which are used as wound cleaners [23–25].

TABLE 16.1 Major companies marketing hydrogel and their flagship products.

3M Healthcare (United States)	Tegaderm15 and 25 g tubes	Wound filler	Pressure ulcer and wound care [19]
3M Healthcare	Tegagel	Bioactive hydrogel (alginate based)	Wound care [20]
Johnson and Johnson (United States)	NU-GEL	Wound rehydration (bioactive hydrogel)	Debridement and hydration of eschar [21]
B. Braun Melsungen (Germany)	Prontosan Wound Gel	Cleaning and dressing of infected wounds	Acute, chronic, and burn wounds [22]
Smith & Nephew (United Kingdom)	ALGISITE M	Wound dressing	Wound care and foot ulcers [23]
DermaRite Industries	Derma film	Hydrocolloid wound dressing	Wound care
3M Healthcare	Tegasorb	Activated charcoal cloth alginate	Bioactive wound dressing
Smith & Nephew	Intrasite	Bioactive hydrogel	Wound care
ConvaTec	Granuflex	Activated charcoal cloth alginate	Deodorizing wound care

It is apparent from Table 16.1 that among the commercially available hydrogel products, wound dressings are the most common. Development of an ideal wound healing product is a demanding job because an ideal dressing should have properties similar to the human skin. It should be able to generate an environment of high humidity at the wound site, permit gaseous exchange, provide bacterial protection, be nontoxic and biocompatible, as well as allow easy application and removal. It should also control pain and tissue necrosis. Based on the mode of action, wound dressings are of three types: passive, interactive, and bioactive products. Passive products simply generate a mechanical barrier between the wound and the external environment, whereas interactive products act as an interface between the wound and the environment. The interactive types are permeable to oxygen but prevent bacterial entry into the wound. Bioactive dressings participate in the process of wound healing through delivery of the bioactive substances. Of the three types, the last is preferred for treatment of large and difficult to heal wounds. Although fulfilling all these criteria is a tall order, hydrogel dressings come close to the ideal.

The chief ingredient of most of the healing hydrogel products is natural alginate because alginate has certain properties that are desirable in wound healing. Alginate dressings are highly versatile and come with various mechanical strengths. A natural copolymer of glucuronic acid and mannuronic acid, the mechanical strength of alginate varies with the composition, that is, the ratio of glucuronic and mannuronic acid. Whenever the polymer is richer in mannuronic acid, it forms soft gels. If the glucuronic acid block is high in proportion, the gels are firm. Alginates have bacteriostatic property, which makes them suitable for use in chronic wounds (infected foot ulcers). They have high absorbency and act as thermal insulators. Some dressings contain both alginate and chitosan to increase absorbability. Being occlusive, they promote autolytic debridement and long duration of action. Hydrogel-based wound healing products are available in three forms. First, free-flowing amorphous hydrogels with packaging in tubes or sprays; second, impregnated hydrogel saturated onto gauge pads or sponges, third, sheet hydrogels supported by fiber mesh [20]. Hydrocolloid dressings are similar to hydrogels in many ways. Here, the gel forming materials are laminated on a thin layer of water-repellent polymers.

16.2 Hydrogels in drug delivery

Hydrogels have been used in several forms of drug delivery, as described in the following sections.

16.2.1 Hydrogels in oral drug delivery

Oral delivery is considered to be the most affordable and convenient route of drug delivery for small molecules. The site of absorption for most drugs in the oral route is small intestine, but gastrointestinal (GI) mucosa is practically impermeable to big molecules. Moreover, this route is not suitable for protein and peptide drugs, which get degraded in the harsh acidic conditions of human stomach. Recently, an option has come to protect these drugs from the GI degradation by entrapping them in a layer of protective hydrogels. The hydrogels are designed in such a way that they remain shrunken in the stomach and open up only at the site of absorption. Polymers with pendant anionic groups are specifically designed for this purpose by grafting acrylic acid derivatives onto them [26]. Because ionization of the anionic polymer is suppressed in acidic media, they remain in unswollen state in the stomach, which retards the entry of stomach fluid into the dosage form, thereby preventing their degradation in the earlier part of the GI tract.

Some of the important hydrogel products for oral drug delivery have been represented in Table 16.2.

16.2.2 Natural hydrogels in buccal delivery

Oral cavity of the humans, having a surface area of around $100\,cm^2$, can be used as a site for drug administration because of certain unique advantages. It allows easy administration as well as removal and helps to avoid the first pass elimination. A variety of drugs can reach the systemic circulation through the buccal mucosa, gingival and sublingual mucosa, which makes the floor and sides of the oral cavity. However, one difficulty associated with the buccal delivery is leakage of the drugs through the GI route. Only a dosage form that sticks to the buccal mucosa and dissolves slowly at that site can ensure selective permeation through the buccal mucosa. Bioadhesive hydrogels fulfill these criteria. Some hydrogel-based products for buccal delivery are mentioned in Table 16.3 [26].

16.2.3 Vaginal drug delivery

Although a gender-specific delivery system, vaginal deliveries have some interesting advantages over and above that of the oral delivery. In addition, it can bypass the first pass metabolism. It has good surface area and vascularity, which makes it a better site of absorption for protein drugs. It can accommodate different types of dosage forms such as tablets, capsules, liquids gels, and vaginal films. However, vaginal route has some shortcomings too. Vaginal permeability is affected by estrogen concentration and the fluid content and allows low residence time. This problem can

TABLE 16.2 Hydrogel (natural and semisynthetic)-based commercial products for oral delivery [26].

Product	Company	Polymer	Drug delivered	Dosage form	Indication
Advil	Pfizer Inc.	Hydroxypropyl methyl cellulose	Ibuprofen	Liquid-gel	Fast pain relief
Lopid	Pfizer Inc.	Hydroxypropyl methyl cellulose	Zemfibrogil	Film-coated tablet	Lipid regulating agent (lowers VLDL and triglycerides)
Toviaz	Pfizer Inc.	Hydroxypropyl methyl cellulose and polyvinyl alcohol	Fesoterodine fumarate	Extended release tablets	Overactive bladder syndrome
Aplenzin	Valent Pharmaceuticals Internationals	Ethyl cellulose and polyvinyl alcohol	Bupropion hydrobromide	Tablet	Manic depressive disorder
Belviq XR	Esai Inc.	Polyvinyl alcohol, hydroxyl propyl methyl cellulose, polyethylene glycol	Lorcaserin hydrochloride	Tablet	Antiobesity and binds to serotonin
Voltaren	Glaxo SmithKline	Hydroxyl propyl methyl cellulose and polyethylene glycol	Diclofenac sodium	Enteric-coated tablet	Osteoarthritis and rheumatoid arthritis
Concerta	Alza Corporation	Hypromellose and polyethylene oxide	Methylphenidate	Osmotic tablet	Attention deficit hyperactivity disorder
Gaviscon	Reckitt Benckiser Healthcare Ltd.	Sodium alginate and carbomer 974	Aluminum hydroxide, magnesium carbonate, aluminum-magnesium-alginate…	Chewable tablet/ oral suspension	Heartburn and indigestion

Levora	Mayne Pharmaceuticals	Croscarmellose sodium	Levonorgestrel and ethinylestradiol	Tablet	Oral contraceptive
Portia	Teva pharmaceutical Industries Ltd.	Hypromellose	Levonorgestrel and ethinylestradiol	Tablet	Oral contraceptive
Ranexa	Gilead Sciences	Polyvinyl alcohol and hydroxyl propyl methyl cellulose	Ranolazine	Prolonged release tablets	Antianginal (used in chronic chest pain)
Suprax	Sanofi Aventis	Hydroxyl propyl methyl cellulose	Cefixime	Oral suspension	Antibiotic and treatment of urinary and chest infections
Vicoprofen	AbbVie Ltd.	Hydroxypropyl methyl cellulose	Hydrocodone bitartrate with ibuprofen	Tablet	To reduce the sensation of severe pain (opioid)
Xartemis XR	Mallinckrodt Pharmaceuticals	Polyvinyl alcohol	Oxycodone and acetaminophen	Extended release tablets	Analgesic

TABLE 16.3 Hydrogel-based products for buccal delivery.

Product	Manufacturer	Polymer used	Drug delivered	Indication
Buccastem M	Alliance Drug delivery	Xanthan gum	Prochlorperazine maleate 3 mg, equivalent to 1.85 mg prochlorperazine base (antipsychotic drug)	For treatment of nausea and vomiting associated with migraine
Gengigel	Oraldent Ltd.	Hyaluronan	Hyaluronic acid	For treating oral lesions
Nicotinell	GlaxoSmithKline	Xanthan gum and gelatin	Nicotine	Nicotine replacement therapy
SCHALI Dental care hydrogel	SCHALI Product	Cellulose gum and hydrogenated starch	Hydrated silica	For management of gingivitis and plaque
Imdur	Key Pharmaceuticals	Hydroxyl propyl cellulose and hydroxyl propyl methyl cellulose	Isosorbide mononitrate	Prevention of chest pain in patients with angina
Zilactin-B gel	Zila Pharmaceuticals	Hydroxypropyl cellulose	Benzocaine	Local anesthetic to reduce pain from minor mouth problems

be overcome by using the technology of external stimuli-sensitive gelling, which converts sols to gel in the vaginal microenvironment. As vaginitis, a bacterial infection of the vagina is a common problem, antibacterial and antiviral agents are administered through this route. It can also be used as a noninvasive administration site for protein drugs such as insulin, growth hormone, and some steroids. Hydrogels used in vaginal delivery are tabulated in Table 16.4 [26].

16.2.4 Topical and transdermal delivery

Skin allows permeation of very few drugs, that is, drugs of high lipophilicity, low molecular weight, and very low minimum effective plasma concentration. However, delivering the drugs as hydrogels expands this range. Hydrogels can moisturize the skin and enhance topical delivery. They are used to facilitate the delivery of liposomes and nanoparticles too [27]. Below is a list of hydrogel-based products that are delivered by the topical and transdermal routes (Table 16.5). Transdermal iontophoresis makes the use of electric potentials to drive the ionic drugs into the systemic circulation through the intact skin. Because the main driving force is electrical, the drug reservoir should be made of a conductive medium. Hydrogels because of their water-holding capacity can conduct electricity while retaining their distinct three-dimensional structures. Patents demonstrating the use of hydrogels in drug reservoirs for iontophoretic drug delivery were also noted [28].

16.2.5 Hydrogels for targeted drug delivery

Formation of gel right at the site of action has many benefits. In the treatment of tissue injury, this brings dual benefit of filling the damaged area as well as preventing fluid leakage. The in situ hydrogels would accumulate the serofibrinous exudates to build a fibrin bridge. Fibroblasts would be naturally drawn to this bridge to secrete collagen

TABLE 16.4 Hydrogels for vaginal delivery.

Product	Manufacturer	Polymer used	Drug delivered	Indication
Hyalogyn	Fidia Pharma USA Inc.	Hyaluronic acid	Hydeal-D (hyaluronic acid derivative)	Lubricant activity
Vagisil	Combe Inc.	Hyaluronic acid	Hyaluronic acid	Prevents dryness of vagina
Zestica Moisture	Searchlight Pharma Inc.	Hyaluronic acid	Hyaluronic acid	Prevents vaginal dryness

TABLE 16.5 Table for topical and transdermal drug delivery [26, 28].

Product	Manufacturer	Polymer used	Delivery route	Drug delivered	Indication
Granugel	ConvaTec	Pectin, carboxymethylcellulose, and propylene glycol	Topical	–	Applied on wounds to prevent dryness and promote autolytic debridement
Collagen Hydrogel Mask	Skin Republic	Collagen and sodium hyaluronate	Facial	Collagen, argan oil, and sea water	Hydration, nourishment and reduction of signs of aging in skin
Flector Patch	IBSA Farmaceutici Italia	Gelatin and carboxymethylcellulose	Transdermal	Diclofenac epolamine	Treatment of acute pain in minor strains
Neutrogena	Johnson & Johnson	Hyaluronic acid	Facial	Hyaluronic acid	Hydration of skin
Algisite M	Smith & Nephew	Alginate	Topical	Calcium alginate	Treatment of skin abrasions, lacerations, tears, and burns
Medihoney Adhesive Dressings	Derma Sciences Inc.	Alginate	Topical	Leptospermum honey	Supports wound healing and removal of necrotic tissue
Ca-alginate Dressing	Gentell Corp.	Alginate	Topical	Calcium alginate	Wound healing
NU-Derm Hydrogel	Systagenix	Alginate	Topical	Hydrocolloids	Management of lightly exuding wounds
Kaltostat	Convatec	Alginate	Topical	Sodium and calcium salts of alginic acid	Wound dressing

TABLE 16.6 Hydrogels for targeted delivery [30].

Product	Polymer used	Therapeutic application	Drug delivered
Sericin	Dextran	Optically trackable drug delivery system for malignant melanoma	Doxorubicin
Regranex	Carboxymethyl cellulose	Diabetic foot ulcer	Recombinant human-platelet derived growth factor
Hyalofemme/ Hyalo Gyn	Carbomer propylene glycol and hyaluronic acid derivative	Vaginal dryness	Estrogen alternative to hyaluronic acid derivative

that accelerates wound healing. Based on this concept, Lih et al. had fabricated chitosan-polyethylene glycol-tyramine hydrogels that showed good bioadhesiveness [29]. Some of the hydrogels for targeted drug delivery are tabulated in Table 16.6.

16.2.6 Ocular delivery

The use of hydrogels in ocular drug delivery was also investigated. A patent describes the development of a system meant to be plugged into the lacrimal canal or punctum. Soft, flexible, and biodegradable hydrogels were used for this work (US patent 8409606) [31]. One example is dexamethasone punctum plug to control inflammation after ocular surgery. Table 16.7 represents some hydrogels for ocular drug delivery [30].

TABLE 16.7 Hydrogels for ocular drug delivery.

Product	Polymer used	Therapeutic application	Drug delivered
Hylo Gel (CandorPharm Inc.)	Sodium hyaluronate	Used for dry eye syndrome	Sodium hyaluronate
Ocusert (Alza Corporation)	Alginic acid	Glaucoma management	Pilocarpine
Sericin	Dextran	Optically trackable drug delivery system for malignant melanoma	Doxorubicin

16.2.7 Hydrogels for specialized applications

16.2.7.1 Bioengineered hydrogels

Often the properties of natural hydrogels fall short to meet requirements for therapy and systems need to be tuned or engineered. Bioengineered hydrogels are mainly of three types: implantable hydrogels, injectable hydrogels, and sprayable hydrogels. They are used for postsurgical local drug delivery as well as in wound healing, cancer treatment, spinal, and periodontal surgeries. Although most of them use synthetic polymers, some natural biomolecules are also used. Recurrence of cancer after surgery is a common incident. A number of injectable hydrogels have been developed as a sustained drug delivery vehicle for management of postsurgical recurrence [32, 33]. Chitosan, a biodegradable polysaccharide obtained by deacetylation of chitin, has inherent pH responsiveness. Its pH responsiveness results from protonation-deprotonation equilibrium of its amino groups, which have a pK_a around 6 in aqueous media. Thermosensitive chitosan hydrogels can be used in surgical implantation with in situ gelation. A pH-sensitive chitosan-based hydrogel carrying doxorubicin has been developed for hepatocellular carcinoma [34, 35].

16.2.7.2 Thermoresponsive hydrogel

Thermoresponsive polymers exhibit critical solution temperature at which they achieve sol/gel transition. Poly N-isopropylacrylamide (PNIPAAm) is an FDA-approved thermoresponsive polymer that can be used in the development of thermoresponsive hydrogels [36]. Recently, an injectable thermoresponsive hydrogel containing alginate-gelatin-PNIPAAMm was developed. The gel was loaded with doxorubicin with the intent of improving the killing rate of drug-resistant cancer.

16.2.7.3 Sprayable hydrogels

Another innovation in the field of hydrogel technology is sprayable hydrogel where the polymer chains are cross-linked in situ. They are considered to have high curative potential in postsurgery treatments.

A spray hydrogel, as described by Kim et al., makes use of the polymer hyaluronic acid. The phenolic group of the hyaluronic acid was oxidized by recombinant tyrosinase protein that acts as the cross-linker. Tyrosinase was generated by *Streptomyces avermitilis*, which also produces avermectin, the lead in an antianthelmintic drug. Because tyrosinase-driven oxidation of hyaluronic acid is fast, it leads to the very rapid production of hydrogels [37].

16.2.7.4 Supramolecular hydrogels

One of the limitations associated with hydrogels is their lack of affinity for hydrophobic moieties [38]. This is a big constraint because most of the recently developed drugs are hydrophobic in nature. As such, the small-sized drugs could be loaded in the pores of covalently cross-linked preformed hydrogels, but the loading efficiency in such cases are not high [30]. Moreover, such preformed systems because of their comparatively larger size could only be introduced into the human body as implants. To load the hydrophobic drug into hydrogels, special techniques are needed. The system should be made in such a way as to have a hydrophobic zone (for hydrophobic drugs), a hydrophilic part (to attract and bind water), as well as functional groups that may enter into a physical cross-linking with the adjacent molecules to form a gel structure. Such a system can only be composed of many molecules with different physicochemical characteristics and would be known as supramolecular hydrogels. Such systems can also be introduced into target tissue directly for prolonged therapeutic effect (Fig. 16.1).

Cyclodextrins are cyclic oligosaccharides, composed of 6, 7, or 8 D(+) glucose units named as α-, β-, and γ-CD, respectively. The glucose units are linked in such a way that they take the form of a bucket. The inner cavity of the buckets are hydrophobic in nature with a depth of ca. 7.0 Å with internal diameters of ca. 4.5, 7.0, or 8.5 Å (α-, β-, and γ-CD, respectively) [39]. In alpha cyclodextrin, six primary hydroxyl groups are available on the narrow side, whereas 12 secondary hydroxyl groups

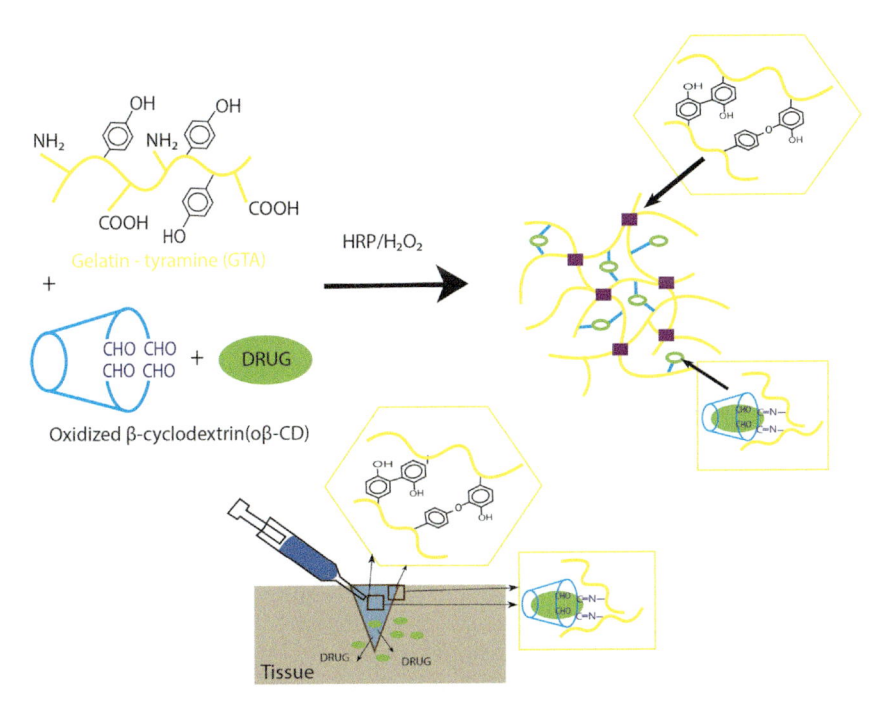

FIG. 16.1 Administration of cyclodextrin hydrogels into tissue by injection.

are there on the wide side [40]. Hence various molecules can be attached to the cyclodextrins through these groups to form supramolecular inclusion complexes.

A study had demonstrated the formation of a glycol-conjugate in which L-glucuronic acid block (extracted from sodium alginate) was treated with mono-6-amino β-cyclodextrin. Lipophilic nonhydroxylated coumarin, a trypanocidal drug, was loaded into the hydrophobic cavity of the β-cyclodextrin. The carboxylate groups of the unconjugated α-L glucuronate residues were made to interact with calcium ions to produce supramolecular hydrogels [41]. The drug delivered as inclusion complex showed better solubility and bioavailability compared with that of free amido-coumarin.

16.2.7.5 Sericin/dextran hydrogel: A hydrogel that allows optical tracking and targeted drug delivery

Release at the targeted site seems to be the recent focus of drug delivery and is immensely desirable for cytotoxic drugs. This can be achieved by simply immobilizing the dosage form at the desired site [42]. In cancer chemotherapy, one more attribute is sought. Monitoring of the dynamic status of the drug within the body improves the treatment significantly.

One of the options to achieve this traceability is to include an externally trackable fluorescent dye in the dosage form. However, the benefit comes with significant disadvantage of cytotoxicity [43].

Silk sericin is a glycoprotein containing high amounts of hydrophilic amino acids, especially serine. The constituent amino acids of silk sericin have polar side chains such as hydroxyl, carboxyl or amino groups that can be reacted with other functional groups to develop customized molecules that can be easily included in a hydrogel system [44].

Sericin has all the properties desirable in a vehicle for injectable drug. It is immunologically inert and is considered to be a biocompatible biopolymer. It can serve as an antioxidant, antielastic, antityrosinase, moisturizing, and mitogenic agent [45]. Its high moisture absorptivity as well as long in vivo half-life makes it an ideal candidate for hydrogel dosage forms. Recently, it has become known that sericin, extracted from a fibroin-deficient mutant silkworm cocoon, is gifted with an intrinsic photoluminescence property [46]. On the flip side, this type of sericin is not of much use because it lasts only for several days and gets degraded by common methods of sterilization. A cheap alternative was procured from a waste.

The prime product of the silk industry is silk fiber, which is composed of a fibrous protein called fibroin, but this delicate fiber is surrounded by several layers of sticky protein called silk sericin. During the processing of silk fibers, this sticky protein is washed out, giving it the lowly status of waste. This sericin is partially degraded by rigorous processing but also inherits the property of photoluminescence [47]. However, because of the rigorous degumming process, it contains a large quantity of low molecular weight soluble polypeptides which makes the cross-linking difficult. The problem could be overcome by forming a composite hydrogel using two biocompatible backbone components. Liu et al. in their pioneering work had developed a composite hydrogel using two components—sericin and dextran—which retained the photoluminescence property of sericin and helped to track the dynamic status of drug noninvasively. Sericin-ADH was prepared by introducing the hydrazide group to sericin through adipohydrazide conjugation (Fig. 16.2). Vicinal hydroxyl groups of dextran were oxidized using $NaIO_4$ to create aldehyde functionalities [48].

For developing drug-loaded hydrogels, drug was dissolved in sericin-ADH and mixed with equal volume of dextran aldehydes. The mixture was incubated for 2 h at 4°C. The researchers studied the drug release profile for both small molecule as well as a macromolecular drug. After injection into mice, the system became semisolid from which drug

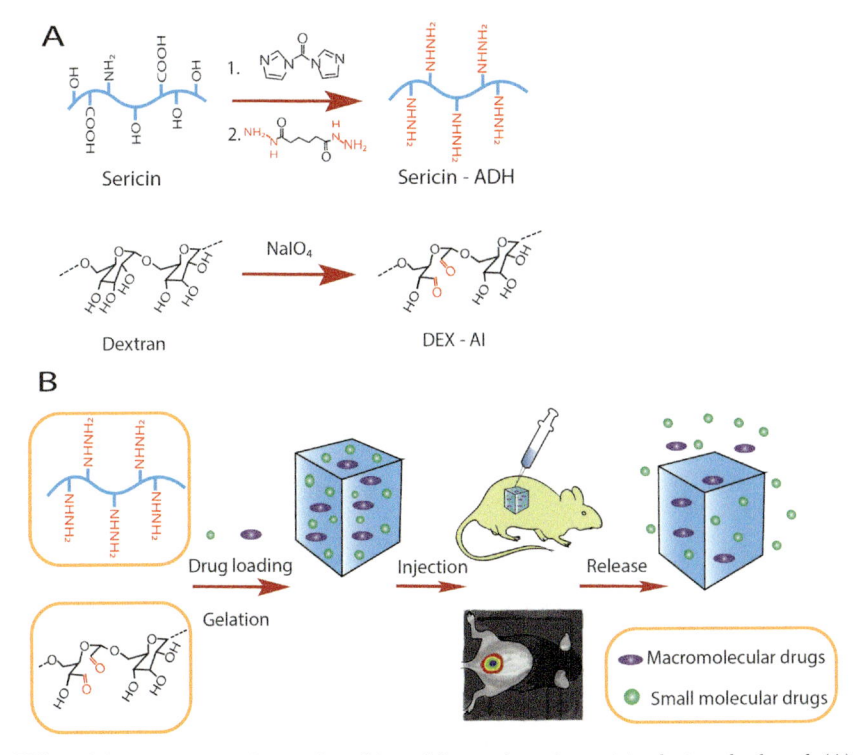

FIG. 16.2 Procedure of optical tracking of drug release by sericin-dextran hydrogel. (A) Preparation of sericin-dextran hydrogel. (B) Drug loading and tracking of drug release by photoluminescence.

got released at differential rates. The photoluminescence property of the hydrogels was analyzed by a PC spectrofluorometer with excitation wavelength ranging from three 320 to 600 nm [48].

16.2.7.6 DNA hydrogels

Quantum dots are tiny particles of a semiconducting material with diameters in the range of 2–10 nm (10–50 atoms), which fluoresce when exposed to light. When strands of DNA are attached to the surface of these particles, we get DNA-functionalized quantum dots. DNA hydrogels make use of complementary strands of DNA hybridized to form a cross-linked network that swells in an aqueous environment. Usually, a fluorescent molecule is attached to the hydrogel for tracing the system through imaging. Zhang et al. had demonstrated a quantum dot-based hydrogel system using the DNA-binding drug doxorubicin. The system had the dual advantage of targeted delivery of drugs and allowed in vivo bioimaging for monitoring tumor growth, demonstrated in Fig. 16.3 [49]. Aptamers such as siRNA can be used to target specific cell types to deliver drug specifically and modulate protein expression during the course of treatment.

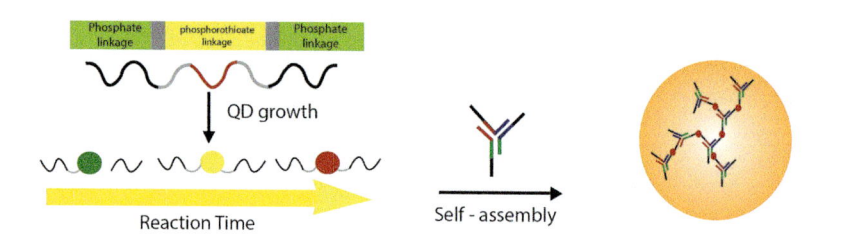

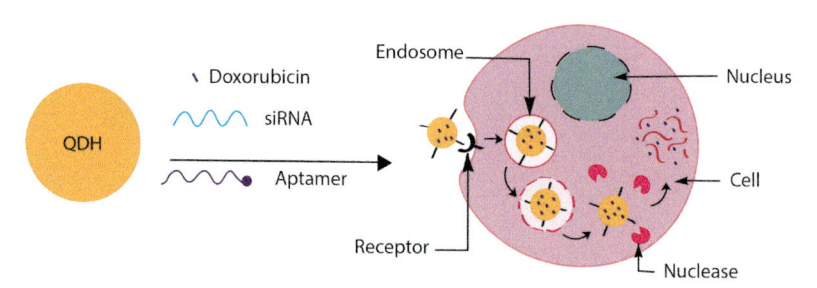

FIG. 16.3   Top: Formation of the QD hydrogel through hybridization with DNA functionalized QDs. Bottom: QD hydrogel specifically targeting the cell using aptamer for drug delivery. Release of doxorubicin and siRNA happens after uptake into the cell through endocytosis (adapted). *Redrawn with some modifications from Zhang L., Jean S.R., Ahmed S., Aldridge P.M., Li X., et al. Multifunctional quantum dot DNA hydrogels. Nat Commun 2017;8:381.*

16.3 Problems related to clinical translation of hydrogel-based drug delivery system

From the above account, it can be observed that some important milestones have already been reached in the usage of natural hydrogels in the field of drug delivery and tissue engineering. But compared to the volume of research, the clinical success is rather low [50, 51]. The sterilization and pyrogen-related problems may be the primary cause baulking their success [52].

Currently, the sterility assurance level for materials that come in direct contact with the blood is limited to 10^{-6} [53, 54]. The presence of water in the hydrogels makes it sensitive to heat-related changes. The alternative option of aseptic sterilization is time-consuming and costly [55]. Moreover, aseptic processing does not guarantee the level of safety achievable by terminal sterilization [55].

Natural polymers resemble the physiological matrix more closely than their synthetic counterparts, but they are more likely to show batch variation [56]. The viscosity, hardness, and adhesiveness of the cellulose derivatives (hydroxypropyl methylcellulose, methyl cellulose, and carboxymethyl cellulose) were significantly reduced by conventional steam sterilization [57]. The viscosity of the carrageenan and xanthan gum hydrogels also decrease by the heat treatment. A new method is now being experimented, which proposes simultaneous sterilization and synthesis of hydrogels [58]. This has generated interest because the problematic chemical initiators used for cross-linking can be avoided with the simultaneous reduction of the microbial load. This was successfully demonstrated in developing drug-loaded chitosan/glycerol phosphate disodium salt-based controlled release hydrogels. For the time being, sterilization is a case to case study because the drugs and additives loaded into the hydrogels also affect sterilization condition [59].

Recently, Nguyen et al. attempted fabrication of hydrogels to deliver dopamine for neural regeneration. They developed a triblock hydrogel of hyaluronic acid (Hy), -dopamine (DA), and -3-(4-Hydroxyphenyl) propionic acid (HPA), that is, HY-DA-HPA, which could have a wide range of storage moduli ~ 100 to ~ 20,000 Pa (at $f = 2000$ rad/s). The developed hydrogel was biocompatible with the mesenchymal stem cells as well as human-induced pluripotent stem cell-derived neural stem cells. Because dopamine can help in regenerating the dopaminergic neuron, use of this novel gel is being investigated in CNS repair and regeneration [60]. Similarly, to deliver curcumin at the site of hepatocellular carcinoma, glycyrrhetinic acid (GA)-modified curcumin-based hydrogel has been developed [61].

16.4 Applications of hydrogels in tissue engineering

The credit for first use of natural hydrogels in the field of tissue engineering goes to Lim and Sun, who in 1980 demonstrated that cells can be encapsulated in calcium alginate hydrogels [62]. Alginic acid is mainly obtained from cell walls of brown sea weed. It is a highly water-soluble anionic polysaccharide, which is well-tolerated in humans. Alginate is an irreversible hydrocolloid because it exists in gelatinous (colloidal) state in water but never returns to a liquid state once it is gelled [63].

Physicochemically, alginate can be described as an anionic polysaccharide with a strong gelation capability. It has the advantage of biocompatibility and low toxicity [1]. Alginic acid could instantly form a gel in combination with calcium ions, which can be used as drug carrier [64]. It is a constituent of a number of tissue engineering devices too. Table 16.8 shows some polysaccharide-based hydrogel devices that serve important purposes in the field of tissue engineering.

16.4.1 Algisyl-LVR

Algisyl-LVR(R), a hydrogel product from LoneStar, has been approved for treatment in advanced heart failure. Classified as a medical device, this implant is directly injected into the heart muscle in people with weakened and enlarged left ventricle. After injection, the hydrogel immediately forms internal scaffolds, which strengthens the heart muscle and causes improvement in cardiac output.

In progressive heart failure, cardiac tissue is initially damaged by a variety of factors such as infection or infarction, which compromise its contractility, thereby reducing its ability to supply the blood throughout the body leading to ischemia in vital organs. To remedy this damage, the weak cardiac tissues continue pumping blood causing further damage to it. So with time, there is increased damage to the tissue and irreversible loss of cardiac function. Algisyl-LVR helps in increasing the strength of the cardiac muscle and allows it to recover from the stress.

Alginate, a complex polysaccharide of glucuronic acid and mannuronic acid, is the basic components of Algisyl-LVR. Basically anionic in nature, it makes complexes with divalent cations that give rise to the three-dimensional structure that is biodegradable. Alginate hydrogel is one of the few natural hydrogels that met the success of commercial application.

16.4.2 OP-1 Putty (Stryker Biotech)

Across the world, life expectancy of humans has increased significantly in the past 50 years [66]. But there is a cost too. World has seen a sharp increase in age-related diseases such as osteoarthritis, sciatica, intervertebral disk degeneration.

The intervertebral disk is composed of two layers: annulus fibrosus (the outer shell) and nucleus pulposus (the inner gelatinous core). Disk

TABLE 16.8 Hydrogels devices in tissue engineering sourced from plant and algal polysaccharides [65].

Name (sponsor company/ university)	Hydrogel material/payload (gelation mechanism)	Site of administration	Indications	http://clinicaltrials.gov identifier (phase)
Algisyl-LVR device (LoneStar Heart, Inc.)	Alginate (physical interaction)	Intramyocardial area	Heart failure and dilated cardiomyopathy	NCT01311791(Ph II/III
Gut Guarding Gel (National Cheng-Kung University Hospital)	Sodium alginate/calcium lactate (physical interaction)	Submucosal area	Gastroenterological tumor and polyps	NCT03321396 (NA)
Radiesse (+) (Merz Pharmaceuticals)	Hydroxylapatite, carboxymethyl cellulose with Lidocaine (physical interaction	Dermis	Correction of wrinkles and folds and stimulation of natural collagen production	FDA (2015)
Radiesse (BioForm Medical, Inc.)	Hydroxylapatite, carboxymethyl cellulose (physical interaction)	Dermis	For correction of facial folds and wrinkles and signs of facial fat loss and volume loss	EMA (2004) FDA (2006) for first indication
Osteogenic protein 1 (OP-1) implant, OP-1 Putty (Stryker Biotech)	Collagen, carboxymethyl cellulose, and recombinant OP-1 (physical interaction)	Spine	Posterolateral lumbar spinal fusion	FDA (2001)
Coaptite (BioForm Medical, Inc.)	Calcium hydroxylapatite, sodium carboxymethyl cellulose and glycerin (physical interaction)	Submucosal area	Female stress urinary incontinence	EMA (2001) FDA (2005)
Promedon	Hydroxyethyl cellulose (physical interaction	Knee	Osteoarthritis	NCT04061733 (NA)
Naofumi Takehara	Gelatin with basic fibroblast growth factor	Myocardium	Ischemic cardiomyopathy	NCT00981006 (Ph I)
Neo-Kidney Augment (InRegen)	Gelatin with selected renal cells	Kidney	Type 2 diabetes and chronic kidney disease	NCT02525263 (Ph II)

degeneration is a complex process that starts at the nucleus pulposus and gradually spreads to surrounding parts [67]. This causes excruciating back pain compromising the quality of life. Treatment options include surgery, which is often beyond the reach of lower-income and middle-income strata [68, 69]. Intervertebral disks are shock absorbers. In some forms of lumbar degenerative disk disease, the intervertebral disks dry out. When this happens, the cushioning effect is compromised and joint flexibility reduces. The regular movements of life may cause stress tears in the outer shell, which affect the nerves leading to pain and inflammation.

Currently, the best treatment for correcting this malady is bone grafting. In lumbar disk degeneration, a surgical procedure called "posterolateral fusion" is performed. In this, the arthritic bone is removed, a bone graft is placed between the transverse processes, and treatment is done so that they heal into a single solid bone [70]. However, it hinders natural movement and often accelerates the degenerative process in adjacent disks. Replacement of the nuclear pulposus with water-retaining hydrogels was thought to be a better option [71–73], and OP-1 Putty of Stryker Biotech, a hydrogel device containing engineered carboxymethylcellulose, is being used as an alternative to autograft in patients requiring revision posterolateral lumbar spinal fusion.

The main ingredient of the OP-1 Putty is recombinant human osteogenic protein (rhOP-1), which induces new bone formation [74]. The other components are Type I Bovine bone collagen matrix, which is the main component of the organic matrix of the bone, and carboxymethyl cellulose sodium [75]. Carboxymethyl cellulose, an anionic polymer with its reservoir of hydroxy groups (–OH), forms hydrogen bonds with water [76].

OP-1 Putty is packaged in two vials of unequal sizes: OP-1 and bone collagen are contained in the bigger vial, and carboxymethyl cellulose as sterile dry powder is packaged in the smaller vial. OP-1 Putty is reconstituted with sterile saline (0.9%) solution and applied at the desired site by a surgeon. The constituent forms a hydrogel because of physical interaction.

Human body has bone morphogenetic protein (BMP-7), which can induce the mesenchymal stem cells to form new bones through calcium deposition [77]. OP-1 Putty potentially mimics BMP-7 [78]. On placement into fusion site, the engineered protein OP-1 stimulates the bone formation process. OP-1 Putty provides a platform to support the new bone. Stem cells from the surrounding tissues accumulate at the fusion site and participate in the process of bone growth. Presently, the use of this device is approved under Humanitarian Device Exemption of USFDA, which allows the marketing of a medical device without evidence of its effectiveness.

16.4.3 Gut guarding gel

The cancer of the gastrointestinal tract is one of the most frequent cancer types observed throughout the world. According to GLOBOCAN 2018 data, it is the third most deadly cancer that caused around 783,000 deaths in the year 2018 itself [79]. However, not all the cancers of the GI tract are fatal. If detected in the early stage, patients can be saved through minimally invasive surgical procedures called endoscopic mucosal resection and endoscopic submucosal dissection [80].

The development of stomach cancer is a slow process, and the severity of the disease can be categorized into five stages depending on the size of tumors (T), presence of nodes (N), and level of metastasis (M). If the cancerous cells are sessile or confined to the mucosa or submucosa, they can be excised out using the endoscopic mucosal resection (EMR) technique and the area cauterized to prevent the recurrence of lesions [81, 82]. However, when the tumors are flat, excising them completely becomes difficult. Surgeons use submucosal injections to separate the tumor-carrying layer from the underlying muscular tissue. Submucosal hydrogel injections can be used to lift the mucosal layer so that they can be easily caught into the snare attached to the tip of the endoscope [83]. The success of EMR depends on the size of tumor. When the size is less than 2 cm, EMR is quite efficient in curing the disease. However, when the size is bigger than 2 cm, excision cannot be done at one go. The mucosal layers have to be removed in piecemeal manner. And this leaves scope for the recurrence at a later date. Endoscopic submucosal dissection (ESD) is recommended in this case. However, in both the procedures, separation between the layers, that is, the layer to be removed from the layer to be retained is required. In the absence of an intervening layer between the layer carrying lesions and the layer to be retained, the risk of accidental damage to the gut multiplies manifold [84]. Submucosal injections reduce this risk by effecting the separation between the two [85].

Injecting a solution into the thin submucosal layer is a delicate process because the injected solution tends to dissipate quickly. Initially, there was a practice of injecting normal saline/dextrose water for lifting up the mucosal layers. But the lifting effects of these solutions are short-lived. The ideal fluid for submucosal injection should generate a strong fluid cushion and at the same time not damage the tissue specimens in any way to affect the histopathological assessment [86, 87]. Solutions having high viscosity and hydrogelatinization ability are preferred [83].

Recently, the National Cheng-Kung University Hospital of Taiwan have come up with a device for submucosal injection and performed a clinical trial on it (NCT03321396) [88]. The injectable product contains a mixture of sodium alginate and calcium lactate and intended for use in endoscopic submucosal dissection. On mixing, the two prime ingredients interact to produce a calcium-alginate gel, which is named as "Gut Guarding Gel" by the inventors.

Alginate is a linear polysaccharide of alternating blocks of (1-4)-linked α-L-guluronic (G-block) and β-D-mannuronic (M-block) acid residues. In contact with divalent cations such as Ca^{2+}, it can form gels. The divalent cations can bind to the negative charges of the G-blocks resulting in a cross-linked hydrogel matrix. At low pH, alginate forms an insoluble alginic acid skin that changes into a soluble viscous layer when exposed to higher pH conditions of the intestinal tract causing effective separation between the layers [89].

16.4.4 Radiesse

The process of natural aging is accompanied with inevitable changes in facial topography. It is manifested by tissue volume loss, appearance of marionette lines, nasolabial folds, deep furrows, and wrinkles, which make the skin lose its youthful appearance. Mainly, these signs arise due to the loss of subcutaneous tissue and thinning of the dermis [90, 91]. Loss of skin elasticity is one of the major factors contributing to these changes.

Skin elasticity is mainly maintained by an intricate balance of the two major proteins: collagen and elastin. Collagen, a fibrous protein helps skin cells adhere to one another, keeping it strong and elastic [92]. Collagen makes three-fourth of the dry weight of skin [93]. With age, collagen production decreases. So when there is a huge loss of collagen, there are empty spaces in the folds of the skin, which give it a puckered appearance. Collagen is produced by the fibroblasts, which play a central role in wound healing too [94]. Scientists believed that if the fibroblast could be activated in one way or the other, the collagen production will spike up and the skin rejuvenation can take place. Accordingly in the 1970s, Stanford University researchers on the basis of some pioneering research, proposed collagen as a facial filler. FDA approved collagen for medical use almost a decade later [95, 96], which led to the launching of a line of cosmetic products, with collagen as their chief constituent. But the filler effect of collagen was found to be temporary.

The ideal biomaterial to be used as derma filler should be long-acting, nonmigratory, biocompatible, nontoxic, nonimmunogenic, and reasonably cheap [91]. So the gap remained unfulfilled for quite some time [97–100].

Much later, a US company called BioForm Medical Inc. launched a product called Radiesse that did not contain collagen but claimed to stimulate endogenous collagen production [90, 101]. The product was a hydrogel containing calcium hydroxyapatite microspheres (25–45 μm) and carboxymethyl cellulose dispersed in a mixture of water and glycerine. Incorporation of carboxymethyl cellulose gave it a gel structure

[91]. The product was administered as an injection using short fine needle (27 gauge, 6 mm) into the deep dermis or subdermal space [97].

On injection, carboxymethylcellulose dissipated through the subdermal layer and filled the empty spaces with immediate effect of fullness, giving the impression of a younger skin. The hydrogel structure gives it sufficient rigidity to keep it confined around the site of its administration. Because carboxymethylcellulose is biocompatible as well as biodegradable, with passage of time, it gets reabsorbed into the body. But the deposited calcium hydroxyapatite microspheres remained at the site to support the fibroblastic ingrowth for new collagen formation. Their presence in the subdermal layer creates delayed fibrotic reaction. With passage of time, they also break down and get cleared by the kidney, and newly grown soft tissues occupy the space [91]. The controlled inflammation resulting from the injection creates a fibroblastic reaction [102]. In the connective tissue, fibroblasts are one of the chief cells that produce collagen, elastin, and other proteins. The porous microspheres of the hydroxyapatite act as a scaffold into which the fibroblasts get a readymade shelter and start producing type-1 collagen along with other biomolecules [102]. Type-1 collagen, thus produced, improves the mechanical properties of the skin. At the end of the process, hydroxyapatite completely breaks down, and the space is filled with in situ produced type-1 and type-3 collagen. This brings semipermanent derma feeling effect of Radiesse (R)

16.4.4.1 RadiesseR(+)

RadiesseR(+) shares all the features of Radiesse, with an extra component, lidocaine. Lidocaine, a local anesthetic, reduces the pain and discomfort associated with the injection.

16.4.5 Coaptite

Stress urinary incontinence or unintentional loss of urine from the urethra in women is a disorder that brings social embarrassment more than physiological damage. The condition occurs when the urethral sphincter fails to resist the flow of urine during increased intraabdominal pressure [103]. A number of treatment options are available for this disorder, but there is no perfect therapy. In serious cases, surgical intervention is done, but it is an inconvenient and costly option. The next best thing to control the symptoms is injecting some innocuous bulking agents into the wall of the bladder neck to reduce its inner diameter [104, 105]. The desired outcome is coaptation or sealing of the urethral lumen [106], so that the involuntary flow of urine can be resisted.

For this purpose, a number of devices were already available, but most of them were single-use products needing a new device after each void. A US-based pharmaceutical company (BioForm Medical Inc.) had introduced a hydrogel-based device Coaptite to control the stress-induced urinary incontinence. The device is a permanent implant in which a composite hydrogel consisting of calcium hydroxyapatite and sodium carboxymethyl cellulose is injected into the wall of the urethra using an injector [107]. Hydroxyapatite (75–125 μm) is suspended in an aqueous gel made of sodium carboxymethylcellulose and glycerine. The material is injected into the submucosal layer at the bladder neck [108], which bulks up the urethral tissue causing it to tighten and stop the involuntary leakage of urine. The device has been compared with other bulking agents regarding efficacy, according to Stamey grading method (assess incontinence on a 4-level scale (0–3) where "0" represents total continence and 3 total incontinence). Coaptite fared well in this evaluation and showed equal efficacy to that of collagen bulking agents [109, 110].

16.4.6 Promogel OA

Osteoarthritis is a disabling musculoskeletal disease that mainly affects obese and aging population [111]. The disease usually starts with an inflammation of the articular cartilage that gradually becomes thinner and finally breaks down, if allowed to progress untreated [112]. The early symptoms of disease are stiffness and pain caused by the inflammation of cartilage in the joints. The weight-bearing joints are more affected than others, and knee arthritis is the most common osteoarthritis [113].

Articular cartilage consists of chondrocytes and is protected by a surrounding layer of a dense network of proteoglycans and collagen [114]. In normal joints, a balance is maintained between the production and degradation of the extracellular matrix molecules. In osteoarthritis, this balance is disturbed. The overproduction of the proinflammatory cytokines and tumor necrosis factors (TNF-Alpha) initiates a cascade of events, leading to a systemic inflammation particularly in the tissues intimately related to joints, that is, cartilage, synovial membrane, subchondral bone, and ligaments. The process results in chondrocyte apoptosis or net destruction of cartilage [115]. The treatment of osteoarthritis is mainly conservative, that is, exercise to develop the muscles and management of pain and inflammation through antiinflammatory drugs. A strategy for the radical cure should attempt at preventing the cartilage destruction and restore the matrix protein synthesis to the healthy level. Presently, a number of cell-based therapies is under evaluation to restore the synthesis of extracellular matrices.

Simultaneously, investigation is going on viscosupplementation to lubricate the space between the bones. In viscosupplementation, a viscous jelly-like fluid is injected into the knee joint to ease the movement of bones [116]. Recently, Promogel OA, a hydroxyethyl cellulose-based hydrogel injection is undergoing clinical trial for this (NCT04061733) [117]. Hydroxyethyl cellulose is a nonionic cellulose, which when dissolved in water forms a viscous solution. It has good water-retention and flow-regulating properties. Promogel OA is injected into the joint to reduce the osteoarthritic pain. The clinical trial was started only in 2019, and the results are awaited.

16.4.7 Hydrogels based on hyaluronic acid

Hyaluronic acid, a natural polysaccharide possessing unique biological activities such as osteo-conductivity, can serve as a wonderful medium to support the regeneration of bone tissue. Being a constituent molecule of human body, it has intrinsic biocompatibility and biodegradability. Hyaluronan-based hydrogels can mimic the natural extracellular matrix and provide an ideal environment for cell growth. But it has some disadvantages too. Hydrogels made of pure hyaluronic acid would be susceptible to breakdown by the intrinsic hyaluronidase and exhibit the disadvantages of low mechanical strength and extreme hydrophilicity. But this can be easily overcome by chemical modification. Hyaluronic acid, chemically a repeating sequence of disaccharide units of glucuronic acid and N-acetylglucosamine, is rich in free hydroxyl and carboxyl groups, which can be used to develop ester bonds. Other functional groups can also be added to it to modify its physicochemical properties. Composite hydrogels can also be developed by combining hyaluronic acid with collagen [118], gelatin [119], fibrin [120], alginate [121], etc. A number of companies and research groups have exploited its potential to develop hydrogel products for bone regeneration.

Almost 50% of the total hyaluronic acid of human body exists in skin. However, this amount is drastically reduced with aging. It was thought that replacement of the lost hyaluronic acid can restore the fullness of skin. Hence, almost all the reputed cosmetic companies market antiaging products based on hyaluronic acid. It finds extensive application in wound dressing too.

Regeneration of the tissues such as bone and cartilage is difficult because they lack blood vessels. Autologous bone graft, currently the standard procedure for bone repair, is costly, inconvenient, and restricted by the inadequate supply of the bone stock. Equally difficult is the repair of cartilages that are nourished by chondrocytes as well as extracellular matrix.

So hyaluronic acid has become one of the current focuses in the treatment of bone and cartilage tissue engineering. For this, stem cells obtained from one's bone marrow is amplified through tissue culture and implanted into a precast biomaterial that can support the growth of the cells. This hybrid material is implanted into the affected area of the bone, where aided by drug and nourishment, the seeded bone cells keep growing until the defect is repaired. Table 16.9 summarizes the hydrogel products based on hyaluronic acid.

TABLE 16.9 Hyaluronic acid-based hydrogels devices.

Company	Hydrogel with drug	Route of administration	Indication	Approval authority
Belotero balance (+) Lidocaine (Merz Pharmaceuticals)	Hyaluronic acid with lidocaine	Injection through dermis	Moderate to severe facial wrinkles and folds	FDA (2019)
Revanesse Versa +	Hyaluronic acid with lidocaine	Injection through dermis	Moderate to severe facial wrinkles and creases	FDA (2018)(cos)
Teosyal RHA (Teoxane SA)	Hyaluronic acid	Injection through dermis	Facial wrinkles and folds	EMA (2015) FDA (2017)
Revanesse Versa/Revanesse Ultra (Prollenium Medical Technologies Inc.)	Hyaluronic acid	Injection through dermis	Moderate to severe facial wrinkles and creases	FDA (2017)
Restylane Lyft, Restylane Refyne, Restylane Defyne (Galderma Laboratories, L.P.) Restylane Silk (Valeant Pharmaceuticals North America LLC/Medicis)	Hyaluronic acid with lidocaine	Subcutaneous Injectable gel dermis, lips	For correction of volume deficit, facial folds and wrinkles, midface contour deficiencies, and perioral rhytids	EMA (2010) FDA (2012 for first indication)
Belotero balance (Merz Pharmaceuticals)	Hyaluronic acid	Injection through dermis	Moderate to severe facial wrinkles and folds	EMA (2004) cos FDA (2011)
Juvéderm XC (Allergan, Inc.)	Hyaluronic acid with lidocaine	Facial tissue	Correction of facial wrinkles and folds	FDA (2010) cos
Elevess (Anika Therapeutics)	Hyaluronic acid with lidocaine	Dermis	Moderate to severe facial wrinkles and folds	FDA (2006) cos EMA (2007)

Juvéderm/Voluma XC/Ultra XC/Volbella XC/Vollure XC (Allergan, Inc.)	Hyaluronic acid	Facial tissue, cheek, and lips	For correction of facial wrinkles and folds, volume loss, and lip augmentation	EMA (2000) cos FDA (2006 for first indication)
Hylaform (Hylan B gel), Captique Injectable Gel, Prevelle Silk (Genzyme Biosurgery)	Modified hyaluronic acid derived from a bird (avian) source	Dermis	Correction of moderate to severe facial wrinkles and folds	EMA (1995) (cos) FDA (2004)
EUFLEXXA (Ferring Pharmaceuticals Inc.) (physical interaction)	Hyaluronic acid	Intraarticular	Knee osteoarthritis	FDA (2004) (bone) EMA (2005)
Granugel (ConvaTec)	Pectin, carboxymethylcellulose, and propylene glycol	Topical	Fillers for partial- and full-thickness wounds	
HYADD 4 hydrogel (Farmaceutici s.p.a.)	Noncross-linked hyaluronic acid alkylamide	Intraarticular	Knee osteoarthritis	NCT02187549 (NA)
Hymovis Viscoelastic Hydrogel (Fidia Farmaceutici s.p.a.)	Hyaluronan	Intraarticular	Osteoarthritis	NCT01372475 (Ph III)

16.4.7.1 Hymovis

Phase III clinical studies were conducted with 800 volunteers to study the efficacy of Hymovis (a viscoelastic hydrogel) compared with phosphate-buffered saline (placebo) in the symptomatic treatment of knee osteoarthritis. The placebo and hydrogel were administered through intraarticular injections over a time frame of 26 weeks [122].

16.4.7.2 HYADD

The clinical trials sponsored by Fidia Farmaceutici s.p.a. evaluated the efficacy of a hydrogel based on noncross-linked hyaluronic acid alkylamide, HYADD in the symptomatic treatment of knee osteoarthritis. The study was conducted on 332 volunteers who received intraarticular injections of the hydrogel over a duration of 26 weeks [123].

16.5 Conclusion

Although there are tremendous advances in hydrogel research in the field of contact lenses and hygiene products, the clinical translation in the field of drug delivery and tissue engineering is rather moderate. Extensive work had produced hydrogels that can cater to the various needs of drug delivery; intricate three-dimensional structures, that support customized drug release pattern, supramolecules that serve as wonderful vehicles for both controlled and targeted drug delivery, systems that act as a surrogate for normal tissue and initiators of natural tissue formation.

Natural hydrogels have the intrinsic advantage of biocompatibility and biodegradability. But some of the properties such as high water retention and structural intricacy are a deterrent to its sterilization. To qualify for use within the human body, every device and dosage form must pass through the strictest safety regulation. Meeting this criterion is difficult for natural hydrogels because most of them are derived from plant, bacteria, or algal sources. At this moment, there is no standard procedure for sterilization and depyrogenation of hydrogel products. Sterilization is performed as a case-to-case basis, which increases the uncertainty level of success as well as the production cost. Once this problem is solved, much higher number of natural hydrogel products will reach the market.

References

[1] Chirani N, Yahia LH, Gritsch L, Motta FL, Chirani S, Fare S. History and applications of hydrogels. J Biomed Sci 2015;4:13.
[2] Kopecek J. Polymer chemistry: swell gels. Nature 2002;417:388–91.
[3] Kumbar SG, Laurencin CT, Deng M. Natural and Synthetic Biomedical Polymers. 1st ed. Burlington, VT: Elsevier Inc; 2014.

[4] Mann BK, Gobin AS, Tsai AT, Schmedlen RH, West JL. Smooth muscle cell growth in photopolymerized hydrogels with cell adhesive and proteolytically degradable domains: synthetic ECM analogs for tissue engineering. Biomaterials 2001;22:3045–51.

[5] Slaughter BV, Khurshid SS, Fisher OZ, Khademhosseini A, Peppas NA. Hydrogels in regenerative medicine. Adv Mater 2009;21:3307–29.

[6] Li J, Mooney DJ. Designing hydrogels for controlled drug delivery. Nat Rev Mater 2016;1:16071.

[7] Thambi T, Yi L, Lee DS. Injectable hydrogels for sustained release of therapeutic agents. J Control Release 2017;267:57–66.

[8] Mayr J, Saldias C, Diaz DD. Release of small bioactive molecules from physical gels. Chem Soc Rev 2018;47:1484–515.

[9] Vermonden T, Censi R, Hennink WE. Hydrogels for protein delivery. Chem Rev 2012;112:2853–88.

[10] Iqbal S, Blenner M, Alexander-Bryant A, Larsen J. Polymersomes for therapeutic delivery of protein and nucleic acid macromolecules: from design to therapeutic applications. Biomacromolecules 2020;21:1327–50.

[11] Sanandiya ND, Vasudevan J, Das R, Lim CT, Fernandez JG. Stimuli-responsive injectable cellulose thixogel for cell encapsulation. Int J Biol Macromol 2019;130:1009–17.

[12] Segura T, Chung P, Shea LD. DNA delivery from hyaluronic acid-collagen hydrogels via a substrate-mediated approach. Biomaterials 2005;26:1575–84.

[13] Guan X, Avci-Adali M, Alarcin E, Cheng H, Kashaf SS, Li Y, Chawla A, Jang HL, Khademhosseini A. Development of hydrogels for regenerative engineering. Biotechnol J 2017;12:10.

[14] Ghasemiyeh P, Samani SM. Hydrogels as drug delivery systems; pros and cons. Trends Pharm Sci 2019;5:7–24.

[15] Cui X, Lee JJL, Chen WN. Eco-friendly and biodegradable cellulose hydrogels produced from low cost okara: towards non-toxic flexible electronics. Sci Rep 2019;9. https://www.nature.com/articles/s41598-019-54638-5.

[16] Xue K, Wang X, Yong PW, Young DJ, Wu YL, Li Z, Loh XJ. Hydrogels as emerging materials for translational biomedicine. Adv Ther 2018;2, 1800088.

[17] Xiang Y, Oo NNL, Lee JP, Li J, Loh XJ. Recent development of synthetic nonviral systems for sustained gene delivery. Drug Discov Today 2017;22:1318–35.

[18] https://www.marketsandmarkets.com/Market-Reports/hydrogel-market-181614457.html.

[19] https://www.3m.com/3M/en_US/company-us/all-3m-products/~/All-3M-Products/Health-Care/Medical/Tegaderm/.

[20] Paul W. Wound healing dressings and drug delivery. In: Paul W, Sharma CP, editors. Advances in Wound Healing Materials: Science and Skin Engineering. Shawbury, United Kingdom: Smithers Rapra Technology Limited; 2015. p. 79–101.

[21] https://www.amtech.co.nz/wc983.html (last downloaded on 27/06/2020).

[22] https://www.bbraun.com/en/products/b/prontosan-wound-gel.html.

[23] https://www.smith-nephew.com/professional/products/advanced-wound-management/algisite-m/.

[24] Minnich KE, Stolarick R, Wilkins RJ, Chilson G, Pritt SL, Unverdorben M. The effect of a wound care solution containing polyhexanide and betaine on bacterial counts: results of an in vitro study. Ostomy Wound Manage 2012;58:32–6.

[25] López-Rojas R, Fernández-Cuenca F, Serrano-Rocha L, Pascual Á. In vitro activity of a polyhexanide-betaine solution against high-risk clones of multidrug-resistant nosocomial pathogens. Enferm Infecc Microbiol Clin 2017;35(1):12–9.

[26] Cascone S, Lamberti G. Hydrogel-based commercial products for biomedical applications: a review. Int J Pharm 2020;573:118803.

[27] Hussain A, Samad A, Ramzan M, Ahsan MN, Rehman ZU, Ahmad FJ. Elastic liposome-based gel for topical delivery of 5-flurouracil: in vitro and in vivo investigation. Drug Deliv 2016;23:1115–29.

[28] Calo E, Khutoryanskiy VV. Biomedical applications of hydrogels: a review of patentsand commercial products. Eur Polym J 2015;65:252–67.

[29] Lih E, Lee JS, Park KM, Park KD. Rapidly curable chitosan-PEG hydrogels as tissue adhesives for hemostasis and wound healing. Acta Biomater 2012;8:3261–9.

[30] Narayanaswamy R, Torchilin VP. Hydrogels and their applications in targeted drug delivery. Molecules 2019;24:603.

[31] Sawhney AS, Jarrett P, Bassett M, Blizzard C, Incept LLC, assignee. Drug Delivery Through Hydrogel Plugs. US patent 8409606 B2; 2013 April 2.

[32] Askari E, Seyfoori A, Amereh M, Gharaie SS, Ghazali HS, Ghazali Z, Khunjush B, Mohsen AM. Stimuli-responsive hydrogels for local post-surgical drug delivery. Gels 2020;6:14–45.

[33] Li Y, Rodrigues JM, Tomás H. Injectable and biodegradable hydrogels: gelation, biodegradation and biomedical applications. Chem Soc Rev 2012;41:2193–221.

[34] Qu J, Zhao X, Ma PX, Guo B. pH-responsive self-healing injectable hydrogel based on N-carboxyethyl chitosan for hepatocellular carcinoma therapy. Acta Biomater 2017;58:168–80.

[35] Zhou H, Jiang LJ, Cao PP, Li JB, Chen X. Glycerophosphate-based chitosan thermosensitive hydrogels and their biomedical applications. Carbohydr Polym 2015;117:524–36.

[36] Nagase K, Yamato M, Kanazawa H, Okano T. Poly(N-isopropylacrylamide)-based thermo responsive surfaces provide new types of biomedical applications. Biomaterials 2018;153:27–48.

[37] Kim SH, Lee S, Lee JE, Park SJ, Kim K, Kim IS, Lee YS, Hwang NS, Kim BG. Tissue adhesive, rapid forming, and sprayable ECM hydrogel via recombinant tyrosinase crosslinking. Biomaterials 2018;178:401–12.

[38] Pillai J, Thulasidasan AK, Anto R, Chithralekha D, Narayanan A, Kumar GS. Folic acid conjugated cross-linked acrylic polymer (FA-CLAP) hydrogel for site specific delivery of hydrophobic drugs to cancer cells. J Nanobiotechnology 2014;12:25.

[39] Li J. Self-assembled supramolecular hydrogels based on polymer–cyclodextrin inclusion complexes for drug delivery. NPG Asia Mater 2010;2:112–8.

[40] Li J, Akira Harada JA, Kamachi M. Sol-gel transition during inclusion complex formation between cyclodextrin and high molecular weight poly(ethylene glycol)s in aqueous solution. Polym J 1994;26:1020–6.

[41] Moncada-Basualto M. Supramolecular hydrogels of β-cyclodextrin linked to calcium homopoly-l-guluronate for release of coumarins with trypanocidal activity. Carbohydr Polym 2019;204:170–81.

[42] Jia F, Liu X, Li L, Mallapragada S, Narasimhan B, Wang Q. Multifunctional nanoparticles for targeted delivery of immune activating and cancer therapeutic agents. J Control Release 2013;172:1020–34.

[43] Alford R, Simpson HM, Duberman J, Hill GC, Ogawa M, Regino C, Kobayashi H, Choyke PL. Toxicity of organic fluorophores used in molecular imaging: literature review. Mol Imaging 2009;8:341–54.

[44] Dash R, Ghosh SK, Kaplan DL, Kundu SC. Purification and biochemical characterization of a 70 kDa sericin from tropical tasar silkworm, Antheraea mylitta. Comp Biochem Physiol B 2007;147:129–34.

[45] Chlapanidas T, Faragò S, Lucconi G, Perteghella S, Galuzzi M, Mantelli M, Avanzini MA, Tosca MC, Marazzi M, Vigo D, Torre ML, Faustini M. Sericins exhibit ROS-scavenging, anti-tyrosinase, anti-elastase, and in vitro immuno-modulatory activities. Int J Biol Macromol 2013;58:47–56.

[46] Wang Z, Zhang Y, Zhang J, Huang L, Liu J, Li Y, Zhang G, Kundu SC, Wang L. Exploring natural silk protein sericin for regenerative medicine: an injectable, photoluminescent, cell adhesive 3D hydrogel. Sci Rep 2014;4:7064.

[47] Lamboni L, Gauthier M, Yang G, Wang Q. Silk sericin: a versatile material for tissue engineering and drug delivery. Biotechnol Adv 2015;33(8):1855–67.

[48] Liu J, Qi C, Tao K, Zhang J, Zhang J, Xu L, Jiang X, Zhang Y, Huang L, Li Q, Xie H, Gao J, Shuai X, Wang G, Wang Z, Wang L. Sericin/dextran injectable hydrogel as an optically trackable drug delivery system for malignant melanoma treatment. ACS Appl Mater Interfaces 2016;8(10):6411–22.

[49] Zhang L, Jean SR, Ahmed S, Aldridge PM, Li X, et al. Multifunctional quantum dot DNA hydrogels. Nat Commun 2017;8:381.

[50] Lee SC, Kwon IK, Park K. Hydrogels for delivery of bioactive agents: a historical perspective. Adv Drug Deliv Rev 2013;65:17–20.

[51] Razem D, Katusin-Razem B. The effects of irradiation on controlled drug delivery/controlled drug release systems. Radiat Phys Chem 2008;77(3):288–344.

[52] Galante R, Rediguieri CF, Kikuchi IS, Vasquez PAS, Colaço R, Serro AP. About the sterilization of chitosan hydrogel nanoparticles. PLoS One 2016;11(12), e0168862.

[53] Killeen S, McCourt M. Decontamination and sterilization. Surgery 2012;30(12):687–92.

[54] Ratner BD, Hoffman AS, Schoen FJ, Lemons JE. Biomaterials Science: An Introduction to Materials in Medicine. 3rd ed. Amsterdam, Boulevard: Academic Press, Elsevier Science; 2012.

[55] Dick HB, Schwenn O. Aseptic production vs. terminal sterilization. In: Dick HB, Schwenn O, editors. Viscoelastics in Ophthalmic Surgery. Berlin, Heidelberg: Springer; 2000. p. 97–9.

[56] Shi Z, Gao X, Ullah MW, Li S, Wang Q, Yang G. Electroconductive natural polymer-based hydrogels. Biomaterials 2016;111:40–54.

[57] Tichy E, Muranyi A, Psenkov AJ. The effects of moist heat sterilization process and the presence of electrolytes on rheological and textural properties of hydrophilic dispersions of polymers hydrogels. Adv Polym Technol 2016;35(2):198–207.

[58] Ji C, Shi J. Sterilization-free chitosan hydrogels for controlled drug release. Mater Lett 2012;72:110–2.

[59] Galante R, Pinto TJA, Colaco R, Serro AP. Sterilization of hydrogels for biomedical applications: a review. J Biomed Mater Res B Appl Biomater 2018;106:2472–92.

[60] Nguyen LTB, Hsu CC, Ye H, Cui Z. Development of an in situ injectable hydrogel containing hyaluronic acid for neural regeneration. Biomed Mater 2020;15, 055005.

[61] Chen G, Li J, Cai Y, Zhan J, Gao J, Song M, Shi Y, Yang Z. A glycyrrhetinic acid-modified curcumin supramolecular hydrogel for liver tumor targeting therapy. Sci Rep 2017;7:44210.

[62] Lim F, Sun AM. Microencapsulated islets as bioartificial endocrine pancreas. Science 1980;210:908–10.

[63] Hamidi M, Azadi A, Rafiei P. Hydrogel nanoparticles in drug delivery. Adv Drug Deliv Rev 2008;60(15):1638–49.

[64] Yotsuyanagi T, Ohkubo T, Ohhashi T, Ikeda K. Calcium-induced gelation of alginic acid and pH-sensitive reswelling of dried gels. Chem Pharm Bull 1987;35(4):1555–63.

[65] Mandal A, Clegg JR, Anselmo AC, Mitragotri S. Hydrogels in the clinic. Bioeng Transl Med 2020;5, e10158.

[66] WHO Library Cataloguing-in-Publication Data. World Report on Ageing and Health. ISBN 978-92-4-156504-2, Luxembourg: WHO Press; 2015.

[67] Vernon-Roberts B, Moore RJ, Fraser RD. The natural history of age-related disc degeneration: the pathology and sequelae of tears. Spine 2007;32(25):2797–804.

[68] Katz JN. Lumbar disc disorders and low-back pain: socioeconomic factors and consequences. J Bone Joint Surg Am 2006;88(Suppl. 2):21–4.

[69] Luo X, Pietrobon R, Sun SX, Liu GG, Hey L. Estimates and patterns of direct health care expenditures among individuals with back pain in the United States. Spine 2004;29(1):79–86.

[70] Watkins MB. Posterolateral bone grafting for fusion of the lumbar and lumbosacral spine. J Bone Joint Surg 1959;41(3):388–96.

[71] Lewis G. Nucleus pulposus replacement and regeneration/repair technologies: present status and future prospects. J Biomed Mater Res 2012;100(6):1702–20.

[72] Reitmaier S, Wolfram U, Ignatius A, Wilke HJ, Gloria A, Martín-Martínez JM, Silva-Correia J, Miguel Oliveira J, Luís Reis R, Schmidt H. Hydrogels for nucleus replacement-facing the biomechanical challenge. J Mech Behav Biomed Mater 2012;14:67–77.

[73] Peroglio M, Grad S, Mortisen D, Sprecher C, Illien-Junger S, Alini M, Eglin D. Injectable thermoreversible hyaluronan-based hydrogels for nucleus pulposus cell encapsulation. Eur Spine J 2011;21(Suppl. 6):S839–49.

[74] Sampath TK, Maliakal JC, Hauschka PV, Jones WK, Sasak H, Tucker RF, White KH, Coughlin JE, Tucker MM, Pang RH. Recombinant human osteogenic protein-1 (hOP-1) induces new bone formation in vivo with a specific activity comparable with natural bovine osteogenic protein and stimulates osteoblast proliferation and differentiation in vitro. J Biol Chem 1999;267:20352–62.

[75] Bigi A, Boanini E, Gazzano M. Ion substitution in biological and synthetic apatites. In: Apiricio C, Ginebra MP, editors. Biomineralization and Biomaterials. Fundamentals and Applications. Sawston, United Kingdom: Woodhead Publishing; 2016. p. 235–66 [chapter 7].

[76] Kabir SMF, Sikdar PP, Haque B, Bhuiya MAR, Ali A, Islam MN. Cellulose-based hydrogel materials: chemistry, properties and their prospective applications. Prog Biomater 2018;7:153–74.

[77] Narasimhulu CA, Singla DK. The role of bone morphogenetic protein 7 (BMP-7) in inflammation in heart diseases. Cell 2020;9:280.

[78] https://www.ele.uri.edu/courses/bme281/F08/Erin_2.pdf.

[79] Rawla P, Barsouk A. Epidemiology of gastric cancer: global trends, risk factors and prevention. Prz Gastroenterol 2019;14(1):26–38.

[80] Park YM, Jung JY. Endoscopic mucosal resection for upper gastrointestinal neoplasia. In: Chun HJ, Yang SK, Choi MG, editors. Therapeutic Gastrointestinal Endoscopy: A Comprehensive Atlas. Singapore: Springer Nature; 2019. p. 93–114.

[81] Gotoda T. Endoscopic resection of early gastric cancer. Gastric Cancer 2007;10:1–11.

[82] Lee H, Yun WK, Min BH, Lee JH, Rhee PL, Kim KM, Rhee JC, Kim JJ. A feasibility study on the expanded indication for endoscopic submucosal dissection of early gastric cancer. Surg Endosc 2011;25(6):1985–93.

[83] Ishihara M, Kumano I, Hattori H, Nakamura S. Application of hydrogels as submucosal fluid cushions for endoscopic mucosal resection and submucosal dissection. J Artif Organs 2015;18(3):191–8.

[84] Shim CS. Endoscopic mucosal resection: an overview of the value of different techniques. Endoscopy 2001;33:271–5.

[85] Castro R, Libânio D, Inês Pita I, Dinis-Ribeiro M. Solutions for submucosal injection: what to choose and how to do it. World J Gastroenterol 2019;25:777–88.

[86] Uraoka T, Saito Y, Yamamoto K, Fujii T. Submucosal injection solution for gastrointestinal tract endoscopic mucosal resection and endoscopic submucosal dissection. Drug Des Devel Ther 2009;2:131–8.

[87] Fujishiro M, Yahagi N, Kashimura K, Matsuura T, Nakamura M, Kakushima N, Kodashima S, Ono S, Kobayashi K, Hashimoto T, Yamamichi N, Tateishi A, Shimizu Y, Oka M, Ichinose M, Omata M. Tissue damage of different submucosal injection solutions for EMR. Gastrointest Endosc 2005;62:933–42.

[88] https://clinicaltrials.gov/ct2/show/NCT03321396 Hydrogel Injection to Assist Endoscopic Submucosal Dissection.

[89] Lee KY, Mooney DJ. Alginate: properties and biomedical applications. Prog Polym Sci 2012;37:106–26.

[90] Jacovella PF, Peiretti CB, Cunille D, Salzamendi M, Schechtel SA. Long lasting results with hydroxylapatite (Radiesse) facial filler. Plast Reconstr Surg 2006;118:15S–21S.

[91] Jacovella PF. Use of calcium hydroxylapatite (Radiesse®) for facial augmentation. Clin Interv Aging 2008;3(1):161–74.

[92] Somaiah C, Kumar A, Mawrie D, Sharma A, Patil SD, Bhattacharyya J, Swaminathan R, Jaganathan BG. Collagen promotes higher adhesion, survival and proliferation of mesenchymal stem cells. PLoS One 2015;10, PMC4678765.

[93] Aziz J, Shezali H, Radzi Z, Yahya NA, Abu Kassim NH, Czernuszka J, Rahman MT. Molecular mechanisms of stress-responsive changes in collagen and elastin networks in skin. Skin Pharmacol Physiol 2016;29(4):190–203.

[94] Tracy LE, Minasian RA, Caterson EJ. Extracellular matrix and dermal fibroblast function in the healing wound. Adv Wound Care 2016;5(3):119–36.

[95] Kanchwala SL, Holloway L, Bucky LP. Reliable soft tissue augmentation: a clinical comparison of injectable soft-tissue filler for facial-volume augmentation. Ann Plast Surg 2005;55:30–5.

[96] Tzikas TL. Evaluation of the radiance FN soft tissue filler for facial soft tissue augmentation. Arch Facial Plast Surg 2004;6:234–9.

[97] Jansen DA, Graivier MH. Evalution of a calcium hydroxylapatite-based implant (Radiesse) for facial soft-tissue augmentation. Plast Reconstr Surg 2006;118:22S–30S.

[98] Dover JS. The filler revolution has just begun. Plast Reconstr Surg 2006;117:38S–40S.

[99] Felderman LI. Radiesse for facial rejuvenation. Cosmet Dermatol 2005;18:823–6.

[100] Broder KW, Cohen SR. An overview of permanent and semipermanent fillers. Plast Reconstr Surg 2006;118:7S–14S.

[101] Hobar PC, Pantaloni M, Byrd HS. Porous hydroxyapatite granules for alloplastic enhancement of the facial region. Clin Plast Surg 2000;27:557–69.

[102] Berlin AL, Hussain M, Goldberg DJ. Calcium hydroxylapatite filler for facial rejuvenation: a histologic and immunohistochemical analysis. Dermatol Surg 2008;34:S64–7.

[103] Rovner EC, Wein AJ. Treatment options for stress urinary incontinence. Rev Urology 2004;6:S29–47.

[104] Murless MB. The injection treatment of stress incontinence. J Obstet Gynaecol Br Emp 1938;45:67–73.

[105] Mamut A, Carlson KV. Periurethral bulking agents for female stress urinary incontinence in Canada. Can Urol Assoc J 2017;6:S152–4.

[106] Matsuoka PK, Locali RF, Paceta AM, Baracat EC, Haddad JM. The efficacy and safety of urethral injection therapy for urinary incontinence in women: a systematic review. Clinics 2016;71:94–100.

[107] https://www.accessdata.fda.gov/cdrh_docs/pdf4/P040047d.pdf. Information for Patients: Coaptite: For the Treatment of Stress Urinary Continence in Women. Franksville: Bio Formn Medical, Inc.; 2005.

[108] https://www.accessdata.fda.gov/cdrh_docs/pdf4/P040047c.pdf. Instructions for use. Franksville: Bio Formn Medical, Inc.; 2005.

[109] Bano F, Barrington JW, Dyer R. Comparison between porcine dermal implant (Permacol) and silicone injection (Macroplastique) for urodynamic stress incontinence. Int Urogynecol J Pelvic Floor Dysfunct 2005;16(2):147–50.

[110] Mayer RD, Dmochowski RR, Appell RA, Sand PK, Klimberg IW, Jacoby K, Graham CW, Snyder JA, Nitti VW, Winters JC. Multicenter prospective randomized 52-week trial of calcium hydroxylapatite versus bovine dermal collagen for treatment of stress urinary incontinence. Urology 2007;69(5):876–80.

[111] Koh RH, Jin Y, Kim J, Hwang NS. Inflammation-modulating hydrogels for osteoarthritis cartilage tissue engineering. Cell 2020;9:419.

[112] Nelson AE. Osteoarthritis year in review 2017: clinical. Osteoarthr Cartil 2018;26:319–25.

[113] Bliddal H, Christensen R. The treatment and prevention of knee osteoarthritis: a tool for clinical decision-making. Expert Opin Pharmacother 2009;10:1793–804.

[114] Fahy N, Farrell E, Ritter T, Ryan AE, Murphy JM. Immune modulation to improve tissue engineering outcomes for cartilage repair in the osteoarthritic joint. Tissue Eng Part B Rev 2015;21:55–66.

[115] Ulivi V, Giannoni P, Gentili C, Cancedda R, Descalzi F. p38/NF-kB-dependent expression of COX-2 during differentiation and inflammatory response of chondrocytes. J Cell Biochem 2008;104:1393–406.

[116] Bowman S, Awad ME, Hamrick MW, Hunter M, Fulzele S. Recent advances in hyaluronic acid based therapy for osteoarthritis. Clin Transl Med 2018;7:6.

[117] https://clinicaltrials.gov/ct2/show/NCT04061733 hydroxyethyl cellulose hydrogel. Last verified March 2020.

[118] Marquass B, Somerson JS, Hepp P. A novel MSC-seeded triphasic construct for the repair of osteochondral defects. J Orthop Res 2010;28:1586–99.

[119] Yue K, Trujillo-de Santiago G, Alvarez MM, Tamayol A, Annabi N, Khademhosseini A. Synthesis, properties, and biomedical applications of gelatinmethacryloyl (GelMA) hydrogels. Biomaterials 2015;73:254–71.

[120] Snyder TN, Madhavan K, Intrator M, Dregalla RC, Park D. A fibrin/hyaluronic acid hydrogel for the delivery of mesenchymal stem cells and potential for articular cartilage repair. J Biol Eng 2014;8:10.

[121] Mahapatra C, Jin GZ, Kim HW. Alginate-hyaluronic acid-collagen composite hydrogel favorable for the culture of chondrocytes and their phenotype maintenance. Tissue Eng Regen Med 2016;13:538–46.

[122] Anon, https://clinicaltrials.gov/ct2/show/NCT01372475.

[123] Anon, https://clinicaltrials.gov/ct2/show/NCT02187549.

Index

Note: Page numbers followed by *f* indicate figures and *t* indicate tables.

Printed in the United States
by Baker & Taylor Publisher Services